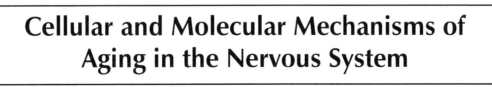

Cellular and Molecular Mechanisms of
Aging in the Nervous System

Cellular and Molecular Mechanisms of Aging in the Nervous System

Editor: Adler Brown

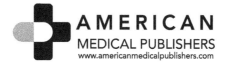

AMERICAN
MEDICAL PUBLISHERS
www.americanmedicalpublishers.com

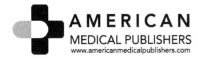

Cataloging-in-Publication Data

Cellular and molecular mechanisms of aging in the nervous system / edited by Adler Brown.
    p. cm.
Includes bibliographical references and index.
ISBN 978-1-63927-970-8
1. Geriatric neurology. 2. Older people--Diseases--Molecular aspects. 3. Older people--Diseases--Cytopathology.
4. Aging--Physiological aspects. 5. Cells--Aging. I. Brown, Adler.
RC346 .C45 2023
616.8--dc23

American Medical Publishers,
41 Flatbush Avenue,
1st Floor, New York,
NY 11217, USA

ISBN 978-1-63927-970-8 (Hardback)

Contents

Preface

This book aims to highlight the current researches and provides a platform to further the scope of innovations in this area. This book is a product of the combined efforts of many researchers and scientists, after going through thorough studies and analysis from different parts of the world. The objective of this book is to provide the readers with the latest information of the field.

The nervous system is a highly complex network of nerves that coordinates actions and sensory information by transmitting signals to and from various parts of the body. Random molecular damage that steadily accumulates with age drives the ageing process at the cellular level. Many molecular mechanisms are involved and exogenous factors, like stress, also play a role in the aging process. The nervous system at the cellular level comprises a special cell called a neuron, which transmits signals to the other cells. Many physical, chemical, or biological changes in the status of neurons characterize brain aging. It is manifested in the form of deterioration in cognitive function and dementia. Dendritic regression in pyramidal neurons, synaptic atrophy, decrease of striatal dopamine receptors, accumulation of fluorescent pigments, cytoskeletal abnormalities, and reactive astrocytes and microglia are the common features of brain aging. The consequence of molecular and cellular alterations in brain aging is characterized by a plethora of anatomical changes, such as significant neuronal loss in hippocampus and neocortex. This book provides comprehensive insights on the molecular and cellular mechanisms of aging. The readers would gain knowledge that would broaden their perspective about this area of study.

I would like to express my sincere thanks to the authors for their dedicated efforts in the completion of this book. I acknowledge the efforts of the publisher for providing constant support. Lastly, I would like to thank my family for their support in all academic endeavors.

Editor

Spectral Variability in the Aged Brain during Fine Motor Control

Fanny Quandt[1], Marlene Bönstrup[1], Robert Schulz[1], Jan E. Timmermann[1], Maximo Zimerman[2, 3], Guido Nolte[4] and Friedhelm C. Hummel[1, 2, 5, 6]*

[1] *BrainImaging and NeuroStimulation Laboratory, Department of Neurology, University Medical Center Hamburg-Eppendorf, Hamburg, Germany,* [2] *Institute of Neuroscience, Favaloro University, Buenos Aires, Argentina,* [3] *Institute of Cognitive Neurology, Buenos Aires, Argentina,* [4] *Department of Neurophysiology, University Medical Center Hamburg-Eppendorf, Hamburg, Germany,* [5] *Clinical Neuroengineering, Brain Mind Institute and Centre of Neuroprosthetics (CNP), Swiss Federal Institute of Technology (EPFL), Geneva, Switzerland,* [6] *Clinique Romande de Réadaptation, Swiss Federal Institute of Technology (EPFL Valais), Sion, Switzerland*

*Correspondence:
Friedhelm C. Hummel
friedhelm.hummel@epfl.ch

Physiological aging is paralleled by a decline of fine motor skills accompanied by structural and functional alterations of the underlying brain network. Here, we aim to investigate age-related changes in the spectral distribution of neuronal oscillations during fine skilled motor function. We employ the concept of spectral entropy in order to describe the flatness and peaked-ness of a frequency spectrum to quantify changes in the spectral distribution of the oscillatory motor response in the aged brain. Electroencephalogram was recorded in elderly ($n = 32$) and young ($n = 34$) participants who performed either a cued finger movement or a pinch or a whole hand grip task with their dominant right hand. Whereas young participant showed distinct, well-defined movement-related power decreases in the alpha and upper beta band, elderly participants exhibited a flat broadband, frequency-unspecific power desynchronization. This broadband response was reflected by an increase of spectral entropy over sensorimotor and frontal areas in the aged brain. Neuronal activation patterns differed between motor tasks in the young brain, while the aged brain showed a similar activation pattern in all tasks. Moreover, we found a wider recruitment of the cortical motor network in the aged brain. The present study adds to the understanding of age-related changes of neural coding during skilled motor behavior, revealing a less predictable signal with great variability across frequencies in a wide cortical motor network in the aged brain. The increase in entropy in the aged brain could be a reflection of random noise-like activity or could represent a compensatory mechanism that serves a functional role.

Keywords: aging, motor control, entropy, oscillations, EEG

INTRODUCTION

Physiological aging is paralleled by a decline of motor performance, most pronounced in demanding fine motor skills. At the higher age (Smith et al., 1999), elderly show a decrease of movement coordination (Stelmach et al., 1988; Wishart et al., 2000) with increasing variability of motor output (Cooke et al., 1989; Darling et al., 1989), along with a general movement slowing (Buckles, 1993). These behavioral changes are accompanied by alterations of the underlying brain network. During movements a more widespread neuronal network is recruited in the aged brain (Sailer et al., 2000; Ward and Frackowiak, 2003; Wu and Hallett, 2005; Naccarato et al., 2006; Rowe et al., 2006; Vallesi et al., 2010; Deiber et al., 2013). Additionally, elderly show higher magnitudes of movement-related desynchronization of oscillatory activity in frequency bands associated with motor control (Sailer et al., 2000). Apart from the larger movement-related power decrease, few studies so far have observed differences in the frequency patterns with age. When reviewing lifespan changes in the alpha peak, Klimesch reported a drop of peak frequency with age (Klimesch, 1999). Moreover, previous studies found shifts of the most reactive peak frequency during rest (Gaál et al., 2010) and attention (Deiber et al., 2013). Hong and Rebec hypothesize that in order to compensate for a non-uniform decrease of nerve conduction in the aged brain, individual neurons increase their firing rate with a non-uniform pattern, leading to an irregular firing pattern which subsequently might lead to an unspecific broadband large-scale oscillatory response (Hong and Rebec, 2012). Such a broadening of the neuronal response has, to our knowledge, not been analytically addressed before and is rather difficult to detect when analyzing the data using movement specific narrow frequency bands as previously suggested in healthy young, such as the alpha or upper beta band (Pfurtscheller, 1989; Crone et al., 1998). In the healthy young, spectral changes in the mu ($\sim$8–13 Hz) and beta band ($\sim$14–30 Hz) are associated with voluntary movements (Pfurtscheller and Lopes da Silva, 1999). Their definite functional role still remains under debate, however, mu and beta rhythms are thought to represent separate functional processes with different time courses and distributions over the scalp. While the mu rhythm dominantly localizes to the post-central hand area, the beta rhythm localizes to pre-central areas (for a review please refer to (Cheyne, 2013; Brittain and Brown, 2014). Here, we investigate movement-related power changes over a broad frequency band from 8 to 25 Hz and aim to determine whether the implementation of motor tasks in the aged brain is in similar frequency bands compared to the young brain. One measure to characterize differences in the distribution of the spectral content is the spectral entropy H. Spectral entropy is an uncertainty measure borrowed from information theory. We solely employ the mathematical concept of entropy by treating the frequency spectrum as a probability density in order to describe the flatness and peaked-ness of a frequency spectrum (Inouye et al., 1991). An oscillatory activity with a flat frequency distribution and large variability results in a high spectral entropy, whereas a peaked signal such as a confined alpha or upper beta movement-related desynchronization would result in a lower spectral entropy. It was our primary objective to mathematically quantify changes of the spectral content of oscillatory movement-related patterns in the aged brain by employing the spectral entropy. Electrophysiological data were recorded from elderly over the age of 60 and young participants while performing different skilled fine motor tasks. So far, most studies investigating the aged motor system have focused on one specific motor task. Here, we assessed different motor tasks, which allows us to make inferences on more generalized age-dependent motor network changes. The magnitude and spatial extent of movement-related power decrease was analyzed. Importantly, we characterized the distribution of the spectral content by spectral entropy. We hypothesized that the aged brain shows larger variability of oscillatory activation patterns with a broadening of the movement-related frequency band and higher spectral entropy.

MATERIALS AND METHODS

Participants

Sixty-six healthy volunteers participated in different EEG experiments, consisting of an elderly group with 32 participants over the age of 60 (mean age 72.2 y/o $\pm$ 5.2 SD, range 61–81 y/o, 19 females) as well as a young control group with 34 participants (mean age 25.5 y/o $\pm$ 3.3 SD, range 19–34, y/o, 14 females). A subgroup of 15 elderly and 16 young participants performed two different motor tasks. All participants were right-handed as confirmed by the Edinburgh handedness inventory (Oldfield, 1971), did not have a history of neurologic disorder and gave written informed consent. All elderly subjects were seen by a neurologist and did not show any cognitive impairment. Elderly subjects participating in the Finger Sequence Task, requiring learning of a digit sequence, all presented with a mini-mental state examination $\geq$28. The study conforms to "The Code of Ethics" of the World Medical Association (Declaration of Helsinki) and was approved by the local ethics committee of the Medical Association of Hamburg.

Motor Tasks

Participants performed a motor task during EEG recording. All motor tasks required a movement in response to an external visual cue. In every participant, a 2–5 min pre- and post-experimental baseline was recorded at unconstrained rest with eyes open.

Finger Sequence Task

Seventeen elderly (range 61–81 y/o) and 18 young (range 19–33 y/o) participants trained a sequence of 10 consecutive button presses [2 4 3 2 5 4 5 2 5 3, with (2) = index finger, (3) = middle, (4) = ring, (5) = little]. The sequence was trained until performance reached a stable level and participants were able to play the sequence at least ten times in a row without any mistakes at a pace of 1 Hz (Gerloff et al., 1997). Hence, the sequence was considered overlearned, ensuring constant baseline performance during the EEG session. Training was conducted either on the day prior or on the day of the experiment. During the following EEG experiment participants sat in front of a computer screen with the right arm positioned on a keyboard. Visual cues without any relation to the learned sequence ("#," "&," "+," "$") were presented on a computer screen. The symbols paced the execution of the memorized, well-trained sequence at a frequency of 1 Hz and participants were asked to enter the finger sequence at the pace of the visual cues. The sequence was played with the right hand, using the index-, middle-, ring,- and little finger. Each participant performed 40 repetitions of the 10-digit sequence.

Pinch Grip and Whole Hand Grip Task

Fifteen elderly (range 67–79 y/o) and 16 young (range 20–34 y/o) participants performed repetitive pinch as well as whole hand grips lifting a weight positioned on a table in front of them. Participants were seated in front of a monitor with their arms placed on a custom-made platform. The right hand was placed on a socket installed on the platform with the elbow 90°Flexed. The 200 g weight was lifted 10–20 cm of the table using the right thumb and index finger and reset immediately after. Instructions were visually presented on a screen, consisting of the word "pinch grip" or "whole hand grip," followed by a "GO!" cue 2–3 s later. Condition "pinch" and condition "whole" were presented in a random, counterbalanced order. The next trial was initiated 8–10 s later. Each participant performed 80 pinch and 80 whole hand grips.

Recording Systems and Preprocessing

Data were sampled at 1000 Hz using a 63-channel EEG system positioned according to the 10–10 System of the American Electroencephalographic Society (using actiCAP®, Brain Products GmbH, Germany, Gilching; Electro-Cap International, Inc., Eaton, OH, USA) and referenced to the Cz electrode. The impedance of the EEG electrodes was kept below 25 kΩ. Data were filtered from 0.2 to 256 Hz with a bandpass-filter of third order. Datasets were segmented into one second epochs for further analysis. Specifically, finger sequence data were segmented ± 500 ms around the visual cue and lifting task data were segmented from 300 to 1300 ms after the "GO" cue. Eye-movement artifacts were removed employing an independent component analysis (Makeig et al., 1996). Epochs containing electrode artifacts, muscle artifacts, head movements, or incompletely rejected blink artifacts were removed manually by visual inspection. In participants with great muscle artifacts a blind source separation-canonical correlation analysis was applied in order to correct these artifacts (De Clercq et al., 2006) as implemented in the eeglab-plugin *meegpipe* (https://github.com/meegpipe/meegpipe/). Subsequently, data were re-referenced to a common average reference. Artifact rejection resulted in an overall number of μ = 117/260, SD = 63/44 trials (elderly/young; Finger Sequence Task), μ = 64/63, SD = 5/6 trials (elderly/young; Pinch Grip Task), and μ = 74/73, SD = 4/8 trials (elderly/young; Whole Hand Grip Task).

Pre- and post-experimental baselines were pooled and subsequently divided into 2000 ms segments and preprocessed jointly as described above. The Fieldtrip toolbox (Oostenveld et al., 2011) as well as custom written software using MATLAB Version 8.2.0 (R2013b, Mathworks Inc. Massachusetts) were used for EEG data analysis.

EEG Data Analysis

Frequency Analysis

Power spectra were calculated from 8 to 25 Hz in steps of 1 Hz applying a fast Fourier transformation using one Hanning taper for each electrode and trial. In order to account for inter-subject variability and decreasing power in higher frequencies, spectral power was expressed as the relative power (Pow$_{rel}$) defined by the percentage of power change during movement (Pow$_{move}$) compared to baseline (Pow$_{baseline}$; Gerloff et al., 1998; Pfurtscheller et al., 2003). Pow$_{baseline}$, was obtained from the preprocessed baseline data and averaged across segments afterwards. Subsequently, Pow$_{rel}$ was computed by:

$$Pow_{rel} = 100 \times \frac{Pow_{move} - Pow_{baseline}}{Pow_{baseline}} \quad (1)$$

Afterwards trials were averaged for each participant.

Spectral Entropy

Spectral entropy is an uncertainty measure borrowed from information theory. Here, we apply the entropy as a mathematical concept to describe the flatness of the frequency spectrum, which is treated as a probability density after appropriate normalization. A uniform flat signal with a high variability and a broad spectral content results in a high spectral entropy (H~1), whereas a more predictable signal with a narrow, peaked power spectrum in a limited number of frequency bins yields a low spectral entropy (H~0). The spectral entropy is calculated by:

$$H = \frac{-1}{\ln(N)} \sum p_i \ln(p_i) \quad (2)$$

with

$$p_i = \frac{|Pow_{rel}(i)|}{\sum_i Pow_{rel}(i)|} \quad (3)$$

and with Pow$_{rel}(i)$ being the relative power of frequency bin i and N being equal to the number of frequency bins (Inouye et al., 1991). In order to quantify the distribution of spectral power, we estimated the spectral entropy H in the broad frequency band between 8 and 25 Hz as well as in the frequency band showing greatest differences between the aged and young brain (13–19 Hz). The spatial extent of differences H was evaluated by calculating H for each electrode separately.

Source Analysis

Sensor data in the frequency band from 13 to 19 Hz were projected to source level in each sensor of each participant. The forward solution is constructed with a segmented template MRI brain (Holmes et al., 1998) using the boundary element method and a template grid of 8 mm spacing (Oostenveld et al., 2011). Individual electrode positions were determined using the Zebris localization system (CMS20, Zebris Medical GmbH, Isny, Germany) and realigned to the template MRI brain. A common filter for the frequency range from 13 to 19 Hz of movement period and baseline period was calculated based on the average real part of the cross-spectrum in that range using dynamic imaging of coherent sources (DICS; Gross et al., 2001) with source orientation chosen to maximize power using the Fieldtrip Toolbox. The DICS beamformer uses a frequency domain implementation of a spatial filter. Subsequently, the contrast was computed expressing a relative change of power as described in Equation (1).

Statistics

Firstly, it was the objective to analyze topographic age-group differences of the mean broadband power changes (8–25 Hz) for each motor task separately. Topographic age-group differences were statistically tested using an unpaired student's *t*-test (relative power, normally distributed) or a Wilcoxon rank sum test (entropy, non-normally distributed) corrected for multiple comparisons (63 channels) controlling the false discovery rate (FDR; Benjamini et al., 2001). Secondly, we tested age-group differences of single frequency bins over left sensorimotor cortex for each motor task separately, in order to demonstrate differences of the power distribution. Power distribution age-group differences were statistically tested using an unpaired student's *t*-test corrected for multiple comparisons (18 frequency bins) controlling the FDR (Benjamini et al., 2001).

In addition, we estimated topographic age-group differences combining all participants of all three motor tasks in linear mixed effects models using R (CDT, 2008) and lme4 (Bates et al., 2015). The linear mixed effects models were calculated for entropy and relative power respectively. In order to correct for a potential influence of task, we entered task as a fixed effect. Participants were entered as a random intercept in order to correct for repeated testing. This model was calculated for each channel separately. We then extracted the *p*-value from our main effect of interest "group" and obtained 63 *p*-values (one per channel), which were then FDR corrected. Moreover, for *post-hoc* testing of task differences in young and elderly participants separately, we modeled the interaction of group and task to perform *post-hoc* testing using a pairwise comparison of least-square means.

RESULTS

Power Amplitude Differences between Elderly and Young Participants

The topology of movement-related broadband power changes (8–25 Hz) revealed a more widespread spatial distribution of desynchronization in the elderly compared to young participants in all three tasks (**Figure 1A**). This difference of power was significant in electrodes covering sensorimotor cortex as well as in more frontal electrodes (electrodes as marked in **Figure 1A**, FDR corr., *p* < 0.05). Further probing the distribution in single frequency bins in electrodes covering the left sensorimotor cortex (mean of electrodes: FC3, C3, CP3), elderly participants showed a greater movement-related power decrease in all frequency bins (**Figure 1B**). This difference was significant from 13 to 20 Hz for Task 1, from 15 to 17 Hz in Task 2, and from 13 to 22 Hz in Task 3. Please refer to Supplementary Tables 1, 2 for *t*-test results and Supplementary Figure 1 for data distribution.

In order to identify responsible sources of oscillatory activity in the significant frequency band, we applied a beamforming technique. **Figure 2** displays the difference of movement-related power in the power band from 13 to 19 Hz between the aged and young brain, revealing that the aged brain recruits a more extended motor network of contralateral but also ipsilateral primary sensorimotor and secondary premotor areas including dorsal and ventral premotor cortex as well as the supplementary motor area (**Figure 2**).

Differences in Spectral Entropy of Oscillations in Elderly and Young Participants

The shape of the distribution of the power spectrum in all three motor tasks differed with age (**Figure 1B**). Whereas, in young participants, a clear and peaked modulation of movement-related power decrease in the alpha and upper beta band was evident

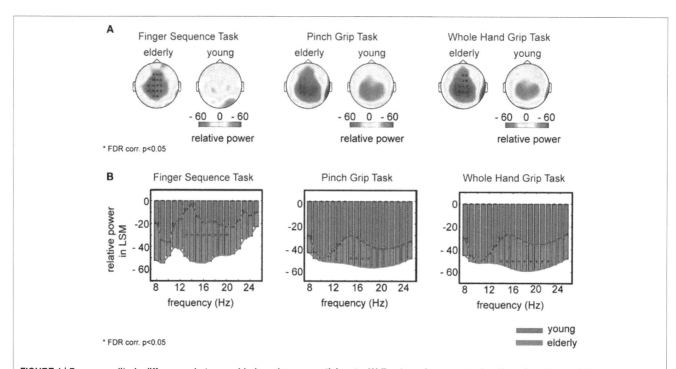

FIGURE 1 | Power amplitude differences between elderly and young participants. (A) Topology of movement-related broadband power (8–25 Hz) for elderly and young participants for each task separately, averaged over participants. Stars mark the significant electrodes (unpaired *t*-test, FDR corr., *p* < 0.05). **(B)** Power in each frequency bin for elderly (red) and young (blue) averaged over electrodes covering the contralateral sensorimotor cortex (as framed by the rectangle in **A**). Black dots mark a significant difference between both groups in the corresponding frequency bin (unpaired *t*-test, FDR corr., *p* < 0.05). The x-axis shows the frequency in Hz, the y-axis displays the relative power (%) to baseline for elderly (red) and young participants (blue) separately.

(**Figure 1B**, blue bars), the aged brain displayed a more uniform flat curve of power decrease (**Figure 1B**, red bars). In order to mathematically quantify this disparity of spectral distribution, we calculated the spectral entropy H for elderly and young participants in each channel.

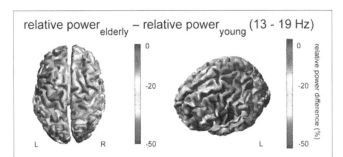

FIGURE 2 | Source localized power. The difference of movement-related source power (relative power$_{elderly}$ − relative power$_{young}$;13–19 Hz) between elderly and young of the Finger Sequence Task and Pinch Grip Task is rendered on the cortical surface, displayed from a top and left-side view, masked by power.

The group difference correcting for tasks and repeated testing of the same participants was assessed in linear mixed effect model for each channel separately. **Figure 3A** displays the estimated mean of the mixed model for each channel over the broadband spectrum from 8 to 25 Hz. Asterisks mark significant models with $p < 0.05$ (FDR corr.; for model results, please refer to Supplementary Tables 3, 4). The aged brain showed a higher spectral entropy H in electrodes covering frontal as well as sensorimotor areas. We further probed the spectral entropy in a more restricted frequency band (13–19 Hz, **Figure 3B**) in which relative power showed greatest differences between groups. Hence, we confirmed a flatter more uniform frequency spectrum with a broader spectral content in the aged population compared to younger people during different fine skilled motor tasks.

When assessing entropy differences in each task separately (mean value of relative power, **Figure 4**), we find a similar pattern in each task, with greater spectral entropy in the aged compared to the young brain in electrodes covering frontal as well as contra- and ipsilateral sensorimotor areas. **Figure 4** revealed that differences between motor tasks were mainly driven by the young participants. Elderly participants showed a similar activation

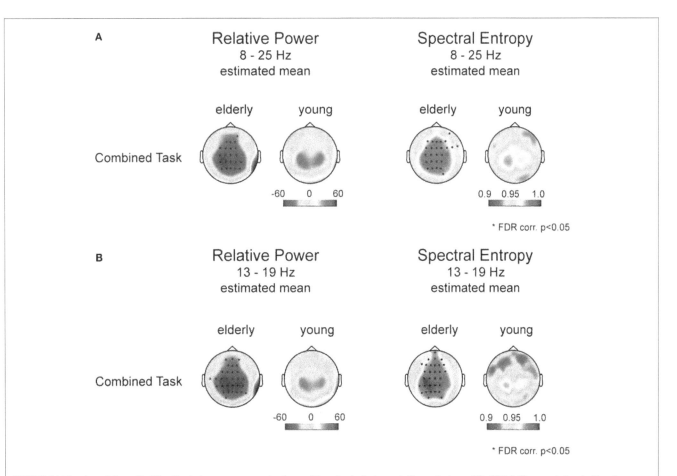

FIGURE 3 | Mixed model results (A) estimated mean power and entropy of the mixed effects model for each channel (8–25 Hz). Stars mark the significant group effect of the mixed model (FDR corr., $p < 0.05$). **(B)** Estimated mean power and entropy of the mixed model for each channel (13–19 Hz). Stars mark the significant group effect of the mixed model (FDR corr., $p < 0.05$).

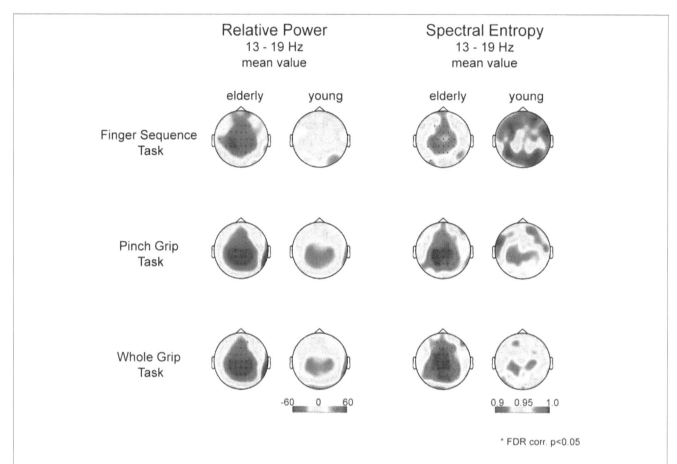

FIGURE 4 | Topology of movement-related power (left) and spectral entropy **(right)** between 13 and 19 Hz respectively for elderly and young participants for each individual task separately. Stars mark the significant electrodes between groups (unpaired t-test, FDR corr., $p < 0.05$).

pattern in all three tasks, whereas in young participants the neuronal activation pattern differs depending on motor tasks' complexity.

Post-hoc testing of task differences in the mixed effects model for the elderly and young group pointed toward differences in entropy between the Finger Sequence Task and the Pinch Grip and Whole Hand Grip Task in the young but not in the elderly participants (**Figure 5**).

DISCUSSION

This study characterizes differences in the spectral content of motor control in healthy aging. By using the concept of entropy, we quantified differences in the spectral distribution between the aged and young brain and found a higher spectral entropy with a flat, uniform distribution of power in the aged brain in various fine skilled motor tasks. Whereas, the young brain showed lower entropy and a distinct peaked movement-related power decrease in the alpha and upper beta band, the aged brain exhibited a larger movement-related decrease of power most pronounced in the low beta frequency band along with a wider recruitment of the cortical motor network involving premotor areas.

Reduced Frequency Specificity of the Aged Brain

Movement execution leads to distinct event-related desynchronization in the alpha and upper beta band over contra- and ipsilateral sensorimotor areas (Pfurtscheller, 1989; Crone et al., 1998). In task-related studies, these frequency bands have been often used for analysis of movement specific oscillatory changes. These motor-task-related frequency bands, however, have been determined based on data in the young brain. In contrast, these bands might not correspond to movement-related changes in the aged brain, as supported by previous studies, indicating changes in oscillatory activity patterns across the lifespan. Apart from a larger magnitude of the movement-related desynchronization within sensorimotor areas (Sailer et al., 2000; Mattay et al., 2002), age-related changes comprise shifts in resting state peak alpha frequency (Klimesch, 1999; Cottone et al., 2013), a decrease of alpha reactivity (Gaál et al., 2010), as well as changes of the dominant oscillator with age (Deiber et al., 2013). Hence, a priori knowledge on frequency specific bands as determined in the young brain might be arbitrary in the aged brain and might hinder the detection of distinct age-related oscillatory changes. For this reason, we characterized oscillatory changes by using the concept of spectral entropy allowing us to

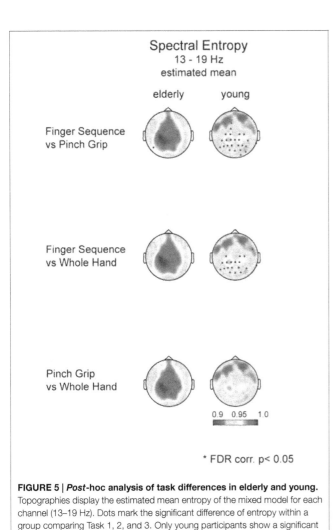

FIGURE 5 | *Post*-hoc analysis of task differences in elderly and young. Topographies display the estimated mean entropy of the mixed model for each channel (13–19 Hz). Dots mark the significant difference of entropy within a group comparing Task 1, 2, and 3. Only young participants show a significant difference between the Finger Sequence Task and the Pinch Grip as well as Whole Hand Grip task (FDR corr., $p < 0.05$).

Computational models of neuromodulation postulate that the aged brain exhibits deficient neuromodulatory mechanisms and consequently less distinctive neural pattern representations (Li and Sikström, 2002). Therefore, the increased spectral entropy could be a result of reduced coordination of enhanced synaptic activity of neuronal assemblies leading to greater variability of the neuronal responses. Correspondingly, increasing variability resulting in less consistent motor actions has been observed during healthy aging (Cooke et al., 1989; Darling et al., 1989; Contreras-Vidal et al., 1998; Sosnoff and Newell, 2011). On the one hand, the signal could be a result of inaccurate interregional neuronal communication leading to a breakdown of the frequency specificity, where the aged brain is not capable of keeping a certain frequency. Hence, the increased variability could be in line with the dedifferentiation of the aging brain (Deiber et al., 2013). On the other hand, the broadening of the frequency band could ensure to preserve the balance between energy consumption and entropy of the neural signal. Tsubo et al. have postulated that with higher uncertainty of the neural responses, the brain reduces the amount of energy necessary (Tsubo et al., 2012). Moreover, high variability of a signal has been suggested to result in an increase of performance and might be beneficial (Garrett et al., 2013). Hence, the increase of entropy could be a compensating mechanism to account for a decline of motor performance. In line Hanslmayr et al. speculated that higher neuronal desynchronization presents a greater richness of information, measured by the entropy and consider it as one mechanism serving memory encoding (Hanslmayr et al., 2012). We cannot, however, definitely infer whether a higher entropy is a reflection of random noise-like activity or if the irregular pattern is a compensatory mechanism that serves a functional role. Hence, higher entropy could mean that either more information is sent, or that more noise-like random activity is produced and sent. Further research will have to address this important issue, especially to determine its functional implication on behavior.

Enhanced Spatial Recruitment in the Aged Brain

Several functional imaging and EEG studies have reported a more extended recruitment of brain areas during movement in the aged brain (Sailer et al., 2000; Mattay et al., 2002; Wu and Hallett, 2005; Naccarato et al., 2006; Rowe et al., 2006; Vallesi et al., 2010; Deiber et al., 2013). In line, we found activations in an extended motor network including bilateral primary motor and sensory areas as well as ipsilateral premotor areas, namely, dorsal and ventral premotor cortex, pre- and supplementary motor areas (**Figure 2**), most pronounced in the lower beta frequency band. The over-recruitment of brain areas might lead to more potential network configurations with higher noise interferences and hence greater variability of states giving rise to the unspecific frequency distribution of movement-related power changes determined here. The cause of this over-recruitment could be either compensation with greater recruitment of secondary motor areas, because of the subjective increase of task-related complexity, in order to achieve the same motor output (Zimerman et al., 2014), or an increase of the attentional load (Reuter-Lorenz and Cappell,

circumvent the analysis of restricted frequency bands predefined from the young brain. Thereby, we observed differences in the spectral distribution of movement-related desynchronization over a broad frequency band (8–25 Hz) and found a widespread increase of spectral entropy during movement in the elderly compared to young, indicating that the movement-related broadband changes in the elderly are more variable and less predictable. This phenomenon was observed in three different fine motor skill tasks. The present finding underlines the notion that the increase of spectral entropy is a rather task unspecific phenomenon occurring during fine skilled motor control in the aged brain. Even though spectral entropy topographies showed differences in-between the Finger Sequence compared to the Pinch Grip and Whole Hand Grip task, these differences were solely derived from the young group. The aged brain on the other hand showed a uniform increase of entropy in all three tasks that did not statistically differ between tasks. One has to keep in mind, however, that in order to explicitly test, whether this difference of entropy over tasks was solely derived from the young group, one would have to conduct a crossover study, which includes execution of all three tasks in each participant.

2008), or due to inefficient activations with reduced selectivity of neuronal networks and less distinct activation patterns (Li and Lindenberger, 1999; Riecker et al., 2006). However, this question cannot be definitely answered by this study, mostly because it lacks a functional outcome parameter (for a review see Grady, 2012).

Possible Mechanisms of Dynamical Changes during Healthy Aging

The high variability of the spectral content along with the over-recruitment of secondary motor areas might be, on the one hand, a result of a decrease in selective local inhibition with greater background activity. On the other hand, a reduced selectivity of the network could be the consequence of a more general inhibition deficiency due to age-related structural and functional changes of the frontal cortex (Tisserand and Jolles, 2003; Rajah and D'Esposito, 2005). Moreover, a reduction of specific regulatory thalamic input could result in less distinct cortical activations. In Parkinson patients research has demonstrated the modulating influence of the basal ganglia-thalamocortical network on cortical oscillation patterns and motor control (de Hemptinne et al., 2013, 2015). These influences can be either of structural nature or can be evoked by intrinsic changes of synaptic properties. Furthermore, disrupted network dynamics might be a result of more subtle changes (McCarthy et al., 2012; Kopell et al., 2014; Voytek and Knight, 2015), such as neurochemical shifts and changes in synaptic binding potentials and receptor density. Future studies will have to further determine the underlying cause of oscillatory alterations in the aged brain.

In summary, the aged brain exhibits a broadband, frequency-unspecific power desynchronization during movement as reflected by an increase of spectral entropy, revealing a less predictable signal with great variability across frequencies in a wide cortical motor network.

AUTHOR CONTRIBUTIONS

FQ conducted the research, analyzed the data, and drafted the manuscript. MB conducted the research, was involved in data analysis, revised the manuscript. RS, JT, MZ, GN were involved in data acquisition and analysis, revision of the manuscript. FH developed the experimental idea, involved in drafting and revising of the manuscript.

FUNDING

This research was supported by the German Research Foundation (DFG, SFB 936-C4 to FH and Z3 to GN) and the German Ministry of Science (BMBF, 01GQ1424B to FH).

ACKNOWLEDGMENTS

We thank Meike Mund for her help on data collection.

REFERENCES

Bates, D., Mächler, M., Bolker, B., and Walker, S. (2015). Fitting linear mixed-effects models using lme4. *J. Stat. Soft.* 67, 1–48. doi: 10.18637/jss.v067.i01

Benjamini, Y., Drai, D., Elmer, G., Kafkafi, N., and Golani, I. (2001). Controlling the false discovery rate in behavior genetics research. *Behav. Brain Res.* 125, 279–284. doi: 10.1016/S0166-4328(01)00297-2

Brittain, J.-S., and Brown, P. (2014). Oscillations and the basal ganglia: motor control and beyond. *Neuroimage* 85, 637–647. doi: 10.1016/j.neuroimage.2013.05.084

Buckles, V. D. (1993). "Age-related slowing," in *Sensorimotor Impairment in the Elderly*, eds G. E. Stelmach and V. Hömberg (Dordrecht: Springer), 73–87.

CDT, R. (2008). *R: A Language and Environment for Statistical Computing*. Vienna: R Foundation for Statistical Computing.

Cheyne, D. O. (2013). MEG studies of sensorimotor rhythms: a review. *Exp. Neurol.* 245, 27–39. doi: 10.1016/j.expneurol.2012.08.030

Contreras-Vidal, J. L., Teulings, H. L., and Stelmach, G. E. (1998). Elderly subjects are impaired in spatial coordination in fine motor control. *Acta Psychol.* 100, 25–35. doi: 10.1016/S0001-6918(98)00023-7

Cooke, J. D., Brown, S. H., and Cunningham, D. A. (1989). Kinematics of arm movements in elderly humans. *Neurobiol. Aging* 10, 159–165. doi: 10.1016/0197-4580(89)90025-0

Cottone, C., Tomasevic, L., Porcaro, C., Filligoi, G., and Techio, F. (2013). Physiological aging impacts the hemispheric balances of resting state primary somatosensory activities. *Brain Topogr.* 26, 186–199. doi: 10.1007/s10548-012-0240-3

Crone, N. E., Miglioretti, D. L., Gordon, B., Sieracki, J. M., Wilson, M. T., Uematsu, S., et al. (1998). Functional mapping of human sensorimotor cortex with electrocorticographic spectral analysis. I. Alpha

and beta event-related desynchronization. *Brain* 121(Pt 12), 2271–2299. doi: 10.1093/brain/121.12.2271

Darling, W. G., Cooke, J. D., and Brown, S. H. (1989). Control of simple arm movements in elderly humans. *Neurobiol. Aging* 10, 149–157. doi: 10.1016/0197-4580(89)90024-9

De Clercq, W., Vergult, A., Vanrumste, B., Van Paesschen, W., and Van Huffel, S. (2006). Canonical correlation analysis applied to remove muscle artifacts from the electroencephalogram. *IEEE Trans. Biomed. Eng.* 53, 2583–2587. doi: 10.1109/TBME.2006.879459

de Hemptinne, C., Ryapolova-Webb, E. S., Air, E. L., Garcia, P. A., Miller, K. J., Ojemann, J. G., et al. (2013). Exaggerated phase-amplitude coupling in the primary motor cortex in Parkinson disease. *Proc. Natl. Acad. Sci. U.S.A.* 110, 4780–4785. doi: 10.1073/pnas.1214546110

de Hemptinne, C., Swann, N. C., Ostrem, J. L., Ryapolova-Webb, E. S., San Luciano, M., Galifianakis, N. B., et al. (2015). Therapeutic deep brain stimulation reduces cortical phase-amplitude coupling in Parkinson's disease. *Nat. Neurosci.* 18, 779–786. doi: 10.1038/nn.3997

Deiber, M.-P., Ibañez, V., Missonnier, P., Rodriguez, C., and Giannakopoulos, P. (2013). Age-associated modulations of cerebral oscillatory patterns related to attention control. *Neuroimage* 82, 531–546. doi: 10.1016/j.neuroimage.2013.06.037

Gaál, Z. A., Boha, R., Stam, C. J., and Molnár, M. (2010). Age-dependent features of EEG-reactivity-spectral, complexity, and network characteristics. *Neurosci. Lett.* 479, 79–84. doi: 10.1016/j.neulet.2010.05.037

Garrett, D. D., Kovacevic, N., McIntosh, A. R., and Grady, C. L. (2013). The modulation of BOLD variability between cognitive states varies by age and processing speed. *Cereb. Cortex* 23, 684–693. doi: 10.1093/cercor/bhs055

Gerloff, C., Corwell, B., Chen, R., Hallett, M., and Cohen, L. G. (1997). Stimulation over the human supplementary motor area interferes with the organization of future elements in complex motor sequences. *Brain* 120(Pt 9), 1587–1602. doi: 10.1093/brain/120.9.1587

Gerloff, C., Richard, J., Hadley, J., Schulman, A. E., Honda, M., and Hallett, M. (1998). Functional coupling and regional activation of human cortical motor areas during simple, internally paced and externally paced finger movements. *Brain* 121(Pt 8), 1513–1531. doi: 10.1093/brain/121.8.1513

Grady, C. (2012). The cognitive neuroscience of ageing. *Nat. Rev. Neurosci.* 13, 491–505. doi: 10.1038/nrn3256

Gross, J., Kujala, J., Hämäläinen, M., Timmermann, L., Schnitzler, A., and Salmelin, R. (2001). Dynamic imaging of coherent sources: studying neural interactions in the human brain. *Proc. Natl. Acad. Sci. U.S.A.* 98, 694–699. doi: 10.1073/pnas.98.2.694

Hanslmayr, S., Staudigl, T., and Fellner, M.-C. (2012). Oscillatory power decreases and long-term memory: the information via desynchronization hypothesis. *Front. Hum. Neurosci.* 6:74. doi: 10.3389/fnhum.2012.00074

Holmes, C. J., Hoge, R., Collins, L., Woods, R., Toga, A. W., and Evans, A. C. (1998). Enhancement of MR images using registration for signal averaging. *J. Comput. Assist. Tomogr.* 22, 324–333. doi: 10.1097/00004728-199803000-00032

Hong, S. L., and Rebec, G. V. (2012). A new perspective on behavioral inconsistency and neural noise in aging: compensatory speeding of neural communication. *Front. Aging Neurosci.* 4:27. doi: 10.3389/fnagi.2012.00027

Inouye, T., Shinosaki, K., Sakamoto, H., Toi, S., Ukai, S., Iyama, A., et al. (1991). Quantification of EEG irregularity by use of the entropy of the power spectrum. *Electroencephalogr. Clin. Neurophysiol.* 79, 204–210. doi: 10.1016/0013-4694(91)90138-T

Klimesch, W. (1999). EEG alpha and theta oscillations reflect cognitive and memory performance: a review and analysis. *Brain Res. Brain Res. Rev.* 29, 169–195. doi: 10.1016/S0165-0173(98)00056-3

Kopell, N. J., Gritton, H. J., Whittington, M. A., and Kramer, M. A. (2014). Beyond the connectome: the dynome. *Neuron* 83, 1319–1328. doi: 10.1016/j.neuron.2014.08.016

Li, S. C., and Lindenberger, U. (1999). "Cross-level unification: a computational exploration of the link between deterioration of neurotransmitter systems and dedifferentiation of cognitive abilities in old age," *Cognitive Neuroscience of Memory*, eds L. G. Nilsson and H. Markowitsch (Seattle, WA: Hogrefe & Huber Publishers), 103–146.

Li, S.-C., and Sikström, S. (2002). Integrative neurocomputational perspectives on cognitive aging, neuromodulation, and representation. *Neurosci. Biobehav. Rev.* 26, 795–808. doi: 10.1016/S0149-7634(02)00066-0

Makeig, S., Bell, A. J., Jung, T.-P., and Sejnowski, T. J. (1996). "Independent component analysis of electroencephalographic data," in *Advances in Neural Information Processing Systems 8*, eds D. Touretzky, M. Mozer, and M. Hasselmo (Cambridge, MA: MIT Press), 145–151.

Mattay, V. S., Fera, F., Tessitore, A., Hariri, A. R., Das, S., Callicott, J. H., et al. (2002). Neurophysiological correlates of age-related changes in human motor function. *Neurology* 58, 630–635. doi: 10.1212/WNL.58.4.630

McCarthy, M. M., Ching, S., Whittington, M. A., and Kopell, N. (2012). Dynamical changes in neurological diseases and anesthesia. *Curr. Opin. Neurobiol.* 22, 693–703. doi: 10.1016/j.conb.2012.02.009

Naccarato, M., Calautti, C., Jones, P. S., Day, D. J., Carpenter, T. A., and Baron, J.-C. (2006). Does healthy aging affect the hemispheric activation balance during paced index-to-thumb opposition task? An fMRI study. *Neuroimage* 32, 1250–1256. doi: 10.1016/j.neuroimage.2006.05.003

Oldfield, R. C. (1971). The assessment and analysis of handedness: the Edinburgh inventory. *Neuropsychologia* 9, 97–113. doi: 10.1016/0028-3932(71)90067-4

Oostenveld, R., Fries, P., Maris, E., and Schoffelen, J.-M. (2011). FieldTrip: open source software for advanced analysis of MEG, EEG, and invasive electrophysiological data. *Comput. Intell. Neurosci.* 2011:156869. doi: 10.1155/2011/156869

Pfurtscheller, G. (1989). Functional topography during sensorimotor activation studied with event-related desynchronization mapping. *J. Clin. Neurophysiol.* 6, 75–84. doi: 10.1097/00004691-198901000-00003

Pfurtscheller, G., Graimann, B., Huggins, J. E., Levine, S. P., and Schuh, L. A. (2003). Spatiotemporal patterns of beta desynchronization and gamma synchronization in corticographic data during self-paced movement. *Clin. Neurophysiol.* 114, 1226–1236. doi: 10.1016/S1388-2457(03)00067-1

Pfurtscheller, G., and Lopes da Silva, F. (1999). Event-related EEG/MEG synchronization and desynchronization: basic principles. *Clin. Neurophysiol.* 110, 1842–1857. doi: 10.1016/S1388-2457(99)00141-8

Rajah, M. N., and D'Esposito, M. (2005). Region-specific changes in prefrontal function with age: a review of PET and fMRI studies on working and episodic memory. *Brain* 128, 1964–1983. doi: 10.1093/brain/awh608

Reuter-Lorenz, P. A., and Cappell, K. A. (2008). Neurocognitive aging and the compensation hypothesis. *Curr. Dir. Psychol. Sci.* 17, 177–182. doi: 10.1111/j.1467-8721.2008.00570.x

Riecker, A., Gröschel, K., Ackermann, H., Steinbrink, C., Witte, O., and Kastrup, A. (2006). Functional significance of age-related differences in motor activation patterns. *Neuroimage* 32, 1345–1354. doi: 10.1016/j.neuroimage.2006.05.021

Rowe, J. B., Siebner, H., Filipovic, S. R., Cordivari, C., Gerschlager, W., Rothwell, J., et al. (2006). Aging is associated with contrasting changes in local and distant cortical connectivity in the human motor system. *Neuroimage* 32, 747–760. doi: 10.1016/j.neuroimage.2006.03.061

Sailer, A., Dichgans, J., and Gerloff, C. (2000). The influence of normal aging on the cortical processing of a simple motor task. *Neurology* 55, 979–985. doi: 10.1212/WNL.55.7.979

Smith, C. D., Umberger, G. H., Manning, E. L., Slevin, J. T., Wekstein, D. R., Schmitt, F. A., et al. (1999). Critical decline in fine motor hand movements in human aging. *Neurology* 53, 1458–1461. doi: 10.1212/WNL.53.7.1458

Sosnoff, J. J., and Newell, K. M. (2011). Aging and motor variability: a test of the neural noise hypothesis. *Exp. Aging Res.* 37, 377–397. doi: 10.1080/0361073X.2011.590754

Stelmach, G. E., Amrhein, P. C., and Goggin, N. L. (1988). Age differences in bimanual coordination. *J. Gerontol.* 43, P18–P23. doi: 10.1093/geronj/43.1.P18

Tisserand, D. J., and Jolles, J. (2003). On the involvement of prefrontal networks in cognitive ageing. *Cortex* 39, 1107–1128. doi: 10.1016/S0010-9452(08)70880-3

Tsubo, Y., Isomura, Y., and Fukai, T. (2012). Power-law inter-spike interval distributions infer a conditional maximization of entropy in cortical neurons. *PLoS Comput. Biol.* 8:e1002461. doi: 10.1371/journal.pcbi.1002461

Vallesi, A., McIntosh, A. R., Kovacevic, N., Chan, S. C. C., and Stuss, D. T. (2010). Age effects on the asymmetry of the motor system: evidence from cortical oscillatory activity. *Biol. Psychol.* 85, 213–218. doi: 10.1016/j.biopsycho.2010.07.003

Voytek, B., and Knight, R. T. (2015). Dynamic network communication as a unifying neural basis for cognition, development, aging, and disease. *Biol. Psychiatry* 77, 1089–1097. doi: 10.1016/j.biopsych.2015.04.016

Ward, N. S., and Frackowiak, R. S. (2003). Age-related changes in the neural correlates of motor performance. *Brain* 126, 873–888. doi: 10.1093/brain/awg071

Wishart, L. R., Lee, T. D., Murdoch, J. E., and Hodges, N. J. (2000). Effects of aging on automatic and effortful processes in bimanual coordination. *J. Gerontol. B Psychol. Sci. Soc. Sci.* 55, P85–P94. doi: 10.1093/geronb/55.2.P85

Wu, T., and Hallett, M. (2005). The influence of normal human ageing on automatic movements. *J. Physiol.* 562(Pt 2), 605–615. doi: 10.1113/jphysiol.2004.076042

Zimerman, M., Heise, K. F., Gerloff, C., Cohen, L. G., and Hummel, F. C. (2014). Disrupting the ipsilateral motor cortex interferes with training of a complex motor task in older adults. *Cereb. Cortex* 24, 1030–1036. doi: 10.1093/cercor/bhs385

2

Dissecting the Molecular Mechanisms of Neurodegenerative Diseases through Network Biology

Jose A. Santiago, Virginie Bottero and Judith A. Potashkin*

Department of Cellular and Molecular Pharmacology, The Chicago Medical School, Rosalind Franklin University of Medicine and Science, North Chicago, IL, United States

*Correspondence:
Judith A. Potashkin
judy.potashkin@rosalindfranklin.edu

Neurodegenerative diseases are rarely caused by a mutation in a single gene but rather influenced by a combination of genetic, epigenetic and environmental factors. Emerging high-throughput technologies such as RNA sequencing have been instrumental in deciphering the molecular landscape of neurodegenerative diseases, however, the interpretation of such large amounts of data remains a challenge. Network biology has become a powerful platform to integrate multiple omics data to comprehensively explore the molecular networks in the context of health and disease. In this review article, we highlight recent advances in network biology approaches with an emphasis in brain-networks that have provided insights into the molecular mechanisms leading to the most prevalent neurodegenerative diseases including Alzheimer's (AD), Parkinson's (PD) and Huntington's diseases (HD). We discuss how integrative approaches using multi-omics data from different tissues have been valuable for identifying biomarkers and therapeutic targets. In addition, we discuss the challenges the field of network medicine faces toward the translation of network-based findings into clinically actionable tools for personalized medicine applications.

Keywords: Alzheimer's disease, Parkinson's disease, Huntington's disease, network biology, molecular mechanisms

INTRODUCTION

Neurodegenerative diseases are usually sporadic in nature and commonly influenced by a wide range of genetic, epigenetic and environmental factors. With the advent of new high-throughput technologies such as RNA sequencing, it has become essential to develop methods beyond the classical pathway analysis to systematically interpret large amounts of data in the context of health and disease. Despite the progress of high-throughput genomic studies the precise pathogenic mechanisms leading to the most prevalent neurodegenerative diseases remain elusive. To this end, the applications of network biology have been successful to provide biological insight and to decipher the molecular underpinnings of neurodegenerative diseases. Network biology is based on the premise that complex diseases, like neurodegenerative diseases, are frequently caused by alterations in many genes comprising multiple biological pathways. A network consists of nodes and edges that may represent genes, proteins, miRNAs, noncoding RNAs, drugs, or diseases connected through a wide range of interactions including, but not limited to physical, genetic, co-expression and colocalization. An example of network analysis of Alzheimer's disease (AD) that identifies central hubs is shown in **Figure 1**. Integration of multi-omic information coupled with network-based approaches is becoming

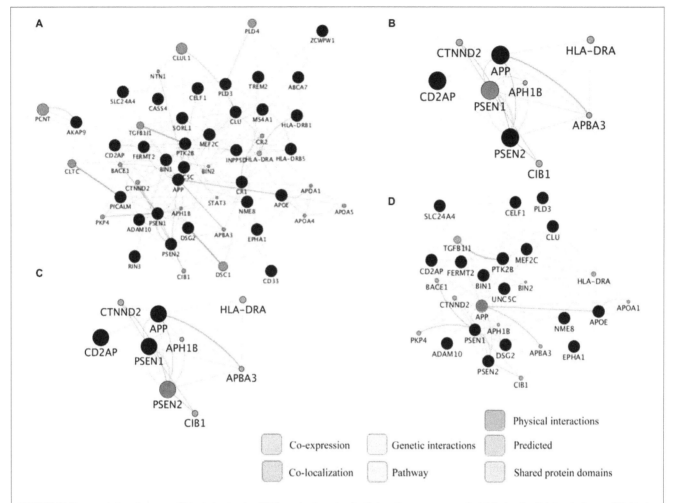

FIGURE 1 | Representation of common biological networks. **(A)** Example of a network of interactions among genetic risk factors for Alzheimer's disease (AD; black circles) and other related genes (gray circles). The color of the lines represents the type of interaction and the thickness is proportional to the strength of the association. **(B–D)** Presenilin 1 (PSEN1), PSEN2 and amyloid precursor protein (APP; red circles) are highly connected genes (hub genes) identified in the network. Hub genes usually play a central role in the disease. These networks were retrieved by GeneMANIA application in Cytoscape 3.1.1 as of September 2016 using the default settings to include the top 20 related genes and automatic weighting.

an essential step towards the advancement of personalized medicine (**Figure 2**). Some of the frequently used terms in network biology approaches are defined in **Table 1**.

Seminal work in network biology including the construction of the human disease network (Goh et al., 2007), the human functional linkage network (Linghu et al., 2009), the discovery of causal genes of obesity (Chen et al., 2008), and clinical biomarkers for cancer (Taylor et al., 2009), prompted efforts to study many different diseases using network-based approaches. In the last few years, there has been a steady growth in studies exploiting the concepts of network biology to understand neurodevelopmental and neurodegenerative diseases (Santiago and Potashkin, 2014a). For example, network approaches have successfully identified putative diagnostic biomarkers for Parkinson's disease (PD; Santiago and Potashkin, 2013a, 2015; Santiago et al., 2014, 2016), and progressive supranuclear palsy (Santiago and Potashkin, 2014b) reviewed in Santiago and Potashkin (2013b, 2014a,c).

In addition, network-based approaches have provided insights into the molecular mechanisms underlying co-morbid diseases associated with PD including diabetes (Santiago and Potashkin, 2013a) and cancer (Ibáñez et al., 2014). In this review article, we highlight the most recent advances in network biology applications to understand the most common neurodegenerative diseases with an emphasis on brain specific networks.

NETWORK-BASED APPROACHES IDENTIFIES PATHWAYS SPECIFIC TO ALZHEIMER'S DISEASE (AD)

AD is the most prevalent neurodegenerative disease, responsible for the majority of the cases of dementia, affecting more than 44 million people worldwide with an estimated global cost of more than 600 billion dollars[1]. Although the exact mechanism

---

[1]http://www.alzheimers.net/resources/alzheimers-statistics/

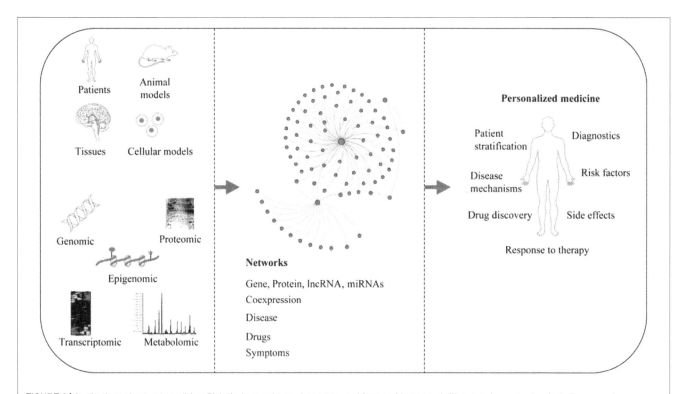

FIGURE 2 | Applications of network medicine. Biological networks can be constructed from a wide range of different omic approaches including genomic, transcriptomic, epigenomic, metabolomic and proteomic datasets. In protein-protein interaction (PPI) networks, proteins are the nodes and their interactions are the edges. Network-based approaches have advanced the field of personalized medicine by providing novel mechanisms of disease, diagnostics and therapeutic targets.

of disease remains unclear, a complex combination of genetic, epigenetic, lifestyle, environmental factors and aging are believed to be responsible for most of the cases. Pathological features of AD include the accumulation of amyloid beta (Aβ) plaques and protein tau in neurofibrillary tangles (NFT). While most of the AD cases are late onset (LOAD) and sporadic, some genetic mutations in the amyloid precursor protein (*APP*), presenilin 1 (*PSEN1*) and presenilin 2 (*PSEN2*) are documented to cause early onset AD, which accounts for approximately 2% of the cases with symptoms appearing before the age of 65 (Goate et al., 1991; Levy-Lahad et al., 1995; Janssen et al., 2003). The apoliporotein E-ε4 (APOEε4) is the only genetic factor identified in more than 60% of the sporadic AD cases, however, it has also been found in healthy individuals thus suggesting that other genetic factors may be responsible for the disease (Coon et al., 2007). To date, emerging high-throughput genomic technologies have reported more than 2900 genetic variations associated with AD[2].

Although these studies have been valuable to understand the genetic diversity associated with AD, the multi-factorial mechanisms leading to the disease are unclear. Network-based approaches have been successful to systematically interpret these results and to gain insight into the mechanisms of disease. In particular, integrative approaches combining multi-omic data in networks have been employed to identify

susceptibility genes and pathways in AD. For example, combinatorial network analysis of proteomic and transcriptomic data revealed subnetworks enriched in pathways associated with the pathogenesis of AD including the downregulation of genes associated with the *MAPK/ERK* pathway and the upregulation of genes associated to the clathrin-mediated receptor endocytosis pathway (Hallock and Thomas, 2012; **Table 2**). In this regard, disruption of the clathrin-mediated receptor pathway can lead to increased levels of APP thereby contributing to disease progression (Schneider et al., 2008; Hallock and Thomas, 2012). Integrative approaches have led to the identification of potential additional genetic risk factors and biomarkers for AD. For instance, integration of genome wide association studies (GWAS), linkage analysis and expression profiling in a protein-protein interaction (PPI) network yielded a 108 potential risk factors for AD including EGFR, ACTB, CDC2, IRAK1, APOE, ABCA1 and AMPH. Among these genes, EGFR, APOE and ACTB were found to overlap with proteomic data from cerebrospinal fluid of AD patients (Talwar et al., 2014) thus providing potential biomarker candidates. Collectively, these studies reinforce the power of integrative network approaches to identify pathways, genetic risk factors and biomarkers for AD.

Weighted gene coexpression networks analysis (WGCNA) are increasingly being used to find highly co-expressed gene modules associated with a particular biological pathway or a clinical trait of interest (Langfelder and Horvath, 2008).

---

[2]http://www.alsgene.org/

TABLE 1 | Frequently used terms in network biology.

Term	Definition
Epigenetic	Epigenetic studies genetic effects not encoded in the DNA sequence of an organism.
Gene ontology (GO)	Gene ontology is a major bioinformatics initiative to unify the representation of gene and gene product attributes across all species.
Genome wide association study (GWAS)	A genome wide association study is an examination of the entire genome that is useful to identify genetic variants (SNPs) associated with a trait of interest.
Module	Module is defined as a group of physically or functionally linked molecules that work together to achieve a relatively distinct function. Modules are also called groups, clusters or communities. Examples of modules are co-regulation, co-expression, membership of a protein complex, of a metabolic or signaling pathway.
Network analysis	Network analysis is a method to systematically analyze a group of interconnected components. Nodes and edges are the basic components of a network. Nodes represent units in the network and edges represent the interactions between the units. Hubs are nodes with high connectivity.
Network medicine	Network medicine is an emerging field of network biology that applies the principles that govern cellular and molecular networks in the context of health and disease.
-omes	-omes are large scale networks. Interactome refers to the entire set of interactions in a particular cell. These interactions could represent, for example, protein-protein interactions (PPI) or interactions between messenger RNA molecules, also known as the transcriptome.
Single nucleotide polymorphism (SNP)	A single nucleotide polymorphism is a variation in a single nucleotide that occurs at a specific position in the genome. They are the most common type of genetic variation among people.
Weighted gene co-expression network analysis (WGCNA)	Weighted gene co-expression network analysis, also known as weighted correlation network analysis (WCNA), represents a systems biologic method for analyzing microarray data, gene information data, and microarray sample traits (e.g., case control status or clinical outcomes). WGCNA facilitates a network-based gene screening method that can be used to identify candidate biomarkers or therapeutic targets.

For example, construction of gene co-expression networks from 1647 postmortem brain tissues from LOAD patients highlighted immune and microglia enriched modules, containing a key regulator of the immune system, known as TYROBP (Zhang et al., 2013). Likewise, WGCNA analysis uncovered astrocyte-specific and microglia-enriched modules in vulnerable brain regions that associated with early tau accumulation (Miller et al., 2013). Implementation of WGCNA in RNA-sequencing data using brain samples obtained from the temporal lobe of subjects with dementia with Lewy body (DLB), LOAD and cognitively normal patients, identified network modules specific to each disease. For example, two network modules enriched in myelination and innate immune response correlated with LOAD whereas network modules associated with synaptic transmission and the generation of precursor metabolites correlated with DLB and LOAD (Humphries et al., 2015). Further, genes previously implicated in LOAD including *FRMD4B* and *ST18* (Miller et al., 2008; Zhang et al., 2013) were prominent hubs within the myelination network (Humphries et al., 2015). Together, these findings suggested the involvement of microglia and myelination in the pathogenesis of AD and established differences in biological pathways between LOAD and DLB. Besides innate immunity pathways, network analysis of transcriptomic data from the brain hippocampus of normal aged and AD subjects identified key transcriptional regulators related to insulin (*INS1, INS2*) and brain derived neurotrophic factor (*BDNF*) interacting with the retinoic acid receptor related orphan receptor (*RORA*, Acquaah-Mensah et al., 2015) previously

implicated in autoimmunity and diabetes (Solt and Burris, 2012).

With the growing interest in personalized medicine, it has become essential to develop tools to stratify patients according to symptoms, prognosis, and disease stage. This is highly important due to the fact that some subgroups of patients within a specific disease may experience a faster disease progression or respond to therapy differently. There are several documented examples on how networks could accelerate individualized treatment. For instance, analysis of protein interaction networks identified unstable network modules in different brain regions, in particular, in the entorhinal cortex of AD patients. Specifically, several protein interactions were present or absent at different Braak stages thus providing network modules characteristic of disease progression in AD (Kikuchi et al., 2013). Interestingly, the network modules with the largest number of disappearing protein interactions at late stage were associated with the histone acetyltransferase and the proteasome complexes. These modules were interacting *via* UCHL5 thereby indicating the perturbation of the ubiquitin-proteosome system in AD. Likewise, network analysis of six relevant brain regions affected in AD uncovered 136 hub genes of which 72 correlated with the Mini Mental State Examination (MMSE) and NFT scores, both widely utilized indicators of disease severity in AD (Liang et al., 2012). Among these genes, there were important transcription factors and kinases associated with AD including *LEF1, SOX9, YY1, TCF3, TFDP1, CDK5, CSK* and *MAP3K3*. Among these

TABLE 2 | Brain network-based analysis of the most common neurodegenerative diseases.

Disease	Networks identified	Reference
AD	*MAPK/ERK* and clathrin-mediated receptor endocytosis	Hallock and Thomas (2012)
	Immune system and microglia	Zhang et al. (2013)
	Astrocyte-specific and microglia-enriched modules	Miller et al. (2013)
	Myelination and innate immune response	Humphries et al. (2015)
	Network modules of AD progression	Kikuchi et al. (2013)
	Co-expression modules based on *APOEε4* stratification	Jiang et al. (2016)
	Downregulated network of genes corresponding to metastable proteins prone to aggregation	Ciryam et al. (2016)
	Hypomethylation patterns in a myelination network	Humphries et al. (2015)
PD	Stress response and neuron survival/degeneration mechanisms	Corradini et al. (2014)
	Key protein targets including p62, GABARAP, GBRL1 and GBRL2 that modulated 1-methyl-4-phenylpyridinium (MPP$^+$) toxicity	Keane et al. (2015)
	Alvespimycin neuroprotective agent for PD	Gao et al. (2014)
	RGS2 as a key regulator of LRRK2 function	Dusonchet et al. (2014)
	Downregulation of RNA and protein expression of a network of transcription factors *FOXA1, NR3C1, HNF4A* and *FOSL2*	Fernández-Santiago et al. (2015)
HD	Modules associated with *Htt* CAG length and toxicity	Langfelder et al. (2016)
	Metalloprotein, stress response, angiogenesis, mitochondrion, glycolysis, intracellular protein transport, proteasome, synaptic vesicle	Neueder and Bates (2014)
	Protein modification, vesicles transport, cell signaling and synaptic transmission	Mina et al. (2016)
	Astrocyte module associated with TGF**β** -FOXO3 signaling, stress and sleep phenotype	Scarpa et al. (2016)
Aging, neurodegeneration	DNA repair, RNA metabolism, and glucose metabolism shared in AD and PD	Calderone et al. (2016)
	242 genes enriched in pathways related to neuron differentiation, apoptosis, gap junction trafficking, and cellular metabolic processes in AD and HD	Narayanan et al. (2014)
	Inflammation, mitochondrial dysfunction, and metal ion homeostasis in aging and PD	Glaab and Schneider (2015)
	Chaperome critical to maintain protein homeostasis in aging and neurodegeneration	Brehme et al. (2014)

genes, overactivation of *CDK5* is a major trigger of tau hyperphosphorylation and NFT formation in AD suggesting it may be a target for therapeutic intervention (Wilkaniec et al., 2016).

Since some genetic risk factors have a stronger influence in the disease than others, patient categorization and stratification according to the genetic basis would be advantageous in personalized medicine. In the context of AD, *APOEε4* is the strongest risk factor for LOAD accounting for more than 50% of the cases. *APOEε4* carriers display different clinical and pathological features than those of non-carriers. For example, *APOEε4* carriers perform worse on memory tasks (Marra et al., 2004) and have a higher amyloid beta deposition than non-carriers (Kandimalla et al., 2011; Jack et al., 2015). Moreover, *APOEε4* carriers respond to treatment differently than non-carriers. For instance, a neuroprotective agent improved MMSE scores in *APOEε4* carriers but not in non-carriers (Richard et al., 1997). WGCNA on a transcriptomic dataset from human cerebral cortex of LOAD identified distinct co-expression modules based on *APOEε4* stratification (Jiang et al., 2016). Co-expression modules of *APOEε4* carriers were enriched in hereditary disorders, neurological diseases, and nervous system development and function whereas modules of non-carriers were enriched in immunological and cardiovascular diseases thus suggesting that different biological processes could play a role in LOAD with different APOEε4 status (Jiang et al., 2016).

NETWORK-BASED APPROACHES IN PARKINSON'S DISEASE (PD)

PD is the second most prevalent neurodegenerative disease after AD, affecting more than 10 million people worldwide. Pathological features include the accumulation of aggregated alpha synuclein (SNCA) in intraneuronal cytoplasmic inclusion known as Lewy bodies and the progressive loss of dopaminergic neurons in the substantia nigra pars compacta. Dopamine restorative drugs and deep brain stimulation are current therapies to treat patients, however, these treatments only alleviate motor symptoms but do not impact disease progression. Mutations in the *LRRK2, PARK2, PARK7, PINK1* and *SNCA* genes are known to cause familial PD. Most of the PD cases, however, are sporadic resulting from a complex interplay between genetics and environmental factors. In fact, some of the same genetic variants including *SNCA* and *LRRK2* implicated in familial PD have been also associated with sporadic PD (Satake et al., 2009; Simón-Sánchez et al., 2009; Lin and Farrer, 2014). To date, advances in genomics have identified 28 genes associated with PD (Lin and Farrer, 2014).

Several pathways have been linked to the pathogenesis of PD including mitochondrial dysfunction, endoplasmic reticulum stress, autophagy, inflammation and impaired insulin signaling (Mercado et al., 2013; Nolan et al., 2013; Santiago and Potashkin, 2013b; Lin and Farrer, 2014). Despite this progress, the precise disease-causing mechanisms of PD are not fully understood. Complementation of genomic and transcriptomic studies with system biology approaches have provided insights into some novel mechanisms of disease. For instance, differential co-expression network analysis (DCA) performed on transcriptomic data from PD substantia nigra at autopsy, uncovered a transcript isoform of *SNCA* with an extended 3′ untranslated region, termed aSynL, which influenced SNCA accumulation (Rhinn et al., 2012). Interestingly, the pattern of expression of the long aSynL isoform relative to the short isoforms was also observed in unaffected individuals harboring a PD risk variant in the *SNCA* locus (Rhinn et al., 2012).

Understanding the molecular events associated with the progression of PD could help delineate a timeline for effective therapeutic intervention. Gene co-expression network analysis showed differences in gene modules between PD and controls for different anatomic brain regions (Corradini et al., 2014). In PD, hub modules in the motor vagal nucleus, locus coeruleus, and substantia nigra were enriched in pathways related to stress response and neuron survival/degeneration mechanisms whereas in control samples gene modules were associated with neuroprotection and aging homeostasis. Interestingly, one of the main hubs in the substantia nigra of control samples was *SIRT1*, which has been widely implicated in neuroprotection in several neurodegenerative diseases (Donmez and Outeiro, 2013; Herskovits and Guarente, 2013). Analysis of PPI networks representing autophagy and mitochondrial dysfunction pathways identified key protein targets including p62, GABARAP, GBRL1 and GBRL2 that modulated 1-methyl-4-phenylpyridinium (MPP$^+$) toxicity (Keane et al., 2015), a widely used toxin to mimic PD in animal and cellular models. Strikingly, overexpression of these proteins combined, but not each one alone, provided rescue of MPP$^+$ toxicity. This result further strengthens the notion that targeting a cluster of genes rather than a single gene may be the route to an effective treatment.

Integrative system biology approaches incorporating network analyses have been valuable in identifying potential therapeutic targets in PD. For instance, construction of networks integrating genetic information from Gene expression Omnibus (GEO), the Parkinson's disease database (ParkDB) and the Comparative Toxicogenomics Database (CTD), identified alvespimycin (17-DMAG) as a candidate neuroprotective agent for PD (Gao et al., 2014). Experimental validation showed that 17-DMAG attenuated rotenone-induced toxicity *in vitro*. Another approach combined human brain and blood transcriptomic data and identified RGS2 as a key regulator of LRRK2 function (Dusonchet et al., 2014), one of the most common genetic risk factor of PD. Of note, RGS2 protected against neuronal toxicity in a *Caenorhabditis elegans* model expressing wild type *LRRK2*. Combination of -omics data from different tissues, for example brain and blood, may be advantageous to understand neurodegeneration in light of the recent finding that demonstrated that cell types outside the brain contain genetic risk factors associated with PD (Coetzee et al., 2016) and thus may help uncover new putative therapeutic targets.

NETWORK ANALYSIS IN HUNTINGTON'S DISEASE (HD)

Huntington's disease (HD) is one of the most common dominantly inherited neurodegenerative disorders. The symptoms include some motor symptoms, such as chorea and dystonia, as well as non-motor symptoms, including psychological changes, and cognitive decline leading to dementia (Ross et al., 2014). These symptoms are correlated with a selective degeneration of the striatal and cortical neurons (Ehrlich, 2012). Currently, there are no therapies to prevent the onset or slow the progression of HD.

This progressive and fatal disease is caused by abnormal extension of the CAG repeat coding for a polyglutamine (polyQ) tail in the huntingtin gene (*HTT*, MacDonald et al., 1993). Unaffected individuals have fewer than 36 repeats, whereas affected patients can have as many as 250 CAG repeats. It has been shown that the length of the polyQ extension is inversely proportional to the age of the disease onset (Orr and Zoghbi, 2007). Vesicle and mitochondrial transport, transcription regulation, neurogenesis and energy metabolism are among the cellular functions of the normal HTT protein (Borrell-Pagès et al., 2006). Both lost of function of the normal protein and gain of toxic properties of mutant HTT leads to HD pathology. In fact, it has been shown that whereas the normal HTT protein is neuroprotective, the mutant HTT is neurotoxic. Despite this progress, the molecular mechanisms involved in the complex phenotype of the disease are still largely unknown.

In order to understand the role of HTT in HD pathology, (Langfelder et al., 2016) expressed HTT with different CAG length in a mice model. They demonstrated that the length of the CAG repeats modified the transcriptome of the striatum, and to a lesser extent, the cortex. WGCNA allowed the identification of 13 striatal and five cortical gene coexpression modules that were strongly associated with *Htt* CAG length. Interestingly, cadherin and protocadherin (*Pcdh*) genes expression were dysregulated in four of the modules, indicating that regulatory factors of these genes, such as *Rest*, *Ctcf* and *Rad21*, could be involved in HTT toxicity in mice (Langfelder et al., 2016).

Similarly, WGCNA was performed on transcriptomic HD post mortem tissues including the frontal cortex, cerebellum and caudate nucleus regions. The authors found that genes involved in metalloprotein, stress response and angiogenesis were positively regulated in all the networks whereas genes involved in mitochondrion, glycolysis, intracellular protein transport, proteasome and synaptic vesicle were downregulated (Neueder and Bates, 2014). Analysis of the human transcriptome from HD patients compared to healthy samples confirmed that protein modification, vesicles transport, cell signaling and synaptic transmission are important pathways involved in HD (Mina et al., 2016). Interestingly, these modules were also found in a blood transcriptomic study (Mina et al., 2016). Despite the fact that dysregulation of similar pathways was observed in the blood and brain, there was no overlap in any of the individual genes common between the two tissues (Mina et al., 2016).

A system-based approach performed on human transcriptomic datasets from post mortem human cerebellum, frontal cortex and caudate nucleus from HD patients and controls showed that an astrocyte module is the network whose connectivity and expression is most altered in HD (Scarpa et al., 2016). This astrocyte module was located downstream of TGFβ -FOXO3 signaling. In this regard, the TGFβ pathway was upregulated in neural stem cell differentiated from HD patient induced pluripotent stem cells (iPSC; Ring et al., 2015). Analysis of corrected iPS cells expressing shorter polyQ tails showed a downregulation of TGFβ pathway target genes, including cyclin-dependent kinase inhibitor 2B (*CDKN2B*), inhibitor of DNA binding 2 (*ID2*), inhibitor of DNA binding 4 (*ID4*), paired-like homeodomain transcription factor 2 (*PITX2*), thrombospondin 1 (*THBS1*), and left-right determination factor 2 (*LEFTY2*, An et al., 2012). In addition, valproic acid and lithium, both affecting TGFβ signaling, have been shown to improve mood in HD patients (Grove et al., 2000; Liang et al., 2008; Watanabe et al., 2011; Scheuing et al., 2014; Raja et al., 2015).

HD non-motor symptoms such as stress-related psychiatric and sleep disturbances often precede the onset of motor symptoms (Duff et al., 2007) and system-based approaches have proposed that sleep and stress traits emerge from shared genetic and transcriptional networks (Jiang et al., 2015). Interestingly, the astrocyte network expression described by Scarpa et al also correlated with stress and sleep phenotype in a chronically stressed mouse model (Scarpa et al., 2016). Collectively, these results suggest that targeting components of the TGFβ signaling pathway may provide novel therapeutics for HD.

NETWORK APPROACHES TO UNDERSTAND THE CONNECTION AMONG NEURODEGENERATIVE DISEASES

Widespread protein misfolding and aggregation is a hallmark of neurodegenerative diseases. Despite the fact that neurodegerative diseases are defined by a set of characteristic pathological and clinical features, there is some overlap in pathology, genetic risk factors, and mechanisms of disease. For example, accumulation of SNCA and Lewy body pathology, central in the pathogenesis of PD, are present in the brains of human AD and implicated in aberrant synapse formation (Hamilton, 2000; Kim et al., 2004). Several studies have identified Single nucleotide polymorphisms (SNPs) in the *MAPT* locus associated with PD and AD thus suggesting that a common genetic factor may put an individual at risk for both diseases (Desikan et al., 2015). In addition to *MAPT*, other genetic variants including *PON1*, *GSTO*, and *NEDD9* have been associated with the risk of PD and AD thus strengthening the genetic overlap between both diseases (Xie et al., 2014). Not surprisingly, shared mechanisms related to oxidative stress, neuroinflammation, impaired insulin signaling, mitochondrial dysfunction, iron dyshomeostasis and nicotinic receptors have been implicated in the pathogenesis of AD and PD (Xie et al., 2014). Therefore, a system-level understanding of the disease-disease connections could accelerate the discovery of novel treatments for both neurodegenerative diseases.

A systems-based approach combining expression quantitative trait loci (eQTL) studies from cerebellum and frontal cortex of AD patients, GWAS from AD and PD and PPI networks indicated that some PD variants (cisSNPs, cis-acting SNPs) were associated with the expression of *CRHR1*, LRRC37A4 and *MAPT* located at 17q21 and suggestive of AD risk (Liu et al., 2015). Similarly, shortest path analysis on a network constructed from literature mining identified known genes that already have an association with AD and PD and seven previously unknown genes including *ROS1*, *FMN1*, *ATP8A2*, *SNORD12C*, *ERVK10*, *PRS* and *C7ORF49* that may link both diseases (Kim et al., 2016). Besides finding shared genetic associations, network analysis employing the computation of a similarity matrix identified gene clusters related to DNA repair, RNA metabolism, and glucose metabolism shared in AD and PD (Calderone et al., 2016). Importantly, these pathways were not detected using the conventional gene ontology (GO) analysis thus highlighting the power of networks to uncover novel pathways.

In addition to the studies focused on AD and PD, recent network-based approaches have been applied to understand the molecular networks shared among other neurodegenerative diseases. One study focused on the dorsolateral prefrontal cortex (DLPFC) which is commonly affected in both AD and HD to construct coexpression networks using genome wide expression data from 600 postmorterm DLPFC tissues from AD, HD, and non-dementia controls. Differential coexpression analysis revealed a subnetwork of 242 genes enriched in pathways related to neuron differentiation, apoptosis, gap junction trafficking, and cellular metabolic processes (Narayanan et al., 2014). Interestingly, the 242 gene subnetwork overlapped with genes downregulated in postmortem brains of major depressive disorder, a condition that is associated with other neurodegenerative disorders including PD (Aarsland et al., 2012). Further inspection of this subnetwork identified a gained/lost gene coexpression patterns associated with chromatin organization and neural differentiation.

NETWORK-BASED APPROACHES TO UNDERSTAND AGING-ASSOCIATED NEURODEGENERATION

Aging is one of the most common risk factors associated with neurodegeneration. With an average age of onset of 60 for the most common neurodegenerative diseases, the risk of developing PD or AD significantly increases with age. Dopamine synthesis, a crucial neurotransmitter that becomes depleted in the brain of PD, declines with age (Ota et al., 2006) and amyloid deposits, characteristic pathology in AD, are found in the aging brain of non-demented individuals (Pike et al., 2007). Beyond the overlap in pathological features, aging and neurodegenerative disorders share several dysregulated pathways. A system-based approach that identifies molecular networks shared between aging and neurodegeneration should reveal shared mechanisms, some of which may be targets for slowing disease progression. Discovering unique dysregulataed pathways that are not aging-associated could pinpoint potential therapeutics targets unique for a particular neurodegenerative disease.

Several studies have employed system biology tools to better understand age-related neurodegeneration. For example, a comparative pathway and network analysis of the brain transcriptome revealed shared networks and pathways between aging and PD including inflammation, mitochondrial dysfunction and metal ion homeostasis (Glaab and Schneider, 2015). Interestingly, the expression of the most significant shared gene, NR4A2, gradually declined with aging and PD. They found that this aging-associated gene expression changes in NR4A2 might increase the risk of PD by mechanisms similar to gene mutations linked to PD (Glaab and Schneider, 2015).

Proteostasis functional decline is common in aging and neurodegenerative diseases. In fact, several studies have proposed a mechanistic link between aging and loss of protein homeostasis leading to protein aggregation and toxicity. In this context, chaperones play a pivotal role in protein assembly and folding and its dysregulation may lead to protein aggregation and proteotoxicity. A recent study identified a chaperone subnetwork that exhibited concordant repression and induction expression patterns in brain tissues from human aging, AD, HD and PD patients. Subsequent investigation led to the discovery of a subnetwork comprising HSC70, HSP90, the CCT/TRiC complex and HSP40 and TPR-domain related co-chaperones with aberrant expression that were required to prevent Aβ and polyQ-associated proteotoxicity in C. elegans (Brehme et al., 2014). This shared chaperome subnetwork in aging and neurodegeneration, which is critical to maintain protein homeostasis, provides new targets for therapeutic intervention in neurodegenerative diseases. Similarly, a recent meta-analysis of about 1600 microarrays from brain tissue of AD patients revealed a set of downregulated genes corresponding to metastable proteins prone to aggregation (Ciryam et al., 2016). Thus, targeting components of the proteome homeostasis network may enable novel therapeutic opportunities for neurodegenerative diseases.

EPIGENETICS, AGING AND NEURODEGENERATIVE DISORDERS

Gene expression is temporally and spatially regulated by DNA methylation or histone modifications. These epigenetic changes could influence a global gene expression or target some specific genes. A role for epigenetic changes in gene expression has been proposed in aging and neurodegenerative disorders. Interestingly, many studies have reported a genome-wide tendency to DNA hypomethylation with age in different organs including the brain in aging animal models (Wilson et al., 1987; Brunet and Berger, 2014). These changes are proposed to play a role in the progression of aging (Benayoun et al., 2015; Zampieri et al., 2015). Interestingly, Humphries et al. (2015) has shown that hypomethylation

was observed in a myelination network dysregulated in AD.

DNA methylation has been proposed as a biomarker for aging in cells, tissues and organs (Horvath, 2013). An acceleration of the epigenetic clock has been proposed in different neurodegenerative disorders. In this context, epigenetic age acceleration correlated with AD neuropathological markers such as neuritic plaques and amyloid load (Levine et al., 2015). In addition, an association between epigenetic age acceleration with episodic memory, working memory and cognitive decline was observed among individuals with AD (Levine et al., 2015). Histones modifications, such as acetylation and methylation, have been observed in AD models and patients (for review see Fischer, 2014). Interestingly, the epigenetic clock is also accelerated in brain regions from HD patients (Horvath et al., 2016).

Epigenetic modification is also proposed to contribute to neurodegeneration in PD. A genome wide DNA methylation and transcriptomic study in iPSC-derived dopaminergic neurons from LRRK2-associated PD patients identified common DNA methylation changes in LRRK2 and sporadic PD (Fernández-Santiago et al., 2015). DNA methylation changes in PD dopaminergic neurons correlated with the downregulation of RNA and protein expression of a network of transcription factors FOXA1, NR3C1, HNF4A and FOSL2, which have been implicated in PD. For instance, FOXA1 is a key determinant in the molecular and physiological properties of dopaminergic neurons (Pristerè et al., 2015) and HNF4A expression in blood has correlated with disease progression in PD (Santiago and Potashkin, 2015).

Several computational tools have been developed to facilitate the integration of epigenetic data in networks. For example, EpiRegNet is a publicly available web server that allows the construction of epigenetic regulatory networks from human transcriptomic data (Wang et al., 2011). Another model, the Artificial Epigenetic Regulatory Network (AERN) incorporated DNA methylation and chromatin modification in addition to genetic factors for the analysis of epigenetic networks (Turner et al., 2013). More recently, another computational model, the Biological Expression Language (BEL)[3], enabled the analysis of functional consequences of epigenetic modifications in the context of disease mechanisms (Khanam Irin et al., 2015). Because BEL integrates literature-derived cause and effect relationships into networks, researchers can formulate novel hypotheses of disease mechanisms. Notably, BEL network modeling has been used to integrate epigenetic and genetic factors in a functional context in PD. Using this approach, SNCA, MAPT, DNMT1, CYP2E1, OLFR151, PRKAR2A and SEPW1, were found to be hypomethylated in PD and suggested to cause overexpression of genes that disrupt normal biological functions. Further, two SNPs, rs3756063 and rs7684318, were associated with hypomethylation of SNCA in PD patients (Khanam Irin et al., 2015). Collectively, these models demonstrate that the integration of epigenetic factors into networks can uncover novel mechanisms of disease.

---

[3]http://www.openbel.org/

CHALLENGES AND FUTURE DIRECTIONS IN NETWORK MEDICINE APPLICATIONS TOWARDS PERSONALIZED TREATMENT

The field of network medicine has undoubtedly accelerated the understanding of the molecular mechanisms leading to neurodegeneration. The most significant brain network-based studies of the most common neurodegenerative diseases are summarized in **Table 2**. While network-based methods provide an unbiased approach to decode complex diseases and generate novel hypothesis, experimental validation is essential for network findings to be translated into useful diagnostics and therapeutic applications. In this regard, a growing number of studies have successfully identified blood-based biomarkers with potential clinical applicability. For instance, network analysis identified *SOD2, APP, HNF4A, PTBP1* and *NAMPT* as useful to distinguish PD patients from HC in blood samples obtained from two independent cohorts (Santiago and Potashkin, 2013a, 2015; Santiago et al., 2014, 2016). Among these biomarkers, *HNF4A* and *PTBP1*, showed a dynamic expression pattern in longitudinal samples thus showing potential to track the clinical course of PD patients. Likewise, network analysis identified *PTPN1* as a useful blood biomarker to distinguish PD from progressive supranuclear palsy, an atypical parkinsonian disorder commonly misdiagnosed as PD (Santiago

and Potashkin, 2014b). Despite the success in PD studies, experimental validation of network-based findings in AD and HTT studies in clinically relevant studies is mostly lacking. For example, a systems medicine approach identified TYROBP as a promising target for therapeutic intervention in AD but to the best of our knowledge there are no follow-up studies (Zhang et al., 2013). Similarly, the involvement of *RORA* (Acquaah-Mensah et al., 2015) and other potential targets in AD are yet to be validated.

Besides experimental validation, another aspect for consideration is the cell-type and tissue specific analysis. This is important since the analysis of gene expression studies from whole brain sections might lead to misleading results that are not relevant to the specific cell type affected in the disorder. To circumvent this problem, recent studies have successfully employed high-throughput technologies that enable a single-cell resolution. A notable example studied the changes in astrocyte and microglia reactivity in AD. They observed that genes within the immune response pathway were more pronounced in astrocytes than in microglia thus demonstrating that cell-type specific characterization of the molecular changes may be more informative (Orre et al., 2014). More details about limitations in system-biology approaches in the context of neurodegenerative diseases have been well described recently (De Strooper and Karran, 2016).

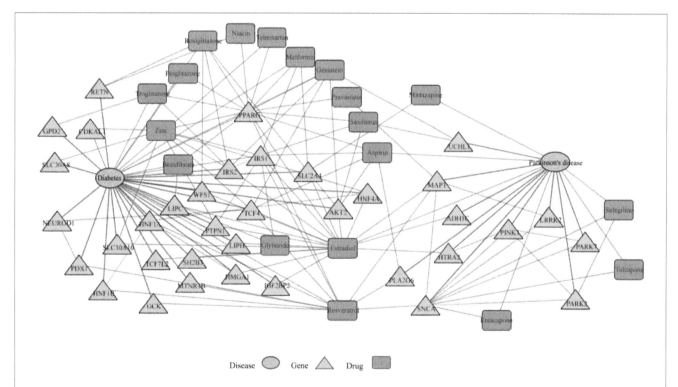

FIGURE 3 | Disease-drugs networks. Interaction among different diseases, drugs and genes can be represented in a multi-level network model. For example, network-based approaches have been used to understand shared dysregulated pathways in Parkinson's disease (PD) and diabetes. For instance, some drugs to treat diabetes patients have shown neuroprotective effects in PD and the observed neuroprotection may be mediated through their interaction with the peroxisome proliferator-activated receptor gamma (PPARG). Blue and gray lines represent drug interactions and disease interactions, respectively. This network was retrieved by iCTNet application in Cytoscape v3.1.1. using genetic associations from genome wide association studies (GWAS) and drug interactions from the Comparative Toxicogenomics Database (CTD) as of September 2016.

Another emerging area of research in the network biology field is the study of disease comorbidities. Several conditions including, diabetes, cancer, major depressive disorder and cardiovascular disease, for example, have been associated with neurodegenerative diseases. For example, insulin resistance and diabetes have been linked to AD and PD and drugs to treat diabetic patients have shown promising results in both disorders (Santiago and Potashkin, 2013b). In addition, analyses of shared networks between PD and diabetes have elucidated potential blood biomarkers for PD (Santiago and Potashkin, 2013a, 2014c; Santiago et al., 2014). More recently, an integrative transcriptomic meta-analysis of PD and major depression identified *NAMPT* as a potential blood biomarker for *de novo* PD patients (Santiago et al., 2016). Furthermore, treatment with an enzymatic product of NAMPT elicited neuroprotective effects via activation of SIRT1 in an *in vitro* model of PD (Zou et al., 2016). Therefore, understanding the molecular networks shared between comorbid diseases could reveal novel diagnostics and therapeutic targets. Network analysis of gene-drug interactions in PD and diabetes demonstrates that some drugs may be beneficial for treating both diseases (**Figure 3**). In this context, treatment with commonly prescribed drugs to treat diabetes including rosiglitazone, metformin, pioglitazone and exenatide have shown neuroprotective effects in PD models (Santiago and Potashkin, 2013b, 2014c; Aviles-Olmos et al., 2014; Carta and Simuni, 2015). In particular, treatment with exenatide improved motor and cognitive function in PD patients (Aviles-Olmos et al., 2013, 2014). Treatment with pioglitazone, however, did not result in disease-modifying benefits in PD patients (NINDS Exploratory Trials in Parkinson Disease (NET-PD) FS-ZONE Investigators, 2015; Simon et al., 2015). Nonetheless, it has been noted that a longer exposure to pioglitazone may have been required to observe an improvement in PD patients (Brundin and Wyse, 2015). As shown in **Figure 3**, interaction of these drugs with the peroxisome proliferator-activated receptor gamma (PPARG) may provide a mechanistic explanation to their neuroprotective effect. Some of these drugs are currently in clinical trials to determine if they are neuroprotective.

Nutrition is also recognized as an important component in the development and treatment of neurodegenerative diseases (Seidl et al., 2014). Given the promise of neuroprotective agents, the field of nutrigenomics is gaining interest among neuroscientists that are seeking to understand the complex nutrient-genetic interactions underlying neurodegeneration and neuroprotection. A recent example conducted a transcriptomic and epigenomic sequencing of the hypothalamus and hippocampus from a rodent model exposed to fructose consumption, which has been shown to contribute to the metabolic syndrome (Meng et al., 2016). Gene network analysis identified *Bgn* and *Fmod* as key genes involved in the observed metabolic alterations induced by fructose in mice. Strikingly, administration of docosahexaeonic acid (DHA) reversed the gene network changes elicited by fructose (Meng et al., 2016). This study provides evidence that integration of nutrigenomics coupled with network analysis can facilitate the identification of neuroprotective agents. Likewise, resveratrol, an antioxidant present in red wine, may also provide neuroprotection in PD patients and thus, could be tested in clinical trials (**Figure 3**).

In addition to a nutrient-rich diet, both physical exercise and cognitive training promote healthy aging (Kraft, 2012; Bamidis et al., 2014). It has been proposed that a combination of both together may be best to prevent cognitive decline and pathological aging (Kraft, 2012; Bamidis et al., 2014). In this regard, network analysis could be a useful tool to characterize the effects of physical exercise and cognitive training in the aging brain. Future studies directed at identifying gene expression changes associated with these lifestyle changes would be advantageous. Collectively, a multidimensional network approach that includes information about symptoms, drug treatments, comorbidities, nutrigenomics, physical exercise and cognitive training will be valuable to accelerate personalized treatment.

AUTHOR CONTRIBUTIONS

JAS and VB wrote the first draft of the manuscript. JAS, VB and JAP edited and reviewed the final draft of the manuscript.

ACKNOWLEDGMENTS

This work was funded by the US Army Medical Research and Materiel Command under awards number W81XWH-09-0708 and W81XWH13-1-0025 and the National Institute of Neurological Disorders and Stroke grant number U01NS097037 to JAP. The funding agencies had no role in study design, data collection and analysis, decision to publish, or preparation of the manuscript.

REFERENCES

Aarsland, D., Påhlhagen, S., Ballard, C. G., Ehrt, U., and Svenningsson, P. (2012). Depression in Parkinson disease—epidemiology, mechanisms and management. *Nat. Rev. Neurol.* 8, 35–47. doi: 10.1038/nrneurol.2011.189

Acquaah-Mensah, G. K., Agu, N., Khan, T., and Gardner, A. (2015). A regulatory role for the insulin- and BDNF-linked RORA in the hippocampus: implications for Alzheimer's disease. *J. Alzheimers Dis.* 44, 827–838. doi: 10.3233/JAD-141731

An, M. C., Zhang, N., Scott, G., Montoro, D., Wittkop, T., Mooney, S., et al. (2012). Genetic correction of Huntington's disease phenotypes in induced pluripotent stem cells. *Cell Stem Cell* 11, 253–263. doi: 10.1016/j.stem.2012.04.026

Aviles-Olmos, I., Dickson, J., Kefalopoulou, Z., Djamshidian, A., Ell, P., Soderlund, T., et al. (2013). Exenatide and the treatment of patients with Parkinson's disease. *J. Clin. Invest.* 123, 2730–2736. doi: 10.1172/JCI68295

Aviles-Olmos, I., Dickson, J., Kefalopoulou, Z., Djamshidian, A., Kahan, J., Ell, P., et al. (2014). Motor and cognitive advantages persist 12 months after exenatide exposure in Parkinson's disease. *J. Parkinsons Dis.* 4, 337–344. doi: 10.3233/JPD-140364

Bamidis, P. D., Vivas, A. B., Styliadis, C., Frantzidis, C., Klados, M., Schlee, W., et al. (2014). A review of physical and cognitive interventions in aging. *Neurosci. Biobehav. Rev.* 44, 206–220. doi: 10.1016/j.neubiorev.2014.03.019

Benayoun, B. A., Pollina, E. A., and Brunet, A. (2015). Epigenetic regulation of ageing: linking environmental inputs to genomic stability. *Nat. Rev. Mol. Cell Biol.* 16, 593–610. doi: 10.1038/nrm4048

Borrell-Pagès, M., Zala, D., Humbert, S., and Saudou, F. (2006). Huntington's disease: from huntingtin function and dysfunction to therapeutic strategies. *Cell. Mol. Life Sci.* 63, 2642–2660. doi: 10.1007/s00018-006-6242-0

Brehme, M., Voisine, C., Rolland, T., Wachi, S., Soper, J. H., Zhu, Y., et al. (2014). A chaperome subnetwork safeguards proteostasis in aging and neurodegenerative disease. *Cell Rep.* 9, 1135–1150. doi: 10.1016/j.celrep.2014.09.042

Brundin, P., and Wyse, R. (2015). Parkinson disease: laying the foundations for disease-modifying therapies in PD. *Nat. Rev. Neurol.* 11, 553–555. doi: 10.1038/nrneurol.2015.150

Brunet, A., and Berger, S. L. (2014). Epigenetics of aging and aging-related disease. *J. Gerontol. A Biol. Sci. Med. Sci.* 69, S17–S20. doi: 10.1093/gerona/glu042

Calderone, A., Formenti, M., Aprea, F., Papa, M., Alberghina, L., Colangelo, A. M., et al. (2016). Comparing Alzheimer's and Parkinson's diseases networks using graph communities structure. *BMC Syst. Biol.* 10:25. doi: 10.1186/s12918-016-0270-7

Carta, A. R., and Simuni, T. (2015). Thiazolidinediones under preclinical and early clinical development for the treatment of Parkinson's disease. *Expert Opin. Investig. Drugs* 24, 219–227. doi: 10.1517/13543784.2015.963195

Chen, Y., Zhu, J., Lum, P. Y., Yang, X., Pinto, S., MacNeil, D. J., et al. (2008). Variations in DNA elucidate molecular networks that cause disease. *Nature* 452, 429–435. doi: 10.1038/nature06757

Ciryam, P., Kundra, R., Freer, R., Morimoto, R. I., Dobson, C. M., and Vendruscolo, M. (2016). A transcriptional signature of Alzheimer's disease is associated with a metastable subproteome at risk for aggregation. *Proc. Natl. Acad. Sci. U S A* 113, 4753–4758. doi: 10.1073/pnas.1516604113

Coetzee, S. G., Pierce, S., Brundin, P., Brundin, L., Hazelett, D. J., and Coetzee, G. A. (2016). Enrichment of risk SNPs in regulatory regions implicate diverse tissues in Parkinson's disease etiology. *Sci. Rep.* 6:30509. doi: 10.1038/srep30509

Coon, K. D., Myers, A. J., Craig, D. W., Webster, J. A., Pearson, J. V., Lince, D. H., et al. (2007). A high-density whole-genome association study reveals that APOE is the major susceptibility gene for sporadic late-onset Alzheimer's disease. *J. Clin. Psychiatry* 68, 613–618. doi: 10.4088/jcp.v68n0419

Corradini, B. R., Iamashita, P., Tampellini, E., Farfel, J. M., Grinberg, L. T., and Moreira-Filho, C. A. (2014). Complex network-driven view of genomic mechanisms underlying Parkinson's disease: analyses in dorsal motor vagal nucleus, locus coeruleus and substantia nigra. *Biomed Res. Int.* 2014:543673. doi: 10.1155/2014/543673

De Strooper, B., and Karran, E. (2016). The cellular phase of Alzheimer's disease. *Cell* 164, 603–615. doi: 10.1016/j.cell.2015.12.056

Desikan, R. S., Schork, A. J., Wang, Y., Witoelar, A., Sharma, M., McEvoy, L. K., et al. (2015). Genetic overlap between Alzheimer's disease and Parkinson's disease at the MAPT locus. *Mol. Psychiatry* 20, 1588–1595. doi: 10.1038/mp.2015.6

Donmez, G., and Outeiro, T. F. (2013). SIRT1 and SIRT2: emerging targets in neurodegeneration. *EMBO Mol. Med.* 5, 344–352. doi: 10.1002/emmm.201302451

Duff, K., Paulsen, J. S., Beglinger, L. J., Langbehn, D. R., Stout, J. C., and Predict-HD Investigators of the Huntington Study Group. (2007). Psychiatric symptoms in Huntington's disease before diagnosis: the predict-HD study. *Biol. Psychiatry* 62, 1341–1346. doi: 10.1016/j.biopsych.2006.11.034

Dusonchet, J., Li, H., Guillily, M., Liu, M., Stafa, K., Derada Troletti, C., et al. (2014). A Parkinson's disease gene regulatory network identifies the signaling protein RGS2 as a modulator of LRRK2 activity and neuronal toxicity. *Hum. Mol. Genet.* 23, 4887–4905. doi: 10.1093/hmg/ddu202

Ehrlich, M. E. (2012). Huntington's disease and the striatal medium spiny neuron: cell-autonomous and non-cell-autonomous mechanisms of disease. *Neurotherapeutics* 9, 270–284. doi: 10.1007/s13311-012-0112-2

Fernández-Santiago, R., Carballo-Carbajal, I., Castellano, G., Torrent, R., Richaud, Y., Sánchez-Danés, A., et al. (2015). Aberrant epigenome in iPSC-derived dopaminergic neurons from Parkinson's disease patients. *EMBO Mol. Med.* 7, 1529–1546. doi: 10.15252/emmm.201505439

Fischer, A. (2014). Targeting histone-modifications in Alzheimer's disease. What is the evidence that this is a promising therapeutic avenue? *Neuropharmacology* 80, 95–102. doi: 10.1016/j.neuropharm.2014.01.038

Gao, L., Zhao, G., Fang, J. S., Yuan, T. Y., Liu, A. L., and Du, G. H. (2014). Discovery of the neuroprotective effects of alvespimycin by computational prioritization of potential anti-Parkinson agents. *FEBS J.* 281, 1110–1122. doi: 10.1111/febs.12672

Glaab, E., and Schneider, R. (2015). Comparative pathway and network analysis of brain transcriptome changes during adult aging and in Parkinson's disease. *Neurobiol. Dis.* 74, 1–13. doi: 10.1016/j.nbd.2014.11.002

Goate, A., Chartier-Harlin, M. C., Mullan, M., Brown, J., Crawford, F., Fidani, L., et al. (1991). Segregation of a missense mutation in the amyloid precursor protein gene with familial Alzheimer's disease. *Nature* 349, 704–706. doi: 10.1038/349704a0

Goh, K. I., Cusick, M. E., Valle, D., Childs, B., Vidal, M., and Barabási, A. L. (2007). The human disease network. *Proc. Natl. Acad. Sci. U S A* 104, 8685–8690. doi: 10.1073/pnas.0701361104

Grove, V. E. Jr., Quintanilla, J., and DeVaney, G. T. (2000). Improvement of Huntington's disease with olanzapine and valproate. *N. Engl. J. Med.* 343, 973–974. doi: 10.1056/NEJM200009283431316

Hallock, P., and Thomas, M. A. (2012). Integrating the Alzheimer's disease proteome and transcriptome: a comprehensive network model of a complex disease. *OMICS* 16, 37–49. doi: 10.1089/omi.2011.0054

Hamilton, R. L. (2000). Lewy bodies in Alzheimer's disease: a neuropathological review of 145 cases using α-synuclein immunohistochemistry. *Brain Pathol.* 10, 378–384. doi: 10.1111/j.1750-3639.2000.tb00269.x

Herskovits, A. Z., and Guarente, L. (2013). Sirtuin deacetylases in neurodegenerative diseases of aging. *Cell Res.* 23, 746–758. doi: 10.1038/cr.2013.70

Horvath, S. (2013). DNA methylation age of human tissues and cell types. *Genome Biol.* 14:R115. doi: 10.1186/gb-2013-14-10-r115

Horvath, S., Langfelder, P., Kwak, S., Aaronson, J., Rosinski, J., Vogt, T. F., et al. (2016). Huntington's disease accelerates epigenetic aging of human brain and disrupts DNA methylation levels. *Aging* 8, 1485–1512. doi: 10.18632/aging.101005

Humphries, C. E., Kohli, M. A., Nathanson, L., Whitehead, P., Beecham, G., Martin, E., et al. (2015). Integrated whole transcriptome and DNA methylation analysis identifies gene networks specific to late-onset Alzheimer's disease. *J. Alzheimers Dis.* 44, 977–987. doi: 10.3233/JAD-141989

Ibáñez, K., Boullosa, C., Tabarés-Seisdedos, R., Baudot, A., and Valencia, A. (2014). Molecular evidence for the inverse comorbidity between central nervous system disorders and cancers detected by transcriptomic meta-analyses. *PLoS Genet.* 10:e1004173. doi: 10.1371/journal.pgen.1004173

Jack, C. R. Jr., Wiste, H. J., Weigand, S. D., Knopman, D. S., Vemuri, P., Mielke, M. M., et al. (2015). Age, sex, and APOE ε4 effects on memory, brain structure, and β-amyloid across the adult life span. *JAMA Neurol.* 72, 511–519. doi: 10.1001/jamaneurol.2014.4821

Janssen, J. C., Beck, J. A., Campbell, T. A., Dickinson, A., Fox, N. C., Harvey, R. J., et al. (2003). Early onset familial Alzheimer's disease: mutation frequency in 31 families. *Neurology* 60, 235–239. doi: 10.1212/01.WNL.0000042088.22694.e3

Jiang, P., Scarpa, J. R., Fitzpatrick, K., Losic, B., Gao, V. D., Hao, K., et al. (2015). A systems approach identifies networks and genes linking sleep and stress: implications for neuropsychiatric disorders. *Cell Rep.* 11, 835–848. doi: 10.1016/j.celrep.2015.04.003

Jiang, S., Tang, L., Zhao, N., Yang, W., Qiu, Y., and Chen, H. Z. (2016). A systems view of the differences between APOE ε4 carriers and non-carriers in Alzheimer's disease. *Front. Aging Neurosci.* 8:171. doi: 10.3389/fnagi.2016.00171

Kandimalla, R. J., Prabhakar, S., Binukumar, B. K., Wani, W. Y., Gupta, N., Sharma, D. R., et al. (2011). Apo-Eε4 allele in conjunction with Aβ42 and tau in CSF: biomarker for Alzheimer's disease. *Curr. Alzheimer Res.* 8, 187–196. doi: 10.2174/156720511795256071

Keane, H., Ryan, B. J., Jackson, B., Whitmore, A., and Wade-Martins, R. (2015). Protein-protein interaction networks identify targets which rescue the MPP+ cellular model of Parkinson's disease. *Sci. Rep.* 5:17004. doi: 10.1038/srep17004

Khanam Irin, A., Kodamullil, A. T., Gündel, M., and Hofmann-Apitius, M. (2015). Computational modelling approaches on epigenetic factors in neurodegenerative and autoimmune diseases and their mechanistic analysis. *J. Immunol. Res.* 2015:737168. doi: 10.1155/2015/737168

Kikuchi, M., Ogishima, S., Miyamoto, T., Miyashita, A., Kuwano, R., Nakaya, J., et al. (2013). Identification of unstable network modules reveals disease modules associated with the progression of Alzheimer's disease. *PLoS One* 8:e76162. doi: 10.1371/journal.pone.0076162

Kim, Y. H., Beak, S. H., Charidimou, A., and Song, M. (2016). Discovering new genes in the pathways of common sporadic neurodegenerative diseases: a bioinformatics approach. *J. Alzheimers Dis.* 51, 293–312. doi: 10.3233/JAD-150769

Kim, S., Seo, J. H., and Suh, Y. H. (2004). α-synuclein, Parkinson's disease, and Alzheimer's disease. *Parkinsonism Relat. Disord.* 10, S9–S13. doi: 10.1016/j.parkreldis.2003.11.005

Kraft, E. (2012). Cognitive function, physical activity, and aging: possible biological links and implications for multimodal interventions. *Neuropsychol. Dev. Cogn. B Aging Neuropsychol. Cogn.* 19, 248–263. doi: 10.1080/13825585.2011.645010

Langfelder, P., Cantle, J. P., Chatzopoulou, D., Wang, N., Gao, F., Al-Ramahi, I., et al. (2016). Integrated genomics and proteomics define huntingtin CAG length-dependent networks in mice. *Nat. Neurosci.* 19, 623–633. doi: 10.1038/nn.4256

Langfelder, P., and Horvath, S. (2008). WGCNA: an R package for weighted correlation network analysis. *BMC Bioinformatics* 9:559. doi: 10.1186/1471-2105-9-559

Levine, M. E., Lu, A. T., Bennett, D. A., and Horvath, S. (2015). Epigenetic age of the pre-frontal cortex is associated with neuritic plaques, amyloid load, and Alzheimer's disease related cognitive functioning. *Aging* 7, 1198–1211. doi: 10.18632/aging.100864

Levy-Lahad, E., Wasco, W., Poorkaj, P., Romano, D. M., Oshima, J., Pettingell, W. H., et al. (1995). Candidate gene for the chromosome 1 familial Alzheimer's disease locus. *Science* 269, 973–977. doi: 10.1126/science.7638622

Liang, D., Han, G., Feng, X., Sun, J., Duan, Y., and Lei, H. (2012). Concerted perturbation observed in a hub network in Alzheimer's disease. *PLoS One* 7:e40498. doi: 10.1371/journal.pone.0040498

Liang, M. H., Wendland, J. R., and Chuang, D. M. (2008). Lithium inhibits Smad3/4 transactivation via increased CREB activity induced by enhanced PKA and AKT signaling. *Mol. Cell. Neurosci.* 37, 440–453. doi: 10.1016/j.mcn.2007.10.017

Lin, M. K., and Farrer, M. J. (2014). Genetics and genomics of Parkinson's disease. *Genome Med.* 6:48. doi: 10.1186/gm566

Linghu, B., Snitkin, E. S., Hu, Z., Xia, Y., and Delisi, C. (2009). Genome-wide prioritization of disease genes and identification of disease-disease associations from an integrated human functional linkage network. *Genome Biol.* 10:R91. doi: 10.1186/gb-2009-10-9-r91

Liu, G., Bao, X., Jiang, Y., Liao, M., Jiang, Q., Feng, R., et al. (2015). Identifying the association between Alzheimer's disease and Parkinson's disease using genome-wide association studies and protein-protein interaction network. *Mol. Neurobiol.* 52, 1629–1636. doi: 10.1007/s12035-014-8946-8

MacDonald, M. E., Ambrose, C. M., Duyao, M. P., Myers, R. H., Lin, C., Srinidhi, L., et al. (1993). A novel gene containing a trinucleotide repeat that is expanded and unstable on Huntington's disease chromosomes. *Cell* 72, 971–983. doi: 10.1016/0092-8674(93)90585-e

Marra, C., Bizzarro, A., Daniele, A., De Luca, L., Ferraccioli, M., Valenza, A., et al. (2004). Apolipoprotein E ε4 allele differently affects the patterns of neuropsychological presentation in early- and late-onset Alzheimer's disease patients. *Dement. Geriatr. Cogn. Disord.* 18, 125–131. doi: 10.1159/000079191

Meng, Q., Ying, Z., Noble, E., Zhao, Y., Agrawal, R., Mikhail, A., et al. (2016). Systems nutrigenomics reveals brain gene networks linking metabolic and brain disorders. *EBioMedicine* 7, 157–166. doi: 10.1016/j.ebiom.2016.04.008

Mercado, G., Valdés, P., and Hetz, C. (2013). An ERcentric view of Parkinson's disease. *Trends Mol. Med.* 19, 165–175. doi: 10.1016/j.molmed.2012.12.005

Miller, J. A., Oldham, M. C., and Geschwind, D. H. (2008). A systems level analysis of transcriptional changes in Alzheimer's disease and normal aging. *J. Neurosci.* 28, 1410–1420. doi: 10.1523/JNEUROSCI.4098-07.2008

Miller, J. A., Woltjer, R. L., Goodenbour, J. M., Horvath, S., and Geschwind, D. H. (2013). Genes and pathways underlying regional and cell type changes in Alzheimer's disease. *Genome Med.* 5:48. doi: 10.1186/gm452

Mina, E., van Roon-Mom, W., Hettne, K., van Zwet, E., Goeman, J., Neri, C., et al. (2016). Common disease signatures from gene expression analysis in Huntington's disease human blood and brain. *Orphanet J. Rare Dis.* 11:97. doi: 10.1186/s13023-016-0475-2

Narayanan, M., Huynh, J. L., Wang, K., Yang, X., Yoo, S., McElwee, J., et al. (2014). Common dysregulation network in the human prefrontal cortex underlies two neurodegenerative diseases. *Mol. Syst. Biol.* 10:743. doi: 10.15252/msb.20145304

Neueder, A., and Bates, G. P. (2014). A common gene expression signature in Huntington's disease patient brain regions. *BMC Med. Genomics* 7:60. doi: 10.1186/s12920-014-0060-2

NINDS Exploratory Trials in Parkinson Disease (NET-PD) FS-ZONE Investigators. (2015). Pioglitazone in early Parkinson's disease: a phase 2, multicentre, couble-blind, randomised trial. *Lancet Neurol.* 14, 795–803. doi: 10.1016/s1474-4422(15)00144-1

Nolan, Y. M., Sullivan, A. M., and Toulouse, A. (2013). Parkinson's disease in the nuclear age of neuroinflammation. *Trends Mol. Med.* 19, 187–196. doi: 10.1016/j.molmed.2012.12.003

Orre, M., Kamphuis, W., Osborn, L. M., Jansen, A. H., Kooijman, L., Bossers, K., et al. (2014). Isolation of glia from Alzheimer's mice reveals inflammation and dysfunction. *Neurobiol. Aging* 35, 2746–2760. doi: 10.1016/j.neurobiolaging.2014.06.004

Orr, H. T., and Zoghbi, H. Y. (2007). Trinucleotide repeat disorders. *Annu. Rev. Neurosci.* 30, 575–621. doi: 10.1146/annurev.neuro.29.051605.113042

Ota, M., Yasuno, F., Ito, H., Seki, C., Nozaki, S., Asada, T., et al. (2006). Age-related decline of dopamine synthesis in the living human brain measured by positron emission tomography with L-[β-^{11}C]DOPA. *Life Sci.* 79, 730–736. doi: 10.1016/j.lfs.2006.02.017

Pike, K. E., Savage, G., Villemagne, V. L., Ng, S., Moss, S. A., Maruff, P., et al. (2007). β-amyloid imaging and memory in non-demented individuals: evidence for preclinical Alzheimer's disease. *Brain* 130, 2837–2844. doi: 10.1093/brain/awm238

Pristerè, A., Lin, W., Kaufmann, A. K., Brimblecombe, K. R., Threlfell, S., Dodson, P. D., et al. (2015). Transcription factors FOXA1 and FOXA2 maintain dopaminergic neuronal properties and control feeding behavior in adult mice. *Proc. Natl. Acad. Sci. U S A* 112, E4929–E4938. doi: 10.1073/pnas.1503911112

Raja, M., Soleti, F., and Bentivoglio, A. R. (2015). Lithium treatment in patients With Huntington's disease and suicidal behavior. *Mov. Disord* 30:1438. doi: 10.1002/mds.26260

Rhinn, H., Qiang, L., Yamashita, T., Rhee, D., Zolin, A., Vanti, W., et al. (2012). Alternative α-synuclein transcript usage as a convergent mechanism in Parkinson's disease pathology. *Nat. Commun.* 3:1084. doi: 10.1038/ncomms2032

Richard, F., Helbecque, N., Neuman, E., Guez, D., Levy, R., and Amouyel, P. (1997). APOE genotyping and response to drug treatment in Alzheimer's disease. *Lancet* 349:539. doi: 10.1016/s0140-6736(97)80089-x

Ring, K. L., An, M. C., Zhang, N., O'Brien, R. N., Ramos, E. M., Gao, F., et al. (2015). Genomic analysis reveals disruption of striatal neuronal development and therapeutic targets in human Huntington's disease neural stem cells. *Stem Cell Reports* 5, 1023–1038. doi: 10.1016/j.stemcr.2015.11.005

Ross, C. A., Aylward, E. H., Wild, E. J., Langbehn, D. R., Long, J. D., Warner, J. H., et al. (2014). Huntington disease: natural history, biomarkers and prospects for therapeutics. *Nat. Rev. Neurol.* 10, 204–216. doi: 10.1038/nrneurol.2014.24

Santiago, J. A., Littlefield, A. M., and Potashkin, J. A. (2016). Integrative transcriptomic meta-analysis of Parkinson's disease and depression identifies NAMPT as a potential blood biomarker for de novo Parkinson's disease. *Sci. Rep.* 6:34579. doi: 10.1038/srep34579

Santiago, J. A., and Potashkin, J. A. (2013a). Integrative network analysis unveils convergent molecular pathways in Parkinson's disease and diabetes. *PLoS One* 8:e83940. doi: 10.1371/journal.pone.0083940

Santiago, J. A., and Potashkin, J. A. (2013b). Shared dysregulated pathways lead to Parkinson's disease and diabetes. *Trends Mol. Med.* 19, 176–186. doi: 10.1016/j.molmed.2013.01.002

Santiago, J. A., and Potashkin, J. A. (2014a). A network approach to clinical intervention in neurodegenerative diseases. *Trends Mol. Med.* 20, 694–703. doi: 10.1016/j.molmed.2014.10.002

Santiago, J. A., and Potashkin, J. A. (2014b). A network approach to diagnostic biomarkers in progressive supranuclear palsy. *Mov. Disord.* 29, 550–555. doi: 10.1002/mds.25761

Santiago, J. A., and Potashkin, J. A. (2014c). System-based approaches to decode the molecular links in Parkinson's disease and diabetes. *Neurobiol. Dis.* 72, 84–91. doi: 10.1016/j.nbd.2014.03.019

Santiago, J. A., and Potashkin, J. A. (2015). Network-based metaanalysis identifies HNF4A and PTBP1 as longitudinally dynamic biomarkers for Parkinson's disease. *Proc. Natl. Acad. Sci. U S A* 112, 2257–2262. doi: 10.1073/pnas. 1423573112

Santiago, J. A., Scherzer, C. R., and Potashkin, J. A. (2014). Network analysis identifies SOD2 mRNA as a potential biomarker for Parkinson's disease. *PLoS One* 9:e109042. doi: 10.1371/journal.pone.0109042

Satake, W., Nakabayashi, Y., Mizuta, I., Hirota, Y., Ito, C., Kubo, M., et al. (2009). Genome-wide association study identifies common variants at four loci as genetic risk factors for Parkinson's disease. *Nat. Genet.* 41, 1303–1307. doi: 10.1038/ng.485

Scarpa, J. R., Jiang, P., Losic, B., Readhead, B., Gao, V. D., Dudley, J. T., et al. (2016). Systems genetic analyses highlight a TGFβ-FOXO3 dependent striatal astrocyte network conserved across species and associated with stress, sleep, and Huntington's disease. *PLoS Genet.* 12:e1006137. doi: 10.1371/journal.pgen. 1006137

Scheuing, L., Chiu, C. T., Liao, H. M., Linares, G. R., and Chuang, D. M. (2014). Preclinical and clinical investigations of mood stabilizers for Huntington's disease: what have we learned? *Int. J. Biol. Sci.* 10, 1024–1038. doi: 10.7150/ijbs. 9898

Schneider, A., Rajendran, L., Honsho, M., Gralle, M., Donnert, G., Wouters, F., et al. (2008). Flotillin-dependent clustering of the amyloid precursor protein regulates its endocytosis and amyloidogenic processing in neurons. *J. Neurosci.* 28, 2874–2882. doi: 10.1523/JNEUROSCI.5345-07.2008

Seidl, S. E., Santiago, J. A., Bilyk, H., and Potashkin, J. A. (2014). The emerging role of nutrition in Parkinson's disease. *Front. Aging Neurosci.* 6:36. doi: 10.3389/fnagi.2014.00036

Simon, D. K., Simuni, T., Elm, J., Clark-Matott, J., Graebner, A. K., Baker, L., et al. (2015). Peripheral biomarkers of Parkinson's disease progression and pioglitazone effects. *J. Parkinsons Dis.* 5, 731–736. doi: 10.3233/JPD-150666

Simón-Sánchez, J., Schulte, C., Bras, J. M., Sharma, M., Gibbs, J. R., Berg, D., et al. (2009). Genome-wide association study reveals genetic risk underlying Parkinson's disease. *Nat. Genet.* 41, 1308–1312. doi: 10.1038/ng.487

Solt, L. A., and Burris, T. P. (2012). Action of RORs and their ligands in (patho)physiology. *Trends Endocrinol. Metab.* 23, 619–627. doi: 10.1016/j.tem. 2012.05.012

Talwar, P., Silla, Y., Grover, S., Gupta, M., Agarwal, R., Kushwaha, S., et al. (2014). Genomic convergence and network analysis approach to identify candidate genes in Alzheimer's disease. *BMC Genomics* 15:199. doi: 10.1186/1471-2164-15-199

Taylor, I. W., Linding, R., Warde-Farley, D., Liu, Y., Pesquita, C., Faria, D., et al. (2009). Dynamic modularity in protein interaction networks predicts breast cancer outcome. *Nat. Biotechnol.* 27, 199–204. doi: 10.1038/nbt.1522

Turner, A. P., Lones, M. A., Fuente, L. A., Stepney, S., Caves, L. S., and Tyrrell, A. M. (2013). The incorporation of epigenetics in artificial gene regulatory networks. *Biosystems* 112, 56–62. doi: 10.1016/j.biosystems.2013. 03.013

Wang, L. Y., Wang, P., Li, M. J., Qin, J., Wang, X., Zhang, M. Q., et al. (2011). EpiRegNet: constructing epigenetic regulatory network from high throughput gene expression data for humans. *Epigenetics* 6, 1505–1512. doi: 10.4161/epi.6. 12.18176

Watanabe, T., Tajima, H., Hironori, H., Nakagawara, H., Ohnishi, I., Takamura, H., et al. (2011). Sodium valproate blocks the transforming growth factor (TGF)-β1 autocrine loop and attenuates the TGF-β1-induced collagen synthesis in a human hepatic stellate cell line. *Int. J. Mol. Med.* 28, 919–925. doi: 10.3892/ijmm.2011.768

Wilkaniec, A., Czapski, G. A., and Adamczyk, A. (2016). Cdk5 at crossroads of protein oligomerization in neurodegenerative diseases: facts and hypotheses. *J. Neurochem.* 136, 222–233. doi: 10.1111/jnc.13365

Wilson, V. L., Smith, R. A., Ma, S., and Cutler, R. G. (1987). Genomic 5-methyldeoxycytidine decreases with age. *J. Biol. Chem.* 262, 9948–9951.

Xie, A., Gao, J., Xu, L., and Meng, D. (2014). Shared mechanisms of neurodegeneration in Alzheimer's disease and Parkinson's disease. *Biomed Res. Int.* 2014:648740. doi: 10.1155/2014/648740

Zampieri, M., Ciccarone, F., Calabrese, R., Franceschi, C., Bürkle, A., and Caiafa, P. (2015). Reconfiguration of DNA methylation in aging. *Mech. Ageing Dev.* 151, 60–70. doi: 10.1016/j.mad.2015.02.002

Zhang, B., Gaiteri, C., Bodea, L. G., Wang, Z., McElwee, J., Podtelezhnikov, A. A., et al. (2013). Integrated systems approach identifies genetic nodes and networks in late-onset Alzheimer's disease. *Cell* 153, 707–720. doi: 10.1016/j.cell.2013. 03.030

Zou, X. D., Guo, S. Q., Hu, Z. W., and Li, W. L. (2016). NAMPT protects against 6-hydroxydopamine-induced neurotoxicity in PC12 cells through modulating SIRT1 activity. *Mol. Med. Rep.* 13, 4058–4064. doi: 10.3892/mmr.2016.5034

3

A Triple Network Connectivity Study of Large-Scale Brain Systems in Cognitively Normal APOE4 Carriers

Xia Wu [1,2], Qing Li [1], Xinyu Yu [1], Kewei Chen [3], Adam S. Fleisher [3,4], Xiaojuan Guo [1], Jiacai Zhang [1], Eric M. Reiman [3], Li Yao [1,2] and Rui Li [5]*

[1] College of Information Science and Technology, Beijing Normal University, Beijing, China, [2] State Key Laboratory of Cognitive Neuroscience and Learning, Beijing Normal University, Beijing, China, [3] Banner Alzheimer's Institute and Banner Good Samaritan PET Center, Phoenix, AZ, USA, [4] Eli Lilly and Company, Indianapolis, IN, USA, [5] Center on Aging Psychology, Key Laboratory of Mental Health, Institute of Psychology, Chinese Academy of Sciences, Beijing, China

*Correspondence:
Rui Li
lir@psych.ac.cn

The triple network model, consisting of the central executive network (CEN), salience network (SN) and default mode network (DMN), has been recently employed to understand dysfunction in core networks across various disorders. Here we used the triple network model to investigate the large-scale brain networks in cognitively normal apolipoprotein e4 (APOE4) carriers who are at risk of Alzheimer's disease (AD). To explore the functional connectivity for each of the three networks and the effective connectivity among them, we evaluated 17 cognitively normal individuals with a family history of AD and at least one copy of the APOE4 allele and compared the findings to those of 12 individuals who did not carry the APOE4 gene or have a family history of AD, using independent component analysis (ICA) and Bayesian network (BN) approach. Our findings indicated altered within-network connectivity that suggests future cognitive decline risk, and preserved between-network connectivity that may support their current preserved cognition in the cognitively normal APOE4 allele carriers. The study provides novel sights into our understanding of the risk factors for AD and their influence on the triple network model of major psychopathology.

Keywords: Alzheimer's disease, APOE4, Bayesian network, connectivity, fMRI, triple network model

INTRODUCTION

The apolipoprotein e4 (APOE4) gene has been well established as a susceptibility gene for sporadic and late-onset familial Alzheimer's disease (AD; Poirier et al., 1995; Reitz and Mayeux, 2010; Kandimalla et al., 2013; Tai et al., 2014). Epidemiologic evidence has clarified that APOE4 decreases the age-at-onset of AD in a gene dosage-dependent manner (Corder et al., 1993; Breitner et al., 1999). Neuroimaging studies have demonstrated that APOE4 carriers exhibit elevated medial temporal lobe (MTL) atrophy (Agosta et al., 2009; Fleisher et al., 2009a,b; Wolk and Dickerson, 2010), and recent studies have shown that the APOE4 allele is associated with Cerebrospinal fluid (CSF) biomarkers including Aβ42, tau (Kandimalla et al., 2011) and ubiquitin levels (Kandimalla et al., 2014). Thus the APOE4 allele has been suggested as an important factor that leads to lower cognitive performance, or the progression to mild cognitive impairment (MCI) and AD (Barabash et al., 2009; Sasaki et al., 2009).

Functional neuroimaging connectome studies of AD have proposed a disconnection hypothesis of the disease. Many studies have consistently reported that the cognitive impairment in AD and the cognitive decline in its preclinical stage were largely due to the disruptions of the brain networks (Stam et al., 2007; Lo et al., 2010; Wang et al., 2013). For example, as one of the most relevant networks in AD, various studies have shown that the default mode network (DMN) exhibited a disruption in functional connectivity in AD (Greicius et al., 2004; Rombouts et al., 2005; Celone et al., 2006; Petrella et al., 2007; Wu et al., 2011), and even at early stages of the disease such as MCI (Lustig et al., 2003; Rombouts et al., 2005; Celone et al., 2006; Petrella et al., 2007; Qi et al., 2010; Li et al., 2013). In addition to the DMN, other networks have also been found to show alterations in AD. For example, the salience network (SN), whose connectivity showed negative correlation with DMN has been linked to AD (Zhou et al., 2010; Balthazar et al., 2014). These alterations in functionally coordinated brain systems can occur long before disease onset in cognitively normal people with various risk factors for AD (Poirier et al., 1995; Kivipelto et al., 2001; Song et al., 2015). For example, Westlye et al. (2011) demonstrated a negative correlation between DMN synchronization and memory performance in healthy APOE4 carriers. Besides, the functional alterations in the DMN and SN connections were also demonstrated in the elderly APOE4 carriers (Machulda et al., 2011). These evidences suggested that the presence of APOE4 gene is accompanied by brain network alterations that are closely relevant to AD progression.

Recently, a triple network model of major psychopathology has been proposed by Menon (2011). The triple network model consists of the central executive network (CEN), SN and DMN. These three networks are generally referred to as the core neurocognitive networks due to their involvement in an extremely wide range of cognitive tasks (Greicius et al., 2003; Greicius and Menon, 2004; Menon and Uddin, 2010; Menon, 2011). Specifically, the CEN and SN typically show increased activation during stimulus-driven cognitive or affective processing, while the DMN shows decreased activation during tasks in which self-referential and stimulus-independent intellectual activity is not involved (Greicius et al., 2003; Greicius and Menon, 2004). The triple network model suggests that the aberrant internal organization within each functional network and the interconnectivity among them are characteristic of many psychiatric and neurological disorders. Recently the triple network model has been widely applied to elucidate the dysfunction across multiple disorders, including schizophrenia, depression and dementia (Menon and Uddin, 2010; Menon, 2011; Zheng et al., 2015; Yuan et al., 2016). However the triple network interactions in elderly APOE4 carriers who are at high risk to AD have not yet been explored.

In the present study, we investigated the APOE4-mediated modulation of the within-network functional connectivity and the between-network connectivity of the three core networks included in the triple network model in cognitively normal individuals carrying a family history of AD and at least one copy of the APOE4 allele using functional magnetic resonance imaging (fMRI). A group independent component analysis (ICA) approach and Bayesian network (BN) approach were used to separate the functional connectivity networks from the fMRI dataset and to determine the between-network effective connectivity, respectively.

MATERIALS AND METHODS

Participants

fMRI data from 29 cognitively normal right-handed volunteers (8 males and 21 females, ages between 50 and 65 years) who were the subjects in our previous study (Fleisher et al., 2009b) were included in this work. They were divided into two groups: the high-risk group and the low-risk group. The high-risk group included 17 subjects who had a significant family history of dementia in a first-degree relative and at least one copy of the APOE4 allele. The other twelve participants who had neither a family history of dementia nor a copy of the APOE4 gene were regarded as the low-risk group. Notably, there were no significant differences in age, gender and education level between these two groups (all $ps > 0.05$). The two groups were matched on general cognitive function as evaluated by Folstein Mini Mental State Exam ($p = 0.39$). The study was conducted according to Good Clinical Practice, the Declaration of Helsinki and US 21 Code of Federal Regulations (CFR) Part 50-Protection of Human Subjects, and Part 56-Institutional Review Boards and was approved by the Institutional Review Board of the University of California, San Diego. Written informed consent for the study was obtained from all of the participants before protocol-specific procedures were performed, including cognitive testing.

All scans were performed on a General Electric Signa EXCITE 3.0 T short bore, twin speed scanner with a body transmit coil and an 8 channel receive array. High-resolution structural brain images were acquired with a magnetization prepared from three-dimensional fast spoiled gradient sequence acquisition (FSPGR: 124 axial slices, 1 mm×1 mm in-plane resolution, 1.3 mm slice thickness, Field of View (FOV) = 256 mm^2 × 256 mm^2, TR = 7.8 ms, TE = 3.1 ms, flip angle = 12°). Blood oxygen level dependent (BOLD) data were acquired using echo planar imaging sequences (35 slices, perpendicular to the axis of the hippocampus, 6 mm in-plane resolution, 0 spacing, FOV = 220 mm^2 × 220 mm^2, TE = 30 ms, TR = 2500 ms, voxel size = 3.4 mm^3 × 3.4 mm^3 × 6.0 mm^3).

Data Preprocessing

For each participant, the original first five-time functional images were discarded to allow for equilibration of the magnetic field. All of the preprocessing steps were performed using the Statistical Parametric Mapping program (SPM8[1]). They included within-subject inter-scan realignment, between-subject spatial normalization to a standard brain template in the Montreal Neurological Institute (MNI) coordinate space, and smoothing by a Gaussian filter with a full width at a half maximum of 8 mm. Following this, the linear trend with regard to time was removed by linear regression via the Resting-State fMRI Data Analysis Toolkit (REST[2]).

---

[1]http://www.fil.ion.ucl.ac.uk/spm
[2]http://restfmri.net

After the preprocessing, we employed the Group ICA and BN to learn the functional interactions of the triple network model. Group ICA was first used to isolate the three brain networks for examination of the functional connectivity changes within each network in the high risk group. The BN was then used to show the directed causal effects between these three networks in the high risk group. Thus, the study was developed to delineate the influence of APOE4 on the triple networks in both within-network connections and between-network interactions.

Group Independent Component Analysis

Group ICA is widely used to separate patterns of task-activated neural networks, image noises, and physiologically generated independent components (ICs) in a data-driven manner. The preprocessed data of all participants were entered into the Group ICA program in the fMRI Toolbox (GIFT[3]) for the separation of the three networks included in the triple network model and the determination of networks for BN analysis. The Group ICA program included two rounds of principal component analyses (PCA) for reduction of fMRI data dimensions, ICA separation and back-reconstruction of the ICs (Calhoun et al., 2001). The optimal number of principal components, 31, was estimated based on the minimum description length (MDL). In the first round of PCA, the data for each individual subject were dimension-reduced to the optimal number temporally. After concatenation across subjects within groups, the dimensions were again reduced to the optimal numbers via the second round of PCA. Then, the data were separated by ICA using the Extended Infomax algorithm (Lee et al., 1999). After ICA separation, the mean ICs and the corresponding mean time courses over all of the subjects were used for the back-reconstruction of the ICs and time courses for each individual subject (Calhoun et al., 2001).

Finally, the ICs that best matched the CEN, DMN, and SN for both the low- and high-risk groups were selected separately. Following this, one-sample t-test ($p < 0.001$, corrected by family wise error (FWE)) was performed to determine the CEN, DMN, and SN functional connectivity for the low-risk and high-risk groups respectively. Between group within-network functional connectivity difference was determined by two-sample t-test ($p < 0.05$, corrected by false discovery rate (FDR)).

Bayesian Network Analysis

BN analysis can be used to learn the global connectivity pattern for complex systems in a data-driven manner, and has been applied in our previous studies of AD and MCI (Wu et al., 2011; Li et al., 2013). Here, we employed the Gaussian BN method to characterize the large-scale networks in terms of directed effective connectivity among CEN, DMN and SN.

To establish the effective connectivity pattern of the three networks for the low- and high-risk groups separately, we defined the region of interest (ROI) mask as each of the three one-sample t-test network map ($p < 0.001$, FWE corrected).

The averaged time series over these voxels in every subject was extracted and then entered into the BN analysis for the construction of an effective connectivity pattern of the three core networks.

A BN model is a directed acyclic graph that encodes a joint probability distribution over a set of random variables. The directed arcs in the graph denote the conditional dependence relationships between nodes, which are qualified by the conditional probability of each node given its parents in the network. Specific to our BN model, we have three nodes in total, which represent the three core networks in the triple network model, and the arcs connecting them represent the directed effective connectivity between these functional networks. The time series of each node was calculated as the mean time series in each network ROI, and was assumed to follow a linear Gaussian conditional distribution. To learn the effective connectivity of the triple network model, we employed the Bayesian information criterion (BIC)-based learning approach. The BN model that maximized the BIC score among the space of possible candidates was selected as the best fit network. We used the L1-Regularization Paths algorithm (Schmidt et al., 2007) and the Maximum Likelihood Estimation (MLE) implemented in the collections of Matlab functions written by Murphy et al.[4] to learn the structure and parameters of the BN model, respectively, for the high- and low-risk groups.

Effective Connectivity Comparison Between the High- and Low-Risk Groups

To examine the effective connectivity difference of CEN, DMN and SN between the high- and low-risk groups, we adopted the randomized permutation procedure. We used the differences of the connection weight coefficients between the two groups as the statistical measure. The reference distribution is obtained by calculating all possible values of the test statistic under rearrangements of the group labels on the observed fMRI datasets. The statistics for the real two group samples were calculated first. Then, at each iteration of the test process, the subject-group membership was randomly assigned for each subject. A BN model for each rearranged group was constructed, and the differences of the connection weight coefficients between the two rearranged groups were calculated. We ran a total of 1000 permutations and assessed the sample distributions for these statistics. Finally, for each of the connections presented in the BN model for the two risk groups, type I errors of having between-group differences were estimated.

RESULTS

Functional Connectivity of CEN, DMN and SN

Figure 1 shows the three networks included in the triple network model in the low and high-risk groups detected by Group ICA

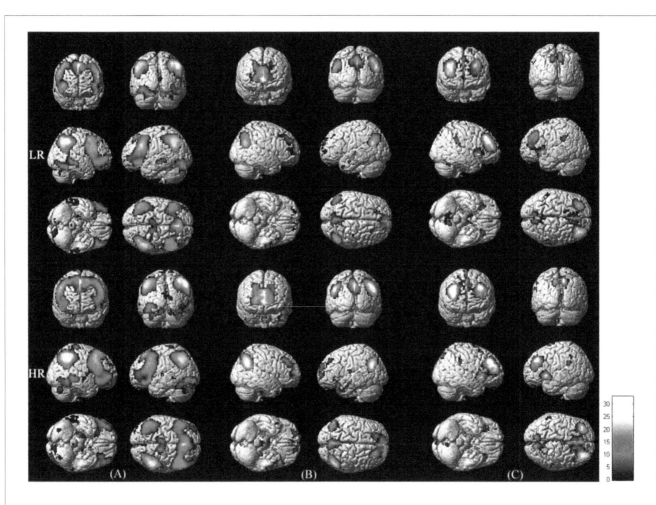

FIGURE 1 | Functional connectivity maps of the central executive network (CEN; A) default mode network (DMN; B) and salience network (SN; C) in **LR (upper panel) and HR (lower panel) groups.** The maps were derived from the one-sample t-test of Group independent component analysis (ICA; $p < 0.001$, corrected by family wise error (FWE)). Bar at the right shows T-values.

(one-sample t-test, $p < 0.001$, FWE corrected). In both groups, the CEN includes the dorsolateral prefrontal cortex and the lateral posterior parietal cortex. The DMN includes the posterior cingulate cortex, medial prefrontal cortex, bilateral inferior parietal cortex, inferior temporal cortex and the hippocampus. The SN includes the dorsal anterior cingulate cortex and the fronto-insular cortex.

Within-Network Functional Connectivity Difference Between Groups

To compare the within-network functional connectivity difference of the CEN, DMN and SN between the low- and high-risk groups, we performed a two-sample t-test ($p < 0.05$, corrected by FDR) on individual maps of the three networks between the two groups. **Figure 2** displays the functional connectivity differences between the low and high-risk groups.

Within the CEN, the angular gyrus displayed increased functional connectivity in the low-risk group compared with the high-risk group ("LR > HR"), whereas the inferior parietal lobule displayed increased functional connectivity in the high-risk group compared with the low-risk group ("HR > LR"). Within the DMN, the right medial frontal gyrus displayed increased functional connectivity in the low-risk group compared with the high-risk group ("LR > HR"), whereas the left middle frontal gyrus displayed increased functional connectivity in the high-risk group compared with the low-risk group ("HR > LR"). Within the SN, the regions including the right middle temporal gyrus, right middle frontal gyrus and the anterior cingulate cortex displayed increased functional connectivity in the low-risk group compared with the high-risk group ("LR > HR"). In contrast, the regions including the left middle temporal gyrus, posterior lobe of the cerebellum and the supplemental motor area displayed increased functional connectivity in the high-risk group compared with the low-risk group ("HR > LR"). Details on these regions with between-group functional connectivity differences are listed in **Table 1**.

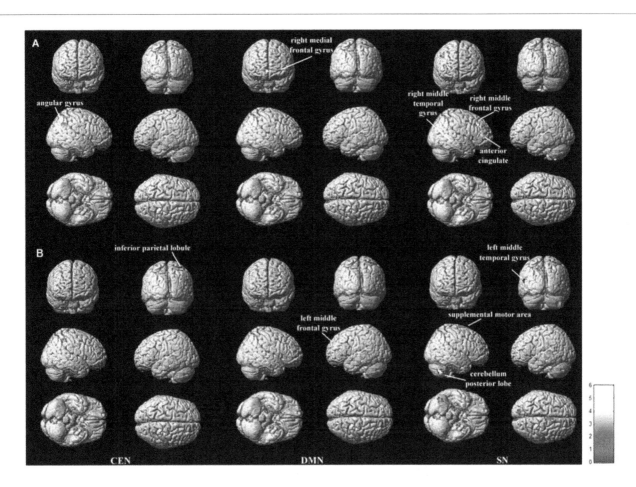

FIGURE 2 | Regions showing between-group functional connectivity difference. The comparison was performed for each of the triple networks by the two-sample *t*-test with *p* < 0.05, false discovery rate (FDR) correction. **(A)** shows the regions in which functional connectivity are stronger in LR group than in HR group (LR > HR), and **(B)** shows the opposite case (HR > LR). Bar at the right shows *T*-values.

BN-Based Effective Connectivity of CEN, DMN and SN

Figure 3 shows the effective connectivity of the CEN, DMN and SN in the low-risk group and high-risk group learned using Gaussian BN approach. In accordance with the triple network model (Menon, 2011), **Figure 3** demonstrates consistently in the two groups that the DMN together with CEN receive connections from SN. It is important to note that the SN plays as a special node that does not receive but only generates connections in the model in both groups. Furthermore, the result of the

TABLE 1 | Brain regions that showed functional connectivity differences between the low and high risk groups (two sample *t*-test, *p* < 0.05, corrected by false discovery rate (FDR)).

Regions	L/R	T value	MNI coordinate			Number of voxels
			x	y	z	
Angular gyrus	R	5.40	30	−54	36	35
Middle frontal gyrus	R	5.90	48	33	44	51
Middle temporal gyrus	R	6.92	48	−15	−16	18
Anterior cingulate	R	5.74	9	30	20	62
Medial frontal gyrus	R	5.25	3	54	−4	15
Inferior parietal lobule	R	5.47	39	−48	60	69
Middle frontal gyrus	L	4.60	−30	45	28	29
Cerebellum posterior lobe	R	5.58	45	−63	−44	71
Middle temporal gyrus	L	5.17	−51	−51	16	21
Supplemental motor area	R	6.16	6	−6	76	42

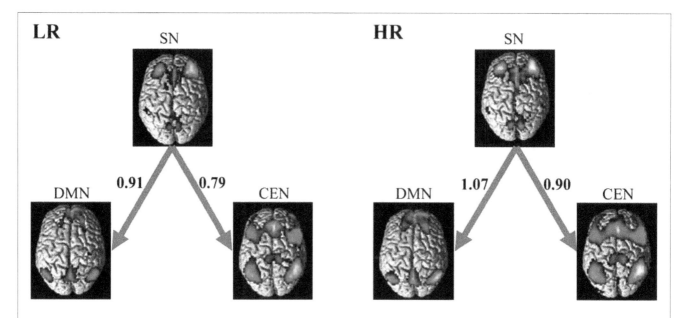

FIGURE 3 | Directed interactions of the triple networks in two groups. The causal interactions were determined based on the Bayesian network (BN) analysis of the triple networks. The LR group and HR group were found to have the same triple network BN connectivity relationships. The SN plays as an influential hub that mediates the activity of the CEN and DMN in both groups. The numbers on the connections represent the BN connectivity weights between brain networks.

random permutation test indicates that there is no significant difference among the effective connectivity coefficients of these three networks between the low- and high-risk groups (all $ps > 0.05$).

DISCUSSION

The focus of the present study was to explore the possible impairment of the within-network functional connectivity and the between-network effective connectivity of the large-scale triple networks in cognitively normal individuals with a family history of AD and at least one copy of the APOE4 allele. Group ICA of the triple network model found that a couple of brain regions in the three networks showed significantly altered functional connectivity in the high-risk individuals, while the BN analysis of the model did not find significant between-group difference in the causal connections among the three functional networks.

We first compared the within-network functional connectivity between the low-risk subjects and the high-risk subjects. The results demonstrated that a number of brain regions, including the medial prefrontal gyrus from the DMN, the angular gyrus from the CEN, the anterior cingulate, the right medial temporal and the right middle frontal gyri from the SN displayed significantly decreased functional connectivity in APOE4 carriers. The medial prefrontal gyrus is a critical area of the DMN (Greicius et al., 2003), and plays a central role in a variety of cognitive functions, especially memory (Euston et al., 2012) and executive function (Dalley et al., 2004) that are vulnerable to cognitive aging and AD (Greicius et al., 2004; Burke and Barnes, 2006; Li et al., 2013). Various studies of the DMN in AD have repeatedly reported functional

connectivity disruption in this region (Greicius et al., 2004; Rombouts et al., 2005; Qi et al., 2010; Wu et al., 2011; Wang et al., 2013). Recently, Song et al. (2015) also demonstrated APOE effect on the medial prefrontal regions in the DMN using seed-based functional connectivity analysis. The angular gyrus is functionally related to associative memory (Ben-Zvi et al., 2015), visuo-spatial attention (Cattaneo et al., 2009), and language ability (Bernal et al., 2015). Agosta et al. (2012) have reported decreased functional connectivity of the angular gyrus from the fronto-parietal CEN in AD. Disrupted functional connectivity of the SN was associated with cognitive and emotional deficits, and has been found in advanced aging and MCI patients (He et al., 2014; Uddin, 2015; Lu et al., 2016). Recently, Joo et al. (2016) and Wang et al. (2015) investigated the functional disruptions in these functional networks, and found that greater reductions of inter-network connectivity were associated with lower cognitive performance in different levels of cognitive impairment. Thus the result here indicated that the functional connectivity in the triple networks was different between the high- and low-risk groups, which may be related to the presence of APOE4 and a family history of dementia. We speculate that these AD-like functional connectivity disruptions in the triple network model may suggest risks of future cognitive decline or the progression to MCI or AD for the APOE4 carriers.

In contrast with the decreased functional activation compared with the low-risk group, we found that the high-risk group also showed increased functional activation in the frontal gyrus, parietal lobe, temporal gyrus and the cerebellum. It is consistent with several recent neuroimaging studies of APOE effects on brain connectivity. For example, Machulda et al. (2011) found increased SN connectivity by calculating the functional connectivity of the anterior cingulate seed in APOE4 carriers. Westlye et al. (2011) and Song et al. (2015) demonstrated increased DMN synchronization in APOE4 carriers. Similarly in AD patients, increased functional activation compared with that in healthy controls has also been reported (Wang et al., 2007; Qi et al., 2010; Zhou et al., 2010; Li et al., 2013). These increases have been usually interpreted as a compensatory reallocation or recruitment of brain resources (Cabeza et al., 2002), which may be a protective factor to keep retain a normal cognitive level in individuals at high risk for AD.

We also employed a BN approach to model and compare the effective connectivity patterns between the CEN, SN and DMN in the low- and high-risk groups. The BN learning approach revealed same-directed connections and network features in these two groups; the SN node does not receive but only generates connections to CEN and DMN. The BN-based directed connectivity pattern in both groups is consistent with the triple network model of major psychopathology suggested by Menon (2011), in which the information transfer occurs only from the SN to the CEN and DMN. It is also consistent with the study of Uddin et al. (2011), in which they employed Granger causality analyses to model the effective connectivity of the triple network with development, and found consistently that the fronto-insular cortex in the SN significantly influence the functional activity of regions in the DMN and CEN. Moreover, a recent study of Liang et al. (2015) demonstrated that the topological organization of the triple network changes with cognitive task loads. By comparing the effective connectivity coefficients between these two risk groups via the random permutation test, however, we found no significant difference in the directed connectivity of the three networks between the low- and high-risk groups. It suggested that although the APOE4 carriers might demonstrate AD-like functional connectivity changes in each of the three networks, the interactions between them could retain a normal process as in non-APOE4 carriers. This interesting finding may be explained first by the methodological difference. The functional connectivity stresses the temporal correlation between different regions, while the effective connectivity refers explicitly to the causal influence that one system exerts over another (Friston, 2011), which is in accordance with the inherent meaning of the triple network model. Second, the BN-based directed connectivity reflects how these three networks in the model cooperate with each other to execute tasks. It essentially demonstrated an organizational architecture of these functional networks. We propose that the stable effective connectivity architecture of the triple networks may be a crucial factor, together with the increased within-network functional connectivity, that enables individuals at high risk for AD to retain a normal cognitive level. Finally, it might be related to the complexity of brain network itself in response to the APOE4 effect. We speculate that the within-network regional connectivity alterations might emerge earlier than between-network changes, and the further deterioration of within-network connectivity may gradually lead to disruptions in interactions between networks for the APOE4 carriers. For example, Zhu et al. (2016) recently reported more changes of within-network connectivity than between-network connectivity in AD and MCI. Further studies would be required to investigate the dynamic changes of the directed connectivity architecture of the triple networks in APOE4 carriers through a longitudinal study.

In summary, we have explored the functional connectivity and effective connectivity of the three networks included in the large-scale triple network model in individuals with low and high risk for AD. The results demonstrated aberrant within-network functional connectivity that suggests future risk of cognitive decline or progression to AD, and preserved between-network effective connectivity that may support their current preserved cognition in the cognitively normal individuals who have a family history of AD and at least one copy of the APOE4 allele.

AUTHOR CONTRIBUTIONS

XW, LY and RL: designed and wrote the article; KC, ASF and EMR: carried out the experiment and collected the data; QL and XY: analyzed the data; XG and JZ: participated in the discussion and criticized the manuscript.

ACKNOWLEDGMENTS

This work was supported by the National Institute on Aging (k23 AG024062), the Funds for International Cooperation and Exchange of the National Natural Science Foundation of China (61210001), the General Program of National Natural Science Foundation of China (61571047, 31200847), and the Key Laboratory of Mental Health, Institute of Psychology, Chinese Academy of Sciences (KLMH2014ZG03, KLMH2015G06).

REFERENCES

Agosta, F., Pievani, M., Geroldi, C., Copetti, M., Frisoni, G. B., and Filippi, M. (2012). Resting state fMRI in Alzheimer's disease: beyond the default mode network. Neurobiol. Aging 33, 1564–1578. doi: 10.1016/j.neurobiolaging.2011.06.007

Agosta, F., Vossel, K. A., Miller, B. L., Migliaccio, R., Bonasera, S. J., Filippi, M., et al. (2009). Apolipoprotein E ε4 is associated with disease-specific effects on brain atrophy in Alzheimer's disease and frontotemporal dementia. Proc. Natl. Acad. Sci. U S A 106, 2018–2022. doi: 10.1073/pnas.0812697106

Balthazar, M. L. F., Pereira, F. R. S., Lopes, T. M., da Silva, E. L., Coan, A. C., Campos, B. M., et al. (2014). Neuropsychiatric symptoms in Alzheimer's disease are related to functional connectivity alterations in the salience network. Hum. Brain Mapp. 35, 1237–1246. doi: 10.1002/hbm.22248

Barabash, A., Marcos, A., Ancín, I., Vázquez-Alvarez, B., de Ugarte, C., Gil, P., et al. (2009). APOE, ACT and CHRNA7 genes in the conversion from amnestic mild cognitive impairment to Alzheimer's disease. Neurobiol. Aging 30, 1254–1264. doi: 10.1016/j.neurobiolaging.2007.11.003

Ben-Zvi, S., Soroker, N., and Levy, D. A. (2015). Parietal lesion effects on cued recall following pair associate learning. Neuropsychologia 73, 176–194. doi: 10.1016/j.neuropsychologia.2015.05.009

Bernal, B., Ardila, A., and Rosselli, M. (2015). Broca's area network in language function: a pooling-data connectivity study. *Front. Psychol.* 6:687. doi: 10.3389/fpsyg.2015.00687

Breitner, J. C. S., Wyse, B. W., Anthony, J. C., Welsh-Bohmer, K. A., Steffens, D. C., Norton, M. C., et al. (1999). APOE-ϵ4 count predicts age when prevalence of AD increases: then declines the cache county study. *Neurology* 53, 321–321. doi: 10.1212/WNL.53.2.321

Burke, S. N., and Barnes, C. A. (2006). Neural plasticity in the ageing brain. *Nat. Rev. Neurosci.* 7, 30–40. doi: 10.1038/nrn1809

Cabeza, R., Anderson, N. D., Locantore, J. K., and McIntosh, A. R. (2002). Aging gracefully: compensatory brain activity in high-performing older adults. *Neuroimage* 17, 1394–1402. doi: 10.1006/nimg.2002.1280

Calhoun, V. D., Adali, T., Pearlson, G. D., and Pekar, J. J. (2001). A method for making group inferences from functional MRI data using independent component analysis. *Hum. Brain Mapp.* 14, 140–151. doi: 10.1002/hbm.1048

Cattaneo, Z., Silvanto, J., Pascual-Leone, A., and Battelli, L. (2009). The role of the angular gyrus in the modulation of visuospatial attention by the mental number line. *Neuroimage* 44, 563–568. doi: 10.1016/j.neuroimage.2008.09.003

Celone, K. A., Calhoun, V. D., Dickerson, B. C., Atri, A., Chua, E. F., Miller, S. L., et al. (2006). Alterations in memory networks in mild cognitive impairment and Alzheimer's disease: an independent component analysis. *J. Neurosci.* 26, 10222–10231. doi: 10.1523/JNEUROSCI.2250-06.2006

Corder, E. H., Saunders, A. M., Strittmatter, W. J., Schmechel, D. E., Gaskell, P. C., Small, G. W., et al. (1993). Gene dose of apolipoprotein E type 4 allele and the risk of Alzheimer's disease in late onset families. *Science* 261, 921–923. doi: 10.1126/science.8346443

Dalley, J. W., Cardinal, R. N., and Robbins, T. W. (2004). Prefrontal executive and cognitive functions in rodents: neural and neurochemical substrates. *Neurosci. Biobehav. Rev.* 28, 771–784. doi: 10.1016/j.neubiorev.2004.09.006

Euston, D. R., Gruber, A. J., and McNaughton, B. L. (2012). The role of medial prefrontal cortex in memory and decision making. *Neuron* 76, 1057–1070. doi: 10.1016/j.neuron.2012.12.002

Fleisher, A. S., Podraza, K. M., Bangen, K. J., Taylor, C., Sherzai, A., Sidhar, K., et al. (2009a). Cerebral perfusion and oxygenation differences in Alzheimer's disease risk. *Neurobiol. Aging* 30, 1737–1748. doi: 10.1016/j.neurobiolaging.2008.01.012

Fleisher, A. S., Sherzai, A., Taylor, C., Langbaum, J., Chen, K., and Buxton, R. B. (2009b). Resting-state BOLD networks versus task-associated functional MRI for distinguishing Alzheimer's disease risk groups. *Neuroimage* 47, 1678–1690. doi: 10.1016/j.neuroimage.2009.06.021

Friston, K. J. (2011). Functional and effective connectivity: a review. *Brain Connect.* 1, 13–36. doi: 10.1089/brain.2011.0008

Greicius, M. D., Krasnow, B., Reiss, A. L., and Menon, V. (2003). Functional connectivity in the resting brain: a network analysis of the default mode hypothesis. *Proc. Natl. Acad. Sci. U S A* 100, 253–258. doi: 10.1073/pnas.0135058100

Greicius, M. D., and Menon, V. (2004). Default-mode activity during a passive sensory task: uncoupled from deactivation but impacting activation. *J. Cogn. Neurosci.* 16, 1484–1492. doi: 10.1162/0898929042568532

Greicius, M. D., Srivastava, G., Reiss, A. L., and Menon, V. (2004). Default-mode network activity distinguishes Alzheimer's disease from healthy aging: evidence from functional MRI. *Proc. Natl. Acad. Sci. U S A* 101, 4637–4642. doi: 10.1073/pnas.0308627101

He, X., Qin, W., Liu, Y., Zhang, X., Duan, Y., Song, J., et al. (2014). Abnormal salience network in normal aging and in amnestic mild cognitive impairment and Alzheimer's disease. *Hum. Brain Mapp.* 35, 3446–3464. doi: 10.1002/hbm.22414

Joo, S. H., Lim, H. K., and Lee, C. U. (2016). Three large-scale functional brain networks from resting-state functional MRI in subjects with different levels of cognitive impairment. *Psychiatry Investig.* 13, 1–7. doi: 10.4306/pi.2016.13.1.1

Kandimalla, R. J., Anand, R., Veeramanikandan, R., Wani, W. Y., Prabhakar, S., Grover, V. K., et al. (2014). CSF ubiquitin as a specific biomarker in Alzheimer's disease. *Curr. Alzheimer Res.* 11, 340–348. doi: 10.2174/1567205011666140331161027

Kandimalla, R. J., Prabhakar, S., Binukumar, B. K., Wani, W. Y., Gupta, N., Sharma, D. R., et al. (2011). Apo-E4 allele in conjunction with Aβ42 and tau in CSF: biomarker for Alzheimer's disease. *Curr. Alzheimer Res.* 8, 187–196. doi: 10.2174/156720511795256071

Kandimalla, R. J., Wani, W. Y., Anand, R., Kaushal, A., Prabhakar, S., Grover, V. K., et al. (2013). Apolipoprotein E levels in the cerebrospinal fluid of north Indian patients with Alzheimer's disease. *Am. J. Alzheimers Dis. Other Demen.* 28, 258–262. doi: 10.1177/1533317513481097

Kivipelto, M., Helkala, E., Laakso, M. P., Hänninen, T., Hallikainen, M., Alhainen, K., et al. (2001). Midlife vascular risk factors and Alzheimer's disease in later life: longitudinal, population based study. *BMJ* 322, 1447–1451. doi: 10.1136/bmj.322.7300.1447

Lee, T.-W., Girolami, M., and Sejnowski, T. J. (1999). Independent component analysis using an extended infomax algorithm for mixed sub-gaussian and supergaussian sources. *Neural Comput.* 11, 417–441. doi: 10.1162/089976699300016719

Li, R., Yu, J., Zhang, S., Bao, F., Wang, P., Huang, X., et al. (2013). Bayesian network analysis reveals alterations to default mode network connectivity in individuals at risk for Alzheimer's disease. *PLoS One* 8:e82104. doi: 10.1371/journal.pone.0082104

Liang, X., Zou, Q., He, Y., and Yang, Y. (2015). Topologically reorganized connectivity architecture of default-mode, executive-control and salience networks across working memory task loads. *Cereb. Cortex* 26, 1501–1511. doi: 10.1093/cercor/bhu316

Lo, C.-Y., Wang, P.-N., Chou, K.-H., Wang, J., He, Y., and Lin, C.-P. (2010). Diffusion tensor tractography reveals abnormal topological organization in structural cortical networks in Alzheimer's disease. *J. Neurosci.* 30, 16876–16885. doi: 10.1523/JNEUROSCI.4136-10.2010

Lu, Y.-T., Chang, W.-N., Chang, C.-C., Lu, C.-H., Chen, N.-C., Huang, C.-W., et al. (2016). Insula volume and salience network are associated with memory decline in parkinson disease: complementary analyses of voxel-based morphometry versus volume of interest. *Parkinsons Dis.* 2016:2939528. doi: 10.1155/2016/2939528

Lustig, C., Snyder, A. Z., Bhakta, M., O'Brien, K. C., McAvoy, M., Raichle, M. E., et al. (2003). Functional deactivations: change with age and dementia of the Alzheimer type. *Proc. Natl. Acad. Sci. U S A* 100, 14504–14509. doi: 10.1073/pnas.2235925100

Machulda, M. M., Jones, D. T., Vemuri, P., McDade, E., Avula, R., Przybelski, S., et al. (2011). Effect of APOE ϵ4 status on intrinsic network connectivity in cognitively normal elderly subjects. *Arch. Neurol.* 68, 1131–1136. doi: 10.1001/archneurol.2011.108

Menon, V. (2011). Large-scale brain networks and psychopathology: a unifying triple network model. *Trends Cogn. Sci.* 15, 483–506. doi: 10.1016/j.tics.2011.08.003

Menon, V., and Uddin, L. Q. (2010). Saliency, switching, attention and control: a network model of insula function. *Brain Struct. Funct.* 214, 655–667. doi: 10.1007/s00429-010-0262-0

Petrella, J. R., Prince, S. E., Wang, L., Hellegers, C., and Doraiswamy, P. M. (2007). Prognostic value of posteromedial cortex deactivation in mild cognitive impairment. *PLoS One* 2:e1104. doi: 10.1371/journal.pone.0001104

Poirier, J., Delisle, M. C., Quirion, R., Aubert, I., Farlow, M., Lahiri, D., et al. (1995). Apolipoprotein E4 allele as a predictor of cholinergic deficits and treatment outcome in Alzheimer disease. *Proc. Natl. Acad. Sci. U S A* 92, 12260–12264. doi: 10.1073/pnas.92.26.12260

Qi, Z., Wu, X., Wang, Z., Zhang, N., Dong, H., Yao, L., et al. (2010). Impairment and compensation coexist in amnestic MCI default mode network. *Neuroimage* 50, 48–55. doi: 10.1016/j.neuroimage.2009.12.025

Reitz, C., and Mayeux, R. (2010). Use of genetic variation as biomarkers for mild cognitive impairment and progression of mild cognitive impairment to dementia. *J. Alzheimers Dis.* 19, 229–251. doi: 10.3233/JAD-2010-1255

Rombouts, S. A. R. B., Barkhof, F., Goekoop, R., Stam, C. J., and Scheltens, P. (2005). Altered resting state networks in mild cognitive impairment and mild Alzheimer's disease: an fMRI study. *Hum. Brain Mapp.* 26, 231–239. doi: 10.1002/hbm.20160

Sasaki, M., Kodama, C., Hidaka, S., Yamashita, F., Kinoshita, T., Nemoto, K., et al. (2009). Prevalence of four subtypes of mild cognitive impairment and APOE in a Japanese community. *Int. J. Geriatr. Psychiatry* 24, 1119–1126. doi: 10. 1002/gps.2234

Schmidt, M., Niculescu-Mizil, A., and Murphy, K. (2007). "Learning graphical model structure using L1-regularization paths," in *Proceedings of the 22nd National Conference on Artificial Intelligence* (Vancouver, BC), 2, 1278–1283.

Song, H., Long, H., Zuo, X., Yu, C., Liu, B., Wang, Z., et al. (2015). APOE effects on default mode network in chinese cognitive normal elderly: relationship with clinical cognitive performance. *PLoS One* 10:e0133179. doi: 10.1371/journal. pone.0133179

Stam, C. J., Jones, B. F., Nolte, G., Breakspear, M., and Scheltens, P. (2007). Small-world networks and functional connectivity in Alzheimer's disease. *Cereb. Cortex* 17, 92–99. doi: 10.1093/cercor/bhj127

Tai, L. M., Mehra, S., Shete, V., Estus, S., Rebeck, G. W., Bu, G., et al. (2014). Soluble apoE/Aβ complex: mechanism and therapeutic target for *APOE4*-induced AD risk. *Mol. Neurodegener.* 9:2. doi: 10.1186/1750-1326-9-2

Uddin, L. Q. (2015). Salience processing and insular cortical function and dysfunction. *Nat. Rev. Neurosci.* 16, 55–61. doi: 10.1038/nrn3857

Uddin, L. Q., Supekar, K. S., Ryali, S., and Menon, V. (2011). Dynamic reconfiguration of structural and functional connectivity across core neurocognitive brain networks with development. *J. Neurosci.* 31, 18578–18589. doi: 10.1523/JNEUROSCI.4465-11.2011

Wang, K., Liang, M., Wang, L., Tian, L., Zhang, X., Li, K., et al. (2007). Altered functional connectivity in early Alzheimer's disease: a resting-state fMRI study. *Hum. Brain Mapp.* 28, 967–978. doi: 10.1002/hbm.20324

Wang, P., Zhou, B., Yao, H., Zhan, Y., Zhang, Z., Cui, Y., et al. (2015). Aberrant intra- and inter-network connectivity architectures in Alzheimer,s disease and mild cognitive impairment. *Sci. Rep.* 5:14824. doi: 10.1038/srep 14824

Wang, J., Zuo, X., Dai, Z., Xia, M., Zhao, Z., Zhao, X., et al. (2013). Disrupted functional brain connectome in individuals at risk for Alzheimer's disease. *Biol. Psychiatry* 73, 472–481. doi: 10.1016/j.biopsych.2012.03.026

Westlye, E. T., Lundervold, A., Rootwelt, H., Lundervold, A. J., and Westlye, L. T. (2011). Increased hippocampal default mode synchronization during rest in middle-aged and elderly APOE ε4 carriers: relationships with memory performance. *J. Neurosci.* 31, 7775–7783. doi: 10.1523/JNEUROSCI.1230-11.2011

Wolk, D. A., Dickerson, B. C., and Alzheimer's Disease Neuroimaging Initiative. (2010). Apolipoprotein E (APOE) genotype has dissociable effects on memory and attentional-executive network function in Alzheimer's disease. *Proc. Natl. Acad. Sci. U S A* 107, 10256–10261. doi: 10.1073/pnas.1001 412107

Wu, X., Li, R., Fleisher, A. S., Reiman, E. M., Guan, X., Zhang, Y., et al. (2011). Altered default mode network connectivity in Alzheimer's disease—a resting functional MRI and Bayesian network study. *Hum. Brain Mapp.* 32, 1868–1881. doi: 10.1002/hbm.21153

Yuan, K., Qin, W., Yu, D., Bi, Y., Xing, L., Jin, C., et al. (2016). Core brain networks interactions and cognitive control in internet gaming disorder individuals in late adolescence/early adulthood. *Brain Struct. Funct.* 221, 1427–1442. doi: 10. 1007/s00429-014-0982-7

Zheng, H., Xu, L., Xie, F., Guo, X., Zhang, J., Yao, L., et al. (2015). The altered triple networks interaction in depression under resting state based on graph theory. *Biomed. Res. Int.* 2015:386326. doi: 10.1155/2015/386326

Zhou, J., Greicius, M. D., Gennatas, E. D., Growdon, M. E., Jang, J. Y., Rabinovici, G. D., et al. (2010). Divergent network connectivity changes in behavioural variant frontotemporal dementia and Alzheimer's disease. *Brain* 133, 1352–1367. doi: 10.1093/brain/awq075

Zhu, H., Zhou, P., Alcauter, S., Chen, Y., Cao, H., Tian, M., et al. (2016). Changes of intranetwork and internetwork functional connectivity in Alzheimer's disease and mild cognitive impairment. *J. Neural Eng.* 13:046008. doi: 10.1088/1741-2560/13/4/046008

tDCS over the Motor Cortex Shows Differential Effects on Action and Object Words in Associative Word Learning in Healthy Aging

Meret Branscheidt[1]*[†], Julia Hoppe[2†], Nils Freundlieb[2,3], Pienie Zwitserlood[4] and Gianpiero Liuzzi[1,2]

[1]Department of Neurology, University Hospital Zurich, Zurich, Switzerland, [2]Department of Neurology, University Medical Center Hamburg-Eppendorf, Hamburg, Germany, [3]Brain Stimulation, Department of Psychiatry and Psychotherapy, University Medical Center Hamburg-Eppendorf, Hamburg, Germany, [4]Department of Psychology, University of Münster, Münster, Germany

*Correspondence:
Meret Branscheidt
mbransc1@jhu.edu

[†] *These authors have contributed equally to this work.*

Healthy aging is accompanied by a continuous decline in cognitive functions. For example, the ability to learn languages decreases with age, while the neurobiological underpinnings for the decline in learning abilities are not known exactly. Transcranial direct current stimulation (tDCS), in combination with appropriate experimental paradigms, is a well-established technique to investigate the mechanisms of learning. Based on previous results in young adults, we tested the suitability of an associative learning paradigm for the acquisition of action- and object-related words in a cohort of older participants. We applied tDCS to the motor cortex (MC) and hypothesized an involvement of the MC in learning action-related words. To test this, a cohort of 18 healthy, older participants (mean age 71) engaged in a computer-assisted associative word-learning paradigm, while tDCS stimulation (anodal, cathodal, sham) was applied to the left MC. Participants' task performance was quantified in a randomized, cross-over experimental design. Participants successfully learned novel words, correctly translating 39.22% of the words after 1 h of training under sham stimulation. Task performance correlated with scores for declarative verbal learning and logical reasoning. Overall, tDCS did not influence associative word learning, but a specific influence was observed of cathodal tDCS on learning of action-related words during the NMDA-dependent stimulation period. Successful learning of a novel lexicon with associative learning in older participants can only be achieved when the learning procedure is changed in several aspects, relative to young subjects. Learning success showed large inter-individual variance which was dependent on non-linguistic as well as linguistic cognitive functions. Intriguingly, cathodal tDCS influenced the acquisition of action-related words in the NMDA-dependent stimulation period. However, the effect was not specific for the associative learning principle, suggesting more neurobiological fragility of learning in healthy aging compared with young persons.

Keywords: associative word learning, healthy aging, transcranial direct current stimulation, motor cortex, language functions

Abbreviations: ANOVA, analysis of variance; ISI, interstimulus interval; MC, motor cortex; MEP, motor evoked potential; MMST, mini-mental status-test; tDCS, transcranial direct current stimulation; TMS, transcranial magnetic stimulation; VAS, visual analog scales; VLMT, verbal learning and memory test.

INTRODUCTION

With increasing life expectancy, quality of life and social participation in older people is more and more dependent on fluid cognitive functioning. However, the ability to acquire new skills, for example to learn a new language, decreases with age (Flöel et al., 2012; Zimerman et al., 2013). The neurobiological aspects underlying language learning in healthy aging constitute a novel research area and are still not well understood. It is known that acquired knowledge and well-trained skills are commonly preserved in healthy aging, while the formation of new memory contents becomes increasingly difficult (Cohen, 1979; Light and Burke, 2009). By consequence, everyday language comprehension shows little abnormalities, whereas linguistic information processing in more challenging situations, for example learning new words, deteriorates with age (Service and Craik, 1993; Light and Burke, 2009).

Associative learning of a new lexicon has been successfully implemented in experimental settings with precise control over stimulus frequency and exposure time (Breitenstein and Knecht, 2002; Dobel et al., 2009; Liuzzi et al., 2010). While these paradigms yielded robust results for different word classes in young adults, testing the suitability and determining learning success in an older population was the scope of the present work.

The framework of embodied semantics is based on the hypothesis that motor areas activated by execution and observation of actions are also involved in processing linguistic information related to these actions (Hauk and Pulvermüller, 2004; Gallese and Lakoff, 2005; Pulvermüller, 2005). Evidence to support this theory comes from fMRI, lesion and electrophysiological studies highlighting a tight functional link between the motor and language systems (Flöel et al., 2003; Kemmerer et al., 2012). Building on this, recent studies have explored the possibility of influencing one system to alter function in the other domain. For instance, it has been shown that listening to food action related sentences results in effector specific excitability changes in the food motor area but not the hand motor area and *vice versa* (Buccino et al., 2005). Also, activation of motor areas (e.g., by allowing manual gestures or suppressing them) can improve certain aspects of language (Rauscher et al., 1996; Pine et al., 2007). Additionally, Liuzzi et al. (2010) could demonstrate that left motor cortex (MC) stimulation was causally involved in learning a novel action word vocabulary. Given the findings for young adults with brain stimulation, we hypothesized an influence of the left MC on the acquisition of a novel action word lexicon. In particular, we explored whether the associative learning principle was specifically altered by brain stimulation in older adults.

Transcranial direct current stimulation (tDCS) is a non-invasive electrical brain stimulation technique, which has been successfully used to improve learning in non-linguistic domains in healthy aging (Hummel et al., 2010; Flöel et al., 2012; Zimerman et al., 2013; Park et al., 2014). While the efficacy of tDCS in improving language function at various levels has been demonstrated in young healthy adults (for an overview see Miniussi et al., 2008; Cotelli et al., 2008), the effect of tDCS on language acquisition in an older population remains an open question. In young people, Liuzzi et al. (2010) demonstrated that tDCS over the left MC affected associative learning of a novel action-word lexicon. tDCS has specific NMDA-dependent and plasticity-related effects that are necessary for the coupling of actions with novel words (Liebetanz et al., 2002; Liuzzi et al., 2010). This allows for a characterization of learning word-to-semantic couplings in a neurobiologically defined way. We here investigated associative word learning of action- and object-related vocabulary applying MC-tDCS in healthy older participants to investigate whether the associative learning principle described in the young is altered in older adults.

We hypothesized that tDCS over the left MC influences associative word learning in healthy, older participants. We were especially interested in whether tDCS has a specific effect on word classes (action- vs. object-related words) and on specific response styles corresponding to Hebbian assumptions.

MATERIALS AND METHODS

Participants

A total of 18 participants were enrolled in the study protocol: 12 females, mean age: 70.6 ± 5.7 years, age range 61–82 years. According to the Edinburgh inventory of handedness, 17 participants were right-handed and one person was born left-handed but retrained to be right-handed during early childhood. All participants were native German speakers and spoke 2.0 ± 1.4 foreign languages. Formal years of education ranged from 8 to 13 years (10.2 ± 1.9).

Participants were not bilingual, had no history of neurological or psychiatric diseases, especially no severe head traumas, seizures, no metal implants in the head/neck region nor pacemaker implantation and did not use neuroactive (e.g., antidepressants, anticonvulsants etc.) or recreational drugs (>6 cups of coffee/day, >50 g of alcohol/day).

To characterize cognitive profiles, participants were screened with a comprehensive battery of neuropsychological tests. Current general cognitive status was assessed with the mini-mental status-test (MMST, Folstein et al., 1975) and the verbal learning and memory test (VLMT, Helmstaedter et al., 2001), verbal fluency with the Regensburg verbal fluency test (Aschenbrenner et al., 2000), visuo-spatial memory and executive abilities with the Rey-Osterrieth complex figure test (Rey, 1959), attention span with the d2-test, working memory with digit spans, and logical reasoning using the Horn Intelligence test (Brickenkamp, 2002). Participants whose performance was more than two standard deviations above or below the age-adjusted mean were to be excluded, but all screened participants were within these boundaries.

This study was carried out in accordance with the recommendations of the local ethics committee at the University of Hamburg and the Deutsche Forschungsgesellschaft (DFG). All subjects gave written informed consent in accordance with the Declaration of Helsinki. The protocol was approved by the ethics committee of the University of Hamburg.

Stimulus Material

Images

An associative word-learning paradigm, previously established and extensively pretested, was used (Breitenstein and Knecht, 2002; Liuzzi et al., 2010; Freundlieb et al., 2012). Participants were presented with spoken pseudowords (e.g., kage, gafo), together with different photographs of actions or objects. For details regarding the generation and compilation of the stimulus material see Liuzzi et al. (2010); Freundlieb et al. (2012).

Actions involving either hands and arms (e.g., knocking or eating), or the whole body (e.g., running or boxing) were taken from a set of photos of everyday actions. Images were previously evaluated regarding quality and suitability for the learning paradigm; assessing naming agreement, quality of depiction, motion association, involvement of a particular body part (head/face/mouth; arm/hand; leg/foot; whole body), daily-life frequency of execution, and frequency of personal everyday performance. Two different pictures were chosen for each action, illustrated by various actors and shot from different perspectives or in different locations (for further details on these images, see Freundlieb et al., 2012).

Object images (e.g., house, tree) were evaluated for recognizability, associations with body parts or motion. Two pictures were selected for each object, depicting the same object concept in two different ways (e.g., different houses). Images were taken from different angles, with different surroundings and without visible human body parts (for details see Freundlieb et al., 2012).

For both visual stimulus sets (action/object images), pictures were converted to grayscale, centered and adjusted for potential distracting features (e.g., text or background objects).

Pseudowords

Thirty-four 4-letter pseudowords were taken from an attested language-learning paradigm (Freundlieb et al., 2012). The spoken stimuli (e.g., binu, gafo) complied with the phonotactics of German, had neutral emotional valence and limited associations with existing words. The novel words had a stimulus duration of 970.3 ± 127.4 ms and the same maximum volume. All stimuli were spoken by the same female voice.

Word Learning Paradigm

During the associative learning task, correct (to be learned) and incorrect picture/pseudoword couplings were presented, with the proportion of correct pairings increasing over time. Participants had to decide intuitively whether word and picture matched or not. Spoken pseudowords were presented over earphones, while pictures were presented on a computer display. The onset of picture presentation was 200 ms after the onset of the spoken pseudoword. Participants answered by left- (correct) or right- (incorrect) clicks on a computer mouse

with their right hand. Single-trial duration was 3000 ms, and only responses obtained within this time window were taken into account for analyses. The interstimulus interval (ISI) was 2000 ms. In contrast to the visual presentation duration used in young healthy participants (Freundlieb et al., 2012), we extended their duration (3000 ms) for our cohort of older participants. Pilot experiments showed that most healthy older participants did not learn with short picture presentation times.

Participants took part in three learning sessions (see description below and **Figure 1**). During each session, they had to learn 34 pseudowords (17 action- and 17 object-related words), with two different images for each concept. Each session was divided into five blocks, separated by 2 min. breaks. Each block consisted of 136 trials, with a total of 680 trials per learning session. Over the course of the five blocks, correct couplings appeared 10 times (five times for each image of the action/object), whilst each pseudoword was also incorrectly paired with 10 different actions/objects (resulting in a correct/incorrect ratio of 10:1). We ensured that the same auditory/visual pair, as well as the same type of coupling (correct/incorrect) did not occur more than two times in a row.

Every participant completed three sessions on three separate days, with anodal, cathodal or sham tDCS and three parallel lexicon versions (lexicon 1, 2 or 3). The order of interventions and lexicon versions was pseudo-randomized and counterbalanced across sessions. Training sessions were separated by at least 2 and maximum 3 weeks. One week prior to the first tDCS training session, participants were familiarized with the learning paradigm, using a small lexicon of five words. Dependent measures were collected within each session: (1) correct responses during each training session; and (b) translation of pseudowords into German after training. No feedback was given on translation performance (for details see **Figure 1**).

Transcranial Direct Current Stimulation

Transcranial magnetic stimulation (TMS) was used to determine the hand region in the left MC in each participant immediately prior to tDCS application. The so-called "hotspot" for the hand region was identified as the position where the highest MEP amplitudes could be consistently evoked in the right first dorsal interosseous muscle (Chen et al., 1998). TMS was delivered by a Magstim 200 stimulator connected to a figure-8 shaped coil (7 cm in diameter, Magstim Co.).

tDCS was administered via two sponge electrodes (Eldith; soaked in 0.9% saline solution) connected to a DC-stimulator (Eldith; serial no. 0006). Either the anode or cathode was placed as stimulating electrode over the left hemispheric "hotspot" of the hand motor area (surface area 25 cm^2). The reference electrode was positioned over the contralateral supraorbital region (surface area 35 cm^2). Stimulation started immediately at the beginning of the learning paradigm, and intensity was increased in a ramp-like fashion over 10 s until 1 mA for verum and sham stimulation. In case of anodal or cathodal tDCS stimulation, the current intensity remained constant for 20 min. In contrast, the

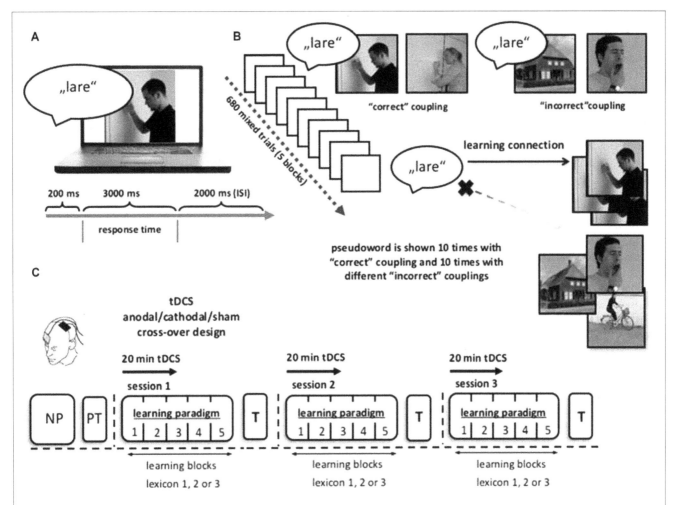

FIGURE 1 | Word learning paradigm. (A) Participants were shown a photographic illustration depicting an action/object paired with a spoken pseudoword. They had to decide intuitively if the presented coupling was a correct or incorrect match. Two-hundred milliseconds after onset of the sound, the picture appeared. Responses had to be given within a time window of 3000 ms. The interstimulus interval (ISI) was 2000 ms between two trials. **(B)** One learning session consisted of 680 single trials, subdivided into five blocks with a 2 min break. Each pseudoword was shown 10 times with the "correct" action/object (depicted by two different images) as well as 10 times with different "incorrect" images. **(C)** Study design: prior to the first learning session participants were screened with a neuropsychological test battery (NP) and were introduced to the learning paradigm with a small lexical pre-test (PT) consisting of five words. Each participant completed three learning sessions on three different days with three different lexicon sets. During the task, participants received anodal, cathodal or sham tDCS in a randomized order across learning sessions (1 mA for 20 min; double blind application). At the start of each session the stimulation side over the left motor cortex (MC) was localized using transcranial magnetic stimulation (TMS). tDCS stimulation and the learning paradigm started simultaneously, the latter exceeding the stimulation for approximately 20 min. After each session, patients were asked to translate the acquired pseudowords into notions of their native language (T). Abbreviations: NP, neuropsychological testing; PT, pre-test; T, translation test.

sham stimulation had a duration period of 30 s during which the intensity was ramped down to zero during the following 10 s. This "fade-in/fade-out" approach is standard best-practise procedure for sham stimulation in tDCS and mimics the cutaneous sensations experienced for verum stimulation (Gandiga et al., 2006). A person not involved in the experiment and data analysis entered the stimulation parameters. Experimenters and participants were blinded for stimulation type.

The neurophysiological effects of tDCS to the MC have been shown to outlast the stimulation period, with effects depending on current intensity and stimulation duration (Nitsche and Paulus, 2000; Nitsche et al., 2003). On this basis, a stimulation period of 20 min was regarded as sufficient for the learning paradigm lasting 40 min.

We evaluated participants' appraisal of attention, unpleasant sensations (i.e., discomfort/pain) and fatigue with questionnaires using visual analog scales (VAS) as control parameters.

Data Analysis

Two outcome measures were selected to determine successful learning: (1) the percentage of correct responses in learning blocks over time; and (2) the translation rate for pseudowords into native language after each training session. In a subanalysis, we also calculated the learning success for different response types in each block over time.

To investigate the influence of tDCS, we performed a three-factorial rmANOVA on the dependent variable percentage of correct decisions, with the within-subject factors "stimulation$_{anodal/cathodal/sham}$", "word class$_{object/action}$" and "blocks$_{1-5}$". We further investigated how stimulation might change response behavior for the word classes differently by two separate three-factorial rmANOVAs for objects and actions, with the within-subject factors "stimulation$_{anodal/cathodal/sham}$", "blocks$_{1-5}$" and "response type$_{hit/miss/corr\_reject/false\_alarm}$". For translation rates, differences between stimulation sessions were analyzed with a two-factorial rmANOVA, with the within-subject factors "stimulation$_{anodal/cathodal/sham}$" and "word class$_{object/action}$".

Performance scores of the neuropsychological test battery were probed for linear association with the translation rate and percentage of correct decisions in block five, using Pearson correlation coefficients. A one-way ANOVA with the within-subject factor "stimulation$_{anodal/cathodal/sham}$" was calculated for the VAS outcomes for attention/fatigue/discomfort/pain.

Before application of parametric tests, normal distribution of the dependent variables was tested using Shapiro-Wilk tests and quantile-quantile plots). All ANOVA results were Greenhouse-Geisser corrected if assumptions of sphericity were violated. Paired two-tailed t-tests were used for the analysis of the predicted effects of stimulation on word class. Results were considered significant at $p < 0.05$ and Cohen's d is reported as a measure of effect size. All data are expressed as mean ± standard error unless stated otherwise. Statistical analyses were done using SPSS 22.0® and GraphPad Prism® Software.

RESULTS

Learning Success

Percentage of Correct Responses

First, we report the effect of tDCS on the performance of associative learning: The number of correct responses increased significantly over the five blocks (blocks$_{1-5}$, $F_{(4,68)} = 30.44$, $p = 0.000$). Averaged over all stimulation conditions, participants started at chance level of 49.33 ± 0.94% and reached 69.32 ± 3.69% in block 5 (see **Figure 2**). However, anodal and cathodal tDCS stimulation over the left MC did not result in significantly different percentages of correct responses (stimulation$_{anodal/cathodal/sham}$ $F_{(2,34)} = 1.51$, $p = 0.235$; stimulation$_{anodal/cathodal/sham}$ *blocks$_{1-5}$: $F_{(8,136)} = 1.16, p = 0.337$), overall mean accuracy in block 5: anodal: 69.61 ± 3.8%; cathodal: 66.54 ± 4.1%; sham: 71.81 ± 4.1%). For all stimulation conditions together, correct responding during learning was better for object- than for action-related words (word class$_{object/action}$, $F_{(1,17)} = 9.59$, $p = 0.007$. There was no significant interaction between blocks and word class (blocks$_{1-5}$* word class$_{object/action}$ $F_{(4,68)} = 1.09$, $p = 0.368$).

Next, we evaluated whether tDCS over the left MC affects word classes differently, as shown in a younger population for cathodal tDCS and action words (Liuzzi et al., 2010). Regarding correct responses, neither the interaction of word class$_{object/action}$ *stimulation$_{anodal/cathodal/sham}$ nor the three-way interaction

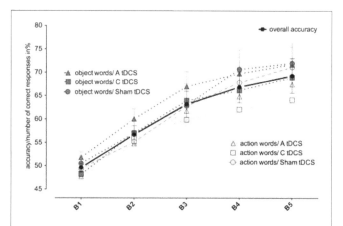

FIGURE 2 | Changes in accuracy depending on stimulation type and word type. Mean accuracy scores over the course of five learning blocks (B1–5) split by type of tDCS stimulation (A = anodal = triangles; C = cathodal = rectangles; Sham = circles). Dashed light gray lines depict action words, dotted dark gray lines depict object words; the bold black line with circles depicts overall mean accuracy.

of blocks$_{1-5}$ *stimulation$_{anodal/cathodal/sham}$ *word class$_{object/action}$ reached significance in the rmANOVA ($F_{(2,34)} = 2.33$, $p = 0.112$, respectively $F_{(8,136)} = 0.73$, $p = 0.661$; see **Figure 2**). However, as predicted from earlier results in young participants, there was a significant effect of cathodal stimulation on reduction of correct responses of action-related, but not of object-related words (cathodal vs. sham stimulation for actions: 64.1 ± 4.2% vs. 71.2 ± 4.1%, $t_{(17)} = 2.21$ $p = 0.02$, $d = 0.41$, cathodal vs. sham stimulation for objects: 69.0 ± 4.3% vs. 72.9 ± 4.2%, $t_{(17)} = 1.53$, $p = 0.144$, $d = 0.22$).

We also looked at the distribution of correct and incorrect response types (see "Materials and Methods" Section) for the different word classes/stimulation types. There was no interaction of response type$_{hit/miss/corr\_reject/false\_alarm}$ *stimulation$_{anodal/cathodal/sham}$ nor a three-way interaction of blocks$_{1-5}$ *response type$_{hit/miss/corr\_reject/false\_alarm}$ *stimulation$_{anodal/cathodal/sham}$ in actions ($F_{(6,102)} = 479.74$, $p = 0.234$, respectively $F_{(24,408)} = 56.10$, $p = 0.221$) or objects ($F_{(6,102)} = 0.75$, $p = 0.507$, respectively $F_{(24,408)} = 1.12, p = 0.358$). Note that cathodal stimulation seemed to lead to lower correct rejection and higher false alarm rates for actions compared to objects.

Translation

We additionally tested whether participants were able to transfer the learnt association between pseudo-word and images to their native language. Across all stimulation conditions, participants were able to translate a mean of 34.32 ± 5.47% pseudowords into German. tDCS stimulation did not significantly influence overall translation rates (stimulation$_{anodal/cathodal/sham}$: $F_{(2,34)} = 2.34$, $p = 0.107$, overall mean translation: anodal: 32.68 ± 5.1%; cathodal: 31.06 ± 5.5%; sham: 39.22 ± 5.6%). Even though the percentage of correct responses differed for word class, there was no significant difference in overall translation rates (word class$_{object/action}$, $F_{(1,17)} = 1.15$, $p = 0.299$; objects: 51.76 ± 8.1%; actions: 48.24 ± 8.9% of all correctly tDCS over the Motor Cortex Shows Differential Effects on Action and Object Words in Associative Word Learning...

37

TABLE 1 | Data for the two outcome measures, as a function of stimulation and word class.

Stimulation	Correct responses (average of last block)		Translation	
	Object	Action	Object	Action
Sham	72.9 ± 4.2%	71.2 ± 4.1%	31.7 ± 6.0%	34.3 ± 6.4%
Anodal	71.7 ± 3.8%	67.5 ± 4.2%	31.7 ± 5.1%	33.7 ± 5.8%
Cathodal	69.0 ± 4.2%	64.1 ± 4.2%	44.1 ± 5.4%	31.4 ± 6.3%

translated object and action words, respectively). The two-way interaction stimulation$_{anodal/cathodal/sham}$ *word class$_{object/action}$ was also not significant ($F_{(2,34)}$ = 2.80, p = 0.075, see also **Table 1**). Our findings suggest that aged-populations might have a limited ability for transfer of associated learning content.

Neuropsychological Evaluation

Finally, we tried to identify cognitive and stimulation-related factors that could potentially influence a participant's performance in the associative learning task. Learning success and translation rates correlated with performance scores in the VLMT (verbal learning and memory ability; r = 0.597, p = 0.009 and r = 0.604, p = 0.008, respectively) and logical reasoning (r = 0.610, p = 0.007 and r = 0.495, p = 0.037, respectively, see **Figure 3**), while the results for visuo-spatial memory and executive abilities, attention and working memory did not correlate with language learning performance.

Stimulation-related factors did not appear to have a noticeable effect on participant performance. Verum and sham tDCS evoked similar minimal painful sensations ($F_{(2,34)}$ = 1.972, p = 0.155; mean VAS 1-10 anodal: 1.56 ± 0.2; cathodal: 2.39 ± 0.5; sham: 1.72 ± 0.3). Ratings for discomfort, fatigue and attention were comparable in all groups (discomfort, $F_{(2,34)}$ = 0.081; mean VAS 1-10 anodal: 4.06 ± 0.6; cathodal: 3.89 ± 0.5; sham: 3.78 ± 0.5; p = 0.923; fatigue, $F_{(2,34)}$ = 1.125, p = 0.336; mean VAS 1-10 anodal: 5.28 ± 0.7; cathodal: 4.61 ± 0.6; sham: 5.22 ± 0.7; attention, $F_{(2,34)}$ = 0.412, p = 0.665; mean VAS 1-10 anodal: 3.78 ± 0.5; cathodal: 4.33 ± 0.6; sham: 3.89 ± 0.6).

DISCUSSION

The aim of this study was to investigate associative word learning and the effect of tDCS over the MC during acquisition of a novel vocabulary in healthy older participants. Using a previously established associative language-learning paradigm (Liuzzi et al., 2010; Freundlieb et al., 2012), older participants acquired a novel vocabulary for everyday objects or actions. No specific effect of anodal or cathodal tDCS application on overall learning success was found, although as predicted there was an impairment of action word acquisition after cathodal tDCS stimulation.

The learning paradigm used here has been applied with some variations in previous studies (Breitenstein and Knecht, 2002; Dobel et al., 2009). Freundlieb et al. (2012) tested the efficiency of the paradigm for learning of novel object and action words in young adults in a single session design, without tDCS stimulation. Paradigm B of their study was similar to our approach except for their shorter visual presentation duration of 1400 ms. Young adults were able to translate 66% of novel words and showed reliable acquisition of the new lexicon, with an overall accuracy rate of 86% in the last block. Performance during the training did not differ between action-related and object-related words, but the translation test revealed significantly better learning of object-related (79%) than of action-related words (53%).

In our study, older participants did not perform as well as the young subjects from Freundlieb et al. (2012) both with respect to translation (66% in young adults, 39% in our older cohort in the sham condition) and correct decisions during training (86% correct decisions in the last block in young adults, 71% in our older population in the sham condition). Additionally, pretesting showed that learning in the older participants was only possible when picture presentation time was more than doubled compared with the duration for young participants. We cannot draw any firm conclusions about which specific process is most compromised in the older participants. Aging may impair both non-linguistic (visuospatial and auditory processing, working memory) as well as linguistic functioning (phonological processes, binding phonological information with semantic context). It can only be concluded that associative word learning is relatively preserved, but is considerably slowed down by aging.

Liuzzi et al. (2010) evaluated the functional role of the MC in action-word acquisition in young healthy participants. Using the same associative learning task that coupled spoken words with action-related pictures only, participants learned one set of 76 pseudowords during four consecutive training sessions. Either anodal, cathodal or sham tDCS stimulation over the MC was administered for 20 min prior to each session. Differences between their and our associative-learning paradigm concerned the number of novel words (76 overall vs. 34 per session), the use of action pictures or action and object pictures, visual presentation time (1400 vs. 3000 ms), the ratio between correct and incorrect couplings (4:2 vs. 10:1), a longer training duration (with training sessions on four consecutive days, with learning success measured on day four vs. three different sets and learning assessments each day) and the design (anodal, cathodal, sham between vs. within subjects). Liuzzi et al. (2010) could demonstrate that cathodal tDCS to the left MC led to a significantly reduced translation of novel action words compared to sham stimulation, whereas no effect was seen for anodal stimulation. Control experiments with object-related pseudowords or stimulation over prefrontal areas indicated a

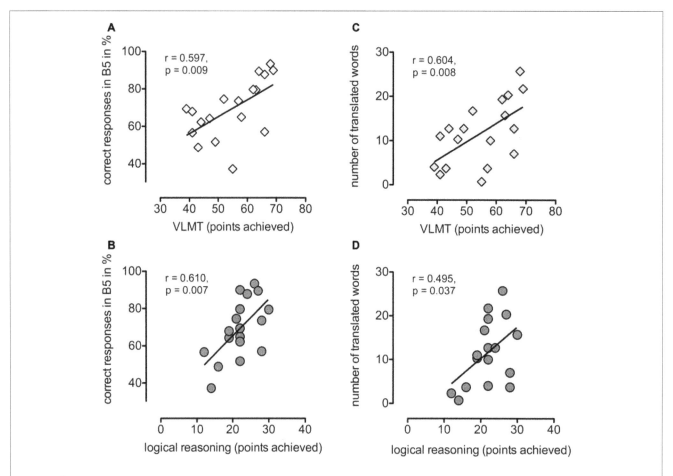

FIGURE 3 | Cognitive task performance and word learning. Left side: correlations between learning success measured as mean percentage of correct responses in block 5 and the performance scores of **(A)** VLMT (verbal learning and memory test) respectively **(B)** logical reasoning. Right side: correlations between number of correctly translated words and performance scores of **(C)** VLMT or **(D)** logical reasoning.

semantic and topographic specificity of the observed effect after cathodal tDCS over the MC (Liuzzi et al., 2010).

In older participants, we also observed that action-word acquisition after cathodal tDCS was significantly lower compared to the sham group. However, the effect was weaker compared with our previous study in young participants. This might be due to the single-session crossover design vs. repeated training over 4 days. Furthermore, while the study design of Liuzzi et al. (2010) allowed for consolidation effects overnight, the older participants were tested on the same day. It has been shown that the time for memory consolidation can have a crucial influence on novel word acquisition in an associative learning paradigm (Geukes et al., 2015). The effect of cathodal tDCS could only be shown in the NMDA-dependent stimulation period, supporting the idea that the MC is functionally connected during learning of novel action words. The pattern of results makes other effects like shifts of membrane polarization during the initial 20 min of stimulation less likely, given that inadvertent general effects on word learning could also not be shown in this study. As in young participants, we could not enhance learning with anodal tDCS over the MC.

In our participant group, verbal-learning ability showed good correlation with successful lexical acquisition. This finding is in line with previous findings in young healthy participants that showed a positive correlation of verbal-memory abilities with associative object word learning (Breitenstein and Knecht, 2002). More intriguing was the finding that logical reasoning and associative word learning were correlated. This is consistent with findings in aphasic patients, suggesting that preservation of executive functions may promote therapeutic outcome (Fillingham et al., 2005, 2006; Nicholas et al., 2005; Fridriksson et al., 2006). Different fMRI studies have shown that besides some task-specific regions decreasing in activity, especially prefrontal activation increases in older adults (Park and Reuter-Lorenz, 2009). The correlation of executive cognitive functions such as logical reasoning with lexical acquisition could hence suggest a compensatory strategy to maintain behavioral performance.

To summarize, associative learning imposes minimal demands on conscious effort compared with declarative vocabulary learning. This makes computer-based associative learning paradigms a promising tool for language learning in healthy aging. The ability for semantic transfer seems to be compromised in older people. Thus, training needs to be more intense in frequency and presentation times in order to build stable word representations.

Non-invasive brain stimulation techniques such as tDCS can be used to probe the interaction of specific brain areas with cognitive performance, to gain a better understanding of age-related changes of learning. Beyond this, the thorough knowledge of age-dependent cognitive skills in healthy older people might help to find predictive factors for language recovery in aphasic patients and to improve speech and language therapy.

AUTHOR CONTRIBUTIONS

GL: study conception and design. MB, JH, GL: acquisition, analysis and interpretation of data. MB, JH, GL: drafting the manuscript. GL, PZ, NF: critical revision. MB, JH, NF, PZ, GL: final approval of the version to be published and agreement to be accountable for all aspects of the work.

FUNDING

The present study was supported by the Deutsche Forschungsgemeinschaft (DFG LI 1892/1-1 to GL).

ACKNOWLEDGMENTS

We thank Annette Baumgärtner, Friedhelm Hummel and Christian Gerloff for their valuable comments on the present study and manuscript.

REFERENCES

Aschenbrenner, A., Chertov, O., and Lange, K. (2000). *RWT Regensburger Wortflüssigkeits-Test. Handanweisung.* Göttingen: Hogreve Verlag für Psychologie.

Breitenstein, C., and Knecht, S. (2002). Development and validation of a language learning model for behavioral and functional-imaging studies. *J. Neurosci. Methods* 114, 173–179. doi: 10.1016/s0165-0270(01)00525-8

Brickenkamp, R. (2002). *Test d2—Aufmerksamkeits-Belastungs-Test.* Göttingen: Hogreve Verlag für Psychologie.

Buccino, G., Riggio, L., Melli, G., Binkofski, F., Gallese, V., and Rizzolatti, G. (2005). Listening to action-related sentences modulates the activity of the motor system: a combined TMS and behavioral study. *Cogn. Brain Res.* 24, 355–363. doi: 10.1016/j.cogbrainres.2005.02.020

Chen, R., Tam, A., Bütefisch, C., Corwell, B., Ziemann, U., Rothwell, J. C., et al. (1998). Intracortical inhibition and facilitation in different representations of the human motor cortex. *J. Neurophysiol.* 80, 2870–2881.

Cohen, G. (1979). Language comprehension in old age. *Cogn. Psychol.* 11, 412–429. doi: 10.1016/0010-0285(79)90019-7

Cotelli, M., Manenti, R., Cappa, S. F., Zanetti, O., and Miniussi, C. (2008). Transcranial magnetic stimulation improves naming in Alzheimer disease patients at different stages of cognitive decline. *Eur. J. Neurol.* 15, 1286–1292. doi: 10.1111/j.1468-1331.2008.02202.x

Dobel, C., Junghöfer, M., Breitenstein, C., Klauke, B., Knecht, S., Pantev, C., et al. (2009). New names for known things: on the association of novel word forms with existing semantic information. *J. Cogn. Neurosci.* 22, 1251–1261. doi: 10.1162/jocn.2009.21297

Fillingham, J. K., Sage, K., and Lambon Ralph, M. A. (2006). The treatment of anomia using errorless learning. *Neuropsychol. Rehabil.* 16, 129–154. doi: 10.1080/09602010443000254

Fillingham, J. K., Sage, K., and Ralph, M. A. L. (2005). Treatment of anomia using errorless versus errorful learning: are frontal executive skills and feedback important? *Int. J. Lang. Commun. Disord.* 40, 505–523. doi: 10.1080/13682820500138572

Flöel, A., Ellger, T., Breitenstein, C., and Knecht, S. (2003). Language perception activates the hand motor cortex: implications for motor theories of speech perception. *Eur. J. Neurosci.* 18, 704–708. doi: 10.1046/j.1460-9568.2003.02774.x

Flöel, A., Suttorp, W., Kohl, O., Kürten, J., Lohmann, H., Breitenstein, C., et al. (2012). Non-invasive brain stimulation improves object-location learning in the elderly. *Neurobiol. Aging* 33, 1682–1689. doi: 10.1016/j.neurobiolaging.2011.05.007

Folstein, M. F., Folstein, S. E., and McHugh, P. R. (1975). "Mini-mental state." A practical method for grading the cognitive state of patients for the clinician. *J. Psychiatr. Res.* 12, 189–198. doi: 10.1016/0022-3956(75)90026-6

Freundlieb, N., Ridder, V., Dobel, C., Enriquez-Geppert, S., Baumgaertner, A., Zwitserlood, P., et al. (2012). Associative vocabulary learning: development and testing of two paradigms for the (re-) acquisition of action- and object-related words. *PLoS One* 7:e37033. doi: 10.1371/journal.pone.0037033

Fridriksson, J., Nettles, C., Davis, M., Morrow, L., and Montgomery, A. (2006). Functional communication and executive function in aphasia. *Clin. Linguist. Phon.* 20, 401–410. doi: 10.1080/02699200500075781

Gallese, V., and Lakoff, G. (2005). The brain's concepts: the role of the sensory-motor system in conceptual knowledge. *Cogn. Neuropsychol.* 22, 455–479. doi: 10.1080/02643290442000310

Gandiga, P. C., Hummel, F. C., and Cohen, L. G. (2006). Transcranial DC stimulation (tDCS): a tool for double-blind sham-controlled clinical studies in brain stimulation. *Clin. Neurophysiol.* 117, 845–850. doi: 10.1016/j.clinph.2005.12.003

Geukes, S., Gaskell, M. G., and Zwitserlood, P. (2015). Stroop effects from newly learned color words: effects of memory consolidation and episodic context. *Front. Psychol.* 6:278. doi: 10.3389/fpsyg.2015.00278

Hauk, O., and Pulvermüller, F. (2004). Neurophysiological distinction of action words in the fronto-central cortex. *Hum. Brain Mapp.* 21, 191–201. doi: 10.1002/hbm.10157

Helmstaedter, C., Lendt, M., and Lux, S. (2001). *Verbaler Lern- und Merkfähigkeitstest.* Göttingen: Beltz Test.

Hummel, F. C., Heise, K., Celnik, P., Floel, A., Gerloff, C., and Cohen, L. G. (2010). Facilitating skilled right hand motor function in older subjects by anodal polarization over the left primary motor cortex. *Neurobiol. Aging* 31, 2160–2168. doi: 10.1016/j.neurobiolaging.2008.12.008

Kemmerer, D., Rudrauf, D., Manzel, K., and Tranel, D. (2012). Behavioral patterns and lesion sites associated with impaired processing of lexical and conceptual knowledge of actions. *Cortex* 48, 826–848. doi: 10.1016/j.cortex.2010.11.001

Liebetanz, D., Nitsche, M. A., Tergau, F., and Paulus, W. (2002). Pharmacological approach to the mechanisms of transcranial DC-stimulation-induced after-effects of human motor cortex excitability. *Brain* 125, 2238–2247. doi: 10.1093/brain/awf238

Light, L. L., and Burke, D. M. (2009). "Patterns of language and memory in old age," in *Language, Memory, and Aging,* eds L. L. Light and D. M. Burke (Cambridge, MA: Cambridge University Press), 244–272.

Liuzzi, G., Freundlieb, N., Ridder, V., Hoppe, J., Heise, K., Zimerman, M., et al. (2010). The involvement of the left motor cortex in learning of a novel action word lexicon. *Curr. Biol.* 20, 1745–1751. doi: 10.1016/j.cub.2010.08.034

Miniussi, C., Cappa, S. F., Cohen, L. G., Floel, A., Fregni, F., Nitsche, M. A., et al. (2008). Efficacy of repetitive transcranial magnetic stimulation/transcranial direct current stimulation in cognitive neurorehabilitation. *Brain Stimul.* 4, 326–336. doi: 10.1016/j.brs.2008.07.002

Nicholas, M., Sinotte, M., and Helm-Estabrooks, N. (2005). Using a computer to communicate: effect of executive function impairments in people with severe aphasia. *Aphasiology* 19, 1052–1065. doi: 10.1080/02687030544000245

Nitsche, M. A., Nitsche, M. S., Klein, C. C., Tergau, F., Rothwell, J. C., and Paulus, W. (2003). Level of action of cathodal DC polarisation induced inhibition of the human motor cortex. *Clin. Neurophysiol.* 114, 600–604. doi: 10.1016/s1388-2457(02)00412-1

Nitsche, M. A., and Paulus, W. (2000). Excitability changes induced in the human motor cortex by weak transcranial direct current stimulation. *J. Physiol.* 527, 633–639. doi: 10.1111/j.1469-7793.2000.t01-1-00633.x

Park, D. C., and Reuter-Lorenz, P. (2009). The adaptive brain: aging and neurocognitive scaffolding. *Annu. Rev. Psychol.* 60, 173–196. doi: 10.1146/annurev.psych.59.103006.093656

Park, S.-H., Seo, J.-H., Kim, Y.-H., and Ko, M.-H. (2014). Long-term effects of transcranial direct current stimulation combined with computer-assisted cognitive training in healthy older adults. *Neuroreport* 25, 122–126. doi: 10.1097/WNR.0000000000000080

Pine, K. J., Bird, H., and Kirk, E. (2007). The effects of prohibiting gestures on children's lexical retrieval ability. *Dev. Sci.* 10, 747–754. doi: 10.1111/j.1467-7687.2007.00610.x

Pulvermüller, F. (2005). Brain mechanisms linking language and action. *Nat. Rev. Neurosci.* 6, 576–582. doi: 10.1038/nrn1706

Rauscher, F. H., Krauss, R. M., and Chen, Y. (1996). Gesture, speech, and lexical access: the role of lexical movements in speech production. *Psychol. Sci.* 7, 226–231. doi: 10.1111/j.1467-9280.1996.tb00364.x

Rey, A. (1959). *Manuel du Test de Copie D'une Figure Complexe de A. Rey.* Paris: Les Editions du Centre de Psychologie Appliquée.

Service, E., and Craik, F. I. M. (1993). Differences between young and older adults in learning A foreign vocabulary. *J. Mem. Lang.* 32, 608–623. doi: 10.1006/jmla.1993.1031

Zimerman, M., Nitsch, M., Giraux, P., Gerloff, C., Cohen, L. G., and Hummel, F. C. (2013). Neuroenhancement of the aging brain: restoring skill acquisition in old subjects. *Ann. Neurol.* 73, 10–15. doi: 10.1002/ana.23761

5

"Cerebellar Challenge" for Older Adults: Evaluation of a Home-Based Internet Intervention

Zoe Gallant and Roderick I. Nicolson[*†]

Department of Psychology, University of Sheffield, Sheffield, United Kingdom

*Correspondence:
Roderick I. Nicolson
rod.nicolson@edgehill.ac.uk

[†]**Present address:**
Roderick I. Nicolson,
Department of Psychology,
Edge Hill University, Ormskirk,
United Kingdom

There is converging evidence that maintenance of function in the multiple connectivity networks involving the cerebellum is a key requirement for healthy aging. The present study evaluated the effectiveness of a home-based, internet-administered "cerebellar challenge" intervention designed to create progressive challenges to vestibular function, multi-tasking, and dynamic coordination. Participants ($n = 98$, mean age 68.2, SD 6.6) were randomly allocated to either intervention (the cerebellar challenge training for 10 weeks) or no intervention. All participants undertook an initial series of pre-tests, and then an identical set of post-tests following the intervention period. The test battery comprised five suites of tests designed to evaluate cognitive-sensori-motor-affective functions, including Physical Coordination, Memory, Language Dexterity, Fluid Thinking and Affect. The intervention group showed significant pre- to post improvements in 9 of the 18 tests, whereas the controls improved significantly on one only. Furthermore, the intervention group showed significantly greater improvement than the controls on the "Physical Coordination" suite of tests, with evidence also of differential improvement on the Delayed Picture Recall test. Frequency of intervention use correlated significantly with the improvement in balance and in peg-moving speed. It is concluded that an internet-based cerebellar challenge programme for older adults can lead to benefits in balance, coordination and declarative memory. Limitations and directions for further research are outlined.

Keywords: declarative memory, cerebellum, hippocampus, sensorimotor, balance, vestibular stimulation, functional networks

INTRODUCTION

The brain and body form a complex, self-regulating system capable of coping with a range of environmental and cognitive challenges, together with the pervasive, age-related progressive impairment in function of many system components. In this article we develop the perspective that the functional networks involving the cerebellum represent a significant part of the degradation in aging. We then briefly review the many interventions that have proved efficacious with older adults, noting the current consensus that multi-component systems designed to maintain a progressive challenge appear to have greater effect than single component systems. On theoretical grounds we argue that interventions designed around "cerebellar challenge", combining coordinative exercise with cerebellar stimulation, should prove particularly effective. We finish by presenting an evaluation of an internet-based cerebellar challenge system, Zing, in terms of its effectiveness compared with a life-as-usual control group.

Traditional approaches to the causes of cognitive decline with aging considered primarily the frontal lobes (Jackson, 1958; Dempster, 1992; Greenwood, 2000). Over the past three decades there has been an explosion of research on all aspects of aging. Early this century extensive research was undertaken on changes in brain structure with aging (Raz et al., 2005), genetics (Deary et al., 2004; Erraji-Benchekroun et al., 2005), together with risk factors including increased white matter (Bartzokis, 2004; Head et al., 2004; Westlye et al., 2010; Sexton et al., 2014); excess homocysteine (Schafer et al., 2005) and reductions in dopamine and acetylcholamine neurotransmitters (Castner and Goldman-Rakic, 2004; Sarter and Bruno, 2004; Erixon-Lindroth et al., 2005).

Following these discoveries, arguably the greatest recent development has been the change of emphasis from these individual components and processes of the aging brain to consideration of the brain as a whole system. A major recent development in cognitive neuroscience has been the development of techniques for determining functional connectivity (Greicius et al., 2003; Fox et al., 2005; Buckner et al., 2008), and the consequent identification of a range of intrinsic networks (Yeo et al., 2011). The approach has great potential for characterizing the connectivity problems that affect brain function. A recent review (Bamidis et al., 2014) highlights the key role of connectivity changes in brain aging, and its implications for assessment and intervention.

It is notable that the cerebellum is also involved in seven of the major intrinsic networks (Buckner et al., 2011; Bernard et al., 2012; Kipping et al., 2013). It is therefore particularly interesting that circuits involving the cerebellum are strongly affected by age (Seidler et al., 2010; Balsters et al., 2013; Bernard et al., 2013; Humes et al., 2013; Bernard and Seidler, 2014; Koppelmans et al., 2015). Furthermore, it appears that the pattern of cerebellar degeneration with age in healthy adults is analogous to that shown by cerebellar patients (Hulst et al., 2015).

It is long established that there are major declines with age in sensory function (Humes et al., 2013; Wayne and Johnsrude, 2015; Roberts and Allen, 2016), in motor function (Seidler et al., 2010) and proprioceptive function (Goble et al., 2009). The cerebellum is centrally involved in sensorimotor processing (Chadderton et al., 2004, 2014; Ramakrishnan et al., 2016) and the involvement of the cerebellum in cognitive function is now fully established (Balsters et al., 2013; Mariën et al., 2014), as are direct, two-way links between the cerebellum and not only motor cortex but also prefrontal and posterior parietal cortex and the basal ganglia (Strick et al., 2009; Bostan et al., 2013).

Taken together, these results converge on the hypothesis (Bernard and Seidler, 2014) that the cerebellum—given its pervasive connectivity, its involvement in multiple sensory, cognitive and motor circuits; and its central role in adapting to internal changes—may be a critical component in the system degradation with age. This new conceptualization offers the promise that interventions designed to maintain or enhance cerebellar function may alleviate the affects of aging on sensori-motor-cognitive performance.

There are many successful interventions for alleviating age-related decline. A recent review (Ballesteros et al., 2015)

focused on three modes of intervention: physical activity, computerized cognitive training and social enhancement and concluded that although single domain interventions were effective the simultaneous training of both cognitive and physical domains offers a greater potential on daily life functioning. One of the key problems identified by the authors was the issue of how to combine different interventions and how to evaluate their effectiveness. The systems approach to healthy aging provides a theoretical perspective on this issue, suggesting that if a major cause if impairment is functional loss in the intrinsic connectivity networks, the optimal intervention should target function in the network as a whole, rather than individual components thereof.

Computerized cognitive training (CCT) approaches, using computer programs to boost core cognitive capabilities such as working memory, speed of processing and visual attention have proved highly effective in some studies, but less so in others. Systematic reviews of brain training programmes with older adults (Gross et al., 2012; Kueider et al., 2012) concluded that computerized training is an effective, less labor intensive alternative to cognitive training. In contrast, a recent analysis (Lampit et al., 2014) concluded that the overall effect size of CCT vs. control was small and statistically significant for nonverbal memory, verbal memory, working memory, processing speed, and visuospatial skills but not for executive functions and attention. A meta-analysis for younger groups (Melby-Lervåg and Hulme, 2013) concluded that WM programs produced reliable short-term improvements in WM skills but that the effects were "short-term, specific training effects that do not generalize".

One of the clear limitations, from a systems view, both of CCT and of direct brain stimulation, is that the intervention is artificial, and isolated from the physical or mental activities involved in normal system functionality. There is strong evidence that natural activities, such as exercise, can improve not only physical fitness but also mental fitness, and even stimulate the growth of new brain neurons and connections (Hillman et al., 2008; Höetting and Röeder, 2013; Kirk-Sanchez and McGough, 2014). An innovative approach, the Long-Lasting Memories intervention, which combines both exercise and CCT approaches ("exergaming") was shown to have beneficial effects for healthy older adults and for those with Mild Cognitive Impairment (MCI; González-Palau et al., 2014).

A recent discovery has been the differential effects of cardiovascular, high intensity, exercise and "co-ordinative exercise" such as balance training or tai-chi. There is strong evidence that exercise can potentiate the brain for new learning, with coordinative balance exercises leading to neural growth in the hippocampus—a core structure for explicit learning and memory (Niemann et al., 2014)—and also in the cerebellar-cortical loop (Burciu et al., 2013)—a core network for implicit learning and coordination. A further study (Nascimento et al., 2014) concluded that multimodal physical exercise was effective in reducing pro-inflammatory cytokines and in improving brain-derived neurotrophic factor (BDNF) peripheral levels, with positive reflexes on cognition in elderly individuals with MCI.

Recent studies of the effects of exercise on rat brains (Kellermann et al., 2012; Abel and Rissman, 2013) reveal strong effects on epigenetic changes and changes in the cerebellar Purkinje cells following a rat vestibular training exercise (Lee et al., 2015). There is also evidence that BDNF is expressed in the cerebellum following environmental enrichment for rats (Angelucci et al., 2009; Vazquez-Sanroman et al., 2013). Of particular interest, there is evidence (though sparse) that Quadrato exercise (like Tai Chi) led to increased creativity and changes in gray matter and white matter in the cerebellum (Ben-Soussan et al., 2015).

There have also been detailed neuroimaging studies of interventions for special groups. Daily clinic-based balance training for 2 weeks in cerebellar patients and age-matched healthy controls (Burciu et al., 2013) led to enhanced balance performance in the patients, with associated increased gray matter volume in the dorsal premotor cortex and within the cerebellum for both groups. A 6 week balance-training study with Parkinson's patients and healthy controls (Sehm et al., 2014) led to improved balance which was maintained for the following year, together with increased gray matter in the hippocampus for the controls and in several brain regions for the patients.

Of particular interest regarding functional connectivity, two recent studies with older adults with MCI have established functional connectivity changes following 8 week interventions. Klados et al. (2016) established that the Long Lasting Memories intervention led to increased beta-band EEG activity (reflecting increased bilateral connections in the occipital, parietal, temporal and prefrontal regions) after the intervention. Chirles et al. (2017) undertook a "walking exercise" intervention, and established that following the intervention the MCI group showed increased connectivity in 10 regions spanning frontal, parietal, temporal and insular lobes, together with the cerebellum.

In summary, current neuroimaging and behavioral research appears to be converging to a view that: (i) a systems approach to aging is the most promising framework for understanding the degradation in multiple functions with age; (ii) there is extensive evidence that the cerebellum is one of the key structures affected, and the multiple intrinsic connectivity networks linking the cerebellum with other brain and body structures may well mediate many of the actual deficits shown; (iii) "single system" interventions can be effective, but generally it is better to have multiple domain interventions; (iv) a range of interventions, from coordinative exercise to direct vestibular stimulation are likely to have beneficial effects on cerebellar function.

The above considerations informed the design of the current study. We wished to evaluate the effectiveness of a novel internet-based "vestibular stimulation" intervention, the Zing intervention[1]. This intervention was originally developed to tune up the coordination abilities of top sporting performers, using a series of graded exercises designed specifically to improve three performance dimensions: sensorimotor coordination, eye movement control and dual tasking. However, extensive feedback had suggested that the programme was valuable for many average performers. Consequently the system was

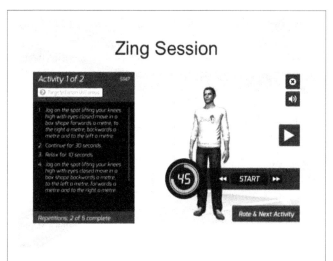

FIGURE 1 | Sample screen from the Zing intervention. This is an example of a screen from the focus strand, at a low level and aimed at developing dual tasking ability.

embedded in an internet-based "game" format designed to challenge and stimulate the user to keep improving their performance. Zing Performance offer a number of courses specifically tailored to each individual user, with applications in sporting areas, organizational development, in education.

The Zing system involves a series of graded activities on three dimensions—dynamic activity (patterned movement sequences), focus activity (developing the ability both to concentrate and to "dual task") and stability activity (coordinative balance). Underpinning the approach is the technique of vestibular stimulation. Rather than cardiovascular exercise, which is designed to have energetic use of highly practised routines, or even coordinative balance such as tai-chi, which does involve learning new actions, vestibular activities are designed to cause abnormal input for the vestibular system, for example by requiring the user to put their head on one side while undertaking tasks. This presents the vestibular system, and the cerebellum, with an immediate challenge, requiring activation of many circuits to cope with the ensuing proprioceptive feedback.

A typical course lasts 6 months and is composed of daily physical activities and digital video games. An example of a low level focus activity (at the time of the study) is given in **Figure 1**. A video is also available for each activity.

The Zing platform therefore provides a user-orientated, motivating framework for delivering a cost-effective cerebellar challenge intervention that satisfies the criteria that have emerged for multimodal, challenging interventions in older adults.

We undertook the study to investigate whether internet-based approaches can indeed be an effective and popular method for older adults, and designed an 8 week intervention. It is important to highlight that although this is a Randomized Control Trial (RCT) study, in that there was a control condition and allocation to condition was random, it is not a full RCT, for which an active intervention condition, matched in time and form to the Zing intervention, would need to be used to counter placebo-type effects. Our view is that this non-equivalent–control RCT (NEC-RCT) design is appropriate for a user-centered trial that has the underlying question "If participants undertake the intervention, will it help them, and, if so, in what ways?" We are not investigating the theoretical issue—is intervention A more effective than intervention B, and if so, why? Each design has its strengths and weaknesses. For the purpose of evaluating whether a low-cost, home-based intervention might be beneficial compared with life-as-usual, the NEC-RCT design is the appropriate one.

A limitation of many previous intervention studies is that the set of tests used from pre-intervention to post-intervention focus on a limited range of performance measures. As noted above, there is reason to expect that a cerebellar challenge intervention might lead to changes in both the sensorimotor domain and in the cognitive domain. There is also longstanding evidence that the cerebellum is involved in emotional processing (Schmahmann and Sherman, 1997), with emerging evidence regarding its involvement in processing emotional salience (Styliadis et al., 2015; Adamaszek et al., 2017). There is also evidence that the resting state networks involving the cerebellum are associated with differences in crystallized intelligence (Pezoulas et al., 2017). Consequently we designed a battery of simple tasks designed to probe sensorimotor, performance, cognitive performance, emotional state and nonverbal reasoning.

The design allows the following hypotheses to be evaluated.

Hypothesis 1. Improvements in balance and sensorimotor coordination. This is the primary applied hypothesis, directly related to attempting to boost balance performance and thus decrease the danger of falling. One in three people of 65 fall at least once per year, with the incidence rising to one half of those over 80 years old (Todd and Skelton, 2004). Falls are a major cost to elderly people and to national health services, estimated to account for 21% of the Dutch health service costs for injuries (Hartholt et al., 2011). Hypothesis 1 states that Zing training will lead to significant improvements in sensorimotor coordination especially balance: (a) for each individual compared with their pre-training; (b) that the intervention group will improve significantly more than a control, no intervention, group.

Hypothesis 2. "Hippocampal" improvements. This hypothesis is derived from the research showing the benefits of coordinative balance training for hippocampal function. Hypothesis 2 states that Zing training will lead to significant improvements in "declarative memory" performance: (a) for each individual compared with their pre-training; (b) that the intervention group will improve significantly more than a control, no intervention, group.

Hypothesis 3. Improvement Specificity. Despite the emerging evidence of cerebellar involvement in affective processing, we would expect any such changes to be of secondary importance in terms of affective state. Consequently, although Zing training may lead to significant "transfer" to other areas, including language, affect and fluid reasoning, any such effects will be minor compared with the specific improvements in hippocampal and sensorimotor skills.

MATERIALS AND METHODS

Participants
Ninety-eight volunteers (30 male, 68 female) aged 50–85 (mean 68.2, SD 6.6) were recruited through advertisements in local newspapers, churches and social groups. An advert also went out on the University of the Third Age Sheffield website. Participants were all without a known diagnosis of dementia. The ethics committee of the Department of Psychology, University of Sheffield, approved the study. Participants gave fully informed prior consent. They were also informed that their information would be anonymised and kept securely. They were also informed that they could withdraw from the study at any time without needing to give any reason. All participants were healthy older adults.

Design
The aim of this study was to test the effectiveness of vestibular stimulation on physical and mental function. Therefore, a repeated measures design was used. Participants were asked to complete a baseline set of tests at the University of Sheffield Department of Psychology before taking part in the 8 week Zing intervention at home. They were then asked to return to the department for a repeat of the baseline tests.

Test Battery
The same tests were used both pre and post-test. While there may be some practice effects here, it would be expected that this would affect both groups equally, and therefore any relative difference in the intervention group's performance is likely to be attributable to the exercises.

We wished to evaluate changes in all the core physical, mental and affective domains, using simple but normed tests where possible. We based the battery on the Dyslexia Adult Screening Test (Fawcett and Nicolson, 1998), which covers the majority of the necessary tests in a 30 min package. We constructed a battery of 14 tests, divided into five suites. Suite 1 was for Physical Coordination and comprised the DAST balance test, the two Purdue pegboard (Tiffin and Asher, 1948) tests (Peg Moving and Peg Assembly), and the DAST writing (copying) test. Suite 2 investigated memory. It included two tests of working memory, the DAST backwards digit span test and the South Yorkshire Ageing Study (Tarmey, 2012) Spatial Memory test which determines spatial memory span for non-verbalizable pictures presented in one of eight locations. There was one declarative memory test, the South Yorkshire Ageing Study (Tarmey, 2012) Picture Memory test which assesses recall for a set of 20 pictures of common objects, presented sequentially for 1 s, including both immediate recall and delayed recall after 20 min. The Language Suite comprised the DAST Rapid Naming, Phonological Processing, Reading, Nonsense Passage and Spelling tests. The Fluid Reasoning suite comprised the DAST Nonverbal Reasoning, Semantic Fluency and Verbal Fluency tests. Finally two tests of affect were administered: the Beck Depression Inventory (BDI; Beck et al., 1996) and the Authentic Happiness Inventory (Seligman, 2002).

Intervention Training

Participants were required to undertake a minimum of 8 weeks and maximum of 10 weeks balance and sensorimotor coordination training using an online set of activities. These were provided by Zing Performance Ltd., and were designed specifically to stimulate brain regions involved in coordinative balance. Initially, participants had to undergo an assessment to determine their strengths and weaknesses. After this a 30 day programme was set for them, specifically designed to target their biggest needs. Participants were required to do two exercises a day, before rating how difficult they found that particular activity. A screen shot is shown in **Figure 1** below. Each week, three exercises were assigned, with two of the three appearing each day. After 30 days, participants were reassessed before continuing onto unit two. It should be noted that a full Zing 360 session programme is designed for 6 months, with two sessions per day. Consequently this study is very much shorter than intended by the Zing designers.

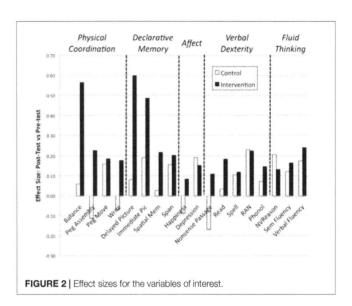

FIGURE 2 | Effect sizes for the variables of interest.

RESULTS

Data were converted to standard scores (mean 100, SD 15) to allow direct comparison across tasks. Where possible, population norms and standard deviations were used to normalize test scores. The population norm for age 55+ was used for all participants, irrespective of age, to represent absolute performance rather than age-adjusted performance.

Effect Sizes

In order to facilitate comparison of the improvements (or otherwise) in performance from pre-test to post-test, effect sizes were calculated using the formula ES = (post-test − pre-test) / SD (all groups on pre-test), which is a form of Cohen, 1988 applied to change analysis. No change would result in an effect size of 0, whereas a score of +1.0 indicates a change of one standard deviation unit. Cohen (1988) suggests that effect sizes of 0.8, 0.5 and 0.2 be labeled large, medium and small, respectively.

Effect sizes for the two groups are shown in **Figure 2**. Tests have been grouped in order of the hypotheses. The Physical Coordination suite—postural stability, peg moving, peg assembly and handwriting speed are on the left, then the Memory Suite—immediate picture recall, delayed picture recall, immediate spatial memory and immediate verbal memory. Group 3 include the affect measures—the BDI (reverse scored such that higher means less depressed) and the Authentic Happiness Index. The remaining tests are the Language Suite and the Fluid Thinking Suite but were not predicted to be affected by the intervention.

Correlations with Zing Usage

Next correlational analyses were undertaken utilizing data collected automatically on "compliance" for the Zing group. Of the 53 participants allocated to the Zing group, 38 completed at least 40 sessions, as requested, but the differential uptake allowed us to investigate the effects both of frequency of Zing use (sessions per week) and the duration (number of weeks). For the frequency of Zing use significant correlations were found for

peg movement ($r = 0.31$, $p < 0.05$), and for postural stability ($r = 0.303$, $p < 0.05$). A significant correlation with number of weeks of the intervention occurred only for nonverbal reasoning ($r = 0.288, p < 0.05$).

Within-Group Statistical Tests

Inferential statistical tests were then undertaken for the 16 tests within the five suites of tests. First repeated measures multivariate analyses of variance were undertaken for each suite separately on the data for pre-test and post-test for each test within the suite.

For the control group, none of the set of MANOVAs approached significance. In fact the only individual comparison to reach the uncorrected 0.05 significance level was for peg moving ($F_{(1,43)} = 6.26, p = 0.016$).

For the Zing group, the MANOVA analyses of the change from pre-test to post-test were highly significant for the suites for Physical Coordination, for Declarative Memory, for Language, and for Fluid Thinking ($F_{(1,47)} = 22.95$, $p < 0.001$; $F_{(1,52)} = 10.71$, $p = 0.002$; $F_{(1,52)} = 15.99$, $p < 0.001$; $F_{(1,52)} = 5.72$, $p = 0.020$ respectively), whereas there was no difference for the Affect suite. It is not sensible to undertake a Bonferroni correction for multiple comparison when all comparisons are significant in the same direction (Moran, 2003), and consequently uncorrected probabilities are reported. The changes for Balance, Peg Assembly and Peg Movement were significant ($F_{(1,50)} = 14.07$, $p < 0.001$; $F_{(1,51)} = 5.53$, $p = 0.023$; $F_{(1,50)} = 4.10$, $p = 0.048$ respectively). The improvements for Delayed Picture Recall, Immediate Picture Recall and Memory Span were also significant ($F_{(1,52)} = 14.44$, $p < 0.001$; $F_{(1,52)} = 15.41$, $p < 0.001$; $F_{(1,52)} = 4.20$, $p = 0.046$ respectively). Two of the improvements for nonsense passage reading, 1 min reading, rapid naming and spelling were significant [$F_{(1,52)} = 3.72$, $p = 0.059$; $F_{(1,52)} = 6.28$, $p = 0.015$; $F_{(1,52)} = 4.73$, $p = 0.034$; $F_{(1,52)} = 3.28$, $p = 0.076$). The improvement for verbal fluency was also significant ($F_{(1,52)} = 5.13, p = 0.028$).

Between-Group Statistical Tests

Finally, in the most stringent test of the changes, a series of multivariate 2-factor analyses of variance was undertaken, with the independent groups factor being the group (Zing vs. Control) and the repeated measure being time-of-test (pre-test vs. post-test. Manovas were undertaken separately for each of the five suites (see **Table 1**). For the MANOVA entry, only the key statistic, the interaction term between time of test (pre vs. post) and Group is reported. A significant interaction would typically indicate that the Intervention led to a significant difference between groups at post-test whereas performance at pre-test was equivalent.

It may be seen that the only suite returning a significant MANOVA result was the Physical Coordination suite. For each of the four tests a univariate two factor mixed measures analysis of variance was undertaken, with the within-group variable being time-of-test (pre-intervention vs. post-intervention) and the between-group variable being group (intervention vs. control). Significant (uncorrected) interactions—all reflecting greater improvement for the intervention group than the control group—were obtained for postural stability and for peg assembly. By contrast, there were no differences for peg moving speed or writing speed.

The MANOVA results for the other four suites of tests were not close to significance. Uncorrected significant differences were obtained for Delayed Picture Memory and for Nonsense Passage Reading.

Correlations with Age

Finally, correlations with age were calculated. Significant correlations were found for performance on the majority of tests, with correlations between age and each dependent variable in descending order being -0.47 (Nonverbal reasoning), -0.40 (peg assembly), -0.38 (immediate picture memory), -0.35 (immediate picture memory), -0.34 (writing), -0.28 (spatial memory), -0.27 (semantic fluency), -0.26 (postural stability) and -0.26 (spelling). Correlations between age and the amount of improvement for the Zing group were also calculated. Few correlations were significant, with only peg assembly (-0.37) being more extreme than -0.25.

DISCUSSION

The primary issue addressed by this study was whether a home-based cerebellar challenge internet-administered intervention was feasible for use with older adults and, if used, whether it would result in better balance, and hence reduce danger of falling (Hypothesis 1). A secondary, theoretical issue, was whether the intervention might also improve cognitive functions previously found to be improved by coordinative balance training (Hypothesis 2).

A set of five "suites" of tests was applied before and after the intervention, allowing comparison with a "life as usual" control group. Comparing individual performances across the intervention period, the control group performance remained roughly constant, with no significant change for 17 of the 18 tests. By contrast, the intervention participants showed significant improvement in their scores for 9 of the 18 tests administered, with only the tests of the Affect suite showing no significant multivariate improvement.

Furthermore, a series of two factor multivariate analyses of variance revealed that the intervention group improved significantly more than the control group on the Physical Coordination suite, but not on the memory suite, the affect suite, the language suite or the fluency suite.

Hypothesis 1 is therefore clearly supported. Not surprisingly—but crucial for applied purposes—the intervention group did improve significantly on balance compared both with their own pre-intervention performance and with the control group's change in balance over the period of the study. There was also transfer of this training effect to manual dexterity (as indicated by the "peg assembly" task).

Clear support is also provided for Hypothesis 2, though the effect is masked by the inclusion of tests of working memory and declarative memory within the memory suite. It is clear from the effect sizes and the between-groups anova data that there was a significant benefit for the Zing group for the tests of declarative memory (especially the key task of delayed picture recall, which is more akin to a realistic memory use task) but not for the tests of working memory. It is therefore legitimate to infer that, consistent with the literature on the benefits of balance training on hippocampal function, there was transfer of this benefit to declarative memory in the delayed picture recall condition (Hypothesis 2).

The specificity of the differential benefit findings to the hypotheses suggests strongly that the changes are not a practice, placebo or Hawthorne effect (Hypothesis 3). Given the null effect on affect, we examined the individual scores on the BDI in order to investigate whether participants more at risk of depression showed differential effects. Of the four participants in the intervention group classifiable as at least mildly depressed, one showed marked improvement. However, the 2 participants

TABLE 1 | Multivariate and univariate analyses of variance for the variables of interest.

(1) Physical coordination	Manova: $F_{(1,87)} = 9.47$, $p = 0.003$
Postural stability	$F_{(1,89)} = 5.24$, $p = 0.024$, $\eta^2 = 0.056$
Peg assembly	$F_{(1,92)} = 4.36$, $p = 0.040$, $\eta^2 = 0.045$
Peg move	$F_{(1,94)} = 0.03$, $p = 0.864$, $\eta^2 = 0.000$
Writing	$F_{(1,92)} = 0.10$, $p = 0.754$, $\eta^2 = 0.001$
(2) Declarative memory	Manova: $F_{(1,93)} = 1.09$, $p = 0.300$
Delayed picture recall	$F_{(1,93)} = 4.58$, $p = 0.035$, $\eta^2 = 0.047$
Immediate picture recall	$F_{(1,93)} = 1.78$, $p = 0.185$, $\eta^2 = 0.019$
Spatial memory	$F_{(1,93)} = 1.05$, $p = 0.308$, $\eta^2 = 0.011$
Verbal memory span	$F_{(1,93)} = 0.15$, $p = 0.703$, $\eta^2 = 0.002$
(3) Language	Manova: $F_{(1,93)} = 2.57$, $p = 0.113$
Nonsense passage reading	$F_{(1,93)} = 4.20$, $p = 0.043$, $\eta^2 = 0.043$
One minute reading	$F_{(1,93)} = 1.72$, $p = 0.193$, $\eta^2 = 0.018$
Rapid naming	$F_{(1,93)} = 0.01$, $p = 0.933$, $\eta^2 = 0.000$
2 min spelling	$F_{(1,93)} = 0.01$, $p = 0.979$, $\eta^2 = 0.000$
Spoonerisms	$F_{(1,93)} = 0.13$, $p = 0.715$, $\eta^2 = 0.001$
(4) Fluid thinking	Manova: $F_{(1,93)} = 0.06$, $p = 0.813$
Nonverbal reasoning	$F_{(1,93)} = 0.11$, $p = 0.742$, $\eta^2 = 0.001$
Semantic fluency	$F_{(1,93)} = 0.06$, $p = 0.805$, $\eta^2 = 0.000$
Verbal fluency	$F_{(1,93)} = 0.32$, $p = 0.571$, $\eta^2 = 0.003$
(5) Affect	Manova: $F_{(1,93)} = 0.99$, $p = 0.755$
Authentic happiness index	$F_{(1,93)} = 2.38$, $p = 0.127$, $\eta^2 = 0.025$
Beck depression inventory	$F_{(1,94)} = 0.02$, $p = 0.890$, $\eta^2 = 0.001$

in the non-intervention group initially showing mild depression also showed marked improvement. We conclude that, at least in this group of heathy older adults, the results do not suggest that there is a direct effect of the cerebellar challenge intervention on affective state.

Of the 52 participants selected for the intervention condition, 38 (73%) completed the requested 40 sessions over 8 weeks. Analyses of the "dose effect" (that is, correlations of performance improvement with number of intervention sessions for the intervention group) revealed significant correlations with intervention frequency for peg movement, reading and balance, with a significant correlation with intervention duration for nonverbal reasoning.

In terms of the participants' response to the intervention, it should be noted that the Zing platform was a prototype version, not yet publicly available and in the process of substantial development and improvement. A sizeable minority of the Zing participants reported difficulties in accessing the system initially, though subsequently problems were relatively small.

It is important to acknowledge the limitations of this study. First, the population sampled was by no means random, involving respondents to a circular. They should therefore be seen as relatively high functioning and with good self efficacy. Furthermore, they represented a spread of ages, with 2 under 55, 27 aged 55–64, 55 aged 65–74 and 15 aged 75 and over. There was a considerable imbalance between the sexes, with 30 male and 68 female. All were living at home in reasonable health. All of these factors reduce the strength of inferences that can be made regarding generalization to the full population of community based older adults, and highlight the need for further research.

CONCLUSION

Prior research has established that home-based balance exercises are among the most cost-effective methods of improving balance ability and hence reducing falls in older adults. Recent developments in cognitive neuroscience have revealed that "coordinative" balance training is likely to have beneficial effects not only on physical coordination but also on hippocampal function. Our theoretical analyses suggested that a multi-component, cerebellar challenge intervention should prove highly effective, combining the effectiveness of coordinative exercise with that of direct cerebellar stimulation, and therefore improving function in the intrinsic connectivity networks involving the cerebellum. The study design did not include brain imaging, and therefore it is not possible to assess directly any underlying neural changes. Furthermore the study design does not permit comparison of the Zing approach with a suitable active control. Nonetheless, the results were encouraging.

The present study is unique in two ways: first we investigated a highly cost-effective internet-based "cerebellar challenge" intervention, "Zing". Second we investigated physical coordination, mental coordination, language, fluid thinking and affect using a specially developed battery of tests. Significant benefits (comparing initial performance with post-intervention performance) were found for the intervention group on the majority of the tests, excluding only those for affect. Furthermore, significantly greater improvements were found for the intervention group (compared with the control group) for balance, for physical coordination and for declarative memory retrieval.

Further research, including research using an active control intervention, would be needed to pinpoint the theoretical causes of the improvements obtained. Nonetheless, given the minimal cost and considerable ease of access of the intervention, it provides a promising approach to improving the overall cerebellar-related function, protecting against subsequent balance problems, and may also benefit declarative memory in older adults.

AUTHOR CONTRIBUTIONS

Both authors contributed to all aspects of the empirical work, the data analysis and the article writing. ZG had a stronger focus on the empirical work, and RIN had a stronger focus on design and theoretical interpretation.

FUNDING

The research was undertaken as part of ZG's doctoral research at the University of Sheffield. This was supported by a fees-only award from the University of Sheffield. The research was undertaken in 2014/15. In 2016 Nicolson was appointed to the scientific advisory board of Zing Performance Outreach, a non-profit charitable organization.

ACKNOWLEDGMENTS

We gratefully acknowledge the support of Samantha Critchley, Mark Manser and Gareth Dore of Zing Performance in helping to resolve any difficulties encountered by the participants. We acknowledge with thanks the contributions made in the pre-test and post-test assessments by Caroline Carta, Penny Jackson, Phil Roughsedge and Laura Scott.

REFERENCES

Abel, J. L., and Rissman, E. F. (2013). Running-induced epigenetic and gene expression changes in the adolescent brain. *Int. J. Dev. Neurosci.* 31, 382–390. doi: 10.1016/j.ijdevneu.2012.11.002

Adamaszek, M., D'Agata, F., Ferrucci, R., Habas, C., Keulen, S., Kirkby, K. C., et al. (2017). Consensus paper: cerebellum and emotion. *Cerebellum* 16, 552–576. doi: 10.1007/s12311-016-0815-8

Angelucci, F., De Bartolo, P., Gelfo, F., Foti, F., Cutuli, D., Bossù, P., et al. (2009). Increased concentrations of nerve growth factor and brain-derived neurotrophic factor in the rat cerebellum after exposure to environmental enrichment. *Cerebellum* 8, 499–506. doi: 10.1007/s12311-009-0129-1

Ballesteros, S., Kraft, E., Santana, S., and Tziraki, C. (2015). Maintaining older brain functionality: a targeted review. *Neurosci. Biobehav. Rev.* 55, 453–477. doi: 10.1016/j.neubiorev.2015.06.008

Balsters, J. H., Whelan, C. D., Robertson, I. H., and Ramnani, N. (2013). Cerebellum and cognition: evidence for the encoding of higher order rules. *Cereb. Cortex* 23, 1433–1443. doi: 10.1093/cercor/bhs127

Bamidis, P. D., Vivas, A. B., Styliadis, C., Frantzidis, C., Klados, M., Schlee, W., et al. (2014). A review of physical and cognitive interventions in aging. *Neurosci. Biobehav. Rev.* 44, 206–220. doi: 10.1016/j.neubiorev.2014.03.019

Bartzokis, G. (2004). Age-related myelin breakdown: a developmental model of cognitive decline and Alzheimer's disease. *Neurobiol. Aging* 25, 5–18. doi: 10.1016/j.neurobiolaging.2003.03.001

Beck, A., Steer, R., and Brown, G. (1996). *Beck Depression Inventory*. San Antonio, TX: The Psychological Corporation.

Ben-Soussan, T. D., Berkovich-Ohana, A., Piervincenzi, C., Glicksohn, J., and Carducci, F. (2015). Embodied cognitive flexibility and neuroplasticity following Quadrato Motor Training. *Front. Psychol.* 6:1021. doi: 10.3389/fpsyg.2015.01021

Bernard, J. A., Peltier, S. J., Wiggins, J. L., Jaeggi, S. M., Buschkuehl, M., Fling, B. W., et al. (2013). Disrupted cortico-cerebellar connectivity in older adults. *Neuroimage* 83, 103–119. doi: 10.1016/j.neuroimage.2013.06.042

Bernard, J. A., and Seidler, R. D. (2014). Moving forward: age effects on the cerebellum underlie cognitive and motor declines. *Neurosci. Biobehav. Rev.* 42, 193–207. doi: 10.1016/j.neubiorev.2014.02.011

Bernard, J. A., Seidler, R. D., Hassevoort, K. M., Benson, B. L., Welsh, R. C., Wiggins, J. L., et al. (2012). Resting state cortico-cerebellar functional connectivity networks: a comparison of anatomical and self-organizing map approaches. *Front. Neuroanat.* 6:31. doi: 10.3389/fnana.2012.00031

Bostan, A. C., Dum, R. P., and Strick, P. L. (2013). Cerebellar networks with the cerebral cortex and basal ganglia. *Trends Cogn. Sci.* 17, 241–254. doi: 10.1016/j.tics.2013.03.003

Buckner, R. L., Andrews-Hanna, J. R., and Schacter, D. L. (2008). The brain's default network—Anatomy, function, and relevance to disease. *Ann. N Y Acad. Sci.* 1124, 1–38. doi: 10.1196/annals.1440.011

Buckner, R. L., Krienen, F. M., Castellanos, A., Diaz, J. C., and Yeo, B. T. T. (2011). The organization of the human cerebellum estimated by intrinsic functional connectivity. *J. Neurophysiol.* 106, 2322–2345. doi: 10.1152/jn.00339.2011

Burciu, R. G., Fritsche, N., Granert, O., Schmitz, L., Spöenemann, N., Konczak, J., et al. (2013). Brain changes associated with postural training in patients with cerebellar degeneration: a voxel-based morphometry study. *J. Neurosci.* 33, 4594–4604. doi: 10.1523/jneurosci.3381-12.2013

Castner, S. A., and Goldman-Rakic, P. S. (2004). Enhancement of working memory in aged monkeys by a sensitizing regimen of dopamine D_1 receptor stimulation. *J. Neurosci.* 24, 1446–1450. doi: 10.1523/jneurosci.3987-03.2004

Chadderton, P., Margrie, T. W., and Häusser, M. (2004). Integration of quanta in cerebellar granule cells during sensory processing. *Nature* 428, 856–860. doi: 10.1038/nature02442

Chadderton, P., Schaefer, A. T., Williams, S. R., and Margrie, T. W. (2014). Sensory-evoked synaptic integration in cerebellar and cerebral cortical neurons. *Nat. Rev. Neurosci.* 15, 71–83. doi: 10.1038/nrn3648

Chirles, T. J., Reiter, K., Weiss, L. R., Alfini, A. J., Nielson, K. A., and Smith, J. C. (2017). Exercise training and functional connectivity changes in mild cognitive impairment and healthy elders. *J. Alzheimers Dis.* 57, 845–856. doi: 10.3233/jad-161151

Cohen, J. (1988). *Statistical Power Analysis for the Behavioral Sciences.* 2nd Edn. New York, NY: Academic Press.

Deary, I. J., Wright, A. F., Harris, S. E., Whalley, L. J., and Starr, J. M. (2004). Searching for genetic influences on normal cognitive ageing. *Trends Cogn. Sci.* 8, 178–184. doi: 10.1016/j.tics.2004.02.008

Dempster, F. N. (1992). The rise and fall of the inhibitory mechanism: toward a unified theory of cognitive development and aging. *Dev. Rev.* 12, 45–75. doi: 10.1016/0273-2297(92)90003-k

Erixon-Lindroth, N., Farde, L., Wahlin, T. B. R., Sovago, J., Halldin, C., and Bäckman, L. (2005). The role of the striatal dopamine transporter in cognitive aging. *Psychiatry Res.* 138, 1–12. doi: 10.1016/j.pscychresns.2004.09.005

Erraji-Benchekroun, L., Underwood, M. D., Arango, V., Galfalvy, H., Pavlidis, P., Smyrniotopoulos, P., et al. (2005). Molecular aging in human prefrontal cortex is selective and continuous throughout adult life. *Biol. Psychiatry* 57, 549–558. doi: 10.1016/j.biopsych.2004.10.034

Fawcett, A. J., and Nicolson, R. I. (1998). *The Dyslexia Adult Screening Test.* London: The Psychological Corporation.

Fox, M. D., Snyder, A. Z., Vincent, J. L., Corbetta, M., Van Essen, D. C., and Raichle, M. E. (2005). The human brain is intrinsically organized into dynamic, anticorrelated functional networks. *Proc. Natl. Acad. Sci. U S A* 102, 9673–9678. doi: 10.1073/pnas.0504136102

Goble, D. J., Coxon, J. P., Wenderoth, N., Van Impe, A., and Swinnen, S. P. (2009). Proprioceptive sensibility in the elderly: degeneration, functional consequences and plastic-adaptive processes. *Neurosci. Biobehav. Rev.* 33, 271–278. doi: 10.1016/j.neubiorev.2008.08.012

González-Palau, F., Franco, M., Bamidis, P., Losada, R., Parra, E., Papageorgiou, S. G., et al. (2014). The effects of a computer-based cognitive and physical training program in a healthy and mildly cognitive impaired aging sample. *Aging Ment. Health* 18, 838–846. doi: 10.1080/13607863.2014.899972

Greenwood, P. M. (2000). The frontal aging hypothesis evaluated. *J. Int. Neuropsycholog. Soc.* 6, 705–726. doi: 10.1017/s1355617700666092

Greicius, M. D., Krasnow, B., Reiss, A. L., and Menon, V. (2003). Functional connectivity in the resting brain: a network analysis of the default mode hypothesis. *Proc. Natl. Acad. Sci. U S A* 100, 253–258. doi: 10.1073/pnas.0135058100

Gross, A. L., Parisi, J. M., Spira, A. P., Kueider, A. M., Ko, J. Y., Saczynski, J. S., et al. (2012). Memory training interventions for older adults: a meta-analysis. *Aging Ment. Health* 16, 722–734. doi: 10.1080/13607863.2012.667783

Hartholt, K. A., van Beeck, E. F., Polinder, S., van der Velde, N., van Lieshout, E. M. M., Panneman, M. J. M., et al. (2011). Societal consequences of falls in the older population: injuries, healthcare costs, and long-term reduced quality of life. *J. Trauma* 71, 748–753. doi: 10.1097/ta.0b013e318 1f6f5e5

Head, D., Buckner, R. L., Shimony, J. S., Williams, L. E., Akbudak, E., Conturo, T. E., et al. (2004). Differential vulnerability of anterior white matter in nondemented aging with minimal acceleration in dementia of the Alzheimer type: evidence from diffusion tensor imaging. *Cereb. Cortex* 14, 410–423. doi: 10.1093/cercor/bhh003

Hillman, C. H., Erickson, K. I., and Kramer, A. F. (2008). Be smart, exercise your heart: exercise effects on brain and cognition. *Nat. Rev. Neurosci.* 9, 58–65. doi: 10.1038/nrn2298

Höetting, K., and Röeder, B. (2013). Beneficial effects of physical exercise on neuroplasticity and cognition. *Neurosci. Biobehav. Rev.* 37, 2243–2257. doi: 10.1016/j.neubiorev.2013.04.005

Hulst, T., van der Geest, J. N., Thürling, M., Goericke, S., Frens, M. A., Timmann, D., et al. (2015). Ageing shows a pattern of cerebellar degeneration analogous, but not equal, to that in patients suffering from cerebellar degenerative disease. *Neuroimage* 116, 196–206. doi: 10.1016/j.neuroimage.2015.03.084

Humes, L. E., Busey, T. A., Craig, J., and Kewley-Port, D. (2013). Are age-related changes in cognitive function driven by age-related changes in sensory processing? *Atten. Percept. Psychophys.* 75, 508–524. doi: 10.3758/s13414-012-0406-9

Jackson, J. H. (1958). *Selected Writings of John Hughlings Jackson.* London: Staples.

Kellermann, T., Regenbogen, C., De Vos, M., Möessnang, C., Finkelmeyer, A., and Habel, U. (2012). Effective connectivity of the human cerebellum during visual attention. *J. Neurosci.* 32, 11453–11460. doi: 10.1523/jneurosci.0678-12.2012

Kipping, J. A., Grodd, W., Kumar, V., Taubert, M., Villringer, A., and Margulies, D. S. (2013). Overlapping and parallel cerebello-cerebral networks contributing to sensorimotor control: an intrinsic functional connectivity study. *Neuroimage* 83, 837–848. doi: 10.1016/j.neuroimage.2013.07.027

Kirk-Sanchez, N. J., and McGough, E. L. (2014). Physical exercise and cognitive performance in the elderly: current perspectives. *Clin. Interv. Aging* 9, 51–62. doi: 10.2147/cia.s39506

Klados, M. A., Styliadis, C., Frantzidis, C. A., Paraskevopoulos, E., and Bamidis, P. D. (2016). Beta-band functional connectivity is reorganized in mild cognitive impairment after combined computerized physical and cognitive training. *Front. Neurosci.* 10:55. doi: 10.3389/fnins.2016.00055

Koppelmans, V., Hirsiger, S., Mérillat, S., Jäencke, L., and Seidler, R. D. (2015). Cerebellar gray and white matter volume and their relation with age and manual motor performance in healthy older adults. *Hum. Brain Mapp.* 36, 2352–2363. doi: 10.1002/hbm.22775

Kueider, A. M., Parisi, J. M., Gross, A. L., and Rebok, G. W. (2012). Computerized cognitive training with older adults: a systematic review. *PLoS One* 7:e40588. doi: 10.1371/journal.pone.0040588

Lampit, A., Hallock, H., and Valenzuela, M. (2014). Computerized cognitive training in cognitively healthy older adults: a systematic review and meta-analysis of effect modifiers. *PLoS Med.* 11:e1001756. doi: 10.1371/journal.pmed.1001756

Lee, R. X., Huang, J.-J., Huang, C., Tsai, M.-L., and Yen, C.-T. (2015). Plasticity of cerebellar Purkinje cells in behavioral training of body balance control. *Front. Syst. Neurosci.* 9:113. doi: 10.3389/fnsys.2015.00113

Mariën, P., Ackermann, H., Adamaszek, M., Barwood, C. H. S., Beaton, A., Desmond, J., et al. (2014). Consensus paper: language and the cerebellum: an ongoing enigma. *Cerebellum* 13, 386–410. doi: 10.1007/s12311-013-0540-5

Melby-Lervåg, M., and Hulme, C. (2013). Is working memory training effective? A meta-analytic review. *Dev. Psychol.* 49, 270–291. doi: 10.1037/a0028228

Moran, D. (2003). Arguments for rejecting the sequential Bonferroni in ecological studies. *Oikos* 100, 403–405. doi: 10.1034/j.1600-0706.2003.12010.x

Nascimento, C. M. C., Pereira, J. R., de Andrade, L. P., Garuffi, M., Talib, L. L., Forlenza, O. V., et al. (2014). Physical exercise in MCI elderly promotes reduction of pro-inflammatory cytokines and improvements on cognition and BDNF peripheral levels. *Curr. Alzheimer Res.* 11, 799–805. doi: 10.2174/156720501108140910122849

Niemann, C., Godde, B., and Voelcker-Rehage, C. (2014). Not only cardiovascular, but also coordinative exercise increases hippocampal volume in older adults. *Front. Aging Neurosci.* 6:170. doi: 10.3389/fnagi.2014.00170

Pezoulas, V. C., Zervakis, M., Michelogiannis, S., and Klados, M. A. (2017). Resting-state functional connectivity and network analysis of cerebellum with respect to crystallized IQ and gender. *Front. Hum. Neurosci.* 11:189. doi: 10.3389/fnhum.2017.00189

Ramakrishnan, K. B., Voges, K., De Proprisl, L., De Zeeuw, C. I., and D'Angelo, E. (2016). Tactile stimulation evokes long-lasting potentiation of purkinje cell discharge *in vivo*. *Front. Cell. Neurosci.* 10:36. doi: 10.3389/fncel.2016.00036

Raz, N., Lindenberger, U., Rodrigue, K. M., Kennedy, K. M., Head, D., Williamson, A., et al. (2005). Regional brain changes in aging healthy adults: general trends, individual differences and modifiers. *Cereb. Cortex* 15, 1676–1689. doi: 10.1093/cercor/bhi044

Roberts, K. L., and Allen, H. A. (2016). Perception and cognition in the ageing brain: a brief review of the short- and long-term links between perceptual and cognitive decline. *Front. Aging Neurosci.* 8:39. doi: 10.3389/fnagi.2016.00039

Sarter, M., and Bruno, J. P. (2004). Developmental origins of the age-related decline in cortical cholinergic function and associated cognitive abilities. *Neurobiol. Aging* 25, 1127–1139. doi: 10.1016/j.neurobiolaging.2003.11.011

Schafer, J. H., Glass, T. A., Bolla, K. I., Mintz, M., Jedlicka, A. E., and Schwartz, B. S. (2005). Homocysteine and cognitive function in a population-based study of older adults. *J. Am. Geriatr. Soc.* 53, 381–388. doi: 10.1111/j.1532-5415.2005.53153.x

Schmahmann, J. D., and Sherman, J. C. (1997). Cerebellar cognitive affective syndrome. *Cereb. Cogn.* 41, 433–440. doi: 10.1016/s0074-7742(08) 60363-3

Sehm, B., Taubert, M., Conde, V., Weise, D., Classen, J., Dukart, J., et al. (2014). Structural brain plasticity in Parkinson's disease induced by balance training. *Neurobiol. Aging* 35, 232–239. doi: 10.1016/j.neurobiolaging.2013.06.021

Seidler, R. D., Bernard, J. A., Burutolu, T. B., Fling, B. W., Gordon, M. T., Gwin, J. T., et al. (2010). Motor control and aging: links to age-related brain structural, functional, and biochemical effects. *Neurosci. Biobehav. Rev.* 34, 721–733. doi: 10.1016/j.neubiorev.2009.10.005

Seligman, M. E. P. (2002). Authentic happiness inventory. Available online at: http://www.authentichappiness.sas.upenn.edu/testcenter

Sexton, C. E., Walhovd, K. B., Storsve, A. B., Tamnes, C. K., Westlye, L. T., Johansen-Berg, H., et al. (2014). Accelerated changes in white matter microstructure during aging: a longitudinal diffusion tensor imaging study. *J. Neurosci.* 34, 15425–15436. doi: 10.1523/JNEUROSCI.0203-14.2014

Strick, P. L., Dum, R. P., and Fiez, J. A. (2009). Cerebellum and nonmotor function. *Annu. Rev. Neurosci.* 32, 413–434. doi: 10.1146/annurev.neuro.31.060407.125606

Styliadis, C., Ioannides, A. A., Bamidis, P. D., and Papadelis, C. (2015). Distinct cerebellar lobules process arousal, valence and their interaction in parallel following a temporal hierarchy. *Neuroimage* 110, 149–161. doi: 10.1016/j.neuroimage.2015.02.006

Tarmey, D. (2012). *Ageing, Cognition, and Sensorimotor Processing: Difficulties in Co-Ordinating Distributed Systems?* Sheffield: University of Sheffield.

Tiffin, J., and Asher, E. J. (1948). The purdue pegboard: norms and studies of reliability and validity. *J. Appl. Psychol.* 32, 243–247. doi: 10.1037/h0061266

Todd, C., and Skelton, D. (2004). "What are the main risk factors for falls among older people and what are the most effective interventions to prevent these falls?," Copenhagen: WHO Regional Office for Europe (Health Evidence Network Report), Available online at: http://www.euro.who.int/document/E82552.pdf. [Accessed May 6, 2010]

Vazquez-Sanroman, D., Sanchis-Segura, C., Toledo, R., Hernandez, M. E., Manzo, J., and Miquel, M. (2013). The effects of enriched environment on BDNF expression in the mouse cerebellum depending on the length of exposure. *Behav. Brain Res.* 243, 118–128. doi: 10.1016/j.bbr.2012.12.047

Wayne, R. V., and Johnsrude, I. S. (2015). A review of causal mechanisms underlying the link between age-related hearing loss and cognitive decline. *Ageing Res. Rev.* 23, 154–166. doi: 10.1016/j.arr.2015.06.002

Westlye, L. T., Walhovd, K. B., Dale, A. M., Bjørnerud, A., Due-Tønnessen, P., Engvig, A., et al. (2010). Life-span changes of the human brain white matter: diffusion tensor imaging (DTI) and volumetry. *Cereb. Cortex* 20, 2055–2068. doi: 10.1093/cercor/bhp280

Yeo, B. T. T., Krienen, F. M., Sepulcre, J., Sabuncu, M. R., Lashkari, D., Hollinshead, M., et al. (2011). The organization of the human cerebral cortex estimated by intrinsic functional connectivity. *J. Neurophysiol.* 106, 1125–1165. doi: 10.1152/jn.00338.2011

6

Greek Traditional Dances: A Way to Support Intellectual, Psychological and Motor Functions in Senior Citizens at Risk of Neurodegeneration

Styliani Douka[1], Vasiliki I. Zilidou[1,2]*, Olympia Lilou[1] and Magda Tsolaki[3]

[1] Laboratory of Sports, Tourism and Recreation Management, School of Physical Education and Sport Science, Aristotle University of Thessaloniki, Thessaloniki, Greece, [2] Laboratory of Medical Physics, Medical School, Aristotle University of Thessaloniki, Thessaloniki, Greece, [3] Department of Neurology, Medical School, Aristotle University of Thessaloniki, Thessaloniki, Greece

*Correspondence:
Vasiliki I. Zilidou
vickyzilidou@gmail.com

One of the major problems that elderly people are facing is dementia. For scientist's dementia is a medical, social and economic problem, as it has been characterized as the epidemic of the 21st century. Prevention and treatment in the initial stages of dementia are essential, and community awareness and specialization of health professionals are required, with the aim of early and valid diagnosis of the disease. Activities are recommended to the senior citizens to improve their physical and mental health. Dance has been suggested as an appropriate recreational activity for the elderly that brings functional adjustments to the various systems of the body, psychological benefits, and makes exercise to seem interesting and entertaining as it combines the performance of multiple animations with musical accompaniment. A Greek traditional dance program was performed where our sample consisted of 30 healthy elderly and 30 with Mild Cognitive Impairment – MCI. It lasted 24 weeks, two times a week for 60 min. Specific traditional dances from all over Greece were selected. The dances were of a moderate intensity at the beginning with a gradual increase in intensity, according to the age and physical abilities of the participants. The results showed a significant improvement in: attention (S4viac-Healthy: $z = -3.085$, $p = 0.002$; MCI: $z = -3.695$, $p < 0.001$, S4viti-Healthy: $z = -2.800$, $p = 0.005$; MCI: $z = -3.538$, $p < 0.001$), anxiety (Healthy: $z = -2.042$, $p = 0.041$; MCI: $z = -2.168$, $p = 0.030$), verbal fluency for MCI (Verflx: $t = -2.396$, $df = 29$, $p = 0.023$, Verfls: $t = -3.619$, $df = 29$, $p = 0.001$, Verfmo: $t = -3.295$, $df = 29$, $p = 0.003$) and in executive functions (FUCAS: $z = -2.168$, $p = 0.030$). Significant improvement also showed in physical condition (Arm curl– Healthy: $z = -3.253$, $p = 0.001$; MCI: $z = -3.308$, $p = 0.001$, Chair stand – Healthy: $t = -3.232$, $df = 29$, $p = 0.003$; MCI: $t = -2.242$, $df = 29$, $p = 0.033$, Back scratch– Healthy: $z = -1.946$, $p = 0.052$; MCI: $z = -2.845$, $p = 0.004$, 2 min step– Healthy:

$z = -2.325, p = 0.020$; MCI: $z = -2.625, p = 0.009$, FootUpandGo– Healthy: $z = -4.289$, $p < 0.001$; MCI: $z = -3.137, p = 0.002$, Sit and Reach: $z = -3.082, p = 0.002$, Balance on One leg: $z = -3.301, p = 0.001$) and Quality of life (Healthy: $z = -1.937, p = 0.053$; MCI: $z = -2.130, p = 0.033$). This study proves that dancing not only improves the cognitive and physical condition of the elderly but also contributes to a better quality of life.

Keywords: Greek traditional dances, dementia, quality of life, physical health, mental health

INTRODUCTION

People living with dementia have poor access to appropriate healthcare, even in most high-income country settings, where only around 50% of people living with dementia receive a diagnosis. In low and middle-income countries, less than 10% of cases are diagnosed. As populations age due to increasing life expectancy, the number of people with dementia is increasing. We estimate that there were 46.8 million people worldwide living with dementia in 2015 and this number will reach 131.5 million in 2050 (World Alzheimer Report 2016; Prince et al., 2016). In Greece, there are more than 200,000 patients with dementia and this figure is expected to exceed to 600,000 patients by 2050, while the annual cost of dementia in Greece is now approaching six billion euros (Alzheimer Athens).

The term "dementia" is generic and refers to a complex group of changes with known or unknown etiology, which occur with widespread disruption of cognitive abilities and social functions of the individual. "Dementia can be reversible or irreversible, with rapid or slow progression, and characterized by multiple deficits of cognitive functions or almost exclusive disorder of emotion, initiative and personality" (Gorelick et al., 2011). The most common type of dementia that mainly occurs in the elderly is Alzheimer's disease type (AD). The rapid increase in dementia ranges from about 2–3% among people aged 70–75 years and from 20–25% among people aged 85 and over (Ferri et al., 2005). The most serious and early cognitive problem in AD is memory loss. This loss is gradual and occurs within the limits of a normal level of consciousness, without any other central nervous system disorder that could explain these symptoms.

Mild Cognitive Impairment (MCI), is an emerging term that encompasses the clinical stage between normal cognitive status and dementia. It is a condition considered to be a transition between normal mental changes due to age and early clinical signs of dementia (Petersen, 2004). Its features, applications, and definitions are controversial. The MCI is now focusing on studies of natural history, biological markers and on the prevention of AD. The stage of the MCI is probably the best stage at which we could intervene with preventive strategies. Despite the conflict, progress has been made in determining the risk factors for progression from MCI to dementia. Now, treatments in order to prevent the development of AD are focusing on the MCI as a treatment group, and neurologists will increasingly be called upon to do this diagnosis. This interest is motivated by patient requests for prognosis and treatment. Therapists-neurologists have at their disposal a wealth of research information, though it is illustrated by the lack of practical suggestions for patient management (Chertkow et al., 2008). MCI is associated with an increasing risk of developing dementia. Patients with this pattern of early deficits develop dementia at a rate of 10–15% per year, while the rate for healthy controls is only 1–2% per year. However, data on the prevalence of MCI and its rate of conversion to dementia vary widely, depending on the different determinants applied.

Also, the functionality is a key area affected by aging. The functional capacity is considered to be an important part of health and wellness. The lack of mobility is the major reason that older people have problems with functionality. During aging, there are some problems in the musculoskeletal system and joints. Strength and muscle mass decrease over time. Physical activity, especially strength training, is very important action to come up against this situation (Keller and Engelhardt, 2013). There exists a small decrease in muscle strength up to 40–50 years and a 30–40% decrease in 70 to 80 years. This reduction is due to sarcopenia, which occurs more in elderly women than in men (Cruz-Jentoft et al., 2010). Genetic factors and lifestyle, such as reduction of physical activity, smoking and the use of alcoholic beverages can contribute also to sarcopenia and dementia. Muscular weakness is associated with increased risk of falls (Soriano et al., 2007; Leveille et al., 2009), resulting in possible fractures (Aniansson et al., 1984; Carpintero et al., 2014).

Physical activity stimulates the physiological functions of the body and can contribute to the stabilization of a good level of cognitive functions making the elderly more energetic. Exercise improves physical health, behavior, mental state, communication and functionality in the elderly with cognitive impairment, especially exercise that is for durability, agility, muscle strength and balance (Garber et al., 2011). The activities proposed for participation by the elderly should lead to the improvement or maintenance of physical, spiritual and mental health (Kim, 2009).

In international literature, dance has been suggested as an appropriate recreational activity for the older adults. Dance is a physical activity that causes functional changes in various systems of the human body. Previous studies have shown that elderly who dance at regular intervals have significant benefits as better balance, stability, flexibility and cognitive status than other elderly who do not dance on a regular interval (Kattenstroth et al., 2011). Dance, also offers psychological benefits and can also make the exercise more interesting and entertaining, as it combines the execution of multiple kinetic tasks with music accompaniment. For elderly, dancing is a pleasure, is exercise capacity, companionship, mental balance, wellness, coordination and muscle tone (Mullen et al., 2012). Music is still an important component of pleasure, as individuals enjoy it and express themselves through it. The rhythmic music, improves the coordination of gait and proprioceptive movement control in people with neuromuscular and skeletal disorders and leads to increased mobility and stability. Mild dance activity can prevent the risk of high blood pressure, of diabetes and the cardiovascular diseases (Gordon et al., 2004). It also helps to prevent falls and loss of bone density (Minne, 2005), improves the flexibility of the joints, especially the lower limbs, as all the muscle groups are exercised through a combination of slow and fast steps. Along with the well-being, it activates the muscles, accelerates the cardiac resistance and blood circulation, increases the burns and thus affects the metabolism, increases the maximum oxygen intake, improves the myocardial contractility, increases the frequency of breathing (Xerakia and Kalogerakou, 2000). It also requires simultaneous operation of both cerebral hemispheres, while at the same time activates kinesthetic, logical, musical and emotional processes. For this reason, dancing as a physical activity helps at a rate of 76% the risk reduction in dementia. The standard steps and specific figures does not help much. Creativity is the special component in dance that offers more results (Powers, 2010).

Greek traditional dances are an activity which offering pleasure, entertainment, education and characterized by diversity, complexity, since the combinations of lower and upper limb movements dominate and differ in intensity and in movements from other types of dance. Apart from the entertainment they offer, they are also classified as an aerobic activity that causes a burden but as part of the physiological adjustments (Galanou, 2003). Also classified as an aerobic leisure activity offering a variety of intensity and rhythm, as there is a pleasant climate during the practice (Pitsi, 2005).

In recent years, there has been growing interest in studying the quality of life. The "quality of life" is a concept with a broad scope, that is something that makes difficult its measure and its integration into the scientific study (Fallowfield, 2007). It includes epidemiological, biomedical, functional, economic and cultural approaches, as well as personal preferences, perceptions and experiences. International organizations such as the Organization of the United Nations (UN) and the World Health Organization (WHO) recognize the importance of quality of life through various declarations and conventions. Participating in properly organized exercise programs, physical education and physical activity programs contributes to positive self-esteem and high self-assessment, factors that lead to the adoption of appropriate and desirable attitudes and behaviors, greatly ensure physical well-being and mental health (Landers and Arent, 2001; Hamill et al., 2011).

The positive contribution of physical exercise to quality of life is well documented, as participation in physical activities and systematic exercise help to enhance mental well-being, increase positive mood, seek pleasurable and intense experiences, improve health and control stress, both in healthy and in clinical populations (Theodorakis, 2010). Continuously new research and work proves that exercise and participation in physical activities are associated with better performance of cognitive functions, self-esteem and self-confidence, reduction of anxiety and depression, mental well-being and an improvement in quality of life.

The aim of this study is to demonstrate the importance of Greek traditional dances in improving both the cognitive and physical health of the senior citizens. Dance is an enjoyable type of aerobic exercise that can cause various changes in the human body. We investigated if the Greek traditional dance can be an important tool for enhancing health status of senior citizens and simultaneously to improve their quality of life. Furthermore, we investigated if dance may delay the beginning of a cognitive impairment or dementia.

MATERIALS AND METHODS

Subjects

The sample consisted of elderly people ($n = 60$) who were self-serving, had good functional and emotional state and normal or non-normal cognitive status. The subjects were divided into two groups depending on their diagnosis. More precisely, thirty participants ($n1 = 30$) were healthy seniors with median age of 65.50 years [Interquartile range (IQR) = (62.00, 68.00)] and median education of 13 years [IQR = (8.75, 16.25)] while thirty participants ($n2 = 30$) had a diagnosis of mild cognitive impairment (MCI). The MCI participants had a median age of 67.50 years [IQR = (63.00, 70.00)] and median education of 6 years [IQR = (6.00, 8.25)]. Participants did not participate in other Greek Traditional Dances programs or at any other cognitive rehabilitation programs. The intervention took place at the Greek Association of Alzheimer Disease and Relative Disorders (Alzheimer Hellas) and at the Day Care Centers of Municipality of Thessaloniki It lasted 24 weeks with a frequency of two times per week in sessions of 60 min.

Inclusion criteria were age ≥60 years, senior citizens with mild cognitive impairment, agreement of a medical doctor and time commitment to the dance protocol. Exclusion criteria were concurrent participation in another study, hypertension, heart and respiratory failure, uncorrectable vision problems, inability to participate at 80% of the hours of the program. The training program was provided at no cost and participants received no compensation. At the beginning of the program and at the end of this, a neuropsychological evaluation was performed by a psychologist to assess the cognitive, functional, and behavioral status of each participant. The fitness and functional capacity evaluated by a fitness instructor and their quality of life was assessed through appropriate questionnaires. The required descriptions were given for the purpose of this research and written consent was requested from the senior citizens to participate. Ethical and Scientific Committee of GAARD approved the protocol of this study.

Outcome Measures
Psychological Evaluation

The neuropsychological assessment was performed before the intervention (initial assessment) and after the intervention of dance (final assessment). Fifteen (15) different tests were used, which examine all cognitive functions (memory, reason, judgment, abstract thinking, complex skills, attention, concentration, orientation, audiovisual perception), activities of daily living behavioral problems and quality of life. The tests that were selected are the following with a reference to what they evaluate: Mini Mental State Examination (MMSE), it is a screening instrument to separate patients with cognitive impairment from those without it (Fountoulakis et al., 2000), Clinical Dementia Rating (CDR), characterize six domains of cognitive and functional performance (Morris, 1993), Functional Cognitive Assessment Scale (FUCAS), assesses executive function in daily life activities directly in patients with dementia (Kounti et al., 2006), Functional Rating Scale for Symptoms of Dementia (FRSSD), assesses the daily functionality (Hutton, 1990), Instrumental Activities of Daily Living (IADL), assesses the independent living skills (Theotoka et al., 2007), Test of Every Day Attention (TEA), assesses the attention (Robertson et al., 1996), Trail-making Test (TMT), assesses the executive function (Vlahou and Kosmidis, 2002), Rey–Osterreith Complex Figure Test (ROCF), assesses the memory (Rey and Osterrieth, 1993), Rey Auditory Verbal Learning Test (RAVLT) and Rivermead Behavioral Memory Test (RBMT), assesses the memory (Efkildes et al., 2002), Verbal Fluency Test (VFT), assesses the cognitive function (Kosmidis et al., 2004), Neuropsychiatric Inventory (NPI), assesses the range of neuropsychiatric symptoms (Politis et al., 2004), Geriatric Depression Scale (GDS), assesses the depression (Fountoulakis et al., 1999), Quality of Life in Alzheimer's Disease (QOL-AD), assesses the quality of life (Logsdon et al., 1999), Beck Anxiety Inventory (BAI), record the anxiety (Beck and Steer, 1988). These tests have been selected on the basis of the validity and reliability and the existence of norms for the Greek population (Kosmidis, 2008; Tsolaki and Kounti, 2010).

Physical Evaluation

In order to assess their physical condition and functional capacity, the Body Mass Index (BMI) was first calculated and then the Senior Fitness Fullerton Test was used, which consists of six tests and evaluates the flexibility of low back and hamstrings, the functional capacity of individuals through the strength of the lower limbs and the dynamic balance, the speed, agility and balance during movement (Jones and Rikli, 2002). In addition, their static equilibrium was evaluated through the Flamingo test (Barabas et al., 1996), the length of time spent on one leg was calculated, the strength of the strong hand was recorded with the use of the dynamometer (Saehan Corp., Masan, South Korea) and the jumping ability (vertical jump) was evaluated using OptoJump system (Microgate, Bolzano, Italy). Specifically, the tests used are: Chair stand, 8 FootUpandGo, Back Scratch, Arm Curl, Chair Sit and Reach, 2 Min Step, Balance One leg, Hand Grip Strength, and Jumping ability.

Quality of Life Evaluation

To evaluate the quality of life, the questionnaire developed by the WHO was used, the WHOQOL, which aims to promote an intercultural Quality of Life assessment system and the use of this questionnaire in the wider health sector. It includes 26 questions and is divided into four thematic sections

(Skevington et al., 2004) where the relevant questions address: (a) physical health; (b) mental health; (c) social relations; and (d) the environment. It also includes two questions, which offer an overall assessment of Quality of Life and Health Status (Ginnieri-Kokkosi et al., 2003). The results with the highest values are an indication of a better quality of life. In general, the multifaceted Quality of Life is examined, as well as a general state of health.

Selection of Greek Traditional Dances

The traditional dances selected from all over Greece. The design of the program held by dividing the dances into three categories depending on the complexity and number of steps, the rate of intensity (slow speed) and the position-movement of the hands. Dances were also classified into three categories: mild, moderate and high intensity. Most of them were in moderate intensity, with progressive and increasing intensity, indicative of the age and physical abilities of the participants.

Statistical Analysis
Demographics

We planned comparisons between the independent variables age and education level between groups, respectively. Initially, demographic data were tested for normality assumption between groups (Healthy, MCI) using visual inspection of histograms, normal Q-Q plots and boxplots, in terms of Skewness and Kurtosis as well as using the normality tests (Shapiro and Wilk, 1965; Razali and Wah, 2011). If the independent variable was approximately normally distributed in both groups, differences between groups were explored using parametric methods (independent samples t-tests). However, if the normality assumption was not met, non-parametric analysis (Mann–Whitney U-Test) was followed. Additionally, the possible association between and the gender (male, female) and the group (Healthy, MCI) was investigated by means of Chi-squared test.

The participants' demographic information was described in tables in terms of mean (standard deviation) or median, interquartile range, respectively, depending on the normality assumption. More precisely, when normality assumption was met, the mean (standard deviation) was used whereas in non-normally distributed variables, median and interquartile range was depicted.

Statistical analysis was performed using the IBM SPSS Statistics (Version 20) and the level of significance was set at $p < 0.05$.

Data

Tasks examining the neuropsychological and somatometric state as well as the quality of life of the participants were performed both before and after the intervention in both groups (Healthy and MCI participants). As assumptions for a Mixed Model Analysis of Variance (or Split-plot ANOVA) were not fulfilled, an alternative analysis was performed. Differences in scores collected from the neuropsychological and somatometric assessment at the two-time points (after training – before training scores) were computed and then tested for normality. The within-group changes, after grouping our data by diagnosis, were explored using either paired t-test or Wilcoxon signed-rank test depending on normality assumption of score differences at the two-time points. Additionally, the between-group differences were explored comparing score differences between the two groups using either independent samples t-test or Mann–Whitney U-test based on normality assumption of score differences. The methodology used has been published elsewhere (Cramer, 1998; Cramer and Howitt, 2004; Doane and Seward, 2011; Arvanitidou-Vagiona and Xaidits, 2013; Athanasiou et al., 2017; Pandria et al., 2018).

RESULTS

Demographics

Both variables age and education were not approximately normally distributed for both groups (Healthy, MCI).

Planned comparisons between groups revealed that the age did not significantly vary between healthy and MCI participants ($U = 333.500$, $p = 0.084$) whereas MCI individuals seem to have significantly fewer educational years compared to healthy participants ($U = 183.500$, $p < 0.001$) (**Table 1**). The proportion of male/female (6/24) participants were equal for both groups and as such no significant association was found between gender and group ($\chi^2 = 0.000$, $df = 1$, $p = 1.000$).

Neuropsychological Data

The performance of healthy and MCI participants significantly changed at the subtests of TEA test, S4viac (Healthy: $z = -3.085$, $p = 0.002$; MCI: $z = -3.695$, $p < 0.001$) and S4viti (Healthy: $z = -2.800$, $p = 0.005$; MCI: $z = -3.538$, $p < 0.001$). More precisely, both healthy and MCI participants showed significant improvement in S4viac test [Healthy – Before training: 9.00 (5.00, 10.00); After training: 10.00 (9.75, 10.00); MCI – Before training: 6.50 (4.00, 10.00); After training: 10.00 (8.00, 10.00)]. However, a significant decrease was observed in S4viti test for both groups [Healthy – Before training: 6.32 (5.20, 9.47); After training: 5.36 (4.36, 6.50); MCI – Before training: 8.58 (6.03, 11.70); After training: 6.39 (5.36, 7.72)].

Additionally, significant decreases were found in RBMT1 and RBMT2 tasks for both groups [RBMT1: Healthy – Before training: 14.00 (11.75, 15.00); After training: 12.00 (9.13, 15.00); $z = -3.176$, $p = 0.001$; MCI – Before training: 11.00 (9.00, 13.00); After training: 8.00 (5.88, 10.00); $z = -3.811$, $p < 0.001$; RBMT2: Healthy – Before training: 12.25 (10.00, 15.00); After training: 12.00 (7.88, 15.00); $z = -1.986$, $p = 0.047$; MCI – Before training: 10.00 (6.00, 13.00); After training: 6.25 (4.00, 10.00); $z = -3.580$, $p < 0.001$]. Moreover, anxiety levels have found to

be considerably altered, as measured by the BAI test (Healthy: $z = -2.042$, $p = 0.041$; MCI: $z = -2.168$, $p = 0.030$). More precisely, MCI individuals showed improvement in anxiety levels based on the scores in BAI test when comparing their scores in two-time conditions [Before training: 7.50 (3.00, 12.25); After training: 4.50 (2.00, 10.25)] whereas anxiety levels in healthy participants were increased [Before training: 2.50 (1.00, 6.50); After training: 4.00 (1.00, 8.50)]. In contrary to this, when comparing the MCI participants' scores in two-time conditions at PSS test they showed significant increase in their scores [Before training: 6.63 (6.75); After training: 9.73 (5.92); $t = -2.168$, $df = 29$, $p = 0.024$].

Healthy individuals seem to improve their immediate memory and delayed recall as they scored higher at RAV test [Before training: 39.77 (9.36); After training: 42.87 (10.08); $t = 2.095$, $df = 29$, $p = 0.045$] in the post-intervention screening (**Figure 1**). On the other hand, MCI participants benefited the most from dancing to verbal fluency scoring higher at tasks Verflx [Before training: 7.97 (3.10); After training: 9.33 (3.19); $t = -2.396$, $df = 29$, $p = 0.023$], Verfls [Before training: 8.03 (3.08); After training: 10.00 (3.33); $t = -3.619$, $df = 29$, $p = 0.001$] and Verfmo [Before training: 8.21 (3.02); After training: 9.54 (2.99); $t = -3.295$, $df = 29$, $p = 0.003$].

Considerable deviations in the performance of MCI individuals at S1map1 [Before training: 25.00 (19.75, 30.25); After training: 21.50 (16.75, 29.00); $z = -2.153$, $p = 0.031$] and S1map2 [Before training: 41.87 (8.11); After training: 37.67 (9.57); $t = 2.508$, $df = 29$, $p = 0.018$] tasks have observed. Marginally significant difference was found in scores of MCI group at NPI task ($z = -1.912$, $p = 0.056$) whereas a statistically significant decrease was reported in their functionality based on FUCAS test [Before training: 42.00 (42.00, 46.00); After training: 44.50 (42.00, 46.00); $z = -2.168$, $p = 0.030$] (**Figure 2**).

Furthermore, we performed comparisons of score differences in two-time conditions (post-pre-scores) between groups resulting in significant interactions time × group at FRSSD [Healthy: 0.9 (2.56); MCI: −0.93 (2.64); $t = 2.729$, $df = 58$, $p = 0.008$], RBMT2 [Healthy: −1.00 (−2.63, 0.25); MCI: −2.00 (−5.00, 0.00); $U = 312.500$, $p = 0.041$] and BAI [Healthy: 0.00 (−0.25, 4.00); MCI: −2.00 (−5.00, 1.00); $U = 262.000$, $p = 0.005$] tests (**Figure 3**). Based on the aforementioned results, MCI participants showed greater improvement in FRSSD and BAI tests.

Somatometric Data

Both groups showed considerable improvement after dancing in their strength of both upper [Arm curl task: Healthy – Before training: 27.00 (22.00, 28.25); After training: 28.00 (25.75, 30.25); $z = -3.253$, $p = 0.001$; MCI – Before training: 24.00 (21.50, 25.00); After training: 25.50 (24.00, 28.00); $z = -3.308$, $p = 0.001$] and lower limbs [Chair stand task: Healthy – Before training: 16.97 (4.80); After training: 18.57 (4.76); $t = -3.232$, $df = 29$, $p = 0.003$; MCI – Before training: 15.73 (4.02); After training: 16.97 (2.46); $t = -2.242$, $df = 29$, $p = 0.033$] as well as in the flexibility of the shoulder belt [Back scratch task: Healthy – Before training: −3.00 (−13.75, 2.00); After training: −2.50 (−14.25, 5.00); $z = -1.946$, $p = 0.052$; MCI – Before training: −13.00

TABLE 1 | Demographic data as age and education of healthy and MCI participants.

Groups	Median, interquartile range (IQR)	
	Age	Education
Healthy (30 elderly)	65.50, 6.00	13.00, 8.00
Mild cognitive impairments-MCI (30 elderly)	67.50, 7.00	6.00, 2.00

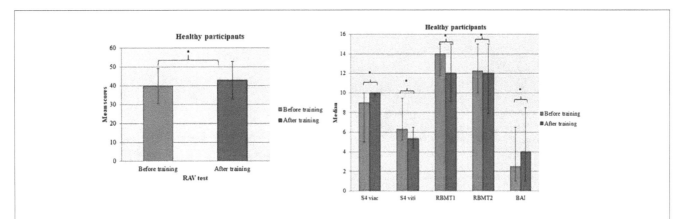

FIGURE 1 | Significant design. differences in the performance of Healthy participants when comparing tests' scores in two-time conditions. Asterisk indicates the p-values that reached statistical significance ($p < 0.05$).

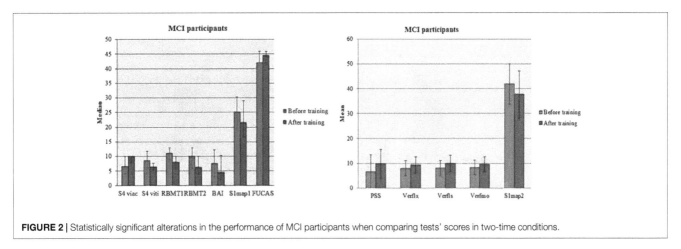

FIGURE 2 | Statistically significant alterations in the performance of MCI participants when comparing tests' scores in two-time conditions.

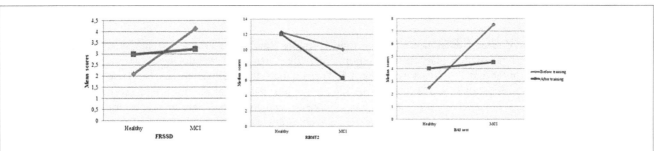

FIGURE 3 | Significant interactions time × group were found when comparing post-pre-differences in scores at FRSSD, RBMT2, and BAI tests between the two groups.

(-20.00, 2.25); After training: -8.00 (-16.25, 4.00); $z = -2.845$, $p = 0.004$]. Additionally, the intervention seems to promote gains in aerobic capacity [2-min step: Healthy – Before training: 96.00 (82.75, 115.25); After training: 102.00 (81.50, 125.00); $z = -2.325$, $p = 0.020$; MCI – Before training: 90.50 (81.75, 104.50); After training: 99.00 (85.50, 113.50); $z = -2.625$, $p = 0.009$] and movement coordination [FootUpandGo task: Healthy – Before training: 4.89 (4.36, 5.78); After training: 4.41 (4.18, 5.16); $z = -4.289$, $p < 0.001$; MCI – Before training: 4.99 (4.53, 5.70); After training: 4.73 (4.13, 5.14); $z = -3.137$, $p = 0.002$] for both

health and MCI individuals (**Figures 4**, **5**). Moreover, healthy participants improved their suppleness of back and the lower femoral back along with their balance achieving higher scores at Sit and Reach task [Before training: 2.00 (-0.25, 5.00); After training: 4.00 (1.50, 9.25); $z = -3.082$, $p = 0.002$] and Balance on One leg task [Before training: 37.28 (13.46, 57.30); After training: 45.76 (19.54, 67.06); $z = -3.301$, $p = 0.001$], respectively. On the other hand, MCI individuals marginally altered their performance at the Handgrip task [Before training: 23.13 (9.27); After training: 24.27 (8.54); $t = 2.014$, $df = 29$, $p = 0.053$].

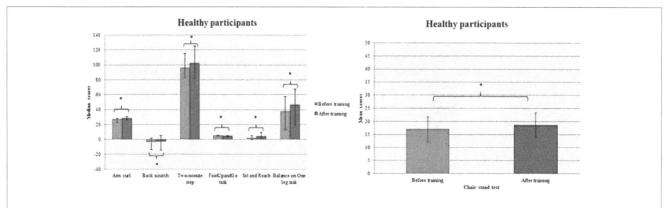

FIGURE 4 | Healthy participants improved their performance in most of the somatometric tests. Asterisk indicates the *p*-values that reached statistical significance (*p* < 0.05).

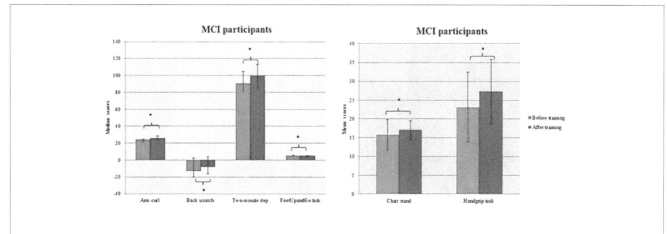

FIGURE 5 | MCI participants benefited most from the intervention in the tasks Chair stand, Handgrip, FootUpandGo, Back scratch, Arm curl, and the Two-Min step. Asterisk indicates the *p*-values that reached statistical significance (*p* < 0.05).

Planned comparisons of score differences in two-time conditions between groups revealed a marginally significant interaction time × group in Sit and Reach task [Healthy: 2.50 (0.75, 6.00); MCI: 1.00 (–1.25, 3.25); $U = 322.000$, $p = 0.057$] (**Figure 6**).

Quality of Life Parameters

Dance seems to promote generally significant gains in the quality of life and health status for both healthy [Before training: 62.63 (57.25, 71.25); After training: 64.88 (62.13, 73.56); $z = -1.937$, $p = 0.053$] and MCI [Before training: 61.25 (54.44, 70.13); After training: 65.00 (57.06, 70.50); $z = -2.130$, $p = 0.033$] individuals (**Figure 7**). Moreover, healthy participants due to the intervention improved their interaction with the environment [Before training: 72.00 (61.25, 81.00); After training: 75.00 (69.00, 81.00); $z = -2.062$, $p = 0.039$].

DISCUSSION

In this research, it is observed that the dance intervention has presented significant benefits to mental and physical health in

healthy elderly and in elderly with MCI, also in their quality of life. Their performance significantly changed in the assay examining the daily attention (selective attention, sustained attention, stirring of attention and execution of dual work in visual and auditory attention). Specifically, in two sub-tests, significant statistical results were observed. It seems that the effect of dance was positive in this particular test. The test requires in terms of the participant not only speed but also good visual competence. Consequently, the effect of dance seems to be particularly beneficial to participants, increasing their alertness and improving their visual perception. In addition, intervention has altered the performance of visual and audio information, and the level of anxiety was found to have changed significantly. In particular, Mild Cognitive Impairment (MCI) individuals showed an improvement in their anxiety levels based on their two-time scores, while healthy participants increased stress levels. Healthy individuals appear to have improved their immediate and delay memory as they were scored higher in the post-intervention test. This increase indicates, that after the dance intervention participants were able to improve their memory levels. The fact that dance intervention has had positive effects on memory improvement is considered to be particularly important

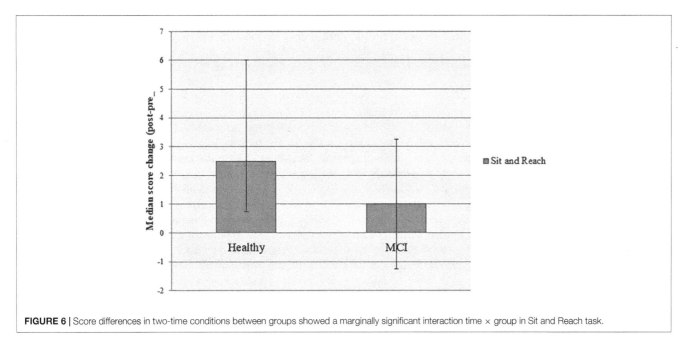

FIGURE 6 | Score differences in two-time conditions between groups showed a marginally significant interaction time × group in Sit and Reach task.

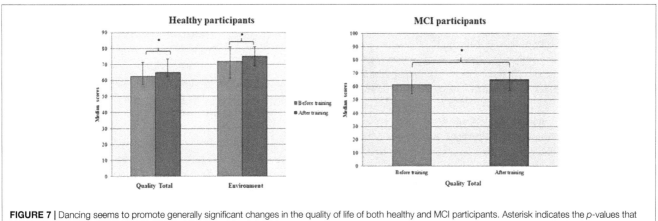

FIGURE 7 | Dancing seems to promote generally significant changes in the quality of life of both healthy and MCI participants. Asterisk indicates the p-values that reached statistical significance ($p < 0.05$).

because the most common form of dementia is AD, which basically decreases the brain hippocampus resulting in memory difficulties. The speech fluency seems to be dwindling as dementia progresses, so patients cannot even say a word in advanced stages of the disease. In the final count, the number of words recalled in each sub-test of the verbal option was significantly larger than the original one. In our research, it was observed that the dance had a positive effect on the healthy group as it improved their performance, but the effects were more admirable in the MCI participants. This shows that dance has produced positive results, which helped them to function and think faster. All of these findings, are based on the effectiveness of dance in elderly people and in particular in their physical and mental health, as shown by other studies (Kim et al., 2011; Kattenstroth et al., 2013).

The criterion for the separation of MCI from dementia is the ability to resolve daily activities, something that patients with MCI can achieve with a potentially relatively slower pace than normal elderly, but they can achieve it with positive results, while

patients with dementia, even at baseline, seems to be unable to do so. After the dance intervention, the price seems to have increased. This could be explained in two ways: (a) Probably the increase in units in the test is a normal increase, as we know that dementia is an evolving disease and therefore over time it is expected that the patient will have more difficulty and (b) dance can maintain the functionality of the patients which would statistically worsen if they did not take the dance intervention. As shown in Hwang and Braun (2015), survey, adding physical activity to one's life is an effective method of preventing, controlling, and alleviating some health conditions. Studies have demonstrated that physical activity has positive effects on depression, anxiety, dementia, heart failure, stroke, cognition and sleep. The harmful effects resulting from physical inactivity and the positive effects of physical activity suggest that further efforts are needed to encourage physical activity, with an emphasis on populations at high risk for inactivity. Maintaining the functional capacity of the elderly at satisfactory levels, is something that leads them to an independent and quality lifestyle, while reducing the risk of various diseases. In our research, the two groups showed a significant improvement after the intervention of the dance in their strength both in the upper and low part of the body, as well as in the flexibility. Moreover, the dance seems to promote significant benefits to their aerobic capacity and coordination of movements, both in healthy and in MCI individuals.

In addition, healthy participants improved their flexibility in the lower back and in femoral back as well as their equilibrium by achieving higher scores. Both teams have improved their functional capacity and body balance, especially the skills that related to day-to-day activities such as luggage or shopping and they have gained more confidence and independence as physical strength and energy allow them to engage in more activities with less fatigue.

Controlling the balance and maintaining the strength of the lower limbs, are considered important in order to reduce the episodes of drastic falls (Buchner et al., 1997). Many investigations have reported the importance of the ankle joint in the entire human body's mechanics, particularly in sensitive groups such as the elderly, in whom the muscles around the joint seem to be more affected by old age. As the strength of the dorsal flexors of the ankle seems to be affected by aging, especially in the elderly with a history of falls, it is likely that the strengthen of this particular muscle group improves the control of the elderly, resulting in falls reduction. Balance is an important functional capacity that influences significantly the ability of human to perform daily activities for their survival, such as maintaining a stable posture, the straight movement from one position to another and maintain the upright posture (Islam et al., 2004).

Quality of life refers not only to one or some particular external features, but rather expresses an existential state of the individual. Its assessment methodology should focus on identifying those factors that have a particular focus on subjective judgment and quality of life assessment. The results of our research showed statistically significant effects in the overall quality of life and the general health status of participants in the Greek traditional dances program. Dance generally seems to promote significant gains in quality of life and health status for both the healthy and for the MCI subjects. In addition, healthy participants due to dance intervention improved their interaction with the environment. It appeared that they began to acquire a sense of security with regard to external dangers, they have also started to engage in various recreational activities in their spare time and to use the means of transport more easily. Cruz-Ferreira et al. (2015), presented the positive effects of dance in different dimensions of functioning and the potential to contribute to healthy aging. This could be related to the integrated mobilization of physical, cognitive, and social skills promoted by creative dance. Also, Sivvas et al. (2015) at his study, shown that dancing helps in many ways to preserve and improve human health, as far as physical health is concerned – as it maintained the physical state in good level, but also concerning mental health – by minimizing stress and depression. Finally, social health also proved to be positively affected as the factors that prevent an individual from socialization were reduced.

Generally, our findings are in line with Teri et al. (2008) study that for long-term participation of dementia patients in exercise programs, it is necessary to be able to perform them, be fun and enjoyable. Thus, the pleasant environment, the effective communication, the feeling of security as well as the entertaining character of the exercise programs, strongly consent to the regular participation of patients in them.

In Greece than in many other countries, there is a "living tradition," i.e., in the villages living tradition continues, evolves and sometimes consciously experienced. This is an element of the inextricable relationship of the Greeks with their traditions that are lost in the depths of the ages. Traditional dances are deeply rooted in the culture of Greece, expressing local history, traditions and customs, express culture. By learning the dances of an area, someone could learn at the same time its peculiarities, history, geographic stories and myths. It is a necessity for the Greek people to remain in tradition, with the result that local dances have a strong expression of emotions but also creativity. We could investigate dances from different countries in a next study in order to evaluate the results that will arise.

CONCLUSION

The participation of the elderly in activities helps them to maintain their physical status, but also gives them the opportunity to interact with other people of all ages. This interaction, removes the feeling of loneliness, which stimulates their psychological state. Also, improves their self-esteem as they realize that they can participate in new skills. Dance as exercise, increases body resistance, helps them to maintain proper posture, stimulates the muscular system and improves physical fitness. Combined with music, helps to express emotions, combat stress and improves mental health. With the repetition of the steps, the movement of the hands and their combined function helps to improve the cognitive functions.

Furthermore, dance seems to be particularly important to protect against dementia and to slow the progression of the disease. Socialization contributes to the maintenance of positive psychology, which can be a protective shield for dementia, and to protect patients with MCI from potential depression, which adds to the situation of a patient with mental problems. It is true that nowadays, the non-pharmaceutical interventions for the treatment of dementia play a particularly important role on the world stage, and our research confirms the studies that have been established so far which mention the importance of dance.

FUTURE DIRECTIONS

The results of our research suggest that the intervention of Greek traditional dances in elderly is effective for their physical and mental health. Future research should focus on an additional diagnostic test such as neuropsychological recordings through an electroencephalography that records the brain's functions and in particular its electrical activity. After the end of interventional assessment will identify any changes that occur in brain activity. Generally, the electroencephalography is a very useful method, because it can non-invasively and painlessly give a complete view of brain function or even brain disorders.

AUTHOR CONTRIBUTIONS

VZ designed and implemented the dance program, collected and analyzed the data, prepared the initial draft of the manuscript, guided the analysis, and revised the manuscript. OL implemented the dance program, collected the data, and revised the manuscript. MT guided the study. SD co-guided the study.

FUNDING

This work was partly supported by the project "Augmentation of the Support of Patients suffering from Alzheimer's Disease and their caregivers (ASPAD/2875)," which is materialized by the Special Account of the Research Committee at Aristotle University of Thessaloniki. The project was funded by the European Union (European Social Fund) and the Ministry of Education, Lifelong Learning and Religious Affairs in the context of the National Strategic Reference Framework (NSRF, 2007–2013).

REFERENCES

Aniansson, A., Zetterberg, C., Hedberg, M., and Henriksson, K. G. (1984). Impaired muscle function with aging. A background factor in the incidence of fractures of the proximal end of the femur. *Clin. Orthop. Rel. Res.* 191, 193–201.

Arvanitidou-Vagiona, T., and Xaidits, A. M. (2013). *Medical Statistical Basic Principles.* Thessaloniki: University Studio Press.

Athanasiou, A., Arfaras, G., Pandria, N., Xygonakis, I., Foroglou, N., Astaras, A., et al. (2017). Wireless brain-robot interface: user perception and performance assessment of spinal cord injury patients. *Wirel. Commun. Mob. Comput.* 2017:2986423. doi: 10.1155/2017/2986423

Barabas, A., Bretz, K., and Kaske, R. (1996). "Stabilometry of the flamingo balance test," in *Proceedings of the 14th International Symposium on Biomechanics in Sports*, Funchal, 162–265.

Beck, A. T, and Steer, R. A. (1988). *Beck Anxiety Inventory, Manual.* San Antonio, TX: Psychological Corporation.

Buchner, D. M., Cress, M. E., de Lateur, B. J., Esselman, P. C., Margherita, A. J., Price, R., et al. (1997). The effect of strength and endurance training on gait, balance, fall risk, and health services use in community-living older adults. *J. Gerontol. A Biol. Sci. Med. Sci.* 52, M218–M224. doi: 10.1093/gerona/52A.4.M218

Carpintero, P., Caeiro, J. R., Carpintero, R., Morales, A., Silva, S., and Mesa, M. (2014). Complications of hip fractures: a review. *World J. Orth.* 5, 402–411. doi: 10.5312/wjo.v5.i4.402

Chertkow, H., Whatmough, C., Saumier, D., and Duong, A. (2008). Cognitive neuroscience studies of semantic memory in Alzheimer's disease. *Prog. Brain Res.* 2008, 393–407. doi: 10.1016/S0079-6123(07)00025-8

Cramer, D. (1998). *Fundamental Statistics for Social Research. Step-by-Step Calculations and Computer Techniques using SPSS for Windows.* . New York, NY: Routledge.

Cramer, D., and Howitt, D. (2004). *The SAGE Dictionary of Statistics.* Thousand Oaks, CA: SAGE Publications. doi: 10.4135/9780857020123

Cruz-Ferreira, A., Marmeleira, J., Formigo, A., Gomes, D., and Fernandes, J. (2015). Creative dance improves physical fitness and life satisfaction in older women. *Res. Aging* 37, 837–855. doi: 10.1177/0164027514568103

Cruz-Jentoft, A. J., Baeyens, J. P., Bauer, J. M., Boirie, Y., Cederholm, T., Landi, F., et al. (2010). European consensus on definition and diagnosis: report of the European working group on sarcopenia in older people. *Age Ageing* 39, 412–423. doi: 10.1093/ageing/afq034

Doane, D. P., and Seward, L. E. (2011). Measuring Skewness: a forgotten statistic? *J. Stat. Educ.* 2011, 1–18. doi: 10.1080/10691898.2011.11889611

Efkildes, A., Yiultsi, E., Kangellidou, T., Kounti, F., Dina, F., and Tsolaki, M. (2002). Wechsler memory scale, rivermead behavioral memory test, and everyday memory questionnaire in healthy adults and Alzheimer's patients. *Eur. J. Psychol. Assess.* 18, 63–77. doi: 10.1027//1015-5759.18.1.63

Fallowfield, L. (2007). Quality of life issues in relation to the aromatase inhibitor. *J. Steroid Biochem. Mol. Biol.* 2007, 168–172. doi: 10.1016/j.jsbmb.2007.05.003

Ferri, C. P., Prince, M., Brayne, C., Brodaty, H., Fratiglioni, L., Ganguli, M., et al. (2005). Res Per Alz. *Lancet* 17, 2112–2117. doi: 10.1016/j.jpsychires.2013.02.001

Fountoulakis, C., Tsolaki, M., Chantzi, H., and Kazis, A. (2000). Mini Mental State Examination (MMSE): a validation study in demented patients from the elderly Greece population. *Am. J. Alzheimers Dis.* 15, 342–347. doi: 10.1177/153331750001500604

Fountoulakis, K. N., Tsolaki, M., Iacovides, A., Yesavage, J., O'Hara, R., Kazis, A., et al. (1999). The validation of the short form of the Geriatric Depression Scale (GDS) in Greece. *Aging Clin. Exp. Res.* 11, 367–372. doi: 10.1007/BF03339814

Garber, C. E., Blissmer, B., Deschenes, M. R., Franklin, B. A., Lamonte, M. J., Lee I. M., et al. (2011). Quantity and quality of exercise for developing and maintaining cardiorespiratory, musculoskeletal, and neuromotor fitness in apparently healthy adults: guidance for prescribing exercise. *Med. Sci. Sports Exerc.* 43, 1334–1359. doi: 10.1249/MSS.0b013e318213fefb

Ginnieri-Kokkosi, M., Triantafyllou, E., Antonopoulou, V., and Tomaras, V. (2003). *Life Quality Manual with Axis Questionnaire WHOQOL-100.* Athens: Publications Beta.

Gordon, N. F., Gulanick, M., Costa, F., Fletcher, G., Franklin, B. A., Roth, E. G., et al. (2004). Physical activity and exercise recommendations for stroke survivors: an American Heart Association scientific statement from the Council on Clinical Cardiology, Subcommittee on Exercise, Cardiac Rehabilitation, and Prevention; the Council on Cardiovascular Nursing; the Council on Nutrition, Physical Activity, and Metabolism; and the Stroke Council. *Circulation* 109, 2031–2041. doi: 10.1161/01.CIR.0000126280.65777.A4

Gorelick, P. B., Scuteri, A., and Black, S. E. (2011). Vascular contributions to cognitive impairment and dementia: a statement for healthcare professionals from the American Heart Association/American Stroke Association. *Stroke* 2011, 2672–2713. doi: 10.1161/STR.0b013e3182299496

Hamill, M., Smith, L., and Röhricht, F. (2011). Dancing down memory lane': circle dancing as a psychotherapeutic intervention in dementia-a pilot study. *Dementia* 11, 709–724. doi: 10.1177/1471301211420509

Hutton, J. T. (1990). "Alzheimer's Disease," in *Conn's Current Therapy*, ed. R. E. Rakel (Amsterdam: Elsevier Health Sciences), 778–781.

Hwang, P. W.-N., and Braun, K. L. (2015). the effectiveness of dance interventions to improve older adults' health: a systematic literature review. *Altern. Ther. Health* 21, 64–70.

Islam, M. S., Kabir, M. S., Khan, S. I., Ekramullah, M., Nair, G. B., Sack, R. B., et al. (2004). Wastewater-grown duckweed may be safely used as fish feed. *Can. J. Microbiol.* 50, 51–56. doi: 10.1139/w03-102

Jones, C. J., and Rikli, R. E. (2002). Measuring functional fitness of older adults. *Int. J. Act. Aging* 1, 25–30.

Kattenstroth, J. C., Kalisch, T., Holt, S., Tegenthoff, M., and Dinse, H. R. (2013). Six months of dance intervention enhances postural, sensorimotor, and cognitive performance in elderly without affecting cardiorespiratory functions. *Front. Aging Neurosci.* 5:5. doi: 10.3389/fnagi.2013.00005

Kattenstroth, J. C., Kalisch, T., Kolankowska, I., and Dinse, H. R. (2011). Balance, sensorimotor, and cognitive performance in long-year expert senior ballroom dancers. *J. Aging Res.* 2011: 176709. doi: 10.4061/2011/176709

Keller, K., and Engelhardt, M. (2013). Strength and muscle mass loss with aging process. Age and strength loss. *Muscles Ligaments Tendons J.* 3, 346–350.

Kim, S. H. (2009). Older people's expectations regarding ageing, health-promoting behaviour and health status. *J. Adv. Nurs.* 65, 84–91. doi: 10.1111/j.1365-2648.2008.04841.x

Kim, S. H., Kim, M., and Ahn, Y. B. (2011). Effect of dance exercise on cognitive function in elderly patients with metabolic syndrome: a pilot study. *J. Sports Sci. Med.* 10, 671–678.

Kosmidis, M. H. (2008). *Clinical Neuropsychological Assessment.* Athens: Parisianou Scientific Publications.

Kosmidis, M. H., Vlahou, C. H., Panagiotaki, P., and Kiosseoglou, G. (2004). The verbal fluency task in the Greek population: Normative data, and clustering and switching strategies. *J. Int. Neuropsych. Soc.* 10, 164–172. doi: 10.1017/S1355617704102014

Kounti, F., Tsolaki, M., and Kiosseoglou, G. (2006). Functional cognitive assessment scale (FUCAS): a new scale to assess executive cognitive function in daily life activities in patients with dementia and mild cognitive impairment. *Human Psychopharmacol. Clin. Exp.* 21, 305–311. doi: 10.1002/hup.772

Landers, D. M., and Arent, S. M. (2001). "Physical activity and mental health," in *Handbook of Sport Psychology*, eds R. N. Singer, H. A. Hausenblas, and C. M. Janelle (New York, NY: Wiley), 740–765.

Leveille, S. G., Jones, R. N., Kiely, D. K., Hausdorff, J. M., Shmerling, R. H., Guralnik, J. M., et al. (2009). Chronic musculoskeletal pain and the occurrence of falls in an older population. *J. Am. Med. Assoc.* 302, 2214–2221. doi: 10.1001/jama.2009.1738

Logsdon, R. G., Gibbons, L. E., McCurry, S. M., and Teri, L. (1999). Quality of life in Alzheimer's disease: patient and caregiver reports. *J. Ment. Health Aging* 1999, 21–32.

Minne, H. W. (2005). *Invest in Your Bones: Move it or Lose it*. Available at: www.bbcbonehealth.org

Morris, C. J. (1993). The Clinical Dementia Rating (CDR). *Neurology* 43, 2412–2414. doi: 10.1212/WNL.43.11.2412-a

Mullen, R., Davis, J. A., and Polatajko, H. J. (2012). Passion in the performing arts: clarifying active occupational participation. *Work* 2012, 15–25. doi: 10.3233/WOR-2012-1236

Pandria, N., Athanasiou, A., Terzopoulos, N., Paraskevopoulos, E., Karagianni, M., Styliadis, C., et al. (2018). Exploring the neuroplastic effects of biofeedback training on smokers. *Behav. Neurol.* 2018, 1–19. doi: 10.1155/2018/4876287

Petersen, R. C. (2004). Mild cognitive impairment as a diagnostic entity. *J. Intern. Med.* 256, 183–194. doi: 10.1111/j.1365-2796.2004.01388.x

Politis, A. M., Mayer, L. S., Passa, M., Maillis, A., and Lyketsos, C. G. (2004). Validity and reliability of the newly translated Hellenic Neuropsychiatric Inventory (H-NPI) applied to Greek outpatients with Alzheimer's disease: a study of disturbing behaviors among referrals to a memory clinic. *Int. J. Geriatr. Psych.* 19, 203–208. doi: 10.1002/gps.1045

Powers, R. (2010). *Use It or Lose It: Dancing Makes You Smarter*. Available at: http://socialdance.stanford.edu/syllabi/smarter.htm [accessed July 30, 2010].

Prince, M., Comas-Herrera, A., Knapp, M., Guerchet, M., and Karagiannidou, M. (2016). *World Alzheimer Report 2016: Improving Healthcare for People Living with Dementia: Coverage, Quality and Costs Now and in the Future*. London: Res per Alz (ADI).

Razali, N. M., and Wah, Y. B. (2011). Power comparisons of Shapiro-Wilk, Kolmogorov-Smirnov, Lilliefors and Anderson-Darling tests. *J. Stat. Model. Anal.* 2, 21–33.

Rey, A., and Osterrieth, P. A. (1993). Translations of excerpts from André Rey's "Psychological exami- nation of traumatic encephalopathy" and P. A. Osterrieth's "The complex figure copy test" (J. Corwin & F. W. Bylsma, Trans.). *Clin. Neuropsychol.* 7, 3–21.

Robertson, I. H., Ward, T., Ridgeway, V., and Nimmo-Smith, I. (1996). The structure of normal human attention: the test of everyday attention. *J. Int. Neuropsychol. Soc.* 2, 525–534. doi: 10.1017/S1355617700001697

Shapiro, S. S., and Wilk, M. B. (1965). An analysis of variance test for normality (complete samples). *Biometrika* 52, 591–611. doi: 10.1093/biomet/52.3-4.591

Sivvas, G., Batsiou, S., Vasoglou, Z., and Filippou, D. A. (2015). Dance contribution in health promotion. *J. Phys. Educ. Sport* 15, 484–489.

Skevington, S. M., Lotfy, M., O'Connell, K. A; WHOQOL Group. (2004). The World Health Organization's WHOQOL-BREF quality of life assessment: psychometric properties and results of the international field trial. A report from the WHOQOL Group. *Qual. Life Res.* 13, 299–310. doi: 10.1023/B:QURE.0000018486.91360.00

Soriano, T. A., DeCherrie, L. V., and Thomas, D. C. (2007). Falls in the community-dwelling older adult: a review for primary-care providers. *Clin. Interv. Aging* 2, 545–553. doi: 10.2147/CIA.S1080

Teri, L., Logsdon, R. G., and McCurry, S. M. (2008). Exercise interventions for dementia and cognitive impairment: the seattle protocols. *J. Nutr. Health Aging* 2008, 391–394. doi: 10.1007/BF02982672

Theodorakis, G. (2010). *Exercise, Mental Health and Quality of Life*, Vol. 16-17. Thessaloniki: Christodoulides Publications, 27–28.

Theotoka, I., Kapaki, E., Vagenas, V., Ilias, I., Paraskevas, G. P., and Liappas, I. (2007). Preliminary report of a validation study of instrumental activities of daily living in a Greek sample. *Percept. Motor Skill* 101, 958–960. doi: 10.2466/pms.104.3.958-960

Tsolaki, M., and Kounti, F. (2010). *Neuropsychological Tests and Diagnostic Criteria for Neurodegenerative Diseases*. Thessaloniki: Giahoudi Publications.

Vlahou, C. H., and Kosmidis, M. H. (2002). The Greek trail making test: preliminary norms for clinical and research use. *Psychol. J. Hellenic Psychol. Soc.* 9, 336–352.

Xerakia, E., and Kalogerakou, T. H. (2000). "The influence of the teaching of Greek traditional dances in the psychosomatic situation of the elderly. Sports & Society (Abstracts)," in *Proceedings of the 8th International Congress of Physical Education and Sports*, Komotini.

7

Acupuncture Modulates the Cerebello-Thalamo-Cortical Circuit and Cognitive Brain Regions in Patients of Parkinson's Disease with Tremor

Zhe Li [1,2†], Jun Chen [3†], Jianbo Cheng [4], Sicong Huang [5], Yingyu Hu [6], Yijuan Wu [1], Guihua Li [1], Bo Liu [3], Xian Liu [3], Wenyuan Guo [1], Shuxuan Huang [1], Miaomiao Zhou [1], Xiang Chen [7], Yousheng Xiao [7], Chaojun Chen [8*], Junbin Chen [9*], Xiaodong Luo [2*] and Pingyi Xu [1*]

[1] Department of Neurology, The First Affiliated Hospital, Guangzhou Medical University, Guangzhou, China, [2] Department of Neurology, The Second Affiliated Hospital, Guangzhou University of Chinese Medicine, Guangzhou, China, [3] Department of Radiology, Guangzhou University of Chinese Medicine, Guangzhou, China, [4] Department of Radiology, The People's Hospital of Gaozhou, Gaozhou, China, [5] Department of Laboratory, The Second Affiliated Hospital, Guangzhou Medical University, Guangzhou, China, [6] Department of Business Development, Zhujiang Hospital, Southern Medical University, Guangzhou, China, [7] Department of Neurology, The First Affiliated Hospital, Sun Yat-sen University, Guangzhou, China, [8] Department of Neurology, Guangzhou Hospital of Integrated Traditional and West Medicine, Guangzhou, China, [9] Department of Neurology, Yuebei People's Hospital, Shaoguan, China

*Correspondence:
Pingyi Xu
pingyixujd@163.com
Xiaodong Luo
luoxiaod@126.com
Junbin Chen
cjbcl0397@163.com
Chaojun Chen
ccjbs@126.com

[†] These authors have contributed equally to this work.

Objective: To investigate the effect of acupuncture on Parkinson's disease (PD) patients with tremor and its potential neuromechanism by functional magnetic resonance imaging (fMRI).

Methods: Forty-one PD patients with tremor were randomly assigned to true acupuncture group (TAG, $n = 14$), sham acupuncture group (SAG, $n = 14$) and waiting group (WG, $n = 13$). All patients received levodopa for 12 weeks. Patients in TAG were acupunctured on DU20, GB20, and the Chorea-Tremor Controlled Zone, and patients in SAG accepted sham acupuncture, while patients in WG received no acupuncture treatment until 12 weeks after the course was ended. The UPDRS II and III subscales, and fMRI scans of the patients' brains were obtained before and after the treatment course. UPDRS II and III scores were analyzed by SPSS, while the degree centrality (DC), regional homogeneity (ReHo) and amplitude low-frequency fluctuation (ALFF) were determined by REST.

Results: Acupuncture improved the UPDRS II and III scores in PD patients with tremor without placebo effect, only in tremor score. Acupuncture had specific effects on the cerebrocerebellar pathways as shown by the decreased DC and ReHo and increased ALFF values, and nonspecific effects on the spinocerebellar pathways as shown by the increased ReHo and ALFF values ($P < 0.05$, AlphaSim corrected). Increased ReHo values were observed within the thalamus and motor cortex of the PD patients ($P < 0.05$, AlphaSim corrected). In addition, the default mode network (DMN), visual areas and insula were activated by the acupuncture with increased DC, ReHo and/or ALFF, while the prefrontal cortex (PFC) presented a significant decrease in ReHo and ALFF values after acupuncture ($P < 0.05$, AlphaSim corrected).

Conclusions: The cerebellum, thalamus and motor cortex, which are connected to the cerebello-thalamo-cortical (CTC) circuit, were modulated by the acupuncture stimulation to alleviate the PD tremor. The regulation of neural activity within the cognitive brain regions (the DMN, visual areas, insula and PFC) together with CTC circuit may contributes to enhancing movement and improving patients' daily life activities.

Keywords: acupuncture, Parkinson's disease, tremor, functional magnetic resonance imaging, neuromechanism

INTRODUCTION

Parkinson's disease (PD) is an age-related neurodegenerative disorder of unknown origin that is characterized by the selective loss of dopaminergic neurons in the substantia nigra pars compacta (Miller and O'Callaghan, 2015). Tremor is usually the first clinical sign of PD, and approximately 70% of PD patients manifest conspicuous tremor at rest and/or during the maintenance of posture (Wang, 2006). The management of PD tremor presents a number of challenges to clinicians (Jiménez and Vingerhoets, 2012). Medication, which is the first line of treatment, often has unpredictable side effects. Stereotactic surgery provides better clinical results than medication but is poorly accepted, due to its invasiveness and high cost (Jiménez and Vingerhoets, 2012). Thus, many physicians and patients desire a complementary alternative strategy for tremor management. Acupuncture is a promising traditional Chinese medicine therapy that can be used to treat PD, and ∼7–10% of Asians choose acupuncture for tremor improvement (Lam et al., 2008). Due to its better adaptability, fewer side effects and lower cost, acupuncture has been widely used. Clinical studies have showed a positive benefit of acupuncture in treating PD tremor (Jiang et al., 2006; Wang et al., 2015). However, the mechanism underlying the effects of acupuncture on tremor associated with PD remains unknown.

Due to advances in brain neuroimaging technologies, recent functional magnetic resonance imaging (fMRI) studies have demonstrated that the basal ganglia (i.e., the pallidum and putamen) are active at the onset of tremor and the cerebellar circuit displays activity that is correlated with the magnitude of the ongoing tremor (Hallett, 2012). Both the basal ganglia and the cerebellum are connected to the motor cortex because the motor cortex is a component of both circuits, indicating the presence of pathology in the cerebello-thalamo-cortical (CTC) circuit in PD patients with tremor (Hallett, 2012).

fMRI is also a versatile tool to investigate the mechanism of acupuncture. According to previous animal studies, acupuncture plays a potential neuroprotective and restorative role in neuron survival (Kim et al., 2011; Sun et al., 2012; Rui et al., 2013; Xiao, 2015). This disease-modifying effect was reported to be similar to the effects of certain neuroprotective agents with anti-oxidative stress, anti-inflammatory and anti-apoptosis effects that improve motor performance in PD patients (Kim et al., 2011; Sun et al., 2012; Rui et al., 2013; Xiao, 2015). However, due to the physiological differences between humans and animals, conclusions based on animal experiments might differ from those based on clinical investigations involving human patients.

fMRI can be used to visually measure the specific impact of acupuncture on the human brain (Deng et al., 2008, 2016; Zhang et al., 2012; Zhou et al., 2014; Zhang Q. et al., 2015; Zhang S. Q. et al., 2015). Although several fMRI studies have investigated the medical effect of acupuncture on PD symptoms, studies investigating tremor are limited (Chae et al., 2009; Su, 2009; Shang, 2010; Ye, 2011; Yeo et al., 2012, 2014). For example, Yeo et al. (2012, 2014) found that acupuncture stimulation on GB34 (Yanglingquan) activated substantia nigra, basal ganglia, precentral gyrus and prefrontal cortex in PD, but the authors were unable to determine the mechanism by which acupuncture decreased tremor.

Based on the abovementioned knowledge, we speculated that acupuncture might alleviate tremor and improve motor function in PD patients by modulating the CTC circuit or other pathways. Thus, here, we investigated the effectiveness of acupuncture paratherapy on PD patients with tremor and explore its underlying neuromechanism by fMRI analyzing the degree centrality (DC), regional homogeneity (ReHo), and amplitudes of low-frequency fluctuation (ALFF). The analytical processes used in these three methods are very similar and, thus, are useful for identifying regions with consistent activity across fMRI studies.

MATERIALS AND METHODS

Subjects

This study was conducted at the 2nd Affiliated Hospital of Guangzhou University of Chinese Medicine between May 2014 and January 2016. The patients included in this study were diagnosed based on the UK PD Society Brain Bank clinical diagnostic criteria, and tremor at rest in at least one upper or lower extremity on either side was assessed by item 20 of the Unified Parkinson's Disease Rating Scale (UPDRS) (Gibb and Lees, 1988; UKNCCF, 2006; Prodoehl et al., 2013). The exclusion criteria included secondary Parkinsonism, atypical parkinsonian disease, advanced PD stage (H-Y $\geq$ 4), age less than 45 or greater than 80 years, history of other neurological disorders or head trauma, left-handedness, cognitive impairment (Mini Mental State Examination (MMSE) score <24), depression tendency (Beck Depression Inventory (BDI) score >4), and any contraindications for fMRI. The subjects were randomly assigned to a true acupuncture group (TAG), sham acupuncture group (SAG), or waiting group (WG) using a computer-generated list based on consecutive numbers that were distributed in sealed, opaque envelopes. All subjects provided written and verbal informed consent before participating in the study. They were informed what the study was about, including the possible risks and benefits to them, and were completely voluntary taking part in this study. They may also leave the study at any time. If they left the study before it was finished, there would be no penalty to them, and they would not lose any benefits to which they were otherwise entitled. This study was approved by the Ethics Committee of the 2nd Affiliated Hospital of Guangzhou University of Chinese Medicine.

Acupuncture

All subjects in the three groups received conventional levodopa treatment for a course of 12 weeks. A single experienced acupuncturist, who was not blinded to the group assignment, performed acupuncture twice weekly. In the TAG, stainless steel needles were inserted to a depth of 2.0–3.0 cm into DU20 (Baihui), GB20 (Fengchi), and the Chorea-Tremor Controlled Zone to alleviate tremor according to traditional Chinese medicine documents. Chorea-Tremor Controlled Zone is located at the scalp above the front of precentral gurus, 1.5 cm before Motor Zone. The reinforcing-reducing method conducted by twirling was performed every 10 min within the 30-min needle retention time. In the SAG, needles were inserted to 0.2 cm deep and 0.5 Chinese cun next to DU20, GB20 and the Chorea-Tremor Controlled Zone, but no manipulation of the needle was performed during the needle retention time. In the WG, true acupuncture was performed for 12 weeks following the completion of the medication course and the acupuncture effect was not evaluated. To guarantee that the patients were blinded during the treatment period, patients in each group received acupuncture treatment in different independent single-rooms; and all patients received bilateral and equivalent number of acupoint each time.

Clinical Evaluation

Clinical evaluators, who remained blinded throughout the study, assessed the UPDRS II and III of all subjects before and after the treatment course. In UPDRS III section, items 20 and 21 are for the tremor score, 22 for the rigidity score, 23, 24, 25, 26, and 31 for the hypokinesia score, and 27, 28, 29, and 30 for the postural instability/gait disorder (PIGD) score (Liu et al., 2011). These four sub-scores represent the four typical motor symptoms of PD. Adverse effects of acupuncture were recorded if they happened.

Image Acquisition

The brains of all subjects were scanned using a 3.0 Tesla MRI (Siemens MAGNETOM Verio 3.0T, Erlangen, Germany) with an 8-channel phased-array head coil at the radiology department of the hospital before and after the treatment course. To eliminate the effect of levodopa on the brain, the fMRI scan was performed at least 4 h after the levodopa administration. During the data acquisition process, all subjects were asked to close their eyes and lie quietly for MR scanning. Resting-state functional images were acquired using a T2-weighted gradient-recalled echo-planar imaging (GRE-EPI) sequence with the following parameters: repetition time = 2,000 ms, echo time = 30 ms, flip angle = 90°, thickness = 3.5 mm, gap = 0.35 mm, field of view = 224 × 224 mm2, matrix = 64 × 64, 31 axial slices, and 240 time points. The structural images were analyzed

using a three-dimensional T1-weighted magnetization-prepared rapid gradient echo (MPRAGE) sequence with the following parameters: repetition time = 1,900 ms, echo time = 2.27 ms, flip angle = 9°, thickness = 1.0 mm, field of view = 256 × 256 mm2, and matrix = 256 × 256.

Data Preprocessing and Calculations

The fMRI data analyser was also blinded to the group assignment. The resting-state fMRI data preprocessing was performed using DPABI based on MATLAB (The Math Works, Natick, MA, USA). After removing the first four volumes of each participant, the functional images were corrected for the intra-volume acquisition time delay using slice-timing and realignment. None of the participants were excluded based on the criteria of displacement >2 mm or angular rotation >2° in any direction. All corrected functional data were then normalized to the Montreal Neurological Institute (MNI) space and resampled to a 3-mm isotropic resolution. The resulting images were further temporally band-pass filtered (0.01–0.08 Hz) to remove the effects of low-frequency drift and high-frequency physiological noise. Finally, 24 head-motion parameters, white matter signals, and cerebrospinal fluid signals were regressed using a general linear model, and linear trends were removed from the fMRI data. Spatial smoothing was also performed before the ALFF analysis using a Gaussian filter (6-mm full-width half-maximum, FWHM), but after the ReHo calculation.

REST (http://resting-fmri.sourceforge.net) (Song et al., 2011) V1.8 was used to calculate the values of the DC, ReHo, and ALFF. The DC represents the large-scale brain intrinsic connectivity related to the global information integration function at the voxel level (Buckner et al., 2009). We applied threshold to the correlation coefficients at $r > 0.25$ to remove the weak correlations caused by noises. ReHo depicts the local synchronization of the time series of neighboring voxels, which is related to the local information integration function (Zang et al., 2004). ALFF measures the amplitude of time series fluctuations at each voxel and is thought to be associated with spontaneous neuronal activity (Zang et al., 2007). Thus, these three fMRI measures probe different aspects of brain activity (Wang et al., 2017).

Statistical Analysis

One-way ANOVA and the chi-squared test were performed to assess the baseline differences in the demographic and clinical data among the three groups, and paired-sample t-test was performed to evaluate UPDRS II and III scores before and after the treatment in each group using SPSS V22.0 (SPSS Inc., Chicago, IL, USA). The level of significance was set as $P < 0.05$.

The statistical analysis of the DC, ReHo and ALFF was conducted using REST V1.8. An ANCOVA was performed on the fMRI data to identify the DC, ReHo and ALFF maps among three groups with the pretreamtment images as covariates. Subsequently, the regions that showed significant differences were extracted as a mask, and the DC, ReHo, and ALFF values were subjected to post hoc analysis. Statistical comparisons of these values between each pair of groups were performed using a two-sample *post-hoc* t-test, and the LSD correction was applied for multiple tests to keep the overall type I error level of 0.05. Voxels with a $P < 0.05$ corrected by AlphaSim and a cluster size $>2,295$ mm^3 (85 voxels) were considered significantly different.

RESULTS

Demographic and Clinical Characteristics

Of the 42 patients who were identified as potential participants, one patient refused the fMRI scanning. The remaining 41 patients were randomized in this study. No patients were withdrawn from the TAG. Two subjects, one in the SAG who was diagnosed with acute ischaemic stroke by fMRI and another in the WG who experienced an accidental fall, were excluded. Four subjects, 2 in the SAG and 2 in the WG, were withdrawn because of poor efficacy, failure to follow up or refusal to re-scan fMRI after the week 4 visit call (**Figure 1**). The baseline demographic and clinical characteristics of the patients in three groups are presented in **Table 1**. All subjects were cognitively normal and free of depression according to the MMSE and the BDI. No statistically significant differences in gender, age, family history, onset age, PD duration, UPDRS (II and III) or levodopa usage were observed among three groups.

Clinical Evaluation

TAG showed significant improvement in UPDRS II and III scores, while WG and SAG didn't. In UPDRS III, tremor score in TAG decreased obviously while in WG increased significantly, but no big change in SAG. However, rigidity, hypokinesia and PIGD scores before and after treatment in each group displayed no significant differences (**Table 2**). No obvious adverse effects of acupuncture in the patients were reported.

DC

An ANCOVA revealed significant differences in the DC index between the TAG, SAG, and WG in the following regions: fusiform gyrus, cuneus, lingual gyrus, superior and middle occipital gyri, insula and cerebellum crus. Compared with the SAG, the TAG showed increased DC in the fusiform gyrus, cuneus, lingual gyrus, superior and middle occipital gyri, and decreases in the cerebellum crus. Compared with the WG, the TAG displayed increased DC in the cuneus and decreased DC in the cerebellum crus. In addition, compared with the WG, the SAG's DC values were significantly elevated in bilateral insula. The details of the peak coordinates and cluster sizes are listed in **Table 3**.

ReHo

An ANCOVA exhibits significant differences in the ReHo index among three groups in the following regions: middle and inferior frontal gyri, rectus gyrus, precentral gyrus, supplement motor area (SMA), inferior parietal lobules, precuneus, cuneus, fusiform gyrus, superior and middle cccipital gyri, anterior cingulate gyrus, hippocampus, thalamus, insula and cerebellum. Compared with the SAG, a significantly increased ReHo values was detected in the SMA, inferior parietal lobules, precuneus, cuneus, fusiform gyrus, superior and middle cccipital gyri, and a significant decrease in the ReHo was observed in the middle and inferior frontal gyri, anterior cingulate gyrus and the cerebellum crus of patients in the TAG (**Figure 2**). Compared to the WG, patients of the TAG had an enhanced ReHo values in the

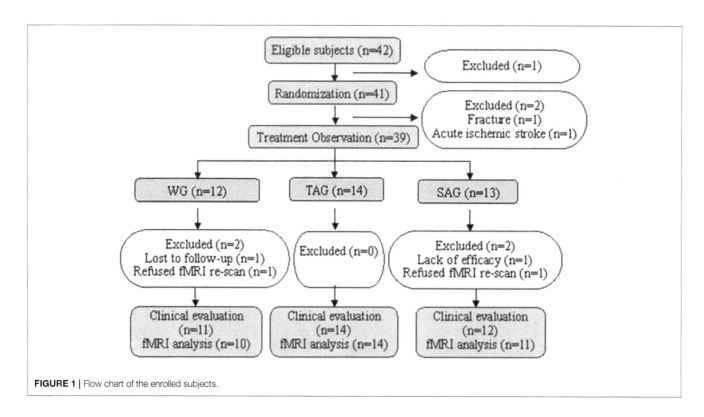

FIGURE 1 | Flow chart of the enrolled subjects.

Acupuncture Modulates the Cerebello-Thalamo-Cortical Circuit and Cognitive Brain Regions in Patients...

65

TABLE 1 | Baseline demographic and clinical data of all subjects.

	WG (n = 12)	TAG (n = 14)	SAG (n = 13)	P-value
Gender (Male/Female)	9/3	8/6	7/6	0.51
Age (Years)	62.17 ± 7.66	65.79 ± 6.07	62.85 ± 5.00	0.30
Family history (Yes/No)	2/10	3/11	1/12	0.75
Onset age (Years)	54.83 ± 9.76	60.64 ± 7.56	57.85 ± 5.43	0.18
PD duration (Years)	7.33 ± 4.62	5.14 ± 3.32	5.03 ± 4.73	0.39
MMSE	27.17 ± 2.82	28.71 ± 1.20	28.69 ± 1.11	0.16
BDI	3.17 ± 1.34	2.36 ± 1.86	1.92 ± 1.66	0.17
UPDRS II score	11.42 ± 6.37	12.64 ± 5.98	11.38 ± 4.41	0.81
UPDRS III score	24.17 ± 13.44	26.00 ± 15.07	20.31 ± 8.64	0.58
Levodopa usage	345.83 ± 173.81	367.86 ± 146.24	338.46 ± 112.09	0.92

TABLE 2 | UPDRS II and III score of all subjects before and after treatment.

		WG (n = 11)	TAG (n = 14)	SAG (n = 12)
UPDRS II score	Pre-treatment	11.09 ± 6.58	12.64 ± 5.98	11.25 ± 4.58
	Post-treatment	12.27 ± 7.90	9.00 ± 4.40	10.33 ± 5.28
	T-value	−1.44	3.40	1.08
	P-value	0.179	0.005*	0.303
UPDRS III score	Pre-treatment	24.36 ± 14.07	26.00 ± 15.07	19.50 ± 8.49
	Post-treatment	26.73 ± 14.03	21.64 ± 13.68	19.25 ± 9.21
	T-value	−1.88	2.96	0.29
	P-value	0.090	0.011*	0.777
Tremor score	Pre-treatment	1.12 ± 0.62	1.17 ± 0.52	0.92 ± 0.49
	Post-treatment	1.31 ± 0.69	0.85 ± 0.43	0.90 ± 0.47
	T-value	−3.75	6.19	0.19
	P-value	0.004*	0.000*	0.851
Rigidity score	Pre-treatment	0.71 ± 0.72	0.89 ± 0.82	0.52 ± 0.54
	Post-treatment	0.80 ± 0.64	0.76 ± 0.79	0.50 ± 0.53
	T-value	−1.46	1.26	0.43
	P-value	0.176	0.229	0.674
Hypokinesia score	Pre-treatment	0.85 ± 0.53	0.84 ± 0.75	0.56 ± 0.32
	Post-treatment	0.91 ± 0.52	0.71 ± 0.77	0.58 ± 0.30
	T-value	−0.69	1.85	−0.39
	P-value	0.506	0.087	0.701
PIGD score	Pre-treatment	0.82 ± 0.66	0.88 ± 0.45	0.79 ± 0.58
	Post-treatment	0.82 ± 0.63	0.82 ± 0.36	0.75 ± 0.62
	T-value	0.00	0.90	0.69
	P-value	1.000	0.385	0.504

*Data are shown as mean ± SD. *P <0.05.*

left precentral gyrus, SMA, precuneus, hippocampus, thalamus, insula and cerebellum 4_5, and a reduced ReHo values in the middle and inferior frontal gyri, rectus gyrus, right precentral gyrus and cerebellum crus (**Figure 3**). What's more, the SAG patients displayed an increased ReHo in the left insula and a decreased regional activity in the right precentral gyrus compared to the WG. The details of the peak coordinates and cluster sizes are listed in **Table 4**.

ALFF

The inferior and medial frontal gyri, fusiform gyrus and the cerebellum revealed significant differences in the ALFF values among the TAG, SAG and WG. Compared to the SAG, an enhanced ALFF in the cerebellum 4_5 and 6, and a reduced ALFF in the orbital inferior frontal gyrus were observed in the patients of TAG. Furthermore, compared to the WG, significantly elevated spontaneous neural activities exhibited in the fusiform

TABLE 3 | Brain regions exhibiting increased and decreased degree centrality among three groups.

Brain regions	Cluster size	Peak intensity	Peak MNI coordinates		
			X	Y	Z
TAG>SAG					
Right Fusiform Gyrus	100	4.68	33	−48	−15
Bilateral Cuneus, Lingual Gyrus, Superior and Middle Occipital Gyri, Fusiform Gyrus	1,181	6.28	−12	−90	15
TAG<SAG					
Left Cerebellum Crus1 and 2	97	−3.96	−36	−78	−27
TAG>WG					
Bilateral Cuneus	116	4.12	3	−81	36
TAG<WG					
Left Cerebellum Crus1 and 2	131	−5.30	−39	−84	−33
SAG>WG					
Left Insula	183	4.42	−27	9	12
Right Insula	110	4.65	42	−9	12

TAG, true acupuncture group; SAG, sham acupuncture group; WG, waiting group. A > B, Compared with B group, A group showed increased DC values; A < B, Compared with B group, A group showed decreased DC values (P < 0.05, AlphaSim corrected).

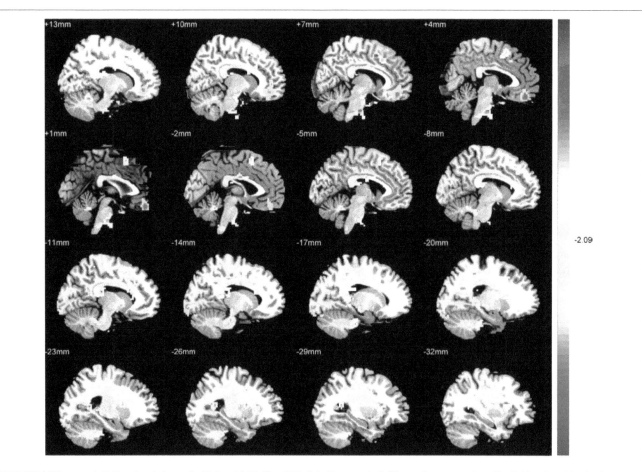

FIGURE 2 | Differences in ReHo values between the TAG and SAG. (P < 0.05, AlphaSim corrected). Warm colors represent positive ReHo values; blue (cold) colors represent negative ReHo values.

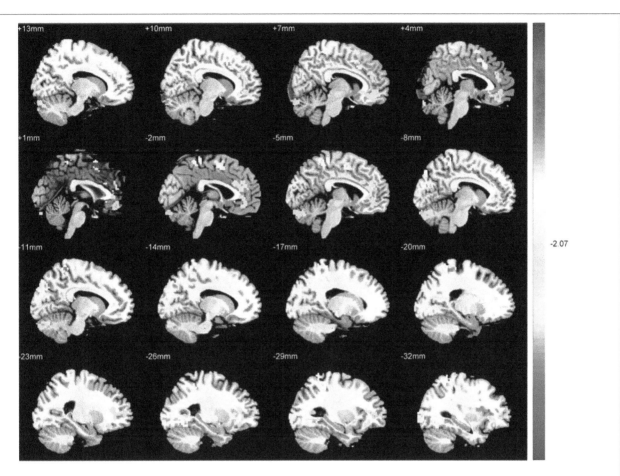

FIGURE 3 | Differences in ReHo values between the TAG and WG. ($P < 0.05$, AlphaSim corrected). Warm colors represent positive ReHo values; blue (cold) colors represent negative ReHo values.

gyrus, cerebellum crus and vermis of the TAG patients, and in the medial frontal gyrus and cerebellum crus of the SAG patients. The details of the peak coordinates and cluster sizes are listed in **Table 5**.

DISCUSSION

In this neural imaging study, we investigated the effect and its neural substrates of acupuncture stimulation on PD patients with tremor by the DC, ReHo and ALFF methods. We proved that acupuncture could improve the daily life activities and motor symptoms in PD patients with tremor without placebo effect, and tremor was the only symptom that had been ameliorated in the four typical motor symptoms of PD. We then analyzed the fMRI data that the DC, ReHo and ALFF analyses were consistent in the spinocerebellum, thalamus, default mode network (DMN), insula, visual areas and prefrontal cortex (PFC), and inconsistent in the cerebrocerebellum and motor cortex.

Interestingly, the acupuncture administration exerted a specific activating effect on the cerebrocerebellum (cerebellum crus1 and 2, and cerebellum 6) with decreased DC and ReHo values and enhanced ALFF signals, and a nonspecific effect on the spinocerebellum (cerebellum 4_5 and vermis) associated with the enhanced ReHo and ALFF values. A significant change of the ReHo value in the thalamus and motor cortex (precentral gyrus and SMA) was also observed. Anatomically, the cerebrocerebellum receives input neural signals from the cerebral cortex and sends output signals mainly to ventrolateral thalamus in turn connected to motor areas of the premotor cortex and the primary motor area of the cerebral cortex, which is thought to be involved in the initiation, planning and coordination of movements (Kandel and Schwartz, 1985; Schmahmann et al., 1999). The conflicting signal changes in the cerebrocerebellum may be due to a compensation by the activated left precentral gyrus and SMA for the function of the cerebellum in integrating information with the motor cortex. The inconsistent ReHo changes in the left and right precentral gyri could be attributed to the fact that all subjects in our study were right-handed; in these patients, the improved function of the left precentral gyrus might be expected to compensate for the decreased function of the right precentral gyrus. The connections of the cerebellum, thalamus and motor cortex to the CTC circuit have been shown to influence patients' functional motor activity (Wu and Hallett, 2013). Thus, our data demonstrate acupuncture improve the motor function and daily life activities of PD patients by a direct stimulatory effect on the CTC circuit. Moreover, several imaging

TABLE 4 | Brain regions exhibiting increased and decreased regional homogeneity among three groups.

Brain regions	Cluster size	Peak intensity	Peak MNI coordinates		
			X	Y	Z
TAG>SAG					
Left Fusiform Gyrus	144	4.13	−24	−75	−6
Left Middle Occipital Gyrus	127	3.96	−39	−93	−3
Left Cuneus and Superior Occipital Gyrus	123	3.98	−15	−78	36
Right Cuneus and Superior Occipital Gyrus	89	5.36	15	−84	48
Bilateral Supplement Motor Area	108	4.18	9	15	39
Left Precuneus	198	5.12	−12	−45	63
Left Inferior Parietal Lobules	91	3.68	−33	−48	51
TAG<SAG					
Bilateral Cerebellum Crus1 and 2	181	−3.99	9	−93	−24
Left Middle and Inferior Frontal Gyri	360	−5.00	−27	27	−18
Bilateral Anterior Cingulate Gyrus	566	−4.57	15	33	18
TAG>WG					
Right Cerebellum_4_5	264	5.10	3	−12	−33
Left Precuneus, Hippocampus and Thalamus	189	4.31	−24	−51	9
Right Hippocampus and Precuneus	377	4.55	18	−45	15
Bilateral Supplement Motor Area	747	5.51	6	9	48
Left Precentral Gyrus	97	4.29	−30	6	30
Left Insula	141	4.14	−30	18	12
TAG<WG					
Right Rectus and Middle Frontal Gyrus	416	−4.77	3	48	−21
Left Cerebellum Crus1	89	−4.04	−27	−90	−24
Right Orbital Inferior Frontal Gyrus	95	−3.95	42	42	−15
Right Precentral Gyrus	98	−5.47	54	0	42
SAG>WG					
Left Insula	107	4.42	−27	9	12
SAG<WG					
Right Precentral Gyrus	162	−5.70	51	0	42

TAG, true acupuncture group; SAG, sham acupuncture group; WG, waiting group. A > B, Compared with B group, A group showed increased ReHo values; A<B, Compared with B group, A group showed decreased ReHo values (P<0.05, AlphaSim corrected).

studies have suggested that PD tremor is strongly associated with the CTC circuit (Helmich et al., 2011, 2012; Zhang J. et al., 2015), which may be the reason that tremor was the only motor symptoms being improved. Although this study may be the first time to elucidate how acupuncture affects PD tremor, evidence for tremor control via the CTC network has been accumulated by deep brain stimulation (DBS) and repetitive transcranial magnetic stimulation (rTMS), and several reports indicate that the stimulating mechanism of DBS or rTMS is potentially similar to that of acupuncture (Fukuda et al., 2004; Mure et al., 2011; Popa et al., 2013; Coenen et al., 2014).

We also observed that acupuncture had a specific effect on brain regions relevant to cognitive activity, such as the DMN (the anterior cingulate gyrus, precuneus, cuneus, medial PFC, inferior parietal lobule and hippocampus), visual areas (the lingual gyrus, superior and middle occipital gyri and the fusiform gyrus), insula and PFC (gyrus rectus, middle and inferior frontal gyri). The effect of DMN and insula on cognitive processing has been confirmed in recent fMRI studies investigating aging

individuals and individuals with neurodegenerative disorders (Tessitore et al., 2012; Zhang S. Q. et al., 2015; Jiang et al., 2016). The visual processing controlled by the visual areas and the executive function managed by the PFC (Yuan and Raz, 2014) are also parts of the cognition. Since the subjects enrolled in this study were cognitively normal, these cognitive brain regions is speculated to participate in the cognitive management of movement, as movement control includes motor and cognitive components (Prevosto and Sommer, 2013). Generally, the cognitive control of movement is achieved by motion perception, movement learning, movement memory, movement planning and motor inhibition (Lu et al., 2012). For instance, in humans, an environmental stimulus related to motion is first perceived by the visual system, and the produced visual information is conveyed from the visual areas to the motor cortex to generate motion perception. Subsequently, an empirical rule is formed from the learning and memory of movement, which results from neural activity in the primary motor cortex, cerebellum, DMN and insula. Then, movement planning is regulated by the

TABLE 5 | Brain regions exhibiting increased and decreased amplitude of low frequency fluctuations among three groups.

Brain regions	Cluster size	Peak intensity	Peak MNI coordinates		
			X	Y	Z
TAG>SAG					
Left Cerebellum 4_5 and 6	94	3.95	−36	−33	−27
TAG<SAG					
Right Orbital Inferior Frontal Gyrus	217	−4.24	27	36	−12
TAG>WG					
Right Fusiform Gyrus	396	4.54	48	−36	−27
Left Fusiform Gyrus	320	4.82	−33	−33	−27
Right Cerebellum_Crus1	176	3.25	33	−57	0
Left Cerebellum_Crus1	273	2.94	−39	−66	−33
Vermis_4_5 and 6	167	3.54	3	−57	−15
SAG>WG					
Right Medial Frontal Gyrus	93	3.89	15	42	12
Right Cerebellum_Crus1	339	4.38	18	−81	−27

TAG, true acupuncture group; SAG, sham acupuncture group; WG, waiting group; A > B, Compared with B group, A group showed increased ALFF values; A < B, Compared with B group, A group showed decreased ALFF values (P < 0.05, AlphaSim corrected).

basal ganglia, SMA and PFC to enable the execution of precise action (Lu et al., 2012). Therefore, the modulation of the neural activity in cognitive regions may contribute to the movement improvement along with the CTC circuit.

Several limitations of this study should be addressed. First, this was a small sample study, and the authors did not continue to assess the clinical symptoms and fMRI after the treatment course was discontinued. Second, there was 6 drop-outs out of 41 randomized patients (15%), which might cause bias in the conclusion. Third, we used MMSE to screen for the cognitive impairments as it's quite specific and easy to complete. Nonetheless, MMSE may not be as sensitive as the Montreal Cognitive Assessment to detect mild cognitive impairments. A study with a larger patient population, long-term follow-up and reliable cognitive tests is needed to more conclusively determine the efficacy and its neuromechanism of acupuncture on PD tremor and find out whether acupuncture could work on the cognition for a longer period of time by modulating the cognitive brain regions.

In conclusion, our findings reveal that acupuncture has specific and nonspecific effects on different brain regions involved in PD tremor, and the motor and cognitive management of movement. The underlying mechanism of the effects of acupuncture on PD tremor may be related to a modification of the CTC circuit, and the modulation of the cognitive functional

regions together with CTC circuit contributes to enhancing movement and improving the daily life activities of PD patients.

AUTHOR CONTRIBUTIONS

ZL, BL, and XDL conceived and designed the experiments. JBC and XL performed the fMRI scans. JC analyzed the fMRI data. GHL performed the acupuncture. WYG and YSX analyzed the clinical data. SCH, SXH, MMZ, and XC collected the clinical data. YJW, CJC, JBC, and XDL recruited potential participants. and ZL, YYH, and PYX wrote the manuscript. All authors read and approved the final manuscript.

ACKNOWLEDGMENTS

This study was supported by the Guangzhou Postdoctoral International Training Program Funding Project, the National Key Research and Development Projects of China (2016YFC1306600, 2017YFC1310300), the National Natural Science Foundation of China (81471292, U1603281, U1503222, 81430021, 81603681), the Science and Technology Project of Guangdong Province (2015A030311021, 2016A020215201), a Science and Technology Planning Project of Guangzhou (201504281820463, 2018-1202-SF-0019) and an international project of science and technology for Guangdong (2016A050502025).

REFERENCES

Buckner, R. L., Sepulcre, J., Talukdar, T., Krienen, F. M., Liu, H., Hedden, T., et al. (2009). Cortical hubs revealed by intrinsic functional connectivity: mapping, assessment of stability, and relation to Alzheimer's disease. *J. Neurosci.* 29, 1860–1873. doi: 10.1523/JNEUROSCI.5062-08.2009

Chae, Y., Lee, H., Kim, H., Kim, C. H., Chang, D. I., Kim, K. M., et al. (2009). Parsing brain activity associated with acupuncture treatment in Parkinson's diseases. *Mov. Disord.* 24, 1794–1802. doi: 10.1002/mds.22673

Coenen, V. A., Allert, N., Paus, S., Kronenbürger, M., Urbach, H., and Mädler, B. (2014). Modulation of the cerebello-thalamo-cortical network in thalamic deep brain stimulation for tremor: a diffusion tensor imaging study. *Neurosurgery* 75, 657–669. doi: 10.1227/NEU.0000000000000540

Deng, D., Duan, G., Liao, H., Liu, Y., Wang, G., Liu, H., et al. (2016). Changes in regional brain homogeneity induced by electro-acupuncture stimulation at the Baihui acupoint in healthy subjects: a functional magnetic resonance imaging study. *J. Altern. Complement. Med.* 22, 794–799. doi: 10.1089/acm.2015.0286

Deng, G., Hou, B. L., Holodny, A. I., and Cassileth, B. R. (2008). Functional magnetic resonance imaging (fMRI) changes and saliva production associated with acupuncture at LI-2 acupuncture point: a randomized controlled study[J]. *BMC Complement. Altern. Med.* 8:37. doi: 10.1186/1472-6882-8-37

Fukuda, M., Barnes, A., Simon, E. S., Holmes, A., Dhawan, V.,Giladi, N., et al. (2004). Thalamic stimulation for parkinsonian tremor: correlation between regional cerebral blood flow and physiological tremor characteristics. *Neuroimage* 21, 608–615. doi: 10.1016/j.neuroimage.2003.09.068

Gibb, W. R., and Lees, A. J. (1988). The relevance of the Lewy body to the pathogenesis of idiopathic Parkinson's disease. *J. Neurol. Neurosurg. Psychiatry* 51, 745–752. doi: 10.1136/jnnp-2012-302969

Hallett, M. (2012). Parkinson's disease tremor: pathophysiology. *Parkinsonism Relat. Disord.* 18(Suppl. 1), S85–S86. doi: 10.1016/S1353-8020(11)70027-X

Helmich, R. C., Hallett, M., Deuschl, G., Toni, I., and Bloem, B. R. (2012). Cerebral causes and consequences of parkinsonian resting tremor: a tale of two circuits?. *Brain* 135, 3206–3226. doi: 10.1093/brain/aws023

Helmich, R. C., Janssen, M. J., Oyen, W. J., Bloem, B. R., and Toni, I. (2011). Pallidal dysfunction drives a cerebellothalamic circuit into Parkinson tremor. *Ann. Neurol.* 69, 269–281. doi: 10.1002/ana.22361.

Jiang, S., Wang, M., Zhang, L., Yuan, Y., Tong, Q., Ding, J., et al. (2016). Regional homogeneity alterations differentiate between tremor dominant and postural instability gait difficulty subtypes of Parkinson's disease. *J. Neural Transm. (Vienna)* 123, 219–229. doi: 10.1007/s00702-015-1490-5

Jiang, X. M., Huang, Y., Zhuo, Y., and Gao, Y. P. (2006). Therapeutic effect of scalp electroacupuncture on Parkinson disease. *Nan Fang Yi Ke Da Xue Xue Bao* 26, 114–116.

Jiménez, M. C., and Vingerhoets, F. J. (2012). Tremor revisited: treatment of PD tremor. *Parkinsonism Relat. Disord.* 18(Suppl. 1), S93–S95. doi: 10.1016/S1353-8020(11)70030-X

Kandel, E. R., and Schwartz, J. H (1985).*Principles of Neural Science, 2nd Edn.* New York, NY: Elsevier, 502–522.

Kim, S. N., Kim, S. T., Doo, A. R., Park, J. Y., Moon, W., Chae, Y., et al. (2011). Phosphatidylinositol 3-kinase/Akt signaling pathway mediates acupuncture-induced dopaminergic neuron protection and motor function improvement in a mouse model of Parkinson's disease. *Int. J. Neurosci.* 121, 562–569. doi: 10.3109/00207454.2011.591515

Lam, Y. C., Kum, W. F., Durairajan, S. S., Lu, J. H., Man, S. C., Xu, M., et al. (2008). Efficacy and safety of acupuncture for idiopathic Parkinson's disease: a systematic review *J. Altern. Complement. Med.* 14, 663–671. doi: 10.1089/acm.2007.0011

Liu, P., Feng, T., Wang, Y. J., Zhang, X., and Chen, B. (2011). Clinical heterogeneity in patients with early-stage Parkinson's disease: a cluster analysis. *J. Zhejiang Univ. Sci. B* 12, 694–703. doi: 10.1631/jzus.B1100069

Lu, Q. Q., Dai, S. F., Gu, K., Zuo, Y. F., and Yu, P. (2012). The role of cortical and subcortical motor areas in the cognitive control of movement. *Adv. Psychol. Sci.* 20, 1794–1802. doi: 10.3724/sp.j.1042.2012.01794

Miller, D. B., and O'Callaghan, J. P. (2015). Biomarkers of Parkinson's disease: present and future. *Metabolism* 64(3 Suppl. 1.), S40–S46. doi: 10.1016/j.metabol.2014.10.030

Mure, H., Hirano, S., Tang, C. C., Isaias, I. U., Antonini, A., Ma, Y., et al. (2011). Parkinson's disease tremor-related metabolic network: characterization, progression, and treatment effects. *Neuroimage* 54, 1244–1253. doi: 10.1016/j.neuroimage.2010.09.028

Popa, T., Russo, M., Vidailhet, M., Roze, E., Lehéricy, S., Bonnet, C., et al. (2013). Cerebellar rTMS stimulation may induce prolonged clinical benefits in essential tremor, and subjacent changes in functional connectivity: an open label trial. *Brain Stimul.* 6, 175–179. doi: 10.1016/j.brs.2012.04.009

Prevosto, V., and Sommer, M. A. (2013). Cognitive control of movement via the cerebellar-recipient thalamus. *Front. Syst. Neurosci.* 7:56. doi: 10.3389/fnsys.2013.00056

Prodoehl, J., Planetta, P. J., Kurani, A. S., Comella, C. L., Corcos, D. M., and Vaillancourt, D. E. (2013). Differences in brain activation between tremor- and nontremor-dominant Parkinson disease. *JAMA Neurol.* 70, 100–106. doi: 10.1001/jamaneurol.2013.582

Rui, G., Guangjian, Z., Yong, W., Jie, F., Yanchao, C., Xi, J., et al. (2013). High frequency electro-acupuncture enhances striatum DAT and D1 receptor expression, but decreases D2 receptor level in 6-OHDA lesioned rats[J]. *Behav. Brain Res.* 237, 263–226. doi: 10.1016/j.bbr.2012.09.047

Schmahmann, J. D., Doyon, J., Mcdonald, D., Holmes, C., Lavoie, K., Hurwitz, A. S., et al. (1999). Three-dimensional MRI atlas of the human cerebellum in proportional stereotaxic space. *Neuroimage* 10, 233–260. doi: 10.1006/nimg.1999.0459

Shang, X. J. (2010). *The fMRI Study on the Influence of Scalp Acupuncture on Central Nervous in Patients with Parkinson's Disease.* Guangzhou University of Chinese Medicine (Guangzhou).

Song, X. W., Dong, Z. Y., Long, X. Y., Li, S. F., Zuo, X. N., Zhu, C. Z., et al. (2011). REST: a toolkit for resting-state functional magnetic resonance imaging data processing. *PLoS ONE* 6:e25031. doi: 10.1371/journal.pone.0025031

Su, C. H. (2009). *The Impact of Electro-acupuncture the Chorea-Trembling Controlled Area of Parkinson's Patients and Preliminary Study of its Efficacy.* Guangzhou University of Chinese Medicine (Guangzhou).

Sun, Z., Jia, J., Gong, X., Jia, Y., Deng, J., Wang, X., et al. (2012). Inhibition of glutamate and acetylcholine release in behavioral improvement induced by electroacupuncture in parkinsonian rats. *Neurosci. Lett.* 520, 32–37. doi: 10.1016/j.neulet.2012.05.021

Tessitore, A., Esposito, F., Vitale, C., Santangelo, G., Amboni, M., Russo, A., et al. (2012). Default-mode network connectivity in cognitively unimpaired patients with Parkinson disease. *Neurology* 79, 2226–2232. doi: 10.1212/WNL.0b013e31827689d6

UKNCCF (2006). *Parkinson's Disease: National Clinical Guideline for Diagnosis and Management in Primary and Secondary Care.* London: Royal College of Physicians (UK).

Wang, F., Sun, L., Zhang, X. Z., Jia, J., Liu, Z., Huang, X. Y., et al. (2015). Effect and potential mechanism of electroacupuncture add-on treatment in patients with Parkinson's Disease. *Evid. Based Complement. Alternat. Med.* 2015:692795. doi: 10.1155/2015/692795

Wang, J. B., Zheng, L. J., Cao, Q. J., Wang, Y. F., Sun, L., Zang, Y. F., et al. (2017). Inconsistency in abnormal brain activity across cohorts of ADHD-200 in children with attention deficit hyperactivity disorder. *Front. Neurosci.* 11:320. doi: 10.3389/fnins.2017.00320

Wang, W. Z. (2006). *Neurology.* Beijing: People's Medical Publishing House, 1093–1102.

Wu, T., and Hallett, M. (2013). The cerebellum in Parkinson's disease. *Brain* 136, 696–709. doi: 10.1093/brain/aws360

Xiao, D. (2015). Acupuncture for Parkinson's Disease: a review of clinical, animal, and functional magnetic resonance imaging studies. *J. Tradit. Chin. Med.* 35, 709–717.

Ye, X. F. (2011). *The Impact of Fang-Acupuncture of Parkinson's Patients on FMRI and Preliminary Study of its Effcacy.* Guangzhou University of Chinese Medicine (Guangzhou).

Yeo, S., Choe, I. H., van den Noort, M., Bosch, P., Jahng, G. H., Rosen, B., et al. (2014). Acupuncture on GB34 activates the precentral gyrus and prefrontal cortex in Parkinson's disease. *BMC Complement. Altern. Med.* 14:336. doi: 10.1186/1472-6882-14-336

Yeo, S., Lim, S., Choe, I. H., Choi, Y. G., Chung, K. C.,Jahng, G. H., et al. (2012). Acupuncture stimulation on GB34 activates neural responses associated with Parkinson's disease. *CNS Neurosci. Ther.* 18, 781–790. doi: 10.1111/j.1755-5949.2012.00363.x

Yuan, P., and Raz, N. (2014). Prefrontal cortex and executive functions in healthy adults: a meta-analysis of structural neuroimaging studies. *Neurosci. Biobehav. Rev.* 42:180–192. doi: 10.1016/j.neubiorev.2014.02.005

Zang, Y. F., He, Y., Zhu, C. Z., Cao, Q. J., Sui, M. Q.,Liang, M., et al. (2007). Altered baseline brain activity in children with ADHD revealed by resting-state functional MRI. *Brain Dev.* 29, 83–91. doi: 10.1016/j.braindev.2006.07.002

Zang, Y., Jiang, T., Lu, Y., He, Y., and Tian, L. (2004). Regional homogeneity approach to fMRI data analysis. *Neuroimage* 22, 394–400. doi: 10.1016/j.neuroimage.2003.12.030

Zhang, G., Yin, H., Zhou, Y. L., Han, H. Y., Wu, Y. H., Xing, W., et al. (2012). Capturing amplitude changes of low-frequency fluctuations in functional magnetic resonance imaging signal: a pilot acupuncture study on NeiGuan (PC6). *J. Altern. Complement. Med.* 18, 387–393. doi: 10.1089/acm.2010.0205

Acupuncture Modulates the Cerebello-Thalamo-Cortical Circuit and Cognitive Brain Regions in Patients...

71

Zhang, J., Wei, L., Hu, X., Xie, B., Zhang, Y., Wu, G.-R., et al. (2015). Akinetic-rigid and tremor-dominant Parkinson's disease patients show different patterns of intrinsic brain activity. *Parkinsonism Relat. Disord.* 21, 23–30. doi: 10.1016/j.parkreldis.2014.10.017

Zhang, Q., Li, A., Yue, J., Zhang, F., Sun, Z., and Li, X. (2015). Using functional magnetic resonance imaging to explore the possible mechanism of the action of acupuncture at Dazhong (KI 4) on the functional cerebral regions of healthy volunteers. *Int. Med. J.* 45, 669–671. doi: 10.1111/imj.12767

Zhang, S. Q., Wang, Y. J., Zhang, J. P., Chen, J. Q., Wu, C. X., Li, Z. P., et al. (2015). Brain activation and inhibition after acupuncture at Taichong and Taixi: resting-state functional magnetic resonance imaging. *Neural Regen. Res.* 10, 292–297. doi: 10.4103/1673-5374.152385

Zhou, Y. L., Xu, H. Z., Duan, Y. L., Zhang, G., Su, C. G., Wu, Y. H., et al. (2014). Effect of acupuncture at pericardium points of amplitude of low frequency fluctuations of healthy people in resting state functional magnetic resonance imaging. *Zhongguo Zhong Xi Yi Jie He Za Zhi* 34, 1197–1201. doi: 10.7661/cjim.2014.10.1197

8

Investigating Focal Connectivity Deficits in Alzheimer's Disease Using Directional Brain Networks Derived from Resting-State fMRI

Sinan Zhao[1], D Rangaprakash[1,2], Archana Venkataraman[3], Peipeng Liang[4,5,6]* and Gopikrishna Deshpande[1,7,8]*

[1] AU MRI Research Center, Department of Electrical and Computer Engineering, Auburn University, Auburn, AL, United States, [2] Department of Psychiatry and Biobehavioral Sciences, University of California, Los Angeles, Los Angeles, CA, United States, [3] Department of Electrical and Computer Engineering, Johns Hopkins University, Baltimore, MD, United States, [4] Department of Radiology, Xuanwu Hospital, Capital Medical University, Beijing, China, [5] Beijing Key Laboratory of Magnetic Resonance Imaging and Brain Informatics, Beijing, China, [6] Key Laboratory for Neurodegenerative Diseases, Ministry of Education, Beijing, China, [7] Department of Psychology, Auburn University, Auburn, AL, United States, [8] Alabama Advanced Imaging Consortium, Auburn University and University of Alabama Birmingham, Auburn, AL, United States

Correspondence:
Peipeng Liang
p.p.liang@163.com
Gopikrishna Deshpande
gopi@auburn.edu

Connectivity analysis of resting-state fMRI has been widely used to identify biomarkers of Alzheimer's disease (AD) based on brain network aberrations. However, it is not straightforward to interpret such connectivity results since our understanding of brain functioning relies on regional properties (activations and morphometric changes) more than connections. Further, from an interventional standpoint, it is easier to modulate the activity of regions (using brain stimulation, neurofeedback, etc.) rather than connections. Therefore, we employed a novel approach for identifying focal directed connectivity deficits in AD compared to healthy controls. In brief, we present a model of directed connectivity (using Granger causality) that characterizes the coupling among different regions in healthy controls and Alzheimer's disease. We then characterized group differences using a (between-subject) generative model of pathology, which generates latent connectivity variables that best explain the (within-subject) directed connectivity. Crucially, our generative model at the second (between-subject) level explains connectivity in terms of local or regionally specific abnormalities. This allows one to explain disconnections among multiple regions in terms of regionally specific pathology; thereby offering a target for therapeutic intervention. Two foci were identified, locus coeruleus in the brain stem and right orbitofrontal cortex. Corresponding disrupted connectivity network associated with the foci showed that the brainstem is the critical focus of disruption in AD. We further partitioned the aberrant connectomic network into four unique sub-networks, which likely leads to symptoms commonly observed in AD. Our findings suggest that fMRI studies of AD, which have been largely cortico-centric, could in future investigate the role of brain stem in AD.

Keywords: Alzheimer's disease, functional MRI, effective connectivity, disease foci, brain stem, orbitofrontal cortex

INTRODUCTION

Alzheimer's disease (AD) is a progressive neurodegenerative disorder with a long pre-morbid asymptomatic period (Caselli et al., 2004) which affects millions of elderly individuals worldwide (Blennow et al., 2006). The disease is initially characterized by the presence of neuronal and synaptic loss, β-amyloid (Aβ) production which results in the formation of intracellular neurofibrillary tangles and senile plaques (Buerger et al., 2006), thereby resulting in memory loss, cognitive decline, etc. Structural and functional decline are inevitable with age and the existing treatment options for AD are highly limited. Therefore, determining neural aberrations underlying AD are an important step in addressing this challenge.

Resting-state functional magnetic resonance imaging (RS-fMRI) is a promising neuroimaging technique that can non-invasively characterize underlying brain networks. This technology has been widely used to identify biomarkers of AD based on brain network alterations (Wang et al., 2007; Agosta et al., 2012; Sui et al., 2015). Seed-based approaches (Fox et al., 2009), independent components analysis (ICA) based approaches (Lee et al., 2015) and graph theory (Zhang et al., 2011) have been the three primary methods used in the study of resting-state functional connectivity (FC) in the brain. The seed-based approach involves predefining a region of interest (ROI) and extracting the BOLD signal from it; then a map of FC is obtained by calculating the cross-correlation between the time series extracted from the seed ROI and all other voxels in the brain. Previous studies in AD employing seed-based FC revealed decreased connectivity between the posterior cingulate cortex seed and regions spread across the whole brain in subjects with AD compared to healthy aging, with the Default Mode Network (DMN) being the most affected system (Zhang et al., 2009; Dennis and Thompson, 2014). Rather than define prior seeds, the ICA approach is model-free, which identifies independent components or co-activation networks throughout the brain. Damoiseaux et al. (2012) examined the components corresponding to the DMN for AD patients, and found significantly decreased FC in the posterior DMN and increased connectivity in ventral and anterior DMN in the AD group. Graph theoretic analysis is typically performed using FC matrices, revealing the topological properties and organization of the underlying brain network. For example, Brier et al. (2014) found that AD impacted the clustering coefficient and modularity in resting-state networks before the onset of the symptoms, suggesting that there might be a network-level pathology even in the preclinical stage. In summary, a profile of decreased connectivity has been consistently observed in AD.

However, most of the existing works on connectivity analyses have relied on FC or co-activation patterns, the literature on directed or effective connectivity (EC) patterns in AD is comparatively limited (more on this in the next paragraph). It is noteworthy that synchronization and causality in fMRI time series both represent distinct mechanisms in the brain (Friston, 2011), hence investigating EC aberrations in AD deserves attention. Motivated by this, we employed EC modeling to investigate aberrations in causal relationships between brain regions in AD. EC is often obtained using either of the two popular approaches, Granger causality (GC) (Granger, 1969; Deshpande et al., 2008, 2010a) and dynamic causal modeling (DCM) (Friston et al., 2003). DCM is highly dependent on prior assumptions concerning the underlying connectomic architecture and is therefore not generally considered suitable for analyses of large graphs. On the other hand, GC is a data-driven approach that does not need a predefined model (Deshpande et al., 2012; Sathian et al., 2013; Grant et al., 2014; Kapogiannis et al., 2014; Lacey et al., 2014; Wheelock et al., 2014; Chattaraman et al., 2016). Recent developments have demonstrated that GC is a viable technique for obtaining EC networks from fMRI data (Katwal et al., 2013; Wen et al., 2013). Therefore, in this study, we used a GC-based analysis framework. Strictly speaking, GC measures directed functional connectivity because it does not appeal to an underlying model of causal influences. In other words, GC tests for temporal precedence, thereby endowing functional connectivity with a direction. However, to emphasize the distinction between directed and non-directed connectivity, we will refer to our GC measures as effective connectivity (see Friston et al., 2013) for further discussion on this issue).

There have been several studies investigating EC-related aberrations in AD (Liu et al., 2012; Li et al., 2013; Chen et al., 2014; Zhong et al., 2014). These studies have reported distributed increases as well as decreases in directed relationships among brain regions in AD compared to healthy controls. However, these studies performing conventional GC analysis assume connectivity to be stationary over time, wherein only one connectivity value is obtained from the whole scan (Hampstead et al., 2011; Krueger et al., 2011; Lacey et al., 2011; Preusse et al., 2011; Sathian et al., 2011; Strenziok et al., 2011). However, connectivity, specifically the non-directed FC, has been shown to be non-stationary across time (Chang and Glover, 2010; Hutchison et al., 2013). Recent works suggests that connectivity varies over time, and that the temporal variability of connectivity is sensitive to human behavior in health and disease (Garrett et al., 2013; Jia et al., 2014; Rashid et al., 2016; Rangaprakash et al., 2017). Therefore, in addition to studying the conventional static effective connectivity (SEC), we also estimated dynamic effective connectivity (DEC; Grant et al., 2015; Hutcheson et al., 2015; Bellucci et al., 2016; Feng et al., 2016; Hampstead et al., 2016) from the resting-state fMRI data acquired from participants with AD as well as healthy controls (HC).

Traditionally, univariate statistical tests are performed for analyzing connectivity differences in population studies. Based on the statistical score, connectivity paths that differ from HC are ascertained. However, it is not straightforward to interpret such connectivity results, because traditionally our knowledge of brain functioning relies more on region-based properties (activations and morphometric changes) than connectivities. Further, from an interventional standpoint, it is easier to modulate the activity of brain regions (using brain stimulation, neurofeedback, etc.) rather than connections. With these viewpoints, Venkataraman et al. (2013) recently introduced a technique for identification of focal regions of functional disruption based on non-directed FC differences between populations. In this work, we extend this technique for identifying focal regions of disruption based on static as well as dynamic directed/effective connectivity aberrations in AD compared to HC.

We constructed brain networks using strength (SEC) and temporal variability (variance of DEC [vDEC]). After certain modifications to the connectivity measures, we fed them into the foci-identification model to obtain disrupted foci. The foci obtained independently from SEC and vDEC networks were then overlapped (intersection) to identify the common foci which exhibited impairments in both static and time-varying EC. Reduced temporal variance in dynamic connectivity is often associated with psychiatric disorders (Miller et al., 2016; Rangaprakash et al., 2017), and a relatively low variability of connectivity has been associated with poor behavioral performance in healthy individuals (Jia et al., 2014). Recall that a profile of decreased static connectivity has been consistently found in AD as discussed above. Taken together, we hypothesized that AD is characterized by dysfunctional disease foci, and that these foci are associated with connectivity paths that exhibit lower strength (SEC) as well as lower variability (vDEC) of effective connectivity.

MATERIALS AND METHODS

Participants

Data used in this study were obtained from the ADNI database (http://www.loni.ucla.edu/ADNI). Resting state fMRI data of 30 participants diagnosed with Alzheimer's disease (AD), along with 39 matched healthy controls (HC) were obtained through ADNI-2 cohort. Participants in this study were recruited between 2011 and 2013 through the ADNI-2 protocol, and we selected participants who had completed both 3D MPRAGE and resting-state fMRI data. Functional MRI data were obtained from a 3.0 Tesla Philips MR scanner with repetition time (TR) = 3,000 ms, echo time (TE) = 30 ms, flip angle (FA) = 80 degrees, field of view (FOV): RL (right-left) = 212, AP (anterior-posterior) = 198.75 mm, FH (foot-head) = 159 mm, voxel size: RL = 3.3125 mm, AP = 3.3125 mm, slices = 48, thickness = 3.3125 mm. 140 temporal volumes were acquired for each participant in a single scanning session. All data available from the ADNI database was acquired in accordance with the recommendations of local IRBs with written informed consent from all subjects. All subjects gave written informed consent in accordance with the Declaration of Helsinki. The protocol was approved by local IRBs. More specific information can be obtained from the ADNI website (http://www.loni.ucla.edu/ADNI). The data was subjected to a standard resting-state preprocessing pipeline using SPM12 (Friston et al., 1995) and DPARSF toolboxes (Chao-Gan and Yu-Feng, 2010), including slice timing correction, realignment and motion correction, normalization to MNI space, and spatial smoothing with a Gaussian kernel of 4 × 4 × 4 mm^3 full width at half maximum (FWHM). Six rotation and translation parameters were first tested individually. Except rotation in Y axis ($P < 0.05$), there were no significant differences between the groups ($P > 0.05$). Then, all the six head motion parameters were aggregated into a single metric (i.e., framewise displacement), and no significant differences in framewise were found between the groups ($P > 0.05$). Nuisance variables such as

the mean white matter signal, mean cerebrospinal fluid signal, and six head motion parameters were regressed out of the BOLD time series. It should be noted that band-pass filtering was not performed during pre-processing since it will likely impact deconvolution. Mean time series were extracted from 200 functionally homogeneous ROIs identified via spectral clustering (Craddock et al., 2012).

Connectivity Analysis

SEC was obtained using Granger causality (GC) analysis. However, before GC analysis is performed, it is necessary to acknowledge the impact of hemodynamic response function (HRF) on connectivity modeling, which is known to vary across different regions within a participant, as well as vary across participants (Handwerker et al., 2004). Previous studies have shown that results obtained by using GC analysis on HRF-corrupted fMRI data can be confounded by the variability of the HRF (David et al., 2008; Deshpande et al., 2010b). Hence, a blind deconvolution technique, proposed by Wu et al. (2013), was employed to minimize the non-neural variability of the HRF and estimate the latent neuronal time series from the observed fMRI data. In brief, the resting-state data was modeled as spontaneous event-related data (Tagliazucchi et al., 2012), and the HRF of each voxel was estimated by Wiener deconvolution (Glover, 1999). The estimated neural time series were then used in further GC analysis.

The underlying concept of GC is that a directed causal influence from time series X to time series Y can be inferred if the past values of time series X improves the prediction of the present and future values of time series Y (Granger, 1969). Let q time series $X(t) = [x_1(t), x_2(t),...,x_q(t)]$ be the latent neural time series obtained after HRF deconvolution of selected ROI fMRI time series, with q being 200 ROIs in this study. Then the multivariate autoregressive (MVAR) model with order p is given by

$$X(t) = A(1)X(t-1) + A(2)X(t-2) + \cdots + A(p)X(t-p) + E(t)$$

(1)

Where $A(1)...A(p)$ are the model parameters, and $E(t)$ is the vector of the residual error.

To remove the zero-lag correlation effect (i.e., ignore co-activations), the time series were input into a modified multivariate autoregressive model which included the zero-lag term used by Deshpande et al. (2009) shown as follows:

$$X(t) = A'(0)X(t) + A'(1)X(t-1) + \cdots + A'(p)X(t-p) + E(t)$$

(2)

The diagonal elements of $A'(0)$ were set to zero, to model only the instantaneous cross-correlation rather than zero-lag auto-correlation. The off-diagonal elements of $A'(0)$ corresponded to the zero-lag cross-correlation (Deshpande et al., 2009). It is to be noted that the coefficients in Equation (1) $A(1),...A(p)$ would not be the same as $A'(1)...A'(p)$ as in Equation (2), because the modified zero-lag term affects other coefficients since it removes the zero-lag cross correlation effects from them. Accordingly, the correlation-purged granger causality (CPGC) from time series i to time series j was obtained using the following equation

$$CPGC_{ij} = \sum_{n=1}^{p} (a'_{ij})^2(n) \qquad (3)$$

Where a'_{ij} are the elements of A'. It is well-known that the coupling among brain areas is time-varying and context-sensitive. Indeed, the most interesting parameters of dynamic causal models are the fluctuations in effective connectivity (induced by experimental manipulations or time). In recent years, the functional connectivity (resting state) community has dubbed these fluctuations in coupling as "dynamic functional connectivity." In our work, we characterized DEC using a temporally adaptive modified MVAR model:

$$X(t) = A'(0,t)X(t) + A'(1,t)X(t-1) + \cdots + A'(p,t)X(t-p)$$
$$+E(t) \qquad (4)$$

In this model, the coefficients $A'(p)$ were allowed to vary over time, thus "dynamically" estimating EC.

The parameters $A'(n,t)$, $n = 0,...,p$ were estimated in a Kalman filter framework using variable parameter regression (Arnold et al., 1998; Büchel and Friston, 1998). The Kalman filtering is a recursive process, where new information is added when it arrives. Thus, estimates taken from early steps are less reliable compared to later ones. A forgetting factor (FF) is introduced to circumvent this problem by taking recent past Kalman filter estimates into account during current estimation in order to control smoothness and enhance stability. The forgetting factor was determined by minimizing the variance of estimated error energy (Havlicek et al., 2010) and was found to be equal to one in our study. In brief, Kalman filtering treats the underlying MVAR coefficients as slowly fluctuating states. This enables the estimation of time varying directed connectivity that was used for subsequent modeling at the between-subject level. The DGC is estimated as:

$$DGC_{ij}(t) = \sum_{n=1}^{p} (a'_{ij}(n,t))^2 \qquad (5)$$

Where $DGC_{ij}(t)$ is the dynamic Granger causality value from time series i to time series j at time point t. Given that the neural delays of interest are of the order of a TR or less (Deshpande et al., 2013), and that previous literature supports using a first order model to capture most relevant causal information (Deshpande and Hu, 2012), we employed a first order model for estimating both SEC and DEC in this work.

Identification of Disease Foci

Connectivity studies often report aberrations in functional connections between brain regions. While this is useful, it does not provide a comprehensive characterization of the underlying connectomics. First, it is likely that several aberrations in connectivity are the after-effects arising from disruptions in certain focal brain regions. Second, our knowledge about brain

functioning is centered on functions of regions rather than connections. Therefore, it is advantageous to identify certain focal regions of disruption using connectivity data. Thus in this study, we sought to identify diseased foci in AD. A recent study introduced a novel technique for the identification of disease foci (Venkataraman et al., 2013) based on non-directed FC differences between populations. Here we generalize this technique to the identification of diseased foci from effective connectivity as well as dynamic connectivity data.

The model proposed by Venkataraman et al. (2012) considers the connectivity measure (C_{ij}^M for HC group and P_{ij}^M for the AD group) as a noisy observation of the latent connectivity (C_{ij}^L for HC group and P_{ij}^L for the AD group). The model is illustrated in **Figure 1** and consists of several parts.

The first part defines a binary indicator vector that selects disrupted regions, and a binary graph characterizes corresponding abnormal connectivity. Let N be the total number of regions in the brain being considered. The model assumes a the random variable $R = [R_1,...,R_N]$ is a binary vector (i.e., brain regions are either healthy with $R_i = 0$ or disrupted with $R_i = 1$, where $i = 1 .. N$) indicates the state of each region in the brain. Elements of R follow an independent, identically distributed (i.i.d.) Bernoulli distribution model $Q^b(R)$ where $Q(\cdot)$ denotes the posterior distribution and superscript b indicates a Bernoulli distribution. Then, an underlying binary graph G which characterizes the network of abnormal connectivity can be defined as follows: a connection between two healthy regions is always healthy with probability equal to 1, a connection between two disrupted regions is always abnormal with probability equal to 1, and a connection between a healthy region and a disrupted region is abnormal with probability η. The second part specifies the latent connectivity for controls (C^L) as a tri-state variable from a multinomial distribution with parameter π_k (k denotes three different states), positive connectivity with probability

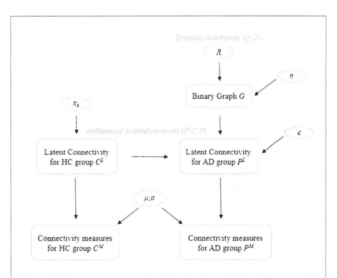

FIGURE 1 | General model of the Foci identification technique. Parameters in circles indicate random variables. Please refer to the text for a description of the variables.

π_1, little or no functional connection (0) with probability π_0, and negative connectivity with probability π_{-1}. Given the binary graph G and latent connectivity for controls C^L, the tri-state latent connectivity of the AD population can be defined. Specifically, the latent connectivity from the control group C_{ij}^L equals to P_{ij}^L with probably ϵ if the binary graph connection between regions i and j is abnormal, C_{ij}^L equals to P_{ij}^L with probably $1 - \epsilon$ if the connection between regions i and j is healthy. The third part characterizes the observed connectivity measures C_{ij}^M and P_{ij}^M as Gaussian random variables whose mean and variance (μ and σ) depend on the value of C_{ij}^L and P_{ij}^L. Then, the joint likelihood of all configurations of latent connections between regions can be modeled as an 9-state multinomial distribution model $Q^m(C, P)$ (superscript m denotes that $Q(\cdot)$ is a multinomial distribution).

The model in Venkataraman et al. (2013) was applied in the case of functional connectivity, i.e., the Pearson's correlation coefficient between regions. However, EC is not a bounded measure, a small number of outliers is to be expected. In our EC data, we found a small portion of connectivity values which were >1 or < -1 (0.3%), wherein these outliers indicate stronger causal information flow between regions. To maintain the importance of those stronger effective connections and minimize its negative impact on model evaluation, inverse Fisher transformation was used to render the EC values as a bounded measure within $[-1\ 1]$. For the variance of dynamic EC, the latent tri-states of variance of connectivity vF_{ij} can be considered as follows: little variability or stationary connection, modest variability and strong variability. It is to be noted that static FC is direction-less, hence only the upper or lower triangle of the symmetric connectivity matrices were needed to fit the model in Venkataraman et al. However, in our case, both SEC and vDEC are directed with asymmetric connectivity matrices, and hence the whole matrices were used in the model. Taken together, these modifications permitted the model to be applied to both static and dynamic EC.

After initiating the prior parameters (such as the Bernoulli prior for binary state vector R, prior for latent connectivity for controls π_k, etc.) for the model, a variational expectation maximization (EM) algorithm (Dempster et al., 1977) was adopted for estimating the latent connectivity and model parameters from the observed connectivity measures (C^M and P^M). Technically, we inverted the (between subject) model of disconnection using variational Bayes. This scheme is formally similar to an EM algorithm that uses a variational update for all the factors of an approximate posterior. These included an approximate posterior distribution over model parameters (π_k, η, ϵ, μ, and σ), latent connectivity for both groups of subjects [$Q^m(C, P)$] and regional pathology [$Q^b(R)$]. In brief, this variational scheme optimizes the sufficient statistics of each marginal distribution or density with respect to variational free energy (FE), under the expected values of the remaining factors. The variational EM alternates between updating the latent posterior distribution and estimating the nonrandom model parameters. Convergence was based on the relative change in free energy of the model of $<10^{-4}$ between consecutive iterations.

Disrupted focal regions and latent abnormal connectivity would then be identified from the posterior probabilities for each region and each connection. **Figure 2** illustrates the flow chart of the algorithm.

The significance of the resulting foci was estimated using nonparametric permutation tests. Specifically, the group label of each participant was randomly permuted for 1,000 times. For each permutation, we fit the data to the model and obtained the posterior probability of disrupted foci for each region. This provided an empirical null distribution from which the p-value of the significance was obtained. The method also identified the affected connections associated with the disrupted foci. Among such connections, we retained those that were also in accordance with our hypothesis (paths exhibit lower SEC, as well as lower vDEC of effective connectivity in AD compared to healthy controls with a threshold of $p < 0.05$).

RESULTS

We identified two disrupted foci which were common to both SEC and vDEC networks: (1) Locus Coeruleus (LC) in the Brainstem ($p = 0.003$ for SEC and 0.006 for vDEC), (2) Right orbitofrontal cortex or R OFC ($p = 0.007$ for SEC and 0.002 for vDEC). Disrupted connectivity paths associated with these foci exhibited higher strength and larger temporal variability in HC as compared to AD (in accordance with our hypothesis). Furthermore, they exhibited a unique pattern of disrupted connectivity—those associated with the LC in the brain stem emanated from it, while connectivity paths associated with R OFC converged onto it (**Figure 3**).

Five of the ten connectivity paths emanating from the LC resulted in connectivity paths terminating in the R OFC, with four of these five paths being indirect pathways via the L MFG, L MTG, R MOG, and L Calcarine, and one path being a direct connection from LC to R OFC. All connectivity paths exhibited lower SEC and lower vDEC in AD compared to HC.

Further clarity on the corresponding aberrant connectomic network was obtained by partitioning the network into four unique subnetworks: (**Figure 4A**) LC-PFC working memory system, (**Figure 4B**) LC-PHG emotional memory system, (**Figure 4C**) LC-visual cortex sensory system, and (**Figure 4D**) LC-MTG language system. Note that this partitioning is based on different functions performed by the locus coeruleus—norepinephrine system and is not based on any analytical strategy. Taken together, the disruption of these networks likely leads to working memory deficits, difficulties in processing emotional memories, and several other symptoms commonly observed in those with AD. The relevance of these subnetworks to AD pathology are discussed in detail in the next section.

DISCUSSION

In this study, we estimated static and dynamic measures of directed influences between 200 ROIs covering the entire brain in both AD and HC participants taken from the ADNI database. SEC and vDEC connectivity data were fed into a

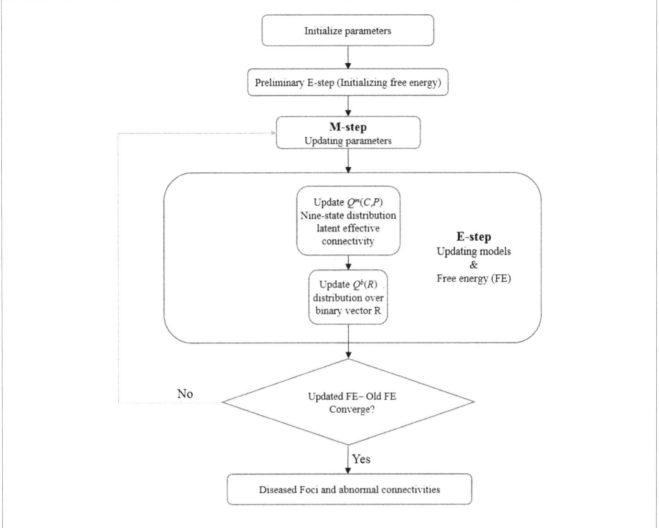

FIGURE 2 | A flow chart of the Foci identification technique. The foci-identification technique posits that the latent connectivities can be stochastically generated from a distribution mode, and that the observed connectivity data are a noisy measurement of the latent unmeasured connectivity. Latent variables of the model were randomly initialized, and the variational EM algorithm was used to obtain the posterior distribution Q (both the nine-state distribution of latent functional connectivity and distribution over binary vector R) and model parameters to minimize the variational free energy. Then the disrupted foci and corresponding dysfunctional connections can be identified.

probabilistic model to identify regions with focal connectivity deficits in AD, with the hypothesis that connections associated with those regions would be weaker in strength and lower in temporal variability (i.e., rigid) in AD. We identified two such foci, brain stem and orbitofrontal cortex, which were affected significantly by the disease. The aberrant connections emanating from LC suggested a widespread dysregulation originating from the brainstem, part of which terminated into the other focus (orbitofrontal cortex).

Interestingly, all connectivity paths corresponded with the directed influence of the LC (in the brain stem) on mostly cortical (and few sub-cortical) regions. This corroborates with previous studies that have shown progressive damage (Kienzl et al., 1999) in the brain stem during early periods of AD. Further, LC in the brain stem is the largest repository of

Norepinephrine (NE) in the human brain (Herregodts et al., 1991). Noradrenergic neurons in LC have projections to several parts of the brain including olfactory, limbic, prefrontal, and other cortical regions (Sara, 2009; Sara and Bouret, 2012). NE is known to suppress neuroinflammation (Weinshenker, 2008). This purported role has been hypothesized to be a protective factor against AD. In fact, Heneka et al. (2010) showed that NE stimulation of mouse microglia suppressed Aβ-induced cytokine and chemokine production and increased microglial migration and phagocytosis of Aβ. Induced degeneration of the brain stem increased the expression of inflammatory mediators in amyloid precursor protein (APP)-transgenic mice and resulted in elevated Aβ deposition. Kelly et al. (2017) suggesting that the decrease of NE in the brainstem facilitates the inflammatory reaction of microglial cells in AD and impairs microglial migration and

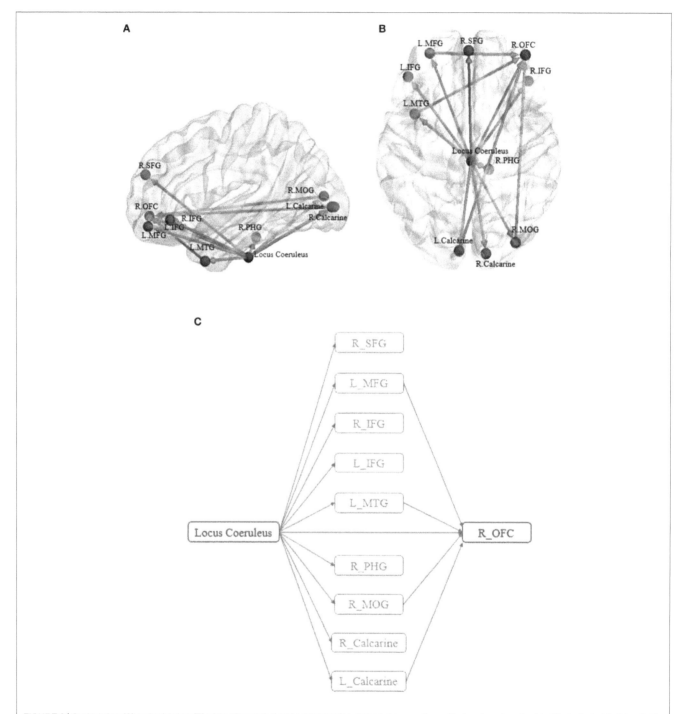

FIGURE 3 | Sagittal view **(A)** and axial view **(B)** of the disease foci and corresponding disrupted connections. Regions in red are the identified affected foci, located in Locus Coeruleus and Right orbitofrontal cortex. Regions in blue are the non-foci regions that were connected from/to the disease foci. A schematic of the identified network is also shown for better visualization of the network architecture **(C)**. The expansions for the abbreviations are as follows: SFG, superior frontal gyrus; MFG, middle frontal gyrus; IFG, inferior frontal gyrus; MTG, middle temporal gyrus; PHG, parahippocampal gyrus; MOG, middle occipital gyrus; OFC, orbitofrontal cortex.

phagocytosis, thereby contributing to reduced Aβ clearance. The Aβ is the critical initiating event in AD, starting with the aberrant clearance of Aβ-peptides followed by consecutive peptide aggregation and disruption of neural activity (Selkoe, 2002). Moreover, a post-mortem study has found significant volume decreases in the LC during AD progression, highlighting the importance of this region in AD (Theofilas et al., 2016). These findings indicate that the depletion of NE in LC is an etiological factor in the development of MCI and progression to AD. The studies discussed above provide some basis for the important

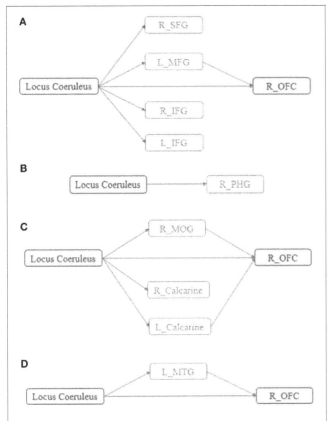

FIGURE 4 | Disrupted networks associated with the diseased foci, showing the entire network partitioned into four unique subnetworks: **(A)** LC-PFC working memory system, **(B)** LC-PHG emotional memory system, **(C)** LC-visual sensory system, and **(D)** LC-MTG language system. SFG, superior frontal gyrus; MFG, middle frontal gyrus; IFG, inferior frontal gyrus; MTG, middle temporal gyrus; PHG, parahippocampal gyrus; MOG, middle occipital gyrus; OFC, orbitofrontal cortex.

role of brainstem in AD. Further, an animal study has found that boosting NE transmission can lead to increased functional connectivity (Guedj et al., 2016), suggesting that the reduction of NE could potentially result in lower connectivity between LC and cortical regions.

Several previous studies have suggested that OFC may be important for understanding the mechanisms for putative spreading of AD pathology in the brain (Van Hoesen et al., 2000; Sepulcre et al., 2013). Robust correlation has been found between Aβ deposition levels and volume in the orbitofrontal area (Ishibashi et al., 2014). In fact, the amyloid precursor protein (APP) gene contains the sequence for the Aβ peptide, which is concentrated in the senile plaques (SPs) (Cras et al., 1991). During AD progression, the SPs appear first in the orbitofrontal and temporal cortices and later extend to the whole cortex (Braak and Braak, 1999). Further, SPs and Aβ deposition has been associated with reduced connectivity at the synaptic level (Yeh et al., 2011), suggesting a potential mechanism that might link SPs and Aβ deposition with directed connectivity estimated from fMRI. While we discuss the role of temporal regions later in this section, the findings

presented above highlight the importance of the role of OFC in AD.

Connectivity paths from LC to the prefrontal cortex (PFC) in general, and OFC in specific (note that OFC is a region in the PFC), can be considered as an aberrant LC-PFC working memory system (**Figure 4A**). Given that many studies have referred to the PFC in general without specifying sub-regions, and hence we are going to use the same nomenclature in the ensuing discussion. Previous studies have indicated that NE is instrumental in enhancing working memory through actions within the prefrontal cortex (PFC). PFC underlies the encoding of task-relevant information in working memory (Baddeley, 2003), and it has been shown that damage to the noradrenergic innervation of the PFC impairs performance in working memory (Brozoski et al., 1979). The stimulation of α_2-adrenergic receptors in the PFC of nonhuman primates has been shown to improve performance in working memory tasks (Li et al., 1999) while α_1-adrenergic receptors impaired the working memory (Arnsten and Jentsch, 1997). α_2-adrenergic receptors have a higher affinity for NE compared to α_1-adrenergic receptors, thus under normal conditions, NE facilitates working memory performance via actions at α_2-adrenergic receptors in general and also in the PFC. However, dysfunction in noradrenergic pathways emanating from LC may result in low PFC NE levels, affecting working memory (O'Rourke et al., 1994).

The connectivity from LC to PHG can be considered as a LC-PHG emotional and spatial memory system (**Figure 4B**). The LC-NE system modulates emotional memories, and studies have suggested that emotional memories induce the activation of LC and subsequent NE release (Weiss et al., 1980). Corticotropin-releasing hormone (CRH) receptors are known play an important role in the coordination of autonomic and electrophysiological responses associated with emotional memories (Koob and Bloom, 1985; Dunn and Berridge, 1990). CRH-immunoreactive fibers were observed in the LC, suggesting that CRH may modulate LC neuronal activity (Merchenthaler et al., 1982; Cummings et al., 1983). In fact, many studies (Valentino et al., 1983; Finlay et al., 1997; Jedema et al., 2001) have shown that CRH administered locally into the LC increases LC discharge activity and NE release in its terminal fields. Moreover, an abundant expression of CRH was found in PHG (Wong et al., 1994). The first sign of emotional memories was also observed in PHG, and was found to then gradually spread to PFC and other cortical regions (Sotiropoulos et al., 2011). On the other hand, PHG is known to be involved in spatial memory (Bohbot et al., 1998). Noradrenergic neurons within LC have widely distributed, ascending projections to the limbic system including PHG (Szabadi, 2013). Thus, the LC-NE system may help trigger the involvement of the PHG in spatial memory. An animal study has indicated that the LC-NE system is necessary for the acquisition of spatial memories (Gertner and Thomas, 2006). These evidence suggest that the decrease of NE in LC could likely cause dysregulation of the emotional and spatial memory system in the LC-PHG network.

Connectivity paths from LC to the frontal cortex, mediated by sensory visual regions, can be considered as a LC-visual sensory system (**Figure 4C**). Previous works in animal models have shown that the LC-NE system can alter receptive field properties such as velocity tuning, direction selectivity, etc. (Waterhouse et al., 1990; McLean and Waterhouse, 1994). Malfunction of the LC-visual sensory network may contribute to deficits in visual assessment (Johnson et al., 2012).

Connectivity paths from LC to the OFC mediated by MTG can be considered as a LC-MTG language system (**Figure 4D**). A previous study has shown decreased regional cerebral blood flow (rCBF) after ingestion of an α_2-adrenergic agonist drug in the MTG (Swartz et al., 2000). Given that the noradrenergic system in the brain originates from LC, this suggests that there might exist a noradrenergic pathway between LC and MTG which is impaired in AD. The malfunction of the LC-MTG language system may cause language impairments often observed in AD (Ferris and Farlow, 2013; Szatloczki et al., 2015).

It is evident that most of the disrupted connectivity paths emanating from the LC in the brain stem drive OFC either directly or via other systems. OFC is known to play a critical role in memory, emotions, reward, as well as decision-making mechanisms (Rolls, 2004; Rempel-Clower, 2007). Disrupted connectivity paths that converge into the OFC were observed in three of the subnetworks, and could potentially underlie behavioral deficits in these domains.

Taken together, we identified LC in the brainstem and OFC as the foci of network disruption in AD. The dysregulation of LC-NE neurotransmission likely contributes to behavioral deficits observed in AD. In corroboration, previous literature has pinpointed the same regions (Heneka et al., 2010; Ishibashi et al., 2014) to be affected in AD. Our identification of the LC in the brain stem as the disease focus in AD supports these previous observations and suggests that functional MRI studies of AD, which have been largely cortico-centric (Dennis and Thompson, 2014; Li et al., 2014), must in future investigate the role of this structure in AD.

Previous studies have also identified some other regions to be crucial to AD pathology (Brier et al., 2014; Dai et al., 2015; Mutlu et al., 2016). In fact, our foci-identification technique did identify some of the regions reported in these papers. Specifically, we also identified parahippocampal gyrus, middle frontal gyrus, and precuneus as foci only considering DEC networks. Further, middle temporal gyrus, lateral occipital cortex and cerebellum posterior lobe were identified as foci in SEC networks. However, these regions were not identified as foci in both DEC and SEC networks. Acknowledging that previous studies reported regions as having significantly different static connectivity between the groups, in this study we only reported the foci and the associated connectomic network that were found as having impairments in both static and dynamic EC.

Next, we report a few noteworthy limitations of this work. We have based our interpretation on the efferent projections of neurotransmitters arising out of LC. We employed this logic since functional imaging studies of the brain stem (and LC) in AD are limited, with the existing literature employing functional imaging in AD being cortico-centric. However, we have not directly measured norepinephrine in the brain, as it is difficult to do so using

MRI. Therefore, our results form the basis for a hypothesis regarding dysfunction in the noradrenergic pathways in AD. Future studies must employ other modalities such as positron emission tomography for *in vivo* imaging of noradrenergic pathways (not just NE deficits) in AD. This could potentially open up possibilities for therapeutic interventions in AD. Further, the proposed methodology of combining static as well as DEC analysis with probabilistic modeling for identifying dysfunctional foci and associated dysfunctional networks could provide novel insights into the pathophysiology of other brain-based disorders.

AUTHOR CONTRIBUTIONS

GD and PL designed the study; AV and DR contributed analysis tools; SZ performed data analysis; All authors interpreted the results and wrote the paper.

FUNDING

The work described in this paper was supported by a grant from the National Natural Science Foundation of China (61473196). The authors also acknowledge support from the Auburn University MRI Research Center. The funders had no role in study design, data collection, and analysis, decision to publish, or preparation of the manuscript.

ACKNOWLEDGMENTS

Data used in this article were obtained from the Alzheimer's Disease Neuroimaging Initiative (ADNI) database (adni.loni.usc.edu). Investigators within ADNI contributed to design and implementation of ADNI and provided data but did not participate in analysis or writing of this report. Complete listing of ADNI investigators: http://adni.loni.usc.edu/wp-content/uploads/how_to_apply/ADNI_Acknowledgement_List.pdf. Data collection and sharing for this work was funded by ADNI (National Institutes of Health Grant U01 AG024904) and DOD ADNI (Department of Defense award number W81XWH-12-2-0012). ADNI is funded by the National Institute on Aging, the National Institute of Biomedical Imaging and Bioengineering, and through generous contributions from the following: AbbVie, Alzheimer's Association; Alzheimer's Drug Discovery Foundation; Araclon Biotech; BioClinica, Inc.; Biogen; Bristol-Myers Squibb Company; CereSpir, Inc.; Eisai Inc.; Elan Pharmaceuticals, Inc.; Eli Lilly and Company; EuroImmun; F. Hoffmann-La Roche Ltd and its affiliated company Genentech, Inc.; Fujirebio; GE Healthcare; IXICO Ltd.; Janssen Alzheimer Immunotherapy Research & Development, LLC.; Johnson & Johnson Pharmaceutical Research & Development LLC.; Lumosity; Lundbeck; Merck & Co., Inc.; Meso Scale Diagnostics, LLC.; NeuroRx Research; Neurotrack Technologies; Novartis Pharmaceuticals Corporation; Pfizer Inc.; Piramal Imaging; Servier; Takeda Pharmaceutical Company; and Transition Therapeutics. The Canadian Institutes of Health Research is providing funds to support ADNI clinical sites in Canada. Private sector contributions are facilitated by the Foundation for NIH (www.fnih.org). The grantee is the Northern California Institute for Research and Education, and the study is coordinated by Alzheimer's Disease Cooperative Study at the University of California, San Diego. ADNI data are disseminated by the Laboratory for Neuro Imaging at the University of Southern California, Los Angeles, USA.

REFERENCES

Agosta, F., Pievani, M., Geroldi, C., Copetti, M., Frisoni, G. B., and Filippi, M. (2012). Resting state fMRI in Alzheimer's disease: beyond the default mode network. *Neurobiol. Aging* 33, 1564–1578. doi: 10.1016/j.neurobiolaging.2011.06.007

Arnold, M., Miltner, W. H. R., Witte, H., Bauer, R., and Braun, C. (1998). Adaptive AR modeling of nonstationary time series by means of kaiman filtering. *IEEE Trans. Biomed. Eng.* 45, 545–552. doi: 10.1109/10.668741

Arnsten, A. F. T., and Jentsch, J. D. (1997). The alpha-1 adrenergic agonist, cirazoline, impairs spatial working memory performance in aged monkeys. *Pharmacol. Biochem. Behav.* 58, 55–59. doi: 10.1016/S0091-3057(96)00477-7

Baddeley, A. (2003). Working memory: looking back and looking forward. *Nat. Rev. Neurosci.* 4, 829–839. doi: 10.1038/nrn1201

Bellucci, G., Chernyak, S., Hoffman, M., Deshpande, G., Dal Monte, O., Knutson, K. M., et al. (2016). Effective connectivity of brain regions underlying third-party punishment: functional MRI and Granger causality evidence. *Soc. Neurosci.* 12, 1–11. doi: 10.1080/17470919.2016.1153518

Blennow, K., de Leon, M. J., and Zetterberg, H. (2006). Alzheimer's disease. *Lancet* 368, 387–403. doi: 10.1016/S0140-6736(06)69113-7

Bohbot, V. D., Kalina, M., Stepankova, K., Spackova, N., Petrides, M., and Nadel, L. (1998). Spatial memory deficits in patients with lesions to the right hippocampus and to the right parahippocampal cortex. *Neuropsychologia* 36, 1217–1238. doi: 10.1016/S0028-3932(97)00161-9

Braak, H., and Braak, E. (1999). Temporal sequence of Alzheimer's disease-related pathology. *Cereb. Cortex* 14, 475–512. doi: 10.1007/978-1-4615-4885-0_14

Brier, M. R., Thomas, J. B., Fagan, A. M., Hassenstab, J., Holtzman, D. M., Benzinger, T. L., et al. (2014). Functional connectivity and graph theory in preclinical Alzheimer's disease. *Neurobiol. Aging* 35, 757–768. doi: 10.1016/j.neurobiolaging.2013.10.081

Brozoski, T. J., Brown, R. M., Rosvold, H. E., and Goldman, P. S. (1979). Cognitive deficit caused by regional depletion of dopamine in prefrontal cortex of rhesus monkey. *Science* 205, 929–932. doi: 10.1126/science.112679

Büchel, C., and Friston, K. J. (1998). Dynamic changes in effective connectivity characterized by variable parameter regression and Kalman filtering. *Hum. Brain Mapp.* 6, 403–408. doi: 10.1002/(SICI)1097-0193(1998)6:5/6<403::AID-HBM14>3.0.CO;2-9

Buerger, K., Ewers, M., Pirttil, T., Zinkowski, R., Alafuzoff, I., Teipel, S. J., et al. (2006). CSF phosphorylated tau protein correlates with neocortical neurofibrillary pathology in Alzheimer's disease. *Brain* 129, 3035–3041. doi: 10.1093/brain/awl269

Caselli, R. J., Reiman, E. M., Osborne, D., Hentz, J. G., Baxter, L. C., Hernandez, J. L., et al. (2004). Longitudinal changes in cognition and behavior in asymptomatic carriers of the APOE e4 allele. *Neurology* 62, 1990–1995. doi: 10.1212/01.WNL.0000129533.26544.BF

Chang, C., and Glover, G. H. (2010). Time-frequency dynamics of resting-state brain connectivity measured with fMRI. *Neuroimage* 50, 81–98. doi: 10.1016/j.neuroimage.2009.12.011

Chao-Gan, Y., and Yu-Feng, Z. (2010). DPARSF: a MATLAB toolbox for "Pipeline" data analysis of resting-state fMRI. *Front. Syst. Neurosci.* 4:13. doi: 10.3389/fnsys.2010.00013

Chattaraman, V., Deshpande, G., Kim, H., and Sreenivasan, K. R. (2016). Form "defines" function: Neural connectivity between aesthetic perception and product purchase decisions in an fMRI study. *J. Consum. Behav.* 15, 335–347. doi: 10.1002/cb.1575

Chen, G., Ward, B. D., Chen, G., and Li, S. J. (2014). Decreased effective connectivity from cortices to the right parahippocampal gyrus in Alzheimer's disease subjects. *Brain Connect.* 4, 702–708. doi: 10.1089/brain.2014.0295

Craddock, R. C., James, G. A., Holtzheimer, P. E., Hu, X. P., and Mayberg, H. S. (2012). A whole brain fMRI atlas generated via spatially constrained spectral clustering. *Hum. Brain Mapp.* 33, 1914–1928. doi: 10.1002/hbm.21333

Cras, P., Kawai, M., Lowery, D., Gonzalez-DeWhitt, P., Greenberg, B., and Perry, G. (1991). Senile plaque neurites in Alzheimer disease accumulate amyloid precursor protein. *Proc. Natl. Acad. Sci. U.S.A.* 88, 7552–7556. doi: 10.1073/pnas.88.17.7552

Cummings, S., Elde, R., Ells, J., and Lindall, A. (1983). Corticotropin-releasing factor immunoreactivity is widely distributed within the central nervous system of the rat: an immunohistochemical study. *J. Neurosci.* 3, 1355–1368.

Dai, Z., Yan, C., Li, K., Wang, Z., Wang, J., Cao, M., et al. (2015). Identifying and mapping connectivity patterns of brain network hubs in Alzheimer's disease. *Cereb. Cortex* 25, 3723–3742. doi: 10.1093/cercor/bhu246

Damoiseaux, J. S., Prater, K. E., Miller, B. L., and Greicius, M. D. (2012). Functional connectivity tracks clinical deterioration in Alzheimer's disease. *Neurobiol. Aging* 33, 828.e19–828.e30. doi: 10.1016/j.neurobiolaging.2011.06.024

David, O., Guillemain, I., Saillet, S., Reyt, S., Deransart, C., Segebarth, C., et al. (2008). Identifying neural drivers with functional MRI: an electrophysiological validation. *PLoS Biol.* 6:e315. doi: 10.1371/journal.pbio.0060315

Dempster, A. P., Laird, N. M., and Rubin, D. B. (1977). Maximum likelihood from incomplete data via the EM algorithm. *J. R. Stat. Soc. Ser. B* 39, 1–38.

Dennis, E. L., and Thompson, P. M. (2014). Functional brain connectivity using fMRI in aging and Alzheimer's disease. *Neuropsychol. Rev.* 24, 49–62. doi: 10.1007/s11065-014-9249-6

Deshpande, G., and Hu, X. (2012). Investigating effective brain connectivity from fMRI data: past findings and current issues with reference to Granger causality analysis. *Brain Connect.* 2, 235–245. doi: 10.1089/brain.2012.0091

Deshpande, G., Hu, X., Lacey, S., Stilla, R., and Sathian, K. (2010a). Object familiarity modulates effective connectivity during haptic shape perception. *Neuroimage* 49, 1991–2000. doi: 10.1016/j.neuroimage.2009.08.052

Deshpande, G., Hu, X., Stilla, R., and Sathian, K. (2008). Effective connectivity during haptic perception: a study using Granger causality analysis of functional magnetic resonance imaging data. *Neuroimage* 40, 1807–1814. doi: 10.1016/j.neuroimage.2008.01.044

Deshpande, G., LaConte, S., James, G. A., Peltier, S., and Hu, X. (2009). Multivariate granger causality analysis of fMRI data. *Hum. Brain Mapp.* 30, 1361–1373. doi: 10.1002/hbm.20606

Deshpande, G., Libero, L. E., Sreenivasan, K. R., Deshpande, H. D., and Kana, R. K. (2013). Identification of neural connectivity signatures of autism using machine learning. *Front. Hum. Neurosci.* 7:670. doi: 10.3389/fnhum.2013.00670

Deshpande, G., Sathian, K., and Hu, X. (2010b). Assessing and compensating for zero-lag correlation effects in time-lagged granger causality analysis of fMRI. *IEEE Trans. Biomed. Eng.* 57, 1446–1456. doi: 10.1109/TBME.2009.2037808

Deshpande, G., Sathian, K., Hu, X., and Buckhalt, J. A. (2012). A rigorous approach for testing the constructionist hypotheses of brain function. *Behav. Brain Sci.* 35, 148–149. doi: 10.1017/S0140525X1100149X

Dunn, A. J., and Berridge, C. W. (1990). Physiological and behavioral responses to corticotropin-releasing factor administration: is CRF a mediator of anxiety or stress responses? *Brain Res. Rev.* 15, 71–100. doi: 10.1016/0165-0173(90)90012-D

Feng, C., Deshpande, G., Liu, C., Gu, R., Luo, Y. J., and Krueger, F. (2016). Diffusion of responsibility attenuates altruistic punishment: a functional magnetic resonance imaging effective connectivity study. *Hum. Brain Mapp.* 37, 663–677. doi: 10.1002/hbm.23057

Ferris, S. H., and Farlow, M. (2013). Language impairment in alzheimer's disease and benefits of acetylcholinesterase inhibitors. *Clin. Interv. Aging* 8, 1007–1014. doi: 10.2147/CIA.S39959

Finlay, J. M., Jedema, H. P., Rabinovic, a, D., Mana, M. J., Zigmond, M. J., and Sved, a F. (1997). Impact of corticotropin-releasing hormone on extracellular norepinephrine in prefrontal cortex after chronic cold stress. *J. Neurochem.* 69, 144–150. doi: 10.1046/j.1471-4159.1997.69010144.x

Fox, M. D., Zhang, D., Snyder, A. Z., and Raichle, M. E. (2009). The global signal and observed anticorrelated resting state brain networks. *J. Neurophysiol.* 101, 3270–3283. doi: 10.1152/jn.90777.2008

Friston, K. J., Holmes, A. P., Worsley, K. J., Poline, J.-P., Frith, C. D., and Frackowiak, R. S. J. (1995). Statistical parametric maps in functional imaging: a general linear approach. *Hum. Brain Mapp.* 2, 189–210. doi: 10.1002/hbm.460020402

Friston, K., Moran, R., and Seth, A. K. (2013). Analysing connectivity with Granger causality and dynamic causal modelling. *Curr. Opin. Neurobiol.* 23, 1–7. doi: 10.1016/j.conb.2012.11.010

Friston, K. J. (2011). Functional and effective connectivity: a review. *Brain Connect.* 1, 13–36. doi: 10.1089/brain.2011.0008

Friston, K. J., Harrison, L., and Penny, W. (2003). Dynamic causal modeling. *Neuroimage* 19, 1273–1302. doi: 10.1016/S1053-8119(03)00202-7

Garrett, D. D., Samanez-Larkin, G. R., MacDonald, S. W. S., Lindenberger, U., McIntosh, A. R., and Grady, C. L. (2013). Moment-to-moment brain signal variability: a next frontier in human brain mapping? *Neurosci. Biobehav. Rev.* 37, 610–624. doi: 10.1016/j.neubiorev.2013.02.015

Gertner, M. J., and Thomas, S. A. (2006). "The role of norepinephrine in spatial reference and spatial working memory," in *CUREJ: College Undergraduate Research Electronic Journal, University of Pennsylvania.* Available online at: http://repository.upenn.edu/curej/18

Glover, G. H. (1999). Deconvolution of impulse response in event-related BOLD fMRI. *Neuroimage* 9, 416–429. doi: 10.1006/nimg.1998.0419

Granger, C. W. J. (1969). Investigating causal relations by econometric models and cross-spectral methods. *Econometrica* 37, 424–438. doi: 10.2307/1912791

Grant, M. M., White, D., Hadley, J., Hutcheson, N., Shelton, R., Sreenivasan, K., et al. (2014). Early life trauma and directional brain connectivity within major depression. *Hum. Brain Mapp.* 35, 4815–4826. doi: 10.1002/hbm.22514

Grant, M. M., Wood, K., Sreenivasan, K., Wheelock, M., White, D., Thomas, J., et al. (2015). Influence of early life stress on intra- and extra-amygdaloid causal connectivity. *Neuropsychopharmacology* 40, 1–12. doi: 10.1038/npp.2015.28

Guedj, C., Monfardini, E., Reynaud, A. J., Farnè, A., Meunier, M., and Hadj-Bouziane, F. (2016). Boosting norepinephrine transmission triggers flexible reconfiguration of brain networks at rest. *Cereb. Cortex.* doi: 10.1093/cercor/bhw262. [Epub ahead of print].

Hampstead, B. M., Khoshnoodi, M., Yan, W., Deshpande, G., and Sathian, K. (2016). Patterns of effective connectivity during memory encoding and retrieval differ between patients with mild cognitive impairment and healthy older adults. *Neuroimage* 124, 997–1008. doi: 10.1016/j.neuroimage.2015.10.002

Hampstead, B. M., Stringer, A. Y., Stilla, R. F., Deshpande, G., Hu, X., Moore, A. B., et al. (2011). Activation and effective connectivity changes following explicit-memory training for face-name pairs in patients with mild cognitive impairment: a pilot study. *Neurorehabil. Neural Repair* 25, 210–222. doi: 10.1177/1545968310382424

Handwerker, D. A., Ollinger, J. M., and D'Esposito, M. (2004). Variation of BOLD hemodynamic responses across subjects and brain regions and their effects on statistical analyses. *Neuroimage* 21, 1639–1651. doi: 10.1016/j.neuroimage.2003.11.029

Havlicek, M., Jan, J., Brazdil, M., and Calhoun, V. D. (2010). Dynamic Granger causality based on Kalman filter for evaluation of functional network connectivity in fMRI data. *Neuroimage* 53, 65–77. doi: 10.1016/j.neuroimage.2010.05.063

Heneka, M. T., Nadrigny, F., Regen, T., Martinez-Hernandez, A., Dumitrescu-Ozimek, L., Terwel, D., et al. (2010). Locus ceruleus controls Alzheimer's disease pathology by modulating microglial functions through norepinephrine. *Proc. Natl. Acad. Sci. U.S.A.* 107, 6058–6063. doi: 10.1073/pnas.0909586107

Herregodts, P., Ebinger, G., and Michotte, Y. (1991). Distribution of monoamines in human brain: evidence for neurochemical heterogeneity in subcortical as well as in cortical areas. *Brain Res.* 542, 300–306. doi: 10.1016/0006-8993(91)91582-L

Hutcheson, N. L., Sreenivasan, K. R., Deshpande, G., Reid, M. A., Hadley, J., White, D. M., et al. (2015). Effective connectivity during episodic memory retrieval in schizophrenia participants before and after antipsychotic medication. *Hum. Brain Mapp.* 36, 1442–1457. doi: 10.1002/hbm.22714

Hutchison, R. M., Womelsdorf, T., Allen, E. A., Bandettini, P. A., Calhoun, V. D., Corbetta, M., et al. (2013). Dynamic functional connectivity: promise, issues, and interpretations. *Neuroimage* 80, 360–378. doi: 10.1016/j.neuroimage.2013.05.079

Ishibashi, K., Ishiwata, K., Toyohara, J., Murayama, S., and Ishii, K. (2014). Regional analysis of striatal and cortical amyloid deposition in patients with Alzheimer's disease. *Eur. J. Neurosci.* 40, 2701–2706. doi: 10.1111/ejn.12633

Jedema, H. P., Finlay, J. M., Sved, A. F., and Grace, A. A. (2001). Chronic cold exposure potentiates CRH-evoked increases in electrophysiologic activity of locus coeruleus neurons. *Biol. Psychiatry* 49, 351–359. doi: 10.1016/S0006-3223(00)01057-X

Jia, H., Hu, X., and Deshpande, G. (2014). Behavioral relevance of the dynamics of the functional brain connectome. *Brain Connect.* 4, 741–759. doi: 10.1089/brain.2014.0300

Johnson, K. A., Fox, N. C., Sperling, R. A., and Klunk, W. E. (2012). Brain imaging in Alzheimer disease. *Cold Spring Harb. Perspect. Med.* 2:a006213. doi: 10.1101/cshperspect.a006213

Kapogiannis, D., Deshpande, G., Krueger, F., Thornburg, M. P., and Grafman, J. H. (2014). Brain networks shaping religious belief. *Brain Connect.* 4, 70–79. doi: 10.1089/brain.2013.0172

Katwal, S. B., Gore, J. C., Gatenby, J. C., and Rogers, B. P. (2013). Measuring relative timings of brain activities using fMRI. *Neuroimage* 66, 436–448. doi: 10.1016/j.neuroimage.2012.10.052

Kelly, S. C., He, B., Perez, S. E., Ginsberg, S. D., Mufson, E. J., and Counts, S. E. (2017). Locus coeruleus cellular and molecular pathology during the progression of Alzheimer's disease. *Acta Neuropathol. Commun.* 5:8. doi: 10.1186/s40478-017-0411-2

Kienzl, E., Jellinger, K., Stachelberger, H., and Linert, W. (1999). Iron as catalyst for oxidative stress in the pathogenesis of Parkinson's disease? *Life Sci.* 65, 1973–1976. doi: 10.1016/S0024-3205(99)00458-0

Koob, G. F., and Bloom, F. E. (1985). Corticotropin-releasing factor and behavior. *Fed. Proc.* 44(1 Pt 2), 259–263. doi: 10.1016/b978-0-12-532102-0.50007-3

Krueger, F., Landgraf, S., Van Der Meer, E., Deshpande, G., and Hu, X. (2011). Effective connectivity of the multiplication network: a functional MRI and multivariate granger causality mapping study. *Hum. Brain Mapp.* 32, 1419–1431. doi: 10.1002/hbm.21119

Lacey, S., Hagtvedt, H., Patrick, V. M., Anderson, A., Stilla, R., Deshpande, G., et al. (2011). Art for reward's sake: visual art recruits the ventral striatum. *Neuroimage* 55, 420–433. doi: 10.1016/j.neuroimage.2010.11.027

Lacey, S., Stilla, R., Sreenivasan, K., Deshpande, G., and Sathian, K. (2014). Spatial imagery in haptic shape perception. *Neuropsychologia* 60, 144–158. doi: 10.1016/j.neuropsychologia.2014.05.008

Lee, Y.-B., Lee, J., Tak, S., Lee, K., Na, D. L., Seo, S., et al. (2015). Sparse SPM: Sparse-dictionary learning for resting-state functional connectivity {MRI} analysis. *Neuroimage* 125, 1032–1045. doi: 10.1016/j.neuroimage.2015.10.081

Li, B. M., Mao, Z. M., Wang, M., and Mei, Z. T. (1999). Alpha-2 adrenergic modulation of prefrontal cortical neuronal activity related to spatial working memory in monkeys. *Neuropsychopharmacology* 21, 601–610. doi: 10.1016/S0893-133X(99)00070-6

Li, H.-J., Hou, X.-H., Liu, H.-H., Yue, C.-L., He, Y., and Zuo, X.-N. (2014). Toward systems neuroscience in mild cognitive impairment and Alzheimer's disease: a meta-analysis of 75 fMRI studies. *Hum. Brain Mapp.* 36, 1217–1232. doi: 10.1002/hbm.22689

Li, R., Wu, X., Chen, K., Fleisher, A. S., Reiman, E. M., and Yao, L. (2013). Alterations of directional connectivity among resting-state networks in Alzheimer disease. *Am. J. Neuroradiol.* 34, 340–345. doi: 10.3174/ajnr.A3197

Liu, Z., Zhang, Y., Bai, L., Yan, H., Dai, R., Zhong, C., et al. (2012). Investigation of the effective connectivity of resting state networks in Alzheimer's disease: a functional MRI study combining independent components analysis and multivariate Granger causality analysis. *NMR Biomed.* 25, 1311–1320. doi: 10.1002/nbm.2803

McLean, J., and Waterhouse, B. D. (1994). Noradrenergic modulation of cat area 17 neuronal responses to moving visual stimuli. *Brain Res.* 667, 83–97. doi: 10.1016/0006-8993(94)91716-7

Merchenthaler, I., Vigh, S., Petrusz, P., and Schally, A. V. (1982). Immunocytochemical localization of corticotropin-releasing factor (CRF) in the rat brain. *Am. J. Anat.* 165, 385–396. doi: 10.1002/aja.1001650404

Miller, R. L., Yaesoubi, M., Turner, J. A., Mathalon, D., Preda, A., Pearlson, G., et al. (2016). Higher dimensional meta-state analysis reveals reduced resting fMRI connectivity dynamism in schizophrenia patients. *PLoS ONE* 11:e0149849. doi: 10.1371/journal.pone.0149849

Mutlu, J., Landeau, B., Tomadesso, C., de Flores, R., Mézenge, F., de La Sayette, V., et al. (2016). Connectivity disruption, atrophy, and hypometabolism within posterior cingulate networks in Alzheimer's disease. *Front. Neurosci.* 10:582. doi: 10.3389/fnins.2016.00582

O'Rourke, M. F., Blaxall, H. S., Iversen, L. J., and Bylund, D. B. (1994). Characterization of [3H]RX821002 binding to alpha-2 adrenergic receptor subtypes. *J. Pharmacol. Exp. Ther.* 268, 1362–1367.

Preusse, F., van der Meer Elke, Deshpande, G., Krueger, F., and Wartenburger, I. (2011). Fluid intelligence allows flexible recruitment of the parieto-frontal network in analogical reasoning. *Front. Hum. Neurosci.* 5:22. doi: 10.3389/fnhum.2011.00022

Rangaprakash, D., Deshpande, G., Daniel, T. A., Goodman, A., Robinson, J., Salibi, N., et al. (2017). Compromised hippocampus-striatum pathway as a potential imaging biomarker of mild traumatic brain injury and posttraumatic stress disorder. *Hum. Brain Mapp.* 38, 2843–2864. doi: 10.1002/hbm.23551

Rashid, B., Arbabshirani, M. R., Damaraju, E., Cetin, M. S., Miller, R., Pearlson, G. D., et al. (2016). Classification of schizophrenia and bipolar patients using static and dynamic resting-state fmri brain connectivity. *Neuroimage* 134, 645–657. doi: 10.1016/j.neuroimage.2016.04.051

Rempel-Clower, N. L. (2007). Role of orbitofrontal cortex connections in emotion. *Ann. N.Y. Acad. Sci.* 1121, 72–86. doi: 10.1196/annals.1401.026

Rolls, E. T. (2004). The functions of the orbitofrontal cortex. *Brain Cogn.* 55, 11–29. doi: 10.1016/S0278-2626(03)00277-X

Sara, S. J. (2009). The locus coeruleus and noradrenergic modulation of cognition. *Nat. Rev. Neurosci.* 10, 211–223. doi: 10.1038/nrn2573

Sara, S. J., and Bouret, S. (2012). Orienting and reorienting: the locus coeruleus mediates cognition through arousal. *Neuron.* 76, 130–141. doi: 10.1016/j.neuron.2012.09.011

Sathian, K., Deshpande, G., and Stilla, R. (2013). Neural changes with tactile learning reflect decision-level reweighting of perceptual readout. *J. Neurosci.* 33, 5387–5398. doi: 10.1523/JNEUROSCI.3482-12.2013

Sathian, K., Lacey, S., Stilla, R., Gibson, G. O., Deshpande, G., Hu, X., et al. (2011). Dual pathways for haptic and visual perception of spatial and texture information. *Neuroimage* 57, 462–475. doi: 10.1016/j.neuroimage.2011.05.001

Selkoe, D. J. (2002). Alzheimer's disease is a synaptic failure. *Science* 298, 789–791. doi: 10.1126/science.1074069

Sepulcre, J., Sabuncu, M. R., Becker, A., Sperling, R., and Johnson, K. A. (2013). *In vivo* characterization of the early states of the amyloid-beta network. *Brain* 136, 2239–2252. doi: 10.1093/brain/awt146

Sotiropoulos, I., Catania, C., Pinto, L. G., Silva, R., Pollerberg, G. E., Takashima, A., et al. (2011). Stress acts cumulatively to precipitate Alzheimer's disease-like tau pathology and cognitive deficits. *J. Neurosci.* 31, 7840–7847. doi: 10.1523/JNEUROSCI.0730-11.2011

Strenziok, M., Krueger, F., Deshpande, G., Lenroot, R. K., Van der meer, E., and Grafman, J. (2011). Fronto-parietal regulation of media violence exposure in adolescents: a multi-method study. *Soc. Cogn. Affect. Neurosci.* 6, 537–547. doi: 10.1093/scan/nsq079

Sui, X., Zhu, M., Cui, Y., Yu, C., Sui, J., Zhang, X., et al. (2015). Functional connectivity hubs could serve as a potential biomarker in alzheimer's disease: a reproducible study. *Curr. Alzheimer Res.* 12, 974–983. doi: 10.2174/1567205012666150710111615

Swartz, B. E., Kovalik, E., Thomas, K., Torgersen, D., and Mandelkern, M. A. (2000). The effects of an alpha-2 adrenergic agonist, guanfacine, on rCBF in human cortex in normal controls and subjects with focal epilepsy. *Neuropsychopharmacology* 23, 263–275. doi: 10.1016/S0893-133X(00)00101-9

Szabadi, E. (2013). Functional neuroanatomy of the central noradrenergic system. *J. Psychopharmacol.* 27, 659–693. doi: 10.1177/0269881113490326

Szatloczki, G., Hoffmann, I., Vincze, V., Kalman, J., and Pakaski, M. (2015). Speaking in Alzheimer's disease, is that an early sign? Importance of changes in language abilities in Alzheimer's disease. *Front. Aging Neurosci.* 7:195. doi: 10.3389/fnagi.2015.00195

Tagliazucchi, E., Balenzuela, P., Fraiman, D., and Chialvo, D. R. (2012). Criticality in large-scale brain fmri dynamics unveiled by a novel point process analysis. *Front. Physiol.* 3, 1–12. doi: 10.3389/fphys.2012.00015

Theofilas, P., Ehrenberg, A. J., Dunlop, S., Di Lorenzo Alho, A. T., Nguy, A., Leite, R. E. P., et al. (2016). Locus coeruleus volume and cell population changes during Alzheimer's disease progression: a stereological study in human postmortem brains with potential implication for early-stage biomarker discovery. *Alzheimer's Dement.* 13, 236–246. doi: 10.1016/j.jalz.2016.06.1776

Valentino, R. J., Foote, S. L., and Aston-Jones, G. (1983). Corticotropin-releasing factor activates noradrenergic neurons of the locus coeruleus. *Brain Res.* 270, 363–367. doi: 10.1016/0006-8993(83)90615-7

Van Hoesen, G. W., Parvizi, J., and Chu, C. C. (2000). Orbitofrontal cortex pathology in Alzheimer's disease. *Cereb. Cortex* 10, 243–251. doi: 10.1093/cercor/10.3.243

Venkataraman, A., Kubicki, M., and Golland, P. (2013). From connectivity models to region labels: identifying foci of a neurological disorder. *IEEE Trans. Med. Imaging* 32, 2078–2098. doi: 10.1109/TMI.2013.2272976

Venkataraman, A., Rathi, Y., Kubicki, M., Westin, C.-F., and Golland, P. (2012). Joint modeling of anatomical and functional connectivity for population studies. *IEEE Trans. Med. Imaging* 31, 164–182. doi: 10.1109/TMI.2011.2166083

Wang, K., Liang, M., Wang, L., Tian, L., Zhang, X., Li, K., et al. (2007). Altered functional connectivity in early Alzheimer's disease: a resting-state fMRI study. *Hum. Brain Mapp.* 28, 967–978. doi: 10.1002/hbm.20324

Waterhouse, B. D., Ausim Azizi, S., Burne, R. A., and Woodward, D. J. (1990). Modulation of rat cortical area 17 neuronal responses to moving visual stimuli during norepinephrine and serotonin microiontophoresis. *Brain Res.* 514, 276–292. doi: 10.1016/0006-8993(90)91422-D

Weinshenker, D. (2008). Functional consequences of locus coeruleus degeneration in Alzheimer's disease. *Curr. Alzheimer Res.* 5, 342–345. doi: 10.2174/156720508784533286

Weiss, J. M., Bailey, W. H., Pohorecky, L. A., Korzeniowski, D., and Grillione, G. (1980). Stress-induced depression of motor activity correlates with regional changes in brain norepinephrine but not in dopamine. *Neurochem. Res.* 5, 9–22. doi: 10.1007/BF00964456

Wen, X., Rangarajan, G., and Ding, M. (2013). Is granger causality a viable technique for analyzing fMRI data? *PLoS ONE* 8:e67428. doi: 10.1371/journal.pone.0067428

Wheelock, M. D., Sreenivasan, K. R., Wood, K. H., Ver Hoef, L. W., Deshpande, G., and Knight, D. C. (2014). Threat-related learning relies on distinct dorsal prefrontal cortex network connectivity. *Neuroimage* 102, 904–912. doi: 10.1016/j.neuroimage.2014.08.005

Wong, M. L., Licinio, J., Pasternak, K. I., and Gold, P. W. (1994). Localization of corticotropin-releasing hormone (CRH) receptor mRNA in adult rat brain by in situ hybridization histochemistry. *Endocrinology* 135, 2275–2278. doi: 10.1210/endo.135.5.7956950

Wu, G., Liao, W., Stramaglia, S., Ding, J.-R., Chen, H., and Marinazzo, D. (2013). A blind deconvolution approach to recover effective connectivity brain networks from resting state fMRI data. *Med. Image Anal.* 17, 365–374. doi: 10.1016/j.media.2013.01.003

Yeh, C., Vadhwana, B., Verkhratsky, A., and Rodríguez, J. J. (2011). Early astrocytic atrophy in the entorhinal cortex of a triple transgenic animal model of Alzheimer's disease. *ASN Neuro* 3, 271–279. doi: 10.1042/AN20110025

Zhang, H. Y., Wang, S. J., Xing, J., Liu, B., Ma, Z. L., Yang, M., et al. (2009). Detection of PCC functional connectivity characteristics in resting-state fMRI in mild Alzheimer's disease. *Behav. Brain Res.* 197, 103–108. doi: 10.1016/j.bbr.2008.08.012

Zhang, T., Wang, J., Yang, Y., Wu, Q., Li, B., Chen, L., et al. (2011). Abnormal small-world architecture of top-down control networks in obsessive-compulsive disorder. *J. Psychiatry Neurosci.* 36, 23–31. doi: 10.1503/jpn.100006

Zhong, Y., Huang, L., Cai, S., Zhang, Y., von Deneen, K. M., Ren, A., et al. (2014). Altered effective connectivity patterns of the default mode network in Alzheimer's disease: an fMRI study. *Neurosci. Lett.* 578, 171–175. doi: 10.1016/j.neulet.2014.06.043

9

Linking Inter-Individual Variability in Functional Brain Connectivity to Cognitive Ability in Elderly Individuals

Rui Li[1,2], Shufei Yin[3], Xinyi Zhu[1,2], Weicong Ren[1,4], Jing Yu[1,5], Pengyun Wang[1,2], Zhiwei Zheng[1,2], Ya-Nan Niu[1,2], Xin Huang[1,2] and Juan Li[1,2,6,7]*

[1] CAS Key Laboratory of Mental Health, Institute of Psychology, Beijing, China, [2] Department of Psychology, University of Chinese Academy of Sciences, Beijing, China, [3] Department of Psychology, Faculty of Education, Hubei University, Wuhan, China, [4] Department of Education, Hebei Normal University, Shijiazhuang, China, [5] Faculty of Psychology, Southwest University, Chongqing, China, [6] Magnetic Resonance Imaging Research Center, Institute of Psychology, Chinese Academy of Sciences, Beijing, China, [7] State Key Laboratory of Brain and Cognitive Science, Institute of Biophysics, Chinese Academy of Sciences, Beijing, China

*Correspondence:
Juan Li
lijuan@psych.ac.cn

Increasing evidence suggests that functional brain connectivity is an important determinant of cognitive aging. However, the fundamental concept of inter-individual variations in functional connectivity in older individuals is not yet completely understood. It is essential to evaluate the extent to which inter-individual variability in connectivity impacts cognitive performance at an older age. In the current study, we aimed to characterize individual variability of functional connectivity in the elderly and to examine its significance to individual cognition. We mapped inter-individual variability of functional connectivity by analyzing whole-brain functional connectivity magnetic resonance imaging data obtained from a large sample of cognitively normal older adults. Our results demonstrated a gradual increase in variability in primary regions of the visual, sensorimotor, and auditory networks to specific subcortical structures, particularly the hippocampal formation, and the prefrontal and parietal cortices, which largely constitute the default mode and fronto-parietal networks, to the cerebellum. Further, the inter-individual variability of the functional connectivity correlated significantly with the degree of cognitive relevance. Regions with greater connectivity variability demonstrated more connections that correlated with cognitive performance. These results also underscored the crucial function of the long-range and inter-network connections in individual cognition. Thus, individual connectivity–cognition variability mapping findings may provide important information for future research on cognitive aging and neurocognitive diseases.

Keywords: individual variability, functional connectivity, cognitive aging, fMRI, brain networks

INTRODUCTION

There is a marked heterogeneity in cognitive functioning during late adulthood and old age (Hedden and Gabrieli, 2004; Lustig et al., 2009; Nyberg et al., 2012). Some older people may display rapid cognitive decline or develop Alzheimer's disease (AD), whereas others may continue to exhibit a superior level of cognitive functioning. One of the main contributions to this heterogeneity originates from the variability of the brain (Hedden and Gabrieli, 2004; Reuter-Lorenz and Lustig, 2005; Bishop et al., 2010; Grady, 2012; Tomasi and Volkow, 2012;

Karama et al., 2014), particularly in regard to functional connectivity (Burke and Barnes, 2006; Andrews-Hanna et al., 2007; Bishop et al., 2010; Grady, 2012; Tomasi and Volkow, 2012; Ferreira and Busatto, 2013; Fornito et al., 2015).

Previous studies demonstrated that preserved functional integration between distributed brain regions supports proficient cognitive function, while functional disruption of the inter-regional neural communication results in cognitive decline and AD (Andrews-Hanna et al., 2007; Eyler et al., 2011; Grady, 2012; Nyberg et al., 2012; Dennis and Thompson, 2014). Much of this evidence comes from direct comparisons of functional connectivity between groups that are pre-defined by neuropsychological questionnaires or clinical classifications of mental states. For instance, elderly individuals who performed better on a verbal fluency test demonstrated stronger connections between the precuneus and prefrontal regions compared to that in individuals with lower verbal fluency test performance (Yin et al., 2015). Similarly, patients with AD exhibited disrupted functional connectivity in the default mode and several fronto-parietal attention networks, compared to that of healthy elderly individuals (Wang et al., 2007, 2015; Buckner et al., 2009; Myers et al., 2014). These "group differences" provide substantial insights into the brain connectivity correlates of cognitive aging. However, a fundamental issue regarding how functional brain connectivity itself differs among older individuals remains to be elucidated. Although many group-based investigations usually included individual-level results, the "individual difference" in functional connectivity remains largely uninvestigated. For example, Betzel et al. (2014) demonstrated the trajectory of individual functional connectivity of resting state networks with age (Betzel et al., 2014). Similarly, there are studies that have largely demonstrated individual-level correlations between functional connectivity and cognitive performance in normal elderly people (Andrews-Hanna et al., 2007; Sala-Llonch et al., 2014; Yin et al., 2015) and patients (Wang et al., 2015). However, it is still not clear how inter-individual variability in functional connectivity can vary in different brain regions and to what extent the inter-individual variability in connectivity impacts cognitive performance at an older age.

An important reason for the bias toward group differences is that traditional task-based neuroimaging studies are limited in their ability to systematically quantify individual brain function differences, given the diverse nature of the tasks used in different studies. Resting-state functional connectivity magnetic resonance imaging (fcMRI) that measures the intrinsic temporal synchronization of the blood oxygen level-dependent (BOLD) signals has been developed to delineate the neural functional architecture in human participants who are not engaged in any specific task. Similar to genomic and phenomic approaches, fcMRI is recognized as a remarkably powerful tool to understand individual variation in brain functioning (Mohr and Nagel, 2010; Buckner, 2013; Mueller et al., 2013; Zatorre, 2013). Mueller et al. (2013) recently measured individual differences of the resting-state connectivity of the cortical regions in 25 healthy adults. The authors reported higher variability in the association cortex and lower variability in the unimodal cortices. Similarly, Gao et al. (2014) examined the inter-individual variability of functional

connectivity during infancy (Gao et al., 2014). However, to our knowledge, there have been no studies to date regarding the distribution of the inter-individual differences in functional connectivity in the brains of elderly individuals.

In the current study, we aimed to investigate two major issues as follows: (1) we sought to delineate the inter-individual variability map of functional brain connectivity during old age. The fcMRI data from 108 healthy older adults were collected during resting-state conditions. The brain was divided into 116 regions of interest (ROIs), including cortical, subcortical, and cerebellar regions, using the automated anatomical labeling (AAL) procedure (Tzourio-Mazoyer et al., 2002). The variation of the individual-to-individual functional connectivity in each ROI of these older adults were then estimated and used to generate the brain variability map. Further, to facilitate the inspection of the brain distribution for the inter-individual variability, the variability was compared in 6 distinct brain systems, including the default mode, fronto-parietal, visual, sensorimotor and auditory, subcortical, and cerebellar networks (Ferrarini et al., 2009; He et al., 2009); and 2) we then linked the inter-individual variability of the connectivity to cognitive function in the elderly. A battery of standardized neuropsychological tests was employed to assess the cognitive function of the older participants. The connectivity–cognition association was first examined by calculating the correlations between each region's connectivity and the cognitive test performance. This allowed us to determine whether the regions that had correlations between connectivity and cognitive ability were concentrated in the areas with large inter-individual variability for functional connectivity. Then, we defined a cognitive relevance index that was calculated as the number of cognition-correlated connections to quantify the role of each region's functional connectivity in cognitive functioning. To examine the cognitive significance of the distribution of inter-individual variability of functional connectivity, a correlation between the value of inter-individual variability and the degree of cognitive relevance was computed across all ROIs. This allowed us to further determine whether regions with larger inter-individual variability in the brain connectivity would play a more important role in cognitive performance of the elderly. Recent studies have suggested that the long-range and inter-network regional connections function critically in cognitive processing and cognitive aging (Tomasi and Volkow, 2012; Park and Friston, 2013; Fjell et al., 2015). Therefore, to better describe the relationship between variability in connectivity to cognitive significance, we also investigated whether this relationship was more specific to the long-range and inter-network connections.

MATERIALS AND METHODS

Participants

A total of 108 cognitively normal, older volunteers (70.3 ± 5.7 years; range: 60–80 years of age; 50 men and 58 women) were recruited from communities near the Institute of Psychology-Chinese Academy of Sciences. All participants met the following inclusion criteria: age ≥60 years; a score ≥ 21 on the Beijing Version of the Montreal Cognitive Assessment

(Yu et al., 2012); a score $\leq$ 16 on the Activities of Daily Living (Lawton and Brody, 1969); right-handed; and free of stroke, heart disease, diabetes mellitus, neurological and psychiatric disorders, and traumatic brain injury. The images were collected under resting-state conditions using a 3.0-T Siemens Trio scanner (Erlangen, Germany), located at the Beijing MRI Center for Brain Research. Functional imaging consisted of 33 T2*-weighted echo-planar image (EPI) slices (time repetition (TR) = 2000 ms, time echo (TE) = 30 ms, flip angle = 90°, field of view (FOV) = 200 mm × 200 mm, thickness = 3.0 mm, gap = 0.6 mm, acquisition matrix = 64 × 64, and in-plane resolution = 3.125 × 3.125). We collected 200 functional volumes for each participant. T1-weighted anatomical images were collected using a magnetization-prepared rapid gradient echo (MPRAGE) sequence (176 slices, acquisition matrix = 256 × 256, voxel size = 1 mm × 1 mm × 1 mm, TR = 1900 ms, TE = 2.2 ms, and flip angle = 9°) for co-registration with the functional images. Of the total number of participants, 85 participants completed a battery of neuropsychological assessments, which included the Digit Forward Span (DFS) and Digit Backward Span (DBS) (Gong, 1992), the Paired Associative Learning Test (PALT) (Xu and Wu, 1986), the Trail Making Test (TMT) Parts A and B (Reitan, 1986), and the Verbal Fluency Test (VFT) (Rosenberg et al., 1984).

Five participants were excluded due to poor image quality or gross structural abnormalities. Six participants were excluded because of excessive head movements (more than 2.0 mm maximum translation or 2.0° rotation) during the scan. Nine participants were excluded because of bad registration quality during the visual inspection for the normalization. Thus, the final statistical analysis included fMRI data from 88 older adults (70.2 ± 5.6 years; range: 60–80 years of age; 40 men and 48 women). Of these, 76 individuals (70.7 ± 5.5 years; range: 60–80 years of age; 35 men and 41 women) completed the neuropsychological assessments and provided behavioral data.

The institutional review board of the Institute of Psychology of Chinese Academy of Sciences approved the current study. All participants provided written informed consent prior to their participation in the experiments.

Image Preprocessing

Data pre-processing was performed using the Statistical Parametric Mapping program[1] (SPM8) and the Data Processing Assistant for Resting-State fMRI[2] (DPARSF). This included the following: removal of the first 5 volumes, corrections for the intra-volume acquisition time differences between the slices using the Sinc interpolation, corrections for the inter-volume geometrical displacement due to head motion using a 6-parameter (rigid body) spatial transformation, a normalization to the standard Montreal Neurological Institute (MNI) space (resampling voxel size, 3 mm × 3 mm × 3 mm) using the DARTEL approach (Ashburner, 2007), spatial smoothing with a 4-mm full width at a half maximum Gaussian kernel to decrease

the spatial noise, and de-trending and temporal band-pass filtering (0.01–0.08 Hz) to reduce the effects of low-frequency drifts and high-frequency physiological noise (Lowe et al., 1998). To remove the head motions for each participant, we performed a nuisance regression of the head motion, using a Friston 24-parameter model (6 head motion parameters, 6 head motion parameters one time point before, and the 12 corresponding squared items) (Friston et al., 1996) with scrubbing (Satterthwaite et al., 2013; Yan et al., 2013a,b; Power et al., 2014). We calculated the mean framewise displacement (FD), which was derived using the Jenkinson's relative root mean square (RMS) algorithm (Jenkinson et al., 2002). This was used as a covariate in the group analyses of the connectivity–cognition correlations to further control for any residual effects of head movement (Yan et al., 2013a,b; Power et al., 2014). In addition, we performed a nuisance regression of the global signal (the average voxel signal within the SPM *apriori* mask (brainmask.nii) thresholded at 50%, and the white matter and cerebrospinal fluid signals, which were calculated by averaging the voxel signals within the SPM *apriori* masks (white.nii and csf.nii, respectively) thresholded at 99%. The residual volumes were retained for use in the following functional connectivity analysis.

Measuring the Inter-Individual Variability of Functional Connectivity

To create the regions for the functional connectivity analyses, we parcellated the brain into 116 ROIs, including 90 cerebral regions and 26 cerebellar regions, based on the AAL atlas (Tzourio-Mazoyer et al., 2002). To ensure that only the gray matter voxels within the AAL ROIs were included in the analyses, these ROIs were multiplied by the SPM's gray matter mask, which was thresholded at 20%, to further remove white matter, cerebrospinal fluid, and other non-brain tissue voxels. The mean time series of each ROI was calculated. Pearson's linear correlation coefficients (r values) were computed between each ROI pair of the averaged time series and subsequently transformed to Fisher z values, which yielded a 116 × 116 correlation matrix for each participant. For a given AAL ROI R_i ($i = 1, 2, \ldots 116$), the functional connectivity of the participant, S_m ($m = 1, 2, \ldots 88$), was denoted as a 1 × 115 correlation coefficient vector, $FC(S_m)_i$, in which each element corresponded to its correlation with each of the remaining 115 regions. To quantify the inter-individual variability at R_i, the inter-individual similarity, FCS_i was first calculated as the mean (E) of the correlation values between any two functional connectivity vectors of the 88 older participants:

$$FCS_i = E[corr(FC(S_m)_i, FC(S_n)_i],$$

where $m, n = 1, 2, \ldots 88$, and $m \neq n$.

The inverted similarity ($1 - FCS_i$) was thus defined as the inter-individual variability (FCV_i) of the functional connectivity at R_i (Mueller et al., 2013). This calculation was repeated for all R_i ROIs to derive the spatial distribution of the inter-individual variability of the functional connectivity across the entire brain.

Further, we investigated the inter-individual variability for distinct functional systems in the older participants. Previous

---

[1]http://www.fil.ion.ucl.ac.uk/spm

[2]http://www.rfmri.org

functional connectome analyses of the brain architecture indicated the existence of a hierarchical modularity, which is typically represented as intrinsic functional networks (Ferrarini et al., 2009; He et al., 2009; Park and Friston, 2013; Turk-Browne, 2013). Here, we associated the 90 cerebrum regions with five networks, including the sensorimotor and auditory network, visual network, fronto-parietal network related to attention and executive function, default-mode network, and the subcortical network (He et al., 2009), and another 26 regions to the cerebellar network. The inter-individual variability values were averaged across the regions from the same functional network. A one-way analysis of variance (ANOVA) with network as a factor (six networks) followed by *post hoc* pair-wise comparisons were performed to investigate the differences in the inter-individual variability between the different functional networks (Bonferroni corrected for 15 comparisons, threshold at $0.05/15 \approx 0.0033$).

Linking Inter-Individual Functional Variability to Cognitive Ability

First, we calculated the correlations between functional connectivity and cognitive ability. Individual cognitive performance was assessed using four functional domains, including working memory (indexed by the average z-score of DFS and DBS), episodic memory (the z-score of PALT), executive function (inverted z-score of TMT B-A), and vocabulary (the z-score of VFT). In addition, the composite average z-score on all tests was considered a measure of individual global cognitive function. Correlation analyses between each functional domain and the global measure and connectivity of all ROI pairs were performed in a subset of participants ($n = 76$). With an emphasis on the overall trend of the connectivity–cognition relationship, we used a liberal threshold of $p < 0.01$ to map the correlation patterns between the cognitive measures and interregional connectivity of all ROI pairs. Age, sex, education level, and the mean head motion FD were considered covariates during the connectivity–cognition correlation analyses. In addition, to further describe the relationship between individual cognition levels to the connectome measures, the number of long-range (Euclidean distance >75 mm between the centroids of the connected regions in stereotactic space), short-range (Euclidean distance ≤ 75 mm) (Achard et al., 2006; Liang et al., 2013), intra-network (connections within the 6 networks mentioned above), and inter-network (connections between the six networks) connections that were significantly related to each cognitive measure were calculated.

Then, to quantify the significance of the functional connectivity of each region with individual cognitive ability in elderly individuals, a cognitive relevance index was defined. It was measured as the number of connections (including the total connections, long-/short-range connections, and inter-/intra-network connections, respectively) that was significantly correlated with all cognitive variables at each ROI.

Finally, to evaluate the cognitive significance of inter-individual variability in connectivity, we examined the correlation between the values of inter-individual variability and the values of cognitive relevance across all the AAL ROIs ($p < 0.05$). We were interested in examining whether a larger inter-individual variability in the brain connectivity would be more cognitively relevant.

Evaluating Potential Confounding Factors

First, global signal regression (GSR) is a controversial step that may significantly affect the results and conclusions. Recent studies have suggested that GSR can decrease dependence on motion, remove artifactual variance, and provide increased tissue sensitivity (Fox et al., 2009; Satterthwaite et al., 2013; Yan et al., 2013a; Power et al., 2014). However, other studies have demonstrated that GSR may introduce undesirable negative correlations (otherwise largely absent from the connectivity data) that alter inter-individual differences (Fox et al., 2009; Gotts et al., 2013; Saad et al., 2013). In view of these conflicting reports, we included the results without GSR (nGSR) as Supplementary Material for the present study.

Second, different AAL regions vary in regional noise and volume, both of which may potentially drive the inter-individual variability distribution. To rule out these possibilities, we calculated the temporal signal-to-noise ratio (SNR), which was measured as the average signal across time divided by standard deviation across time for each voxel, and averaged the SNR of voxels within each ROI. We also calculated the number of voxels for each ROI to index the volume of each AAL region. A correlation analysis ($p < 0.05$) between the SNR/volume and the inter-individual variability values of the ROIs was examined.

Third, although its size in relation to the entire brain is small, recent studies mapping the cerebellar topographical organization suggest that the cerebellum is functionally heterogeneous (Buckner, 2013). Therefore, cerebellar ROIs may be more prone to contain functionally diverse gray matter compared to that of other ROIs. To rule out this potential confound, a connectivity atlas of the cerebellum, which was adopted by a previous study (Buckner et al., 2011) with large data set ($N = 1000$) to calculate the functional connectivity of different cerebellar regions with neocortical network, was used to perform an additional analysis. We chose the 17-network parcellation atlas of the cerebellum. The voxels assigned to the same network were considered as one ROI; thus, the 17 ROIs from Buckner et al. (2011) were used to replace the 26 AAL cerebellar ROIs, and to recalculate the inter-individual functional variability in the brain. This allowed us to rule out the possibility that high functional heterogeneity in the cerebellum may influence the variability estimation.

Finally, to further confirm the robustness of the result with regard to functional inter-individual variability in the elderly, we validated the result by analyzing an independent replication resting-state fMRI dataset ($N = 49$; 12 men and 37 women; 67.1 ± 4.8 years; range: 60–76 years of age). The data were acquired using a Philips Achieva 3.0-T MRI scanner (Philips Healthcare, Andover, MA) at the MRI Center of the First Hospital of Hebei Medical University of China. Functional images were collected using an EPI sequence with TR = 2000 ms, TE = 30 ms, flip angle = 90°, FOV = 200 mm × 200 mm, thickness = 3.6 mm, matrix = 112 × 112; in-plane resolution = 1.786 × 1.786, 33 axial slices, and 200 volumes. T1-weighted MPRAGE image was collected with the following parameters: 176 slices;

matrix $= 256 \times 256$; voxel size $= 1$ mm $\times$ 1 mm $\times$ 1 mm; TR $= 1900$ ms; TE $= 2.2$ ms; flip angle $= 9°$. The individual variability of functional connectivity in this dataset was estimated using the same procedure as described above.

RESULTS

Inter-Individual Variability in Functional Brain Connectivity

The exploration of the whole-brain functional connectivity in 116 AAL regions indicated a highly uneven distribution pattern for inter-individual variability in the 88 older participants (Supplementary Figure 1). There was an overall tendency that the inter-individual functional variability increased from the primary areas to the subcortical structures and association cortex to the cerebellum across the whole brain. The mean variability in the cerebellum (0.72 ± 0.10) was significantly larger (two-sample t-test, $p < 0.0001$) than that in the cerebral regions (0.59 ± 0.07). In the cerebrum (**Figure 1A**), the inter-individual difference in functional connectivity was higher in the frontal and parietal cortices; pre- and post-central gyri; anterior, middle and posterior cingulated gyri; parahippocampus; hippocampus; and amygdala and lower in the occipital, temporal, and other subcortical regions.

The analyses in the six specific functional systems (**Figure 1B**) further highlighted a gradual increase in the functional variability from the visual, subcortical, and sensorimotor and auditory networks to the default and fronto-parietal networks, and to the cerebellar network. The ANOVA revealed a significant main effect of network in the functional variability ($p < 0.001$). The *post hoc* comparisons demonstrated that the mean inter-individual variability in the cerebellar network was significantly larger ($p < 0.001$) than that of each of the other five networks at a Bonferroni-corrected threshold of $p = 0.0033$ (0.05/15). The fronto-parietal network exhibited a trend toward a higher variability compared with the visual network ($p < 0.01$) and subcortical network ($p < 0.05$).

Connectivity–Cognition Correlation

Figure 2 shows the Pearson correlations of the connectivity of all ROI pairs with individual global cognitive function and the four specific cognitive domains ($p < 0.01$, uncorrected). The largest number of connections from the superior and orbital prefrontal cortex and the cerebellum consistently correlated with individual scores in global cognition and in the four specific cognitive domains. Further, the functional connectivity of the following connections were related to the four cognitive measures: (1) from the middle, anterior, and posterior cingulate; hippocampus; parahippocampus; amygdala; and precentral gyrus for working memory (DFS and DBS); (2) from the middle temporal pole, middle temporal gyrus, postcentral gyrus, precuneus, thalamus, parahippocampus, hippocampus, anterior and posterior cingulate, and putamen for episodic memory (PALT); (3) from the middle temporal gyrus, middle temporal pole, anterior cingulate, inferior parietal lobule, and parahippocampus for executive function (TMT B-A); and (4)

from the fusiform, supramarginal gyrus, angular gyrus, middle temporal gyrus, middle temporal pole, and hippocampus for vocabulary (VFT).

Long-range and inter-network connectivity accounted for a considerable proportion of connections that predicted individual cognition (**Figure 2B**). There were more long-range connections than short-range connections (56.7% vs. 43.3% in total), which correlated with both global measures and specific measures, except for the vocabulary score. Moreover, inter-network connections accounted for 87.3% of all the connections that correlated with the cognitive measures in the whole brain, and consistently preponderated over the intra-network connections when the six functional networks were separately analyzed (**Figure 2C**). We also summarized the total number of inter-network connections that correlated with the four specific cognitive measures for each network. Interestingly, we found that the six networks were in the same variability rank order, except for the subcortical network, which moved up to second place (**Figure 3**).

Finally, we calculated the cognitive relevance, which was indexed by the number of connections that were significantly correlated with the cognitive measures, for each AAL ROI. The distribution map for the cognitive relevance (**Figure 4A**) was similar to the inter-individual functional connectivity variability map (**Figure 1A**). The correlation analysis revealed that the value of the inter-individual functional variability was significantly correlated with the cognitive relevance across the 116 ROIs (Pearson correlation $r = 0.29$, $p = 0.001$; **Figure 4B**). Regions with higher inter-individual functional connectivity variability demonstrated more connections that correlated with cognitive performance. More interestingly, when examining the number of long-/short-range and inter-/intra-network connections, the value of the inter-individual variability significantly correlated with the degree of cognitive relevance for the long-range (Pearson correlation $r = 0.32$, $p < 0.001$; **Figure 4C**) and inter-network (Pearson correlation $r = 0.30$, $p = 0.001$; **Figure 4D**) connectivity across all ROIs. There was no significant correlation between the inter-individual variability and the short-range (Pearson correlation $r = 0.10$, $p = 0.27$) or intra-network (Pearson correlation $r = 0.16$, $p = 0.09$) connectivity cognitive relevance measures in the brains of elderly individuals.

Impact of Potential Confounds

First, we re-calculated the functional inter-individual variability without removing the global signal in the preprocessing. Variability maps, estimated with (**Figure 1**) and without (Supplementary Figures 1, 2) GSR, demonstrated a highly similar pattern (Pearson correlation $r = 0.92$, $p < 0.0001$). The cerebellum retained the largest mean inter-individual variability compared to that of cerebral regions (two-sample t-test, $p < 0.0001$). The network-level variability also consistently demonstrated significant statistical difference for the functional variability among the networks ($p < 0.001$), with gradually increased variability occurring in the subcortical network, then the primary networks (i.e., visual, sensorimotor, and auditory networks), to the association networks (i.e., default and fronto-parietal networks), and to the cerebellar network (Supplementary

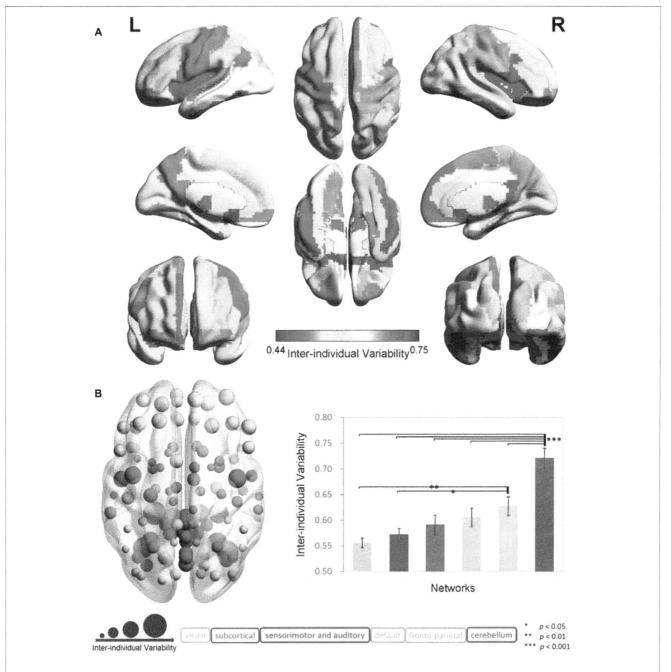

FIGURE 1 | Inter-individual difference in functional brain connectivity in elderly individuals. **(A)** Distribution of inter-individual functional variability in the cerebrum. The inter-individual variability values for the 90-automated anatomical labeling (AAL) cerebral regions were mapped onto the cortical surfaces using varied colors. **(B)** Inter-individual variability in functional networks. The left axial map shows the inter-individual variability in the functional connectivity for 116 AAL regions, which are rendered as color-coded nodes, according to the functional networks (He et al., 2009). The nodes are located at the center of these regions, and the nodal size is proportional to the level of the inter-individual variability. The right histogram plots the averaged inter-individual variability values and the standard errors for the functional networks, which are displayed as color-coded bars in the corresponding color applied to the nodes.

Figure 2B). However, as expected, the GSR largely affected the connectivity–cognition correlations, such that the GSR preprocessing introduced more negative correlations (**Figure 2**) than the nGSR preprocessing (Supplementary Figure 3). As an overall trend, this was consistent with the GSR results regarding the inter-network connectivity, especially for the

connections from the superior and orbital prefrontal cortex, hippocampus, and the cerebellum predominating individual cognitive ability. It is important to note that the retention of the global signal diminished the correlation between the long-range connections and cognition, with a larger proportion of the long-range connections only found in the global measure

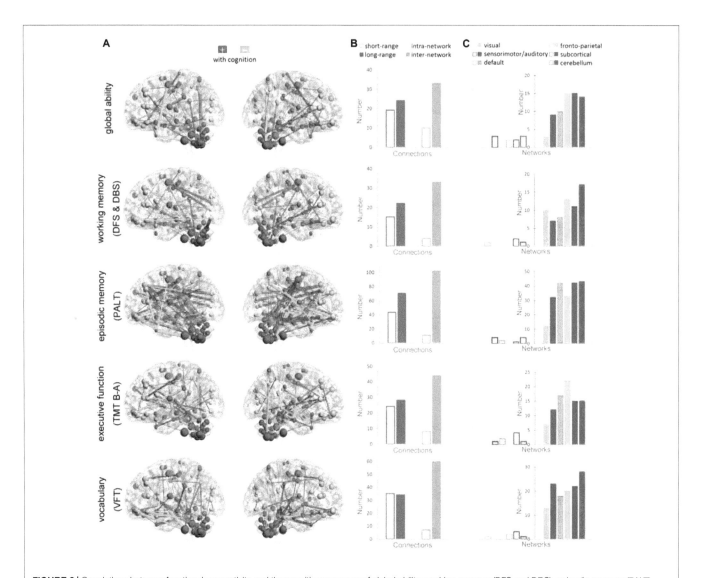

FIGURE 2 | Correlations between functional connectivity and the cognitive measures of global ability, working memory (DFS and DBS), episodic memory (PALT), executive function (TMT B-A), and vocabulary ability (VFT). **(A)** Maps showing significant correlations between the connectivity and cognitive ability ($p < 0.01$). The connections that positively correlated with cognition are shown in red, whereas the connections that negatively correlated with cognition are shown in green. The thickness of the connections is proportional to the connectivity–cognition correlation coefficients. **(B)** The bars show the total number of short-range and long-range connections, as well as the intra-network and inter-network connections that are correlated with each cognitive domain. **(C)** The bars show the total number of connections within each functional network (transparent bars) and the total number of connections with other networks (non-transparent bars) that are correlated with each cognitive domain.

and vocabulary score. In addition, in the nGSR condition, the relationship between the value of the inter-individual functional connectivity variability and the cognitive relevance across all ROIs disappeared (Pearson correlation $r = -0.13$, $p = 0.17$; Supplementary Figure 4).

Next, we calculated the correlation between the regional SNR/size and the inter-individual functional connectivity variability values across all ROIs, to exclude the possibility that the ranking of the regional inter-individual variability was primarily driven by potential noise and size effects. The rank of the inter-individual variability derived with GSR was not influenced by the regional noise or size ($p > 0.05$). The supplementary nGSR result of the inter-individual variability,

however, correlated significantly with the regional SNR (Pearson correlation $r = 0.34$, $p < 0.01$).

Third, to rule out the possibility that high functional heterogeneity in the cerebellar ROIs influenced the variability estimation, we used the 17-network parcellation atlas of the cerebellum (Buckner et al., 2011) to replace the 26 cerebellar AAL ROIs, which allowed us to perform an additional analysis of the inter-individual functional connectivity variability. Consistent with our findings using the cerebellar AAL ROIs, the additional analysis demonstrated that 5 of the 17 cerebellar ROIs ranked highly for the inter-individual functional variability in the brain. The mean variability of the 17 cerebellar ROIs (0.66 ± 0.12) was significantly larger (two-sample t-test, $p = 0.0001$) than that of

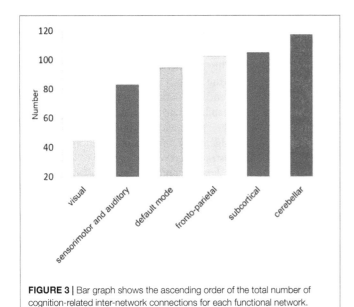

FIGURE 3 | Bar graph shows the ascending order of the total number of cognition-related inter-network connections for each functional network.

the cerebral ROIs (0.58 ± 0.07). No significant differences were found for the inter-individual functional connectivity variability in the cerebellum between the two different atlases (two-sample t-test, $p = 0.09$).

Finally, the robust validation analysis in an independent dataset further confirmed the distribution of inter-individual functional connectivity variability in the brains of elderly people. The distribution patterns in both datasets were highly similar (Pearson correlation $r = 0.61$, $p < 0.0001$). Further, the cerebellum had maximal inter-individual variability (0.72 ± 0.11), and the cerebrum demonstrated gradually increased inter-individual variability from the visual (0.61 ± 0.06), subcortical (0.62 ± 0.05), and sensorimotor and auditory (0.63 ± 0.09) networks to the fronto-parietal (0.64 ± 0.09) and default (0.69 ± 0.09) networks.

DISCUSSION

There is fairly extensive research regarding the relationship between changes in brain connectivity and a broad range of cognitive decline and neuropsychiatric symptoms in aging populations (Hedden and Gabrieli, 2004; Reuter-Lorenz and Lustig, 2005; Andrews-Hanna et al., 2007; Wang et al., 2007, 2015; Bishop et al., 2010; Grady, 2012; Tomasi and Volkow, 2012; Ferreira and Busatto, 2013; Li et al., 2013, 2015; Fornito et al., 2015). Although these studies strongly supported the notion that brain connectivity is an important determinant of cognitive aging, the contribution of person-to-person variation remained unclear. Thus, the present study

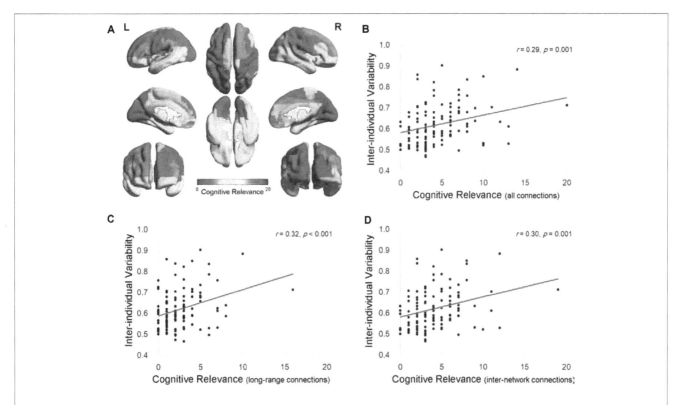

FIGURE 4 | Relationship between inter-individual variability and the cognitive relevance of functional connectivity. **(A)** The cognitive relevance map of AAL cerebral regions. Each AAL regions of interest (ROI) was color coded as the total number of connections that are correlated with four specific cognitive domains. **(B–D)** The scatter plots show the correlation between the inter-individual variability and cognitive relevance as indexed by the total number of cognition-related connections **(B)**, long-range connections **(C)**, and inter-network connections **(D)** across 116 AAL ROIs, respectively. Each dot represents one ROI from AAL.

aimed to bridge the gap in knowledge of how individual variability of functional connectivity and the inter-individual differences affect the cognitive ability of elderly individuals. Our novel study systematically mapped the distribution of individual functional variability on a whole-brain scale, which facilitated understanding of how inter-individual variability differs between different brain areas in the older adults. Further, we demonstrated that the inter-individual variability mapping has important cognitive significance. These findings may thus contribute a valuable reference or evidence for future cognitive aging studies.

Inter-Individual Functional Variability in Elderly Individuals

Functional connectivity in the cerebral cortex indicated that there was higher inter-individual variability in the frontal and parietal cortices, and the pre- and post-central gyri, while there was lower variation in the occipital and temporal regions in elderly individuals. The cortical variability generally aligned with the results from Mueller et al. (2013) who conducted a study of the inter-individual differences in cortical connectivity in 25 healthy adults. In the current study, we expanded this previous work to include a global analysis of the brain in a large sample of older adults. Our findings indicate that inter-individual variability was the largest in the cerebellum, followed by the association regions that largely constitute the fronto-parietal and default mode networks, as well as some subcortical regions, especially the hippocampal formation. Primary regions, including visual and sensorimotor networks, and other subcortical structures exhibited minimal variability among individuals.

It is not surprising that the functional connectivity in the prefrontal and parietal cortices and the relevant fronto-parietal and default mode networks demonstrated major individual variations in the cortex, because extensive evidence suggests these association regions and network connections are the selective targets of aging effects (Andrews-Hanna et al., 2007; Grady, 2012; Tomasi and Volkow, 2012; Ferreira and Busatto, 2013). The cerebellum has not been substantially investigated in most aging studies. However, there is increasingly converging evidence to suggest that the cerebellum is connected to cerebral association regions, including the prefrontal and posterior parietal cortices, and subcortical structures, including the vestibular nuclei and basal ganglia. Therefore, the cerebellum can contribute to a wide variety of functional domains and neuropsychiatric diseases (Stoodley and Schmahmann, 2009; Bostan et al., 2013; Buckner, 2013). Wagner et al. (2017) recently observed that the cerebellar granule cells could encode reward expectation, suggesting that the cerebellum was involved in cognitive processing (Wagner et al., 2017). Further, in a recent review of multidisciplinary findings, Sokolov et al. (2017) suggested a cerebro-cerebellar loop to explain the involvement of the cerebellum in higher cognitive functions, including attention, language, memory, and social cognition (Sokolov et al., 2017). We identified that the largest inter-individual variability resides in the cerebellum, further indicating that it is a noteworthy region for future aging studies. Additional potential studies include the exploration of how the cerebellum is mediated by the prefrontal and parietal regions in the association functional networks, which would provide a better understanding of its role in aging.

Several potential causes may underlie the distribution of the inter-individual variability in the brain functional connectivity of older individuals. First, the hemodynamic MRI signal is triggered by the metabolic demands of neuronal activities (Heeger and Ress, 2002). The variability map of functional connectivity is consistent with the previous metabolic topography of normal aging, as investigated by positron emission tomography; this technique demonstrated covariant metabolic changes in the prefrontal cortex, lateral temporal and parietal cortices, cerebellum, and basal ganglia (Moeller et al., 1996; Chiaravalloti et al., 2014). Thus, we speculated that the inter-individual variability in the functional connectivity had a physiologically reasonable metabolic basis. Second, our findings may be, in part, a functional consequence of the individual heterogeneity in brain structure morphology that occurs with aging. MRI volumetric studies have demonstrated heterogenic aging patterns across structures regarding neuroanatomical volume loss (Jernigan et al., 2001; Walhovd et al., 2005). Jernigan et al. (2001) observed that the cerebellum exhibited the same striking degree of gray matter reduction with aging as the frontal lobes, and exhibited a more accelerated volume loss than the hippocampus (Jernigan et al., 2001). In addition, other anatomical profiles, such as its cortical folding, thickness, and white matter fiber tracts, may also contribute to the individual differences in the functional correlations (Kanai and Rees, 2011; Mueller et al., 2013; Karama et al., 2014). For example, diffusion tensor imaging of white fiber tracts demonstrated that the variability of aging effects was also regionally complex; this was indicated by a gradient increase in the white matter deficits from the posterior to anterior cortex segments, but also by a greater impairment in the cerebellum (Davis et al., 2009; Bennett et al., 2010). Third, the diverse dynamics and heterogeneous distributions of neurons, as well as the selective vulnerability of synapses and neurons during aging, may also promote individual differences in functional connectivity (Morrison and Hof, 1997; Zhao et al., 2008; Bishop et al., 2010; Urban and Tripathy, 2012; Mejias and Longtin, 2014). Although the cerebellum only accounts for approximately 10% of the total brain weight, it accounts for half of its neurons. Thus, the cerebellum would naturally exhibit more variations due to its densely packed neuronal assembly. Finally, genetic and plasticity factors play critical roles in the inter-individual variability in brain connectivity (Mueller et al., 2013; Toro et al., 2014). Genes determine the individual differences in the evolutionarily recent association cortex, specifically in the prefrontal region (Thompson et al., 2001), where the gene expression patterns exhibit substantially greater heterogeneity in middle-old aged populations (Lu et al., 2004; Bishop et al., 2010). Furthermore, the prefrontal cortex and cerebellum are the final structures to achieve maturity, but are also the first structures to undergo involution in later life (Wang and Zoghbi, 2001; Hogan et al., 2011). This protracted development and prolonged degeneration processes can continue to accumulate deeper and more complex inter-individual variations via environment- and lifestyle-dependent neural plasticity.

Cognitive Relevance of the Inter-Individual Connectivity Variability

The connectivity–cognition correlation suggested that the connections that are related to cognitive ability lay mainly in regions with large inter-individual connectivity differences, including the prefrontal cortex, hippocampal formation, inferior parietal gyrus, middle temporal pole, middle temporal gyrus, and cerebellar regions. The prefrontal, parietal, and temporal regions are the uppermost components of the fronto-parietal and default mode networks, which support high-level cognition. Numerous molecular and neuroimaging studies have repeatedly confirmed their role in cognitive aging, such as in memory, attention, and executive function decline (Hedden and Gabrieli, 2004; Burke and Barnes, 2006; Andrews-Hanna et al., 2007; Bishop et al., 2010; Grady, 2012; Nyberg et al., 2012; Tomasi and Volkow, 2012; Ferreira and Busatto, 2013; Karama et al., 2014). The hippocampal formation is also particularly vulnerable to the aging process. Here, we demonstrated that the functional connectivity of the hippocampus and parahippocampus is correlated with all four cognitive measures, including working memory (DFS and DBS), episodic memory (PALT), executive function (TMT B-A), and vocabulary (VFT). Our results are consistent with a recent meta-analysis of 114 fMRI studies of older adults, which suggested a set of regions that are remarkably involved in cognitive aging; these included the frontal gyrus, parahippocampal gyrus, fusiform gyrus, precentral gyrus, and functional networks, especially the fronto-parietal and default networks (Li et al., 2015).

Long-range and inter-network connections appeared to dominate cognitive ability differences among older adults. Long-range connections are well-known for their key role in efficient brain-wide information processing and functional integration of diverse cognitive functions (Jbabdi et al., 2013; Park and Friston, 2013). Previous evidence demonstrated that the long-range connections in the default and fronto-parietal attention networks are selectively vulnerable to aging and are susceptible to early Alzheimer's disease, compared to that of the short-range connections (Andrews-Hanna et al., 2007; Tomasi and Volkow, 2012; Li et al., 2013; Wang et al., 2013; Sala-Llonch et al., 2014). Recently, Fjell et al. (2015) found extensive changes in inter-network functional connectivity across multiple cortical networks that were related to a decline in episodic memory with aging (Fjell et al., 2015). It is also interesting to note that although the subcortical network ranked lower for the average inter-individual variability, some specific regions with larger inter-individual differences, including the hippocampal formation, thalamus, caudate, and amygdala, have considerable connections to regions in other networks that are involved in cognition. Therefore, this may suggest that this network, specifically some specific regions, needs to be considered as having a role in cognitive function through its interactions with other cortical and cerebellar networks.

Importantly, we found larger inter-individual variation of functional connectivity was significantly correlated with higher cognitive relevance, in terms of the number of cognition-correlated connections. This relationship suggested that the functional connectome was a major root of individual behavior differences. Moreover, we demonstrated that the correlation between the inter-individual variability and the cognitive relevance of functional connectivity was specific to long-range and inter-network connections. Given the role of long-range and inter-network connections in cognitive performance, this finding further indicated that regions and networks with large inter-individual variability deserve attention in future studies. Thus, these results provide a new perspective for understanding cognitive aging. Currently, most studies are conducted by first assigning participants to different groups, and then exploring differences in the averaged brain activity signals among the groups. In these studies, inter-individual differences in brain function are essentially neglected, or simplified to group differences (Mohr and Nagel, 2010), limiting the full understanding of cognitive aging. Here, the mapping of the inter-individual functional connectivity variability and its correlation with cognition suggested regions and connections, which are typically overlooked but important to cognitive aging studies. For example, the cerebellum showed the largest inter-individual variability and was correlated with diverse cognitive domains. In fact, several studies investigating the role of the cerebellum in aging has emerged. Increasing evidence has indicated that the cerebellum is involved in frontally based functional decline in elderly individuals (Sullivan and Pfefferbaum, 2006; Hogan et al., 2011; Bernard and Seidler, 2014). Future studies should investigate how the prefrontal cortex interacts with the cerebellum, subcortical areas, and other cortical regions to contribute to the inter-individual differences seen with aging. This would be particularly important to distinguish the connectivity–cognition associations that are specific to aging from the inherent general relationships across the lifespan. For example, previously the prefrontal cortex has been overwhelmingly emphasized in cognitive aging. However, a previous molecular genetic expression study (Erraji-Benchekroun et al., 2005) and a recent cortical thickness study (Karama et al., 2014) have stressed that the prefrontal cortex is in fact linked closely with diverse cognitive abilities throughout the human life-span. The mapping of inter-individual variability thus brings a new perspective to future studies that seek key areas affected by cognitive aging. It will also be exciting to investigate inter-individual connectivity variability and its cognitive importance over time to further understand inter-individual differences in the trajectories of cognitive aging and specific diseases, such as AD.

Limitations

A few limitations of the present study must be noted. First, given the complex and controversial involvement of the GSR in fcMRI studies, we included results both with and without GSR. The GSR was expected to influence the results. The inter-individual variability rank estimated from data with GSR appeared to be more sensitive to the noise than the nGSR results, despite a similar inter-individual ROI variability ranking with both strategies. In addition, the GSR produced negative biased correlations between the individual connectivity and cognitive measures and magnified the proportion of long-range connections that were correlated with performance, compared to that of the nGSR results. However, both suggested an important role for the inter-network connections in cognitive aging. The influence of the regression of global signal in the present result needs to be carefully considered. Second, we noted that as the present study was confined to the estimation of the distribution of inter-individual functional variability of older adults, intra-individual variations were not considered. Variations in the intra-individual functional connectivity may be caused by measurement instability due to technical noise or changes of mental and biological states (Mueller et al., 2013). A recent study conducted by Chen et al. (2015) depicted the pattern of intra-individual functional variability in the brain of young adults with the use of ten repeated fMRI measurements. Another factor is the temporal moment-to-moment variation within an individual's BOLD signal, which has also been suggested to have predictive significance in relation to cognitive function and various clinical conditions (Garrett et al., 2013). It is necessary for future studies to investigate the distribution characteristic of these intra-individual variations and examine their cognitive correlations with aging and to further investigate how these variations may interact with inter-individual variability. Third, we acknowledge that the connectivity–cognition correlation was not corrected for multiple comparisons. This is because the focus of this study was not to report which regional connections were significantly correlated with cognitive performance. We used a threshold of $p < 0.01$ (corresponding to $r > 0.30$) to define the cognitive relevance index for each region, which helped disclose an overall relationship between functional connectivity variability and cognitive association across all brain areas. The definition of "cognitive relevance index" in our study was similar to that of other fMRI connectivity measurements, such as "functional connectivity density" or "degree centrality," which is usually calculated as the number of correlated connections at a liberal correlation coefficient threshold (e.g., $r = 0.25$), without multiple corrections on the correlations between mass voxels (Buckner et al., 2009; Weng et al., 2016). Fourth, the AAL atlas we used to calculate functional connectivity was defined on the basis of anatomical features. Although the use of an alternative connectivity atlas of cerebellum did not change the cerebellar rank in inter-individual variability, the influence of the ROI definition from using the AAL cannot be fully excluded. As the division of brain regions, as well as their functional characteristics, remains controversial, future studies of data-driven parcellation of brain regions and networks would present more precise estimation of inter-individual variability

in elderly individuals. Finally, the current study was focused on mapping a general profile of inter-individual variability in an older population. No attempt was made to examine factors, such as the age of participants, that influence inter-individual variability. Thus, further studies are required to investigate the effect of age, as well as other environmental or genetic factors, that can influence individual functional variability.

CONCLUSION

In the current study, we delineated a map of inter-individual variability in whole-brain functional connectivity for older adults. These results revealed gradually increased variability from the primary regions (including the visual, sensorimotor, and auditory networks), to specific subcortical structures, particularly the hippocampal formation, and the prefrontal and parietal cortices that largely constitute the default mode and fronto-parietal networks, and the cerebellum. The connectivity–cognition results further stressed a crucial function for long-range and inter-network connections in inter-individual cognitive performance. Moreover, the associations between inter-individual variability and the cognition relevance of functional connectivity provide a new perspective for investigating the mechanisms underlying cognitive aging and relevant diseases.

AUTHOR CONTRIBUTIONS

Conceived and designed the experiments: RL, JL. Performed the experiments: SY, XZ, WR, JY, PW, ZZ, Y-NN, XH. Analyzed the data and wrote the paper: RL.

ACKNOWLEDGMENTS

This work was supported by the National Natural Science Foundation of China (31671157, 31470998, 61673374, 31271108, 31200847, 31600904), Beijing Municipal Science and Technology Commission (No. Z171100000117006), the Pioneer Initiative of the Chinese Academy of Sciences, Feature Institutes Program (TSS-2015-06), the National Key Research and Development Program of China (2016YFC1305904), and the CAS Key Laboratory of Mental Health, Institute of Psychology (KLMH2014ZK02, KLMH2014ZG03).

REFERENCES

Achard, S., Salvador, R., Whitcher, B., Suckling, J., and Bullmore, E. T. (2006). A resilient, low-frequency, small-world human brain functional network with highly connected association cortical hubs. *J. Neurosci.* 26, 63–72. doi: 10.1523/jneurosci.3874-05.2006

Andrews-Hanna, J. R., Snyder, A. Z., Vincent, J. L., Lustig, C., Head, D., Raichle, M. E., et al. (2007). Disruption of large-scale brain systems in advanced aging. *Neuron* 56, 924–935. doi: 10.1016/j.neuron.2007.10.038

Ashburner, J. (2007). A fast diffeomorphic image registration algorithm. *Neuroimage* 38, 95–113. doi: 10.1016/j.neuroimage.2007.07.007

Bennett, I. J., Madden, D. J., Vaidya, C. J., Howard, D. V., and Howard, J. H. (2010). Age-related differences in multiple measures of white matter integrity: a diffusion tensor imaging study of healthy aging. *Hum. Brain Mapp.* 31, 378–390. doi: 10.1002/hbm.20872

Bernard, J. A., and Seidler, R. D. (2014). Moving forward: age effects on the cerebellum underlie cognitive and motor declines. *Neurosci. Biobehav. Rev.* 42, 193–207. doi: 10.1016/j.neubiorev.2014.02.011

Betzel, R. F., Byrge, L., He, Y., Goni, J., Zuo, X.-N., and Sporns, O. (2014). Changes in structural and functional connectivity among resting-state networks across the human lifespan. *Neuroimage* 102, 345–357. doi: 10.1016/j.neuroimage.2014.07.067

Bishop, N. A., Lu, T., and Yankner, B. A. (2010). Neural mechanisms of ageing and cognitive decline. *Nature* 464, 529–535. doi: 10.1038/nature08983

Bostan, A. C., Dum, R. P., and Strick, P. L. (2013). Cerebellar networks with the cerebral cortex and basal ganglia. *Trends Cogn. Sci.* 17, 241–254. doi: 10.1016/j.tics.2013.03.003

Buckner, R. L. (2013). The cerebellum and cognitive function: 25 years of insight from anatomy and neuroimaging. *Neuron* 80, 807–815. doi: 10.1016/j.neuron.2013.10.044

Buckner, R. L., Krienen, F. M., Castellanos, A., Diaz, J. C., and Yeo, B. T. T. (2011). The organization of the human cerebellum estimated by intrinsic functional connectivity. *J. Neurophysiol.* 106, 2322–2345. doi: 10.1152/jn.00339.2011

Buckner, R. L., Sepulcre, J., Talukdar, T., Krienen, F. M., Liu, H. S., Hedden, T., et al. (2009). Cortical hubs revealed by intrinsic functional connectivity: mapping, assessment of stability, and relation to Alzheimer's disease. *J. Neurosci.* 29, 1860–1873. doi: 10.1523/jneurosci.5062-08.2009

Burke, S. N., and Barnes, C. A. (2006). Neural plasticity in the ageing brain. *Nat. Rev. Neurosci.* 7, 30–40. doi: 10.1038/nrn1809

Chen, B., Xu, T., Zhou, C., Wang, L., Yang, N., Wang, Z., et al. (2015). Individual variability and test-retest reliability revealed by ten repeated resting-state brain scans over one month. *PLOS ONE* 10:e0144963. doi: 10.1371/journal.pone.0144963

Chiaravalloti, A., Abbatiello, P., Calabria, F., Palumbo, B., Martorana, A., and Schillaci, O. (2014). Cortico-subcortical metabolic changes in aging brain: a 18F FDG PET/CT study. *Int. J. Nuclear Med. Res.* 1, 17–23. doi: 10.15379/2408-9788.2014.01.01.4

Davis, S. W., Dennis, N. A., Buchler, N. G., White, L. E., Madden, D. J., and Cabeza, R. (2009). Assessing the effects of age on long white matter tracts using diffusion tensor tractography. *Neuroimage* 46, 530–541. doi: 10.1016/j.neuroimage.2009.01.068

Dennis, E. L., and Thompson, P. M. (2014). Functional brain connectivity using fMRI in aging and Alzheimer's disease. *Neuropsychol. Rev.* 24, 49–62. doi: 10.1007/s11065-014-9249-6

Erraji-Benchekroun, L., Underwood, M. D., Arango, V., Galfalvy, H., Pavlidis, P., Smyrniotopoulos, P., et al. (2005). Molecular aging in human prefrontal cortex is selective and continuous throughout adult life. *Biol. Psychiatry* 57, 549–558. doi: 10.1016/j.biopsych.2004.10.034

Eyler, L. T., Sherzai, A., Kaup, A. R., and Jeste, D. V. (2011). A review of functional brain imaging correlates of successful cognitive aging. *Biol. Psychiatry* 70, 115–122. doi: 10.1016/j.biopsych.2010.12.032

Ferrarini, L., Veer, I. M., Baerends, E., van Tol, M. J., Renken, R. J., van der Wee, N. J. A., et al. (2009). Hierarchical functional modularity in the resting-state human brain. *Hum. Brain Mapp.* 30, 2220–2231. doi: 10.1002/hbm.20663

Ferreira, L. K., and Busatto, G. F. (2013). Resting-state functional connectivity in normal brain aging. *Neurosci. Biobehav. Rev.* 37, 384–400. doi: 10.1016/j.neubiorev.2013.01.017

Fjell, A. M., Sneve, M. H., Grydeland, H., Storsve, A. B., de Lange, A.-M. G., Amlien, I. K., et al. (2015). Functional connectivity change across multiple cortical networks relates to episodic memory changes in aging. *Neurobiol. Aging* 36, 3255–3268. doi: 10.1016/j.neurobiolaging.2015.08.020

Fornito, A., Zalesky, A., and Breakspear, M. (2015). The connectomics of brain disorders. *Nat. Rev. Neurosci.* 16, 159–172. doi: 10.1038/nrn3901

Fox, M. D., Zhang, D., Snyder, A. Z., and Raichle, M. E. (2009). The global signal and observed anticorrelated resting state brain networks. *J. Neurophysiol.* 101, 3270–3283. doi: 10.1152/jn.90777.2008

Friston, K. J., Williams, S., Howard, R., Frackowiak, R. S. J., and Turner, R. (1996). Movement-related effects in fMRI time-series. *Magn. Reson. Med.* 35, 346–355. doi: 10.1002/mrm.1910350312

Gao, W., Elton, A., Zhu, H., Alcauter, S., Smith, J. K., Gilmore, J. H., et al. (2014). Intersubject variability of and genetic effects on the brain's functional connectivity during infancy. *J. Neurosci.* 34, 11288–11296. doi: 10.1523/jneurosci.5072-13.2014

Garrett, D. D., Samanez-Larkin, G. R., MacDonald, S. W. S., Lindenberger, U., McIntosh, A. R., and Grady, C. L. (2013). Moment-to-moment brain signal variability: a next frontier in human brain mapping? *Neurosci. Biobehav. Rev.* 37, 610–624. doi: 10.1016/j.neubiorev.2013.02.015

Gong, Y. X. (1992). *Manual of Wechsler Adult Intelligence Scale-Chinese Version.* Changsha: Chinese Map Press.

Gotts, S. J., Saad, Z. S., Jo, H. J., Wallace, G. L., Cox, R. W., and Martin, A. (2013). The perils of global signal regression for group comparisons: a case study of Autism Spectrum Disorders. *Front. Hum. Neurosci.* 7:356. doi: 10.3389/fnhum.2013.00356

Grady, C. (2012). The cognitive neuroscience of ageing. *Nat. Rev. Neurosci.* 13, 491–505. doi: 10.1038/nrn3256

He, Y., Wang, J. H., Wang, L., Chen, Z. J., Yan, C. G., Yang, H., et al. (2009). Uncovering intrinsic modular organization of spontaneous brain activity in humans. *PLOS ONE* 4:e5226. doi: 10.1371/journal.pone.0005226

Hedden, T., and Gabrieli, J. D. E. (2004). Insights into the ageing mind: a view from cognitive neuroscience. *Nat. Rev. Neurosci.* 5, 87–96. doi: 10.1038/nrn1323

Heeger, D. J., and Ress, D. (2002). What does fMRI tell us about neuronal activity? *Nat. Rev. Neurosci.* 3, 142–151. doi: 10.1038/nrn730

Hogan, M. J., Staff, R. T., Bunting, B. P., Murray, A. D., Ahearn, T. S., Deary, I. J., et al. (2011). Cerebellar brain volume accounts for variance in cognitive performance in older adults. *Cortex* 47, 441–450. doi: 10.1016/j.cortex.2010.01.001

Jbabdi, S., Behrens, T. E., and New York Academy of Sciences (2013). "Long-range connectomics," in *Conference Reports: Evolutionary Dynamics and Information Hierarchies in Biological Systems: Aspen Center for Physics Workshop and Cracking the Neural Code: Third Annual Aspen Brain Forums,* (New York, NY: The New York Academy of Sciences), 83–93. doi: 10.1111/nyas.12271

Jenkinson, M., Bannister, P., Brady, M., and Smith, S. (2002). Improved optimization for the robust and accurate linear registration and motion correction of brain images. *Neuroimage* 17, 825–841. doi: 10.1006/nimg.2002.1132

Jernigan, T. L., Archibald, S. L., Fennema-Notestine, C., Gamst, A. C., Stout, J. C., Bonner, J., et al. (2001). Effects of age on tissues and regions of the cerebrum and cerebellum. *Neurobiol. Aging* 22, 581–594. doi: 10.1016/s0197-4580(01)00217-2

Kanai, R., and Rees, G. (2011). The structural basis of inter-individual differences in human behaviour and cognition. *Nat. Rev. Neurosci.* 12, 231–242. doi: 10.1038/nrn3000

Karama, S., Bastin, M. E., Murray, C., Royle, N. A., Penke, L., Munoz Maniega, S., et al. (2014). Childhood cognitive ability accounts for associations between cognitive ability and brain cortical thickness in old age. *Mol. Psychiatry* 19, 555–559. doi: 10.1038/mp.2013.64

Lawton, M. P., and Brody, E. M. (1969). Assessment of older people: self-maintaining and instrumental activities of daily living. *Gerontologist* 9, 179–186. doi: 10.1093/geront/9.3_Part_1.179

Li, H.-J., Hou, X.-H., Liu, H.-H., Yue, C.-L., Lu, G.-M., and Zuo, X.-N. (2015). Putting age-related task activation into large-scale brain networks: a meta-analysis of 114 fMRI studies on healthy aging. *Neurosci. Biobehav. Rev.* 57, 156–174. doi: 10.1016/j.neubiorev.2015.08.013

Li, R., Yu, J., Zhang, S., Bao, F., Wang, P., Huang, X., et al. (2013). Bayesian network analysis reveals alterations to default mode network connectivity in individuals at risk for Alzheimer's disease. *PLOS ONE* 8:e82104. doi: 10.1371/journal.pone.0082104

Liang, X., Zou, Q. H., He, Y., and Yang, Y. H. (2013). Coupling of functional connectivity and regional cerebral blood flow reveals a physiological basis for network hubs of the human brain. *Proc. Natl. Acad. Sci. U.S.A.* 110, 1929–1934. doi: 10.1073/pnas.1214900110

Lowe, M. J., Mock, B. J., and Sorenson, J. A. (1998). Functional connectivity in single and multislice echoplanar imaging using resting-state fluctuations. *Neuroimage* 7, 119–132. doi: 10.1006/nimg.1997.0315

Lu, T., Pan, Y., Kao, S. Y., Li, C., Kohane, I., Chan, J., et al. (2004). Gene regulation and DNA damage in the ageing human brain. *Nature* 429, 883–891. doi: 10.1038/nature02661

Lustig, C., Shah, P., Seidler, R., and Reuter-Lorenz, P. A. (2009). Aging, training, and the brain: a review and future directions. *Neuropsychol. Rev.* 19, 504–522. doi: 10.1007/s11065-009-9119-9

Mejias, J. F., and Longtin, A. (2014). Differential effects of excitatory and inhibitory heterogeneity on the gain and asynchronous state of sparse cortical networks. *Front. Comput. Neurosci.* 8:107. doi: 10.3389/fncom.2014.00107

Moeller, J. R., Ishikawa, T., Dhawan, V., Spetsieris, P., Mandel, F., Alexander, G. E., et al. (1996). The metabolic topography of normal aging. *J. Cereb. Blood Flow Metab.* 16, 385–398. doi: 10.1097/00004647-199605000-00005

Mohr, P. N. C., and Nagel, I. E. (2010). Variability in brain activity as an individual difference measure in neuroscience? *J. Neurosci.* 30, 7755–7757. doi: 10.1523/jneurosci.1560-10.2010

Morrison, J. H., and Hof, P. R. (1997). Life and death of neurons in the aging brain. *Science* 278, 412–419. doi: 10.1126/science.278.5337.412

Mueller, S., Wang, D. H., Fox, M. D., Yeo, B. T. T., Sepulcre, J., Sabuncu, M. R., et al. (2013). Individual variability in functional connectivity architecture of the human brain. *Neuron* 77, 586–595. doi: 10.1016/j.neuron.2012.12.028

Myers, N., Pasquini, L., Goettler, J., Grimmer, T., Koch, K., Ortner, M., et al. (2014). Within-patient correspondence of amyloid-beta and intrinsic network connectivity in Alzheimer's disease. *Brain* 137, 2052–2064. doi: 10.1093/brain/awu103

Nyberg, L., Lovden, M., Riklund, K., Lindenberger, U., and Backman, L. (2012). Memory aging and brain maintenance. *Trends Cogn. Sci.* 16, 292–305. doi: 10.1016/j.tics.2012.04.005

Park, H. J., and Friston, K. J. (2013). Structural and functional brain networks: from connections to cognition. *Science* 342:1238411. doi: 10.1126/science.1238411

Power, J. D., Mitra, A., Laumann, T. O., Snyder, A. Z., Schlaggar, B. L., and Petersen, S. E. (2014). Methods to detect, characterize, and remove motion artifact in resting state fMRI. *Neuroimage* 84, 320–341. doi: 10.1016/j.neuroimage.2013.08.048

Reitan, R. M. (1986). *Trail Making Test: Manual for Administration and Scoring.* Tucson, AZ: Reitan Neuropsychology Laboratory.

Reuter-Lorenz, P. A., and Lustig, C. (2005). Brain aging: reorganizing discoveries about the aging mind. *Curr. Opin. Neurobiol.* 15, 245–251. doi: 10.1016/j.conb.2005.03.016

Rosenberg, S. J., Ryan, J. J., and Prifitera, A. (1984). Rey auditory-verbal learning test-performance of patients with and without memory impairment. *J. Clin. Psychol.* 40, 785–787. doi: 10.1002/1097-4679(198405)40:3<785::AID-JCLP2270400325>3.0.CO;2-4

Saad, Z. S., Reynolds, R. C., Jo, H. J., Gotts, S. J., Chen, G., Martin, A., et al. (2013). Correcting brain-wide correlation differences in resting-state FMRI. *Brain Connect.* 3, 339–352. doi: 10.1089/brain.2013.0156

Sala-Llonch, R., Junque, C., Arenaza-Urquijo, E. M., Vidal-Pineiro, D., Valls-Pedret, C., Palacios, E. M., et al. (2014). Changes in whole-brain functional networks and memory performance in aging. *Neurobiol. Aging* 35, 2193–2202. doi: 10.1016/j.neurobiolaging.2014.04.007

Satterthwaite, T. D., Elliott, M. A., Gerraty, R. T., Ruparel, K., Loughead, J., Calkins, M. E., et al. (2013). An improved framework for confound regression and filtering for control of motion artifact in the preprocessing of resting-state functional connectivity data. *Neuroimage* 64, 240–256. doi: 10.1016/j.neuroimage.2012.08.052

Sokolov, A. A., Miall, R. C., and Ivry, R. B. (2017). The cerebellum: adaptive prediction for movement and cognition. *Trends Cogn. Sci.* 21, 313–332. doi: 10.1016/j.tics.2017.02.005

Stoodley, C. J., and Schmahmann, J. D. (2009). Functional topography in the human cerebellum: a meta-analysis of neuroimaging studies. *Neuroimage* 44, 489–501. doi: 10.1016/j.neuroimage.2008.08.039

Sullivan, E. V., and Pfefferbaum, A. (2006). Diffusion tensor imaging and aging. *Neurosci. Biobehav. Rev.* 30, 749–761. doi: 10.1016/j.neubiorev.2006.06.002

Thompson, P. M., Cannon, T. D., Narr, K. L., van Erp, T., Poutanen, V. P., Huttunen, M., et al. (2001). Genetic influences on brain structure. *Nat. Neurosci.* 4, 1253–1258. doi: 10.1038/nn758

Tomasi, D., and Volkow, N. D. (2012). Aging and functional brain networks. *Mol. Psychiatry* 17, 549–558. doi: 10.1038/mp.2011.81

Toro, R., Poline, J. B., Huguet, G., Loth, E., Frouin, V., Banaschewski, T., et al. (2014). Genomic architecture of human neuroanatomical diversity. *Mol. Psychiatry* 20, 1011–1016. doi: 10.1038/mp.2014.99

Turk-Browne, N. B. (2013). Functional interactions as big data in the human brain. *Science* 342, 580–584. doi: 10.1126/science.1238409

Tzourio-Mazoyer, N., Landeau, B., Papathanassiou, D., Crivello, F., Etard, O., Delcroix, N., et al. (2002). Automated anatomical labeling of activations in SPM using a macroscopic anatomical parcellation of the MNI MRI single-subject brain. *Neuroimage* 15, 273–289. doi: 10.1006/nimg.2001.0978

Urban, N., and Tripathy, S. (2012). NEUROSCIENCE: circuits drive cell diversity. *Nature* 488, 289–290. doi: 10.1038/488289a

Wagner, M. J., Kim, T. H., Savall, J., Schnitzer, M. J., and Luo, L. (2017). Cerebellar granule cells encode the expectation of reward. *Nature* 544, 96–100. doi: 10.1038/nature21726

Walhovd, K. B., Fjell, A. M., Reinvang, I., Lundervold, A., Dale, A. M., Eilertsen, D. E., et al. (2005). Effects of age on volumes of cortex, white matter and subcortical structures. *Neurobiol. Aging* 26, 1261–1270. doi: 10.1016/j.neurobiolaging.2005.05.020

Wang, J. H., Zuo, X. N., Dai, Z. J., Xia, M. R., Zhao, Z. L., Zhao, X. L., et al. (2013). Disrupted functional brain connectome in individuals at risk for Alzheimer's disease. *Biol. Psychiatry* 73, 472–481. doi: 10.1016/j.biopsych.2012.03.026

Wang, K., Liang, M., Wang, L., Tian, L., Zhang, X., Li, K., et al. (2007). Altered functional connectivity in early Alzheimer's disease: a resting-state fMRI study. *Hum. Brain Mapp.* 28, 967–978. doi: 10.1002/hbm.20324

Wang, P., Zhou, B., Yao, H., Zhan, Y., Zhang, Z., Cui, Y., et al. (2015). Aberrant intra- and inter-network connectivity architectures in Alzheimer's disease and mild cognitive impairment. *Sci. Rep.* 5:14824. doi: 10.1038/srep14824

Wang, V. Y., and Zoghbi, H. Y. (2001). Genetic regulation of cerebellar development. *Nat. Rev. Neurosci.* 2, 484–491. doi: 10.1038/35081558

Weng, Y., Qi, R., Liu, C., Ke, J., Xu, Q., Wang, F., et al. (2016). Disrupted functional connectivity density in irritable bowel syndrome patients. *Brain Imaging Behav.* doi: 10.1007/s11682-016-9653-z [Epub ahead of print].

Xu, S., and Wu, Z. (1986). The construction of "the clinical memory test". *Acta Psychol. Sin.* 18, 100–108.

Yan, C.-G., Cheung, B., Kelly, C., Colcombe, S., Craddock, R. C., Di Martino, A., et al. (2013a). A comprehensive assessment of regional variation in the impact of head micromovements on functional connectomics. *Neuroimage* 76, 183–201. doi: 10.1016/j.neuroimage.2013.03.004

Yan, C.-G., Craddock, R. C., Zuo, X.-N., Zang, Y.-F., and Milham, M. P. (2013b). Standardizing the intrinsic brain: towards robust measurement of inter-individual variation in 1000 functional connectomes. *Neuroimage* 80, 246–262. doi: 10.1016/j.neuroimage.2013.04.081

Yin, S., Zhu, X., He, R., Li, R., and Li, J. (2015). Spontaneous activity in the precuneus predicts individual differences in verbal fluency in cognitively normal elderly. *Neuropsychology* 29, 961–970. doi: 10.1037/neu0000201

Yu, J., Li, J., and Huang, X. (2012). The Beijing version of the Montreal cognitive assessment as a brief screening tool for mild cognitive impairment: a community-based study. *BMC Psychiatry* 12:156. doi: 10.1186/1471-244x-12-156

Zatorre, R. J. (2013). Predispositions and plasticity in music and speech learning: neural correlates and implications. *Science* 342, 585–589. doi: 10.1126/science.1238414

Zhao, Q. B., Tang, Y. Y., Feng, H. B., Li, C. J., and Sui, D. (2008). The effects of neuron heterogeneity and connection mechanism in cortical networks. *Phys. Statist. Mech. Appl.* 387, 5952–5957. doi: 10.1016/j.physa.2008.07.002

10

Influences of 12-Week Physical Activity Interventions on TMS Measures of Cortical Network Inhibition and Upper Extremity Motor Performance in Older Adults

Keith M. McGregor [1,2]*, Bruce Crosson [1,2], Kevin Mammino [1], Javier Omar [1], Paul S. Garcia [1,3] and Joe R. Nocera [1,2]

[1] VA Rehabilitation R&D Center for Visual and Neurocognitive Rehabilitation, Atlanta VA Medical Center, Decatur, GA, United States, [2] Department of Neurology, Emory University School of Medicine, Atlanta, GA, United States, [3] Department of Anesthesiology, Emory University School of Medicine, Atlanta, GA, United States

*Correspondence:
Keith M. McGregor
keith.mcgregor@emory.edu

Objective: Data from previous cross-sectional studies have shown that an increased level of physical fitness is associated with improved motor dexterity across the lifespan. In addition, physical fitness is positively associated with increased laterality of cortical function during unimanual tasks; indicating that sedentary aging is associated with a loss of interhemispheric inhibition affecting motor performance. The present study employed exercise interventions in previously sedentary older adults to compare motor dexterity and measure of interhemispheric inhibition using transcranial magnetic stimulation (TMS) after the interventions.

Methods: Twenty-one community-dwelling, reportedly sedentary older adults were recruited, randomized and enrolled to a 12-week aerobic exercise group or a 12-week non-aerobic exercise balance condition. The aerobic condition was comprised of an interval-based cycling "spin" activity, while the non-aerobic "balance" exercise condition involved balance and stretching activities. Participants completed upper extremity dexterity batteries and estimates of VO$_2$max in addition to undergoing single (ipsilateral silent period—iSP) and paired-pulse interhemispheric inhibition (pplHI) in separate assessment sessions before and after study interventions. After each intervention during which heart rate was continuously recorded to measure exertion level (load), participants crossed over into the alternate arm of the study for an additional 12-week intervention period in an AB/BA design with no washout period.

Results: After the interventions, regardless of intervention order, participants in the aerobic spin condition showed higher estimated VO$_2$max levels after the 12-week intervention as compared to estimated VO$_2$max in the non-aerobic balance intervention. After controlling for carryover effects due to the study design, participants in the spin condition showed longer iSP duration than the balance condition. Heart rate load was more strongly correlated with silent period duration after the Spin condition than estimated VO_2.

Conclusions: Aging-related changes in cortical inhibition may be influenced by 12-week physical activity interventions when assessed with the iSP. Although inhibitory signaling is mediates both ppIHI and iSP measures each TMS modality likely employs distinct inhibitory networks, potentially differentially affected by aging. Changes in inhibitory function after physical activity interventions may be associated with improved dexterity and motor control at least as evidence from this feasibility study show.

Keywords: aging, motor control, physical fitness, TMS, interhemispheric inhibition, neuroimaging

INTRODUCTION

Aging has been shown to be associated with a loss of interhemispheric inhibition that may negatively affect unimanual motor performance of the dominant hand (McGregor et al., 2012; Fujiyama et al., 2013; Heise et al., 2013, 2014; Levin et al., 2014; see also Spirduso, 1975; Salthouse, 1996; Talelli et al., 2008). Though the motor system is relatively spared as compared to other cognitive domains such as executive function, aging is associated with decreased upper extremity function (Salthouse, 1996). While impaired inhibitory function may not reach clinical significance for diagnostic purpose of motor dysfunction, it may reveal evidence of aging-related alteration of cortical function. This loss of interhemispheric inhibition can be assessed with transcranial magnetic stimulation (TMS). One TMS measure that has shown variability due to aerobic fitness and aging is the ipsilateral silent period (iSP) (McGregor et al., 2011; Davidson and Tremblay, 2013; Coppi et al., 2014). Briefly, the iSP is a stimulation-induced diminution or cessation of oscillation in electromyography (EMG) of a contracted muscle when stimulation is given to the motor cortex ipsilateral to the muscle target. This effect is believed to be mediated by alterations in inhibitory network function (Irlbacher et al., 2007; Lenzi et al., 2007), which may be sensitive to changes in aerobic capacity (Maddock et al., 2016). Previous cross-sectional work has shown that regular aerobic exercise may be associated with changes in interhemispheric inhibition and motor dexterity in older adults (Voelcker-Rehage et al., 2010; McGregor et al., 2011, 2013). This relationship may indicate that aging related motor declines might be mitigated or even reversed by the engagement in aerobic exercise. While the effect of acute exercise has been probed with respect to sensitivity to measures from TMS (Roig et al., 2012; Singh et al., 2014; Lulic et al., 2017), we know of few studies that have assessed the longitudinal effects of a longer-term aerobic exercise program on TMS measures of inhibitory function potentially sensitive to aging and motor control (see Gomes-Osman et al., 2017).

The iSP is a complicated measurement that involves a number of cortical and descending spinal inhibitory connections. The silent period onset is typically ~38 ms after stimulation and can last anywhere from 10 to 70 ms depending on stimulation and level of muscle contraction (Giovannelli et al., 2009; Petitjean and Ko, 2013; Fleming and Newham, 2017; Kuo et al., 2017).

The ipsilateral inhibition seen in the most commonly measured muscle, the first dorsal interosseous (FDI), certainly involves primary motor cortex (M1) callosal transfer, as degradation of the corpus callosum diminishes the measure (Meyer et al., 1995; Li et al., 2013). However, it is likely that inhibitory influences of the reticulospinal and propriospinal tracts provide an additive effect to muscle quiescence (Nathan et al., 1996; Ziemann et al., 1999). In addition to cortically mediated mechanisms the cause of the silent period is also influenced by the dynamics of the alpha-motoneurons themselves (Doherty et al., 1993). Refractory periods of the muscle spindle and the reactive involvement of spinal inhibitory interneurons due to descending ipsilateral corticospinal/corticobulbar/oligospinal input likely contribute to the duration of the iSP if not in its early phase, but later in its delayed resolution to baseline (Jung and Ziemann, 2006). The complexity of the iSP may be of relevance to its possible sensitivity to aging related change. Given that it is a volitional response, in contrast to another measure of interhemispheric using paired pulse parameters, aging related alteration of the iSP may reflect a functional change in motor capacity (Coppi et al., 2014).

A neurotransmitter system with strong influence on cortical inhibition and likely even motor control is the gamma aminobutyric acid system (GABA). The aging process may be responsible for a decrease in GABA tone in the neocortex (Gao et al., 2013; but see also Mooney et al. (2017). However, this decrease may or may not be responsible for changes in motor performance in aging, as GABA receptors can change endogenous sensitivity levels over time (Rozycka and Liguz-Lecznar, 2017). The TMS literature has approached GABA receptor function for many years, particularly in light of aging (Sale and Semmler, 2005; Stagg et al., 2011; Davidson and Tremblay, 2013; Opie et al., 2015). A significant question has arisen as to the role of a particular subtype of GABA receptor (GABAb) in the mediation of interhemispheric inhibition with respect to how it is assessed using TMS. GABAb receptors have been implicated in two distinct measures of interhemispheric inhibition: the iSP (described above) and paired-pulse interhemispheric inhibition (ppIHI). The employ of ppIHI requires the use of two stimulators and reflects the diminution of a motor evoked potential (MEP) in a muscle target when a conditioning pulse to the motor cortex ipsilateral to the target hand precedes a test stimulation pulse (Ferbert et al., 1992). It is yet unknown if these measures involve the same cortical circuitry (inhibitory networks) or reflect complementary findings in the estimation of the effects of pharmacological agents (see Ziemann et al., 2015). That is, the relationship between the two measures may be isolated to the administration of GABAb agents, and may not have a direct relationship with motor behavior. The current work seeks to investigate if physical activity, which has shown been associated with differences in silent period duration in previous cross-sectional work, shows proportional effects on measures of ppIHI.

The present work describes data collected from 21 older participants (60+ years) who engaged a 12-week exercise intervention comprised of either an interval-based aerobic spin program or a non-aerobic, balance and stretching condition. We employed a crossover design to compare the effects of the activity interventions on the same participants in alternate conditions. As such, participants crossed over into the alternate exercise condition for another 12-week intervention. We sought to test motor dexterity and assessments of cortical inhibition using both ppIHI and iSP paradigms that may be associated with improved motor function after increased aerobic activity. Based on our previous cross-sectional data, we hypothesized that participants completing the aerobic spin protocol would show improved upper extremity motor dexterity and increased levels of interhemispheric inhibition. We further hypothesized that changes in iSP after the intervention would indicate greater levels of interhemispheric inhibition as compared to ppIHI potentially due to the volitional and physiologically complex origin of the iSP.

METHODS

Participants

In this 24-week randomized controlled crossover trial (RCT: NCT01787292), participants were randomized and divided into an aerobic, spin cycling exercise group (Spin) or a non-aerobic balance training group (Balance) to equalize contact and monitoring. Each intervention lasted 12-weeks (Arm 1), after which, the participant crossed over into the alternate arm (Arm 2) of the study for an additional, 12-week intervention (e.g., Arm 1, Balance–Arm 2, Spin). The crossover was an AB/BA uniform-within-sequences design with a limited washout period (~1 week). Data from both arms of the intervention are presented in this report.

Study personnel explained the purpose, potential risks of the experiment and completed the informed consent process with each participant following protocols approved by the Emory University's Institutional Review Board (IRB00059193) in compliance with the Helsinki Declaration. All participants gave written informed consent filed with both the Atlanta VA Research and Development Office and Emory University's IRB.

This report includes 21 participants that were recruited from a volunteer database, which included elderly individuals (60 years and over). An additional four older participants enrolled in the study, but chose to withdraw prior to completing the first arm of the intervention. To meet inclusion criteria participants had to (1) be between of 60 and 85 years of age, (2) report being sedentary, defined as not engaging in structured physical activity and/or not accumulating 30 min or more of moderate to strenuous weekly physical activity, assessed with a modified Godin Leisure Time Exercise Questionnaire—LTEQ (Godin and Shephard, 1997), (3) have no history of depression, neurological disease, including Parkinson's disease, Alzheimer's disease, multiple sclerosis or stroke, (4) report being right handed (using the Edinburgh handedness inventory Oldfield, 1971), (5) report being a native English speaker, and (6) obtain primary care physician's approval for study participation. Exclusion criteria included (1) conditions that would contraindicate TMS (e.g., seizure, stroke, tremor, etc.), (2) failure to provide informed consent, (3) hospitalization within the past 6 months, (4) uncontrolled hypertension or diabetes (reported non-compliance with prescribed management program), (5) inability to walk 400 m, and (6) significant cognitive executive impairment, defined as a score on the Montreal Cognitive Assessment (MoCA) of <24, (7) having a TMS measurement of lowest motor threshold (LMT) >66% of maximum stimulator output (MSO) (as stimulation for the paradigm was set to 150% of LMT). Due to the high incidence of prescription of hypertension medications in sedentary older adults ($n = 12$, six per group), we did not exclude individuals on these medications.

During intervention sessions, all participants wore a Polar FT7 chest strap heart rate monitor with paired monitor/wristwatch. Heart rate was taken from each participant every 2–3 min during the sessions and logged on a data sheet. On infrequent occasions (<2% of HR acquisitions), the chest strap monitor would fail to synchronize with the watch during the intervention session. In such instances, we interpolated the heart rate data from adjacent recordings within each session provided they were within reasonable ranges to each other (±~5–10 bpm). If a heart rate monitor failed to synchronize at study outset (a problem with older adults with lower resting galvanic skin responses) we would use a battery-powered pulse oximeter or an Apple Watch (Cupertino, CA) to measure heart rate at the above described intervals. For both interventions, we recorded attendance, attrition, and heart rate. All participants completed the 36 assigned sessions for each intervention though we had to accommodate more absences for individuals in the balance condition.

Aerobic "Spin" Intervention Protocol

Consistent with our previous study (Nocera et al., 2015), the group exercise intervention began with 20 min of Spin aerobic exercise three times a week for 12 weeks on stationary exercise cycles and was led by a qualified instructor. Importantly, the time of each session progressed based on the recommendation of the instructor by 1–2 min as needed to a maximum time of 45 min per session. Heart rate reserve was assessed using the Karvonen method (220 bpm – age = maximum heart rate; heart rate reserve [HRR] = maximum heart rate – resting heart rate). Exercise intensity began at low levels (50% of HRR) and increased by 5% every week (as deemed appropriate by the instructor) to a target maximum of 75% HRR. Participants wishing to exceed this capacity could do so for limited exercise intervals if they so choose. Target exercise intensities were adapted for participants on diuretics, ACE-inhibitors, beta-blockers based on recent recommendations in the literature (Diaz-Buschmann et al., 2014; Taubert et al., 2015) to produce equivalent aerobic capacity improvement as non-medicated individuals. These included the "talk-test" and relative physical exertion estimation using the Borg 6–20 difficulty scale (6 = lowest effort; 20 = maximum effort).

The Spin intervention took place in a climate controlled fitness facility. The instructor guided the participants through a light effort 5-min warm up (not included in data analysis), then a workout phase that included steady up-tempo cadences, sprints (increased rpm), and climbs (increased resistance). As such, the exercise routine employed an interval-based training approach. During the workout phase the target HRR reserve was maintained by averaging increases and decreases in intensity/HR. The goal was to maintain within a 10% offset from the HRR goal during the workout phase. Thus, participants were within target HRR on average across the session despite the intervals of increased and decreased workload. All participants wore HR monitors throughout each session and were instructed to attain their respective HR target range at 5-min intervals. Staff members also monitored and tracked the HR to ensure adequate intensity throughout each session. Brief weekly meetings in which each participant's HR was reviewed served as a way to encourage those with lower attendance or HR measurements to improve their performance for the next week.

Balance/Light Strength Training Intervention Protocol

The main purpose of the Balance and strength training group was to have participants engage in non-aerobic physical activities that may help reduce fall risk. Participants in the balance group were equalized to the Spin group with regards to contact and monitoring frequency. As such they reported to the same facility with the same interventionists; however, instead of progressive aerobic exercise they participated in group balance, stretching and light muscle toning exercises. Beginning at the outset of the intervention, a baseline balance assessment was taken for each individual to titrate task difficulty depending on intake stability risk. This was formally measured using the short physical performance battery (SPPB), which is a measure consisting of a top score of 12 (scores lower than 10 indicate moderate fall risk). All participants in this study had a score of 11 or greater, indicating low fall risk from the SPPB. Participants began the intervention by practicing balance exercises on foam pads using a chair for support (if necessary). Balance exercises included single leg stand, dual-task (counting backwards) and eyes closed conditions lasting about a total of 10 min. Participants increased difficulty when able to perform the balance session without use of the support chair. In place of foam pads, participants stood on less-stable air-filled pads as they advanced through the 12-week intervention. Participants were also challenged to learn to step on moveable friction pads (six-inch diameter "dots") with variable positions on the floor. Instructors changed the positions of these pads as the session progressed to challenge participants to safely deviate center of mass location during foot placement in

order to improve proprioception during gait. In addition, light strength training exercises included instructor-led bodyweight and resistance training using Theraband (Akron, OH) stretch bands. These exercises focused on improving postural support with an emphasis on abdominal engagement and lateral hip abduction. As above, we held brief weekly meetings to discuss progress within the program and workload.

Similar to the aerobic intervention time from the initial 20–45 min over the course of the 12-week intervention with a light 5-min warm up at the onset of each session. Additionally, heart rate was consistently monitored (also using the Polar FT7 chest strap monitors) to assess general intensity during each session and to advise participant to keep HR below aerobic levels (50% of HRR).

Crossover and Attrition

After completing the assessments within a 10-day period following the 12-week intervention, participants crossed over into the opposite arm of the study (e.g., exercise to spin). The participants then completed the second arm of the study for 12-weeks (36 sessions). We did not incorporate a full 12-week "washout" period (to potentially mitigate carryover effects) due to potential attrition of participants. We included a covariate model for carryover effects in our statistical analysis to attempt to account for the lack of washout.

Of note, we enrolled an additional four participants who completed baseline testing, but did not complete the first intervention arm choosing to withdraw from the study. Three of these participants were in the Balance arm, while one was in the Spin. Reasons for attrition were schedule conflicts or exigent family circumstances.

Assessments

All assessments were done no more than 10 days before the start of or 10 days after the conclusion of each 12-week intervention period. In total there was: one baseline measurement and two post-intervention measurements. Assessment sessions did not exceed 2 h to alleviate participant fatigue, so testing was spread across two nearly consecutive days (1–3 days). We assessed behavioral performance and cardiovascular fitness on the first day and TMS measures on the second assessment day. In all cases but two, participants began behavioral assessments during mid-morning hours. All TMS sessions were completed during morning hours.

Cardiovascular Fitness Assessment

To assess aerobic capacity, participants performed a YMCA submaximal fitness test on a Monark 828e (upright) or RC4 (recumbent) cycle ergometer (Vansbro, Sweden). This submaximal test was used to estimate the participant's maximal oxygen uptake (VO_2max) prior to and after interventions. The selected submaximal test is much better tolerated than a maximum exertion treadmill test in the study's population (sedentary older adults). The YMCA-test uses an extrapolation method in which heart rate workload values are obtained at 2–4 points during stages of increasing resistance and extrapolated to predict workload at the estimated maximum heart rate (e.g., 220-age). VO_2max is then calculated from the predicted maximum workload. Prior to beginning the test, the procedures were briefly explained and participants completed a 2-min warm-up consisting of pedaling without load so that they could adapt to the ergometer for the first minute and then pedaling with a 0.5 kg.m load during the second minute. The YMCA submax test has an $R = 0.86$ with VO_2max and a SEE = 10% of the predicted VO_2max (Beekley et al., 2004).

Heart Rate Workload Assessment

As a submaximal exercise estimate may be limited in determining the effectiveness of a physical activity intervention in a smaller sample size, we additionally calculated the average intrasession heart rate as compared to the target goal of 75% HRR. This was done during training intervals physical exertion starting in the sixth week of the spin program where participant HR target zone meet this criteria. Intervals in this zone (75% HRR) increased in frequency as training progressed up to six intervals per session in the final 3 days of the program. To analyze these data, we scaled the HR-values by 75% of HRR (6–10 assessments per session × 16–19 sessions) per participant (with the previously denoted adjustments for BP medications). As such, we divided each HR assessment by 75% of adjusted participant HRR and averaged each assessment across sessions within each participant. For example, if a given participants achieved a HR average of 114 bpm for work intervals their 75% HRR target value was 130 bpm, the score would be 0.87. We completed this HR_{load} analysis for all participant sessions and interventions. For the Balance group HR_{load} assessment, we chose the 75% HRR time blocks in mirror of their Spin intervention ($n = 6$–10 per session × 16–19 sessions). We acknowledge that this estimate may ignore gradual improvement in the Spin intervention as it relies on a single fixed resting HR for baseline.

TMS
EMG

Electromyography (EMG) was taken from the FDI muscle on both hands using Ag-Ag Cl electrodes using BrainSight (BrainSight 2, Rogue Research) EMG pods. EMG is continuously acquired and stimulator driven TTL triggers a 150 ms acquisition window post TTL with 50 ms of pre-trigger baseline. A LabJack U3-LV analog to digital converter acquired amplified EMG traces with a 12-bit dual-channel analog input sampled at 3 kHz. These data were bandpass filtered from 10 to 10,000 Hz. Muscle activation was monitored with oscilloscope software package integrated into a BrainSight 2 neuronavigated positioning system. Motor evoked potential and other EMG data was exported for statistical analysis using ADInstruments LabChart. A MagVenture X100 magnetic stimulator (MagVenture, Alpharetta, GA) and a MagVenture B-60 60 cm butterfly coil were used to stimulate the left primary motor cortex during the initial mapping procedure. Maximum stimulator output (MSO) for this model is 2.2 tesla. All stimulations were biphasic and stimulation and recording devices were synchronized using TTL pulses. The coil was placed tangential

to the scalp with the handle pointing backwards and 45° away from the midline for stimulation. The scalp site corresponding to the lowest stimulator output sufficient to generate a magnetic evoked potential of at least 50 mV in six out of 10 trials was defined as the area of resting motor threshold (RMT), also known as the "hotspot." This was the site that was stimulated for the TMS assessments. It is worthy of note that this threshold determination is different from the currently accepted standard employ of a stimulus response curve analysis for measuring cortical excitability (Chang et al., 2016). We do not report on cortical excitability in the current manuscript as estimation of this according to the previous citation optimally uses more than 10 pulses.

Ipsilateral Silent Period

For iSP, the left FDI muscle was contracted via pinch grip at 25% maximal voluntary contraction (MVC) measured by pinch grip dynamometer and a stimulator output equivalent to 150% RMT was delivered to the left FDI hotspot. Recent work by Fleming and Newham (2017) has shown that these stimulation parameters are reliable in older adults. The highest acceptable RMT for participation in the current study was 66% of MSO. All participants had a RMT of 66% or less in the current study. Twenty silent period assessments were taken with brief rest breaks after every five trials to alleviate potential muscle fatigue. Participants were also instructed to request rest breaks as needed at any time during the stimulation. The iSP was determined using a longstanding visual inspection method (Garvey et al., 2001). Similar to our previous work (McGregor et al., 2011, 2013), we rectified EMG data and we determined silent period onset at background EMG activity during active pinch squeeze dropped below 20% of pinch baseline (assessed with pre-stimulus acquisition of 50 ms).

Paired-Pulse Measures

The long interhemispheric inhibition (LIHI) paired pulse procedure involved interhemispheric inhibition assessment (Ferbert et al., 1992) using a second MagVenture magnetic stimulator (R30) and a matching B-60 (60 cm butterfly coil) for stimulation of the right motor cortex. For this procedure, a conditioning TMS pulse set at 150% of RMT was applied to the right motor cortex FDI hotspot at 40 ms prior to a "test" pulse's administration of 130% of RMT to the left motor cortex. As a result of the conditioning stimulation, the test MEP's response amplitude (in the right FDI muscle) is lowered due to interhemispheric inhibitory processes (denoted as LIHI or long interval interhemispheric inhibition). The inter-trial interval was varied randomly between 4 and 6 s to reduce anticipation of the next trial and mitigate repetitive stimulation effects. Averages of MEP latencies and peak-to-peak amplitudes were calculated for each stimulation condition (baseline, IHI). Twenty baseline stimulations (test pulses without conditioning pulse) were compared with 20 conditioned LIHI stimulations for this procedure. Baseline and conditioned stimulations were interleaved to mitigate systematic cortical modulation.

Behavioral Performance

During behavioral assessment sessions, participants performed a battery of cognitive and upper extremity motor tests. Results from the cognitive battery will be addressed in later report. Participants completed motor assessments of the dominant hand including: grip strength, the Halstead-Reitan Finger Tapping task (Reitan and Wolfson, 2013) simple reaction time, the Purdue Pegboard (peg and assembly) (Tiffin and Asher, 1948), and the Nine-Hole Pegboard task (Mathiowetz et al., 1985). Additionally, to test distal motor dexterity, participants engaged in a coin rotation task with two conditions. In the first condition (unimanual), the participant rotated a coin (U.S. quarter) 20 times as quickly as possible using the index finger, middle finger, and thumb with duration as the outcome measure. This test is used for assessment in routine neurological screening and has been shown to be diagnostic of distal motor function both in cases of suspected pathology and aging in the absence of pathology (Hanna-Pladdy et al., 2002; Hill et al., 2010). In the second condition (bimanual), the participant maintained an isometric pinch force of 20–30% of maximum voluntary force with a Jamar brand pinch grip dynamometer using a lateral grip during the rotations. Coin rotation tasks were performed with both the left and right hands. Both the hand used for coin rotation and trial condition (unimanual or bimanual task) were pseudo-randomized and counterbalanced across participants to account for potential order effects across eight runs (two left unimanual, two left bimanual, two right unimanual, two right bimanual). Accidental coin drops were noted, but excluded from consideration and the trial repeated should a drop occur. Participants were allowed 5 min of practice to acclimate to the rotation task in each task condition. Data acquisition began if the participant reported that they believed that additional practice time would not improve task performance. No participants requested additional time beyond the 5-min practice period. The difference score between the bimanual and unimanual task conditions was calculated to assess the effect of bimanual activity on rotation performance.

Data Analysis

The current study was a uniform-within-sequences mixed-effects 2×2 crossover design with intervention type held as between subjects and intervention sequence (AB/BA) and period (A1B1/A1B2/A2B1/A2B2) as within subjects. A Shapiro-Wilks test was completed across measures to test data for normality. In the event of violation of normality of data, we employed non-parametric Wilcoxon rank sum tests (between subjects) or Mann-Whitney rank sum test (within subjects).

To analyze data from this design, we employed a mixed model approach (PROC MIXED in SAS) using a simple carryover (AB/BA) design with carryover adjustment for session sequence. To account for sequence carryover, we employed analysis of covariance (ANCOVA) in SAS 9.4 (Cary, NC) inclusive of sequence by period covariates against treatment effects. Least square means were adjusted for carryover from the crossover design and Tukey-Kramer mean comparisons for between subjects effects were analyzed with a Kenward-Roger degrees of freedom approximation (Kenward and Roger, 2010). Mauchly's test for sphericity was computed for session

as a within subjects variable, and we applied a Greenhouse-Geisser correction to accommodate any violation. In addition, we completed a significance test for the carryover effect between sequences using a delta G^2 likelihood ratio and Chi-square parameter estimation at alpha of 0.05.

We also performed a mixed-model split-plot ANOVA in JMP 12 (Cary, NC) using a restricted maximum likelihood design holding subjects as random and nested in sequence (i.e., AB/BA) to examine interaction effects of dependent variables based on sequence of presentation. This reduced model did not account for carryover covariates, but was employed to show main effects and interactions of treatments respective of change from each measurement (i.e., intervention at time A vs. intervention at time B; baseline assessment vs. intervention at time A; baseline assessment vs. intervention time at B). Comparisons of intervention effects on dependent variables are shown graphically in Bland-Altman repeated measures plots with t-test for intervention (Altman and Bland, 1983). In addition, we completed correlation analyses on dependent variables across sessions with output statistics reported with the non-parametric Spearman's rho due to the low sample size.

RESULTS

Our screening measure of physical activity (Godin LTEQ) showed a moderate relationship with estimated VO_2 max, $p = 0.42$, $p = 0.06$. Baseline demographic data and neurophysiological correlations at the pre-session across all participants are shown in **Table 1**. Of note, VO_2 was positively correlated with education and inversely correlated with BMI and RMT. Resting motor threshold was also inversely correlated with level of education across all participants in the selected sample. Interestingly, we found no significant correlation between the TMS measures at baseline. There was an effect on gender at baseline with women having slightly longer silent periods $t_{(20)} = 1.99$, $p = 0.05$ as compared to men. Baseline data for TMS and motor performance along with their correlations are shown in **Tables 2–4**, respectively.

Intervention Effects — Spin vs. Balance
VO_2 Measures

Depicted in the repeated measures Bland-Altmann plot in **Figure 1**, change in estimated VO_2max was significant both

---

TABLE 1 | Baseline demographic and exercise metrics: age, education, body mass index (BMI), Handedness (as assessed by Edinburgh Handedness Inventory: Right = 1.0, Left = −1.0, assessed level of oxygen consumption during exercise (VO_2), Modified Godin Leisure Time Exercise Questionnaire (Self-report of physical activity) and Montreal Cognitive Assessment (MoCA).

Metric	Baseline (N = 21, 11 Female)
Age (years)	69.05 (5.98)
Education (years)	16.23 (2.98)
BMI	29.12 (6.01)
Handedness	0.97 (0.06)
VO_2 (ml/min/kg)	24.01 (9.29)
Godin LTEQ	11.62 (5.05)
MoCA	28.12 (2.9)

accounting for carryover covariates $t_{(20)} = 4.90$, $p < 0.001$, and in the reduced model [$t_{(20)} = 5.29$, $p < 0.001$]. Interestingly, there was a significant carryover effects in the Spin First Intervention (AB/BA), $\chi^2_{(0.05, 1)} = 6.89$ ($p < 0.03$) as compared to the Balance First Intervention (BA/AB), which had no carryover effects for VO$_2$ change, $\chi^2_{(0.05, 1)} = 3.28$, ns. We found no gender differences in change measures.

Heart Rate Workload

Heart rate workload (HR$_{load}$) was computed as a function of participants 75% heart rate reserve during intervention sessions. Heart rates in the target interval blocks were expressed as a percentage of the goal of 75% HRR. As expected, HR$_{load}$ was higher for the Spin intervention as compared to the Balance intervention, $Z_{(20)} = 2.27$, $p < 0.04$. A significant carryover effect

was evident for HR$_{load}$ was shown $\chi^2_{(0.05, 2)} = 8.03$ ($p < 0.01$). Interestingly, using a median split within interventions at time A, we determined that individuals who performed with highest HR$_{load}$ when performing Spin first continued to with higher HR$_{load}$ at crossover ($n = 5$), while those performing with the lowest HR$_{load}$ in Balance first had lower HR$_{load}$ at crossover ($n = 5$). No gender effects were evident for heart rate data either (See **Figure 2**).

TMS Measures
Ipsilateral Silent Period

Depicted in repeated measures Bland-Altman plot in **Figure 3** are change scores respective of intervention shown in the **Table 5**

TABLE 2 | Baseline transcranial magnetic stimulation measures between groups—std. dev.

Metric	Baseline (N = 21, 11 Female)
RMT (%MSO)	57.6 (9.55)
iSP (ms)	22.39 (4.73)
pplHI (% baseline)	0.60 (0.19)

No differences were evident in comparisons of resting motor threshold (RMT), ipsilateral silent period (iSP), and paired pulse interhemispheric inhibition (pplHI).

TABLE 3 | Baseline motor comparisons—std. dev.

Metric	Baseline (N = 21, 11 Female)
Purdue Peg	11.19 (1.6)
Purdue assembly	6.77 (0.72)
9-Hole Peg	24.39 (3.41)
Halstead	42.75 (7.09)
Coin rotation	
Right unimanual	16.46 (2.23)
Bimanual difference score	−2.58 (1.89)

Tests were with dominant (right) hand unless otherwise specified. Higher score on Purdue, Halstead are better. Lower scores on 9-Hole peg and coin rotation are better. Bimanual difference score is the difference between unimanual dominant hand coin rotation and dominant coin rotation when non-dominant hand is engaged in 25% maximum voluntary contraction squeeze task.

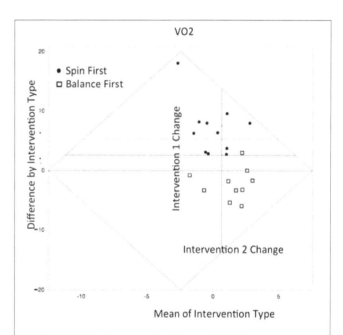

FIGURE 1 | Repeated measures Bland-Altman plot of VO$_2$max estimate comparisons between interventions sessions as plotted in JMP12. Ordinate axis denotes difference score between treatments, while abscissa denotes. The central axis (in red) is offset to depict the mean value between interventions A+B/2. Thus, vertical gain (from red axis) indicates greater improvement in VO$_2$ in Intervention A, while rightward gain indicates greater improvement after crossover. Circles represent Spin participant in Spin first condition while boxes represent participants in balance first (Between groups comparison—means represented by dotted lines: $t = 5.29$, $p < 0.01$).

TABLE 4 | Baseline correlations between VO$_2$, demographic, and TMS measures across all participants with comparison p-value.

Metric	VO$_2$_Pre	BMI	Education	RMT	iSP	pplHI
VO$_2$_Pre	X	X	X	X	X	X
BMI	**−0.54 (p = 0.01)**	X	X	X	X	X
Education	**0.43 (p = 0.04)**	−0.37 ns	X	X	X	X
RMT	**−0.49 (p = 0.04)**	0.36 ns	**−0.54 (p = 0.01)**	X	X	X
iSP	−0.10 ns	−0.02 ns	−0.23 ns	−0.03 ns	X	X
pplHI	−0.11 ns	0.15 ns	0.01 ns	0.18 ns	−0.35 ns	X

Significant correlations were evident between estimated volume of oxygen consumption (VO$_2$), education, resting motor threshold (RMT). Ipsilateral silent period (iSP) and paired pulse interhemispheric inhibition (pplHI) were not correlated with baseline demographics. Correlations use Spearman rho statistic. BOLD denotes statistical significance below p = 0.05.

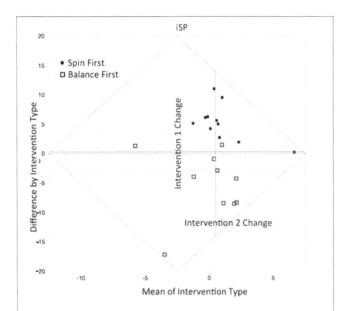

FIGURE 2 | Repeated measures Bland-Altman plot of HR$_{load}$ comparisons between interventions sessions as plotted in JMP12. Ordinate axis denotes difference score between treatments, while abscissa denotes. The central axis (in red) is offset to depict the mean value between interventions A+B/2. Thus, vertical gain (from red axis) indicates higher HR$_{load}$ in Intervention A, while rightward gain indicates greater improvement after crossover. Circles represent Spin participants while boxes represent Balance participants (Between groups comparison—means represented by dotted lines: $t = 2.17$, $p < 0.04$).

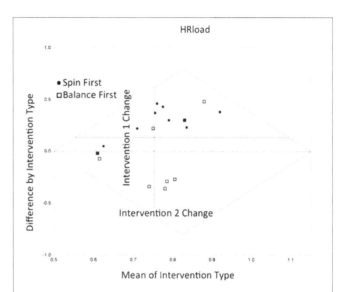

FIGURE 3 | Repeated measures Bland-Altman plot of ipsilateral silent period (iSP) comparisons between interventions sessions as plotted in JMP12. Ordinate axis denotes difference measurement difference between treatments, while abscissa denotes average of both treatments. The central axis (in red) is offset to depict the mean value between interventions A+B/2. Thus, vertical gain (from red axis) indicates higher iSP in Intervention A, while rightward gain indicates greater improvement after crossover. Circles represent Spin participant in Spin first condition while boxes represent participants in balance first (Between groups comparison—means represented by dotted lines: $t = 2.11$, $p < 0.05$).

below, there were significant effects of intervention type on change in iSP duration $t_{(20)} = 2.11$, $p < 0.05$ in the full model (inclusive of carryover), and in the reduced model, $t_{(20)} = 4.93$, $p < 0.01$. Individuals in the Spin intervention had longer iSPs than those in the balance intervention. Significant sequence carryover was present in silent period assessment for both interventions, $\chi^2_{(0.05,\,2)} = 8.89$ ($p < 0.01$). We found no gender effects for change score in silent period duration, though women had a slightly higher baseline duration than men, $t_{(20)} = 1.99$, $p = 0.05$.

Paired Pulse Interhemispheric Inhibition: No significant differences were denoted for ppIHI changes in the full model $t_{(20)} = 2.13$, ns, though a trend was shown in the reduced model with greater interhemispheric inhibition in the spin intervention $t_{(20)} = 1.94$, $p = 0.07$.

Behavioral Changes

Body mass index did not change respective of either intervention. Across a battery of motor indices, individuals completing the Spin Intervention improved on measures of dominant upper extremity, as compared to no change in the Balance condition. These data are shown in **Table 6** and were derived from the reduced model comparison as computed by JMP12. Notably, significant differences were shown in the bimanual coin rotation task, during which the participant actively squeezes a dynamometer while rotating a coin. Participants completing the balance intervention performed the task significantly faster during the bimanual task condition as compared to little change in individuals completing the Spin intervention.

TABLE 5 | TMS change measures after interventions.

Metric	Spin	Balance	p-value
RMT change	−6.60 (4.1)	−7.18 (5.98)	0.54
iSP change	**2.22 (2.96)**	**−0.41 (2.75)**	**0.05**
ppIHI change	−0.01 (0.38)	0.04 (0.11)	0.72

RMT, Resting motor threshold; iSP, ipsilateral silent period; IHI, paired pulse interhemispheric inhibition. iSP is measured in ms, while IHI is percentage change from baseline pulse to preconditioned pulse. BOLD denotes statistical significance below p = 0.05.

Correlations

As there do not exist ideal methods to index aging-related changes in upper extremity motor control, we performed a battery of tests. We were interested in how our TMS measures of interhemispheric inhibition related to these assessments. The data in **Table 7** show significant correlations between the silent period duration and measures of distal dexterity (9-hole pegboard, Purdue, and coin rotation tasks) in aggregate after both interventions. Again, carryover considerations somewhat lessen the extensibility of these results.

In addition, we performed correlations on VO$_2$, HR$_{load}$, TMS measures and motor performance to investigate relationship of the dependent measures. We performed correlations on VO$_2$, HR$_{load}$, TMS measures, and motor performance to investigate relationship of the dependent measures. Interestingly, whereas in the Balance intervention, estimates of VO$_2$ were strongly inversely related to iSP (more so than HR$_{load}$) the strongest predictor of change in iSP was HR_{load}. These data are shown in **Tables 8, 9** for Spin intervention and Balance intervention, respectively. We did not show any relationship between ppIHI and estimates of physical fitness/activity.

It is important to note that these data are underpowered with respect to sample size per intake group. Respective of the change in iSP, the effect size at alpha of 0.05 is 0.6. Ideally, this would require 11 participants per group. As such, we consider these data preliminary.

DISCUSSION

The present study demonstrates that an aerobic spin exercise intervention appears to increase the duration of the iSP in older adults and improve measures of distal upper extremity dexterity. Increased iSP duration was correlated with improved performance across multiple distal dexterity measures. Additionally, we found that the aerobic spin condition had no effect on a paired pulse measure of long interval interhemispheric inhibition (ppIHI).

Previous research has shown that engagement in regular physical activity considered aerobic in nature is associated with increased activity of inhibitory networks within the brain (McGregor et al., 2011, 2013; Nocera et al., 2015). The current

work presents the first evidence that previously sedentary individuals who engage in a relatively short-term (12-week, 36 sessions) aerobic exercise program show changes in a measure of interhemispheric inhibition, the iSP previously shown to be sensitive to aging-related change (Sale and Semmler, 2005; McGregor et al., 2011; Davidson and Tremblay, 2013; Coppi et al., 2014). Moreover, a longer silent period duration was associated with improved unimanual performance on distal dexterity in our study, potentially indicating an association of cortical inhibition with motor dexterity.

Aging-Related Motor Performance and the Ipsilateral Silent Period

One of the most interesting findings in the current study relates to the relationship between iSP duration and motor performance.

TABLE 8 | Post Intervention Correlations accounting for carryover effects after Spin Intervention.

Metric	VO$_2$	HR$_{load}$	iSP	ppIHI % change
VO$_2$	X	X	X	X
HR$_{load}$	0.56 (p = 0.02)	X	X	X
iSP	0.44 (p = 0.05)	0.65 (p = 0.01)	X	X
ppIHI % change	−0.08 ns	−0.36 ns	−0.32 ns	X

Values are Spearman Rho with alpha value in parentheses. BOLD denotes statistical significance below p = 0.05.

TABLE 9 | Post intervention correlations accounting for carryover effects after balance intervention.

Metric	VO$_2$	HR$_{load}$	iSP	ppIHI % change
VO$_2$	X	X	X	X
HR$_{load}$	0.56 (p = 0.02)	X	X	X
iSP	−0.48 (p < 0.05)	−0.50 (p = 0.05)	X	X
ppIHI % change	−0.22 ns	−0.41 ns	−0.41 ns	X

Values are Spearman Rho with alpha significance. BOLD denotes statistical significance below p = 0.05.

TABLE 6 | Change metrics in behavioral performance comparing intervention groups—std. dev.; Purdue Peg—Higher score is better; 9-Hole pegboard and Unimanual coin rotation—lower is better.

Metric	Spin	Balance	p-value
BMI	29.46 (6.85)	28.8 (5.51)	0.75
9-Hole Peg	−2.3 (2.17)	0.95 (3.6)	0.02
Purdue Peg	1.18 (1.4)	−0.3 (1.15)	0.01
Purdue assembly	0.42 (1.4)	0.16 (1.01)	0.01
Coin rotation			
Unimanual	−0.51 (3.72)	−2.21 (5.05)	0.22
Bimanual difference score	−0.24 (2.75)	−3.45 (2.54)	0.02

Bimanual difference is the difference between unimanual and bimanual coin rotation tasks. Data is from reduced model as implemented in JMP12. BOLD denotes statistical significance below p = 0.05.

TABLE 7 | Relationship between TMS measures (iSP change, ppIHI % change) and motor dexterity change across all participants after both interventions regardless of order.

Metric	iSP change	ppIHI % change	9-Hole Peg change	Purdue Peg change	Unimanual coin change	Bimanual coin difference
iSP change	X	X	X	X	X	X
ppIHI % change	0.31 ns	X	X	X	X	X
9-Hole Peg change	−0.80 (p < 0.01)	−0.28 ns	X	X	X	X
Purdue Peg change	0.58 (p = 0.02)	0.34 ns	−0.21 ns	X	X	X
Unimanual coin change	−0.51 (p < 0.03)	0.32 ns	0.25 ns	−0.15 ns	X	X
Bimanual coin difference	0.61 (p < 0.02)	0.48 (p < 0.05)	−0.56 (p < 0.02)	0.43 ns	−0.66 (p < 0.01)	X

Purdue Peg—Higher score is better; 9-Hole pegboard and Unimanual coin rotation—lower is better. Bimanual coin difference is calculated as unimanual coin rotation − bimanual coin rotation. Values are Spearman Rho calculation with df = 20. BOLD denotes statistical significance below p = 0.05.

This work has demonstrated that an aerobic spin exercise program can increase the iSP duration in concert with improving motor performance on dexterity tasks. These findings may relate to previous cross-sectional reports in our lab that found that physically active older adults had longer silent period durations than sedentary individuals in the same age cohort (McGregor et al., 2011, 2013). The question arises as to the functional relationship between the iSP and distal upper extremity dexterity. What does a silent period increase after an intervention actually infer respective of motor capability, particularly for the purposes of rehabilitation? As the iSP is complicated involving alpha motor neuronal dynamics, callosal transfer with multiple inhibitory internetworks (including spinal), and muscular control, determination of the exact mechanism driving the change is not possible in the current work. However, it is likely that cortical changes account for more of the change than changes in the periphery (muscle capacity/tone), as previous work has repeatedly shown that increased levels of exogenous stimulation alters silent period duration more so than increased motor load (Giovannelli et al., 2009; Kuo et al., 2017). Therefore, the silent period may be a reflection of an intrinsic cortical inhibitory framework that serves to regulate interhemispheric transfer.

Toward this, the relationship between the iSP and the coin rotation task is worthy of additional discussion, as it is one the few bimanual motor tasks probed in the current report (a noted limitation). We have previously reported aging-related differences in the coin rotation task when subtracting unimanual performance from bimanual performance. Younger adults complete the coin rotation task faster than sedentary older adults in either the unimanual or bimanual conditions. However, when sedentary older adults engage in the bimanual task condition (i.e., ~25% MVC pinch grip), their coin rotation speed improves. We have previously postulated that aberrant interhemispheric transfer during a unimanual task may interfere with dexterous task performance (McGregor et al., 2012). However, during a bimanual task, the engagement of the ipsilateral motor areas (to the hand performing the rotation) might act to either improve the signal-to-noise dynamics between hemispheres resulting in improved motor dexterity. Additionally, this bimanual performance effect is sensitive to differences in physical activity levels in middle-aged and older adults (McGregor et al., 2011). In the present study, our participants who completed the aerobic spin training showed improved performance on the unimanual coin rotation task. Moreover, the difference score between unimanual and bimanual conditions was lower, particularly for the non-dominant hand. Interestingly, these data were correlated with improved silent period duration. This may indicate that improved interhemispheric inhibition after the aerobic exercise in older adults could restore motor dexterity by improving signal-to-noise characteristics in the task active cortex.

Aerobic Spin Intervention

The main contrast condition in the present crossover study was the type of intervention either aerobic "Spin" or Balance. As a result of our interval-based Spin program our participants,

regardless of sequence of intervention, improved estimated VO_2 as a result of increased workload. The physical performance metrics were highly correlated with both silent period duration and tests of motor dexterity. That individuals improved on motor dexterity is notable in the present study because we did not employ a manual task training component to the study, and indeed, our intervention was largely driven by the activity of the lower extremity. With respect to the mechanism of change, increased levels of brain derived neurotrophic factor (BDNF) has received dominant attention in the literature (Kleim et al., 2006; Tang et al., 2008; Schmolesky et al., 2013; Szuhany et al., 2015). Our lab only recently began to assay serum BDNF levels, but our preliminary data indicates that our aerobic Spin interval training program increases serum BDNF levels by 17% with peaks achieved 15 min post the 45-min spin session (unpublished data). BDNF is believed to promote synaptic plasticity possibly through facilitating signaling cascades after its dimers bind to its preferential receptor, TrkB (Phillips et al., 2014). As a result, multiple proteins associated with cell survival and proliferation are produced if the TrkB receptor has the beneficial Val66Val polymorphism (Kleim et al., 2006). It is unknown what benefit BDNF or other potential modulatory neurotrophins might have on either the TMS or behavioral measures employed in the current study. It is likely that increased HR workload is associated with a higher release of BDNF (Schmolesky et al., 2013) and this would predict greater motor performance and longer silent periods. However, this postulation requires additional study to vet. As such, the specific mechanism by which aerobic exercise alters cortical function remains largely unidentified with respect to both systems physiology and molecular neuroscience. Clearly, much more work is required address this critical issue.

It is important to note that the contrast condition of Balance training was not of detriment to our participants in terms of functional outcome despite a negative correlation between silent period duration and physical activity measures. Indeed, while the participants' aerobic capacity and heart rates were similar at post-assessment as compared to immediately beginning the Balance program, a crossover effect was evident in this condition. That is, participants continued to maintain gains in the currently reported metrics if they crossed over from Spin into this condition. Moreover, beyond the contrast to Spin, the Balance and light strength training condition improved core strength in participants and improved proprioception. As such, the negative correlations to motor dexterity shown in the current study may rather reflect the dominant improvement in the Spin comparison, rather than functional declines in the Balance condition. Respective of this, the Balance condition employed in the current report served as a contact control, but perhaps not an ideal control. We previously attempted to employ a wait-list control and an education-only program and washout periods to this project, but due to the study environment and recruitment dropout, we instead chose to directly enroll participants into the Spin or Balance interventions with immediate crossover. Future work will certainly employ a cleaner study design, though the results from the current, albeit non-ideal design are extremely encouraging.

Differences between iSP and ppIHI

The change in iSP after aerobic exercise is notable insofar that it differed from an alternative measure of interhemispheric inhibition assessed with the paired-pulse LIHI stimulation, which showed no differences after the intervention and was not correlated with motor performance. This is curious and worth some exploration since both the iSP and ppIHI protocols have been reported to involve similar neurotransmitter receptor systems and are considered complementary measures of interhemispheric inhibition (Chen, 2004; Di Lazzaro et al., 2007; Wischnewski et al., 2016). In a recent study, Li et al. (2013) identified patients with callosotomy or callosal agenesis and tested iSP duration and magnitude of ppIHI. The authors reported that both ppIHI and iSP are impaired after lesion of the corpus callosum. The inhibitory effects should not be considered identical, however, as ppIHI and iSP paradigms show different changes during pharmacological manipulations (Siebner et al., 1998; McDonnell et al., 2007; Ziemann et al., 2015) and when employed immediately after or in concert with other TMS paradigms (e.g., LICI, SICI) (Udupa et al., 2010). Based on pharmacologic investigations, it has been suggested that the interhemispheric inhibition underlying both the ppIHI and iSP paradigms involve GABA Type B (metabotropic) receptor (Ziemann et al., 2015). Our results show a difference between iSP and ppIHI and therefore suggest that it is unlikely that GABAb receptor activity is the sole mechanism of this interhemispheric inhibition. Were this true, the iSP and ppIHI measures should have been directly related in the current study. Much more study is required to elucidate the neurophysiological metabolism of inhibition using TMS methodology.

There are some noted limitations with the current work. Carryover effects in the crossover design from one intervention to the other limits the extensibility of these. Future work should employ a more appropriate control condition such as an education-only arm with equivalent frequency of participant contact. As the participants in the current study do not have motor pathology, the extensibility of these findings to clinical populations may be limited. With regard to the TMS procedures, additional metrics such as cortical excitability would have been useful to report. We additionally acknowledge that the motor assessment battery was somewhat limited. Largely due to time considerations for testing, we could only administer a relatively small number of upper extremity tests in our sessions. In addition, most tests involved engagement of the dominant hand. Given the coin rotation findings, intermanual differences should be assessed with better granularity in future work. Finally, we did not track extramural activity and lifestyle habits in the current study. As such, we cannot account for variance from various unmeasured factors (i.e., overall daily activity, inflammatory biomarkers) in our statistical models, which should be tracked closely in future work.

In conclusion, we believe the current work is the first to show that a 12-week aerobic exercise intervention may affect the duration of the iSP duration in older, sedentary adults. In addition, change in silent period duration is correlated with improvements in motor dexterity. These findings are in concert with previous data collected from cross-sectional work involving middle-age and older adults of varying physical fitness levels (McGregor et al., 2011, 2013).

AUTHOR CONTRIBUTIONS

KMM, JN, and BC: conceptualized the experiment; KMM, KM, and JN: completed data collection and handled recruitment of participants. KMM, KM, JO, and PG: analyzed the data for the work. KMM, PG, JN, and BC wrote the manuscript.

ACKNOWLEDGMENTS

The views expressed in this work do not necessarily reflect those of the United States Government or Department of Veterans Affairs. All authors contributed significantly to the production of this work. This work was supported by VA grants: E0956-W, 5IK2RX000744, and C9246C. The authors would like to thank Paul Weiss, MS for statistical consultation.

REFERENCES

Altman, D. G., and Bland, J. M. (1983). Measurement in medicine: the analysis of method comparison studies. *Statistician* 32, 307–317. doi: 10.2307/2987937

Beekley, M. D., Brechue, W. F., Garzarella, L., Werber-Zion, G., and Pollock, M. L. (2004). Cross-validation of the ymca submaximal cycle ergometer test to predict VO2max. *Res. Q. Exerc. Sport* 75, 337–342. doi: 10.1080/02701367.2004.10609165

Chang, W. H., Fried, P. J., Saxena, S., Jannati, A., Gomes-Osman, J., Kim, Y. H., et al. (2016). Optimal number of pulses as outcome measures of neuronavigated transcranial magnetic stimulation. *Clin. Neurophysiol.* 127, 2892–2897. doi: 10.1016/j.clinph.2016.04.001

Chen, R. (2004). Interactions between inhibitory and excitatory circuits in the human motor cortex. *Exp. Brain Res.* 154, 1–10. doi: 10.1007/s00221-003-1684-1

Coppi, E., Houdayer, E., Chieffo, R., Spagnolo, F., Inuggi, A., Straffi, L., et al. (2014). Age-related changes in motor cortical representation and interhemispheric interactions: a transcranial magnetic stimulation study. *Front. Aging Neurosci.* 6:209. doi: 10.3389/fnagi.2014.00209

Davidson, T., and Tremblay, F. (2013). Age and hemispheric differences in transcallosal inhibition between motor cortices: an ispsilateral silent period study. *BMC Neurosci.* 14:62. doi: 10.1186/1471-2202-14-62

Di Lazzaro, V., Pilato, F., Dileone, M., Profice, P., Ranieri, F., Ricci, V., et al. (2007). Segregating two inhibitory circuits in human motor cortex at the level of GABAA receptor subtypes: a TMS study. *Clin. Neurophysiol.* 118, 2207–2214. doi: 10.1016/j.clinph.2007.07.005

Diaz-Buschmann, I., Jaureguizar, K. V., Calero, M. J., and Aquino, R. S. (2014). Programming exercise intensity in patients on beta-blocker treatment: the importance of choosing an appropriate method. *Eur. J. Prev. Cardiol.* 21, 1474–1480. doi: 10.1177/2047487313500214

Doherty, T. J., Vandervoort, A. A., and Brown, W. F. (1993). Effects of ageing on the motor unit: a brief review. *Can. J. Appl. Physiol.* 18, 331–358. doi: 10.1139/h93-029

Ferbert, A., Priori, A., Rothwell, J. C., Day, B. L., Colebatch, J. G., and Marsden, C. D. (1992). Interhemispheric inhibition of the human motor cortex. *J. Physiol.* 453, 525–546. doi: 10.1113/jphysiol.1992.sp019243

Fleming, M. K., and Newham, D. J. (2017). Reliability of transcallosal inhibition in healthy adults. *Front. Hum. Neurosci.* 10:681. doi: 10.3389/fnhum.2016.00681

Fujiyama, H., Hinder, M. R., and Summers, J. J. (2013). Functional role of left PMd and left M1 during preparation and execution of left hand movements in older adults. *J. Neurophysiol.* 110, 1062–1069. doi: 10.1152/jn.00075.2013

Gao, F., Edden, R. A. E., Li, M., Puts, N. A. J., Wang, G., Liu, C., et al. (2013). Edited magnetic resonance spectroscopy detects an age-related decline in brain GABA levels. *Neuroimage* 78, 75–82. doi: 10.1016/j.neuroimage.2013.04.012

Garvey, M. A., Ziemann, U., Becker, D. A., Barker, C. A., and Bartko, J. J. (2001). New graphical method to measure silent periods evoked by transcranial magnetic stimulation. *Clin. Neurophysiol.* 112, 1451–1460. doi: 10.1016/S1388-2457(01)00581-8

Giovannelli, F., Borgheresi, A., Balestrieri, F., Zaccara, G., Viggiano, M. P., Cincotta, M., et al. (2009). Modulation of interhemispheric inhibition by volitional motor activity: an ipsilateral silent period study. *J. Physiol.* 587, 5393–5410. doi: 10.1113/jphysiol.2009.175885

Godin, G., and Shephard, R. J. (1997). Godin leisure-time exercise questionnaire. *Med. Sci. Sports Exerc.* 29, 36–38. doi: 10.1097/00005768-199706001-00009

Gomes-Osman, J., Cabral, D. F., Hinchman, C., Jannati, A., Morris, T. P., and Pascual-Leone, A. (2017). The effects of exercise on cognitive function and brain plasticity - a feasibility trial. *Restor. Neurol. Neurosci.* 35, 547–556. doi: 10.3233/RNN-170758

Hanna-Pladdy, B., Mendoza, J. E., Apostolos, G. T., and Heilman, K. M. (2002). Lateralised motor control: hemispheric damage and the loss of deftness. *J. Neurol. Neurosurg. Psychiatry* 73, 574–577. doi: 10.1136/jnnp.73.5.574

Heise, K. F., Niehoff, M., Feldheim, J. F., Liuzzi, G., Gerloff, C., and Hummel, F. C. (2014). Differential behavioral and physiological effects of anodal transcranial direct current stimulation in healthy adults of younger and older age. *Front. Aging Neurosci.* 6:146. doi: 10.3389/fnagi.2014.00146

Heise, K. F., Zimerman, M., Hoppe, J., Gerloff, C., Wegscheider, K., and Hummel, F. C. (2013). The aging motor system as a model for plastic changes of GABA-mediated intracortical inhibition and their behavioral relevance. *J. Neurosci.* 33, 9039–9049. doi: 10.1523/JNEUROSCI.4094-12.2013

Hill, B. D., Barkemeyer, C. A., Jones, G. N., Santa Maria, M. P., Minor, K. S., and Browndyke, J. N. (2010). Validation of the coin rotation test: a simple, inexpensive, and convenient screening tool for impaired psychomotor processing speed. *Neurologist* 16, 249–253. doi: 10.1097/NRL.0b013e3181b1d5b0

Irlbacher, K., Brocke, J., Mechow, J. V., and Brandt, S. A. (2007). Effects of GABA(A) and GABA(B) agonists on interhemispheric inhibition in man. *Clin. Neurophysiol.* 118, 308–316. doi: 10.1016/j.clinph.2006.09.023

Jung, P., and Ziemann, U. (2006). Differences of the ipsilateral silent period in small hand muscles. *Muscle Nerve* 34, 431–436. doi: 10.1002/mus.20604

Kenward, M. G., and Roger, J. H. (2010). The use of baseline covariates in crossover studies. *Biostatistics* 11, 1–17. doi: 10.1093/biostatistics/kxp046

Kleim, J. A., Chan, S., Pringle, E., Schallert, K., Procaccio, V., Jimenez, R., et al. (2006). BDNF val66met polymorphism is associated with modified experience-dependent plasticity in human motor cortex. *Nat. Neurosci.* 9, 735–737. doi: 10.1038/nn1699

Kuo, Y. L., Dubuc, T., Boufadel, D. F., and Fisher, B. E. (2017). Measuring ipsilateral silent period: effects of muscle contraction levels and quantification methods. *Brain Res.* 1674, 77–83. doi: 10.1016/j.brainres.2017.08.015

Lenzi, D., Conte, A., Mainero, C., Frasca, V., Fubelli, F., Totaro, P., et al. (2007). Effect of corpus callosum damage on ipsilateral motor activation in patients with multiple sclerosis: a functional and anatomical study. *Hum. Brain Mapp.* 28, 636–644. doi: 10.1002/hbm.20305

Levin, O., Fujiyama, H., Boisgontier, M. P., Swinnen, S. P., and Summers, J. J. (2014). Aging and motor inhibition: a converging perspective provided by brain stimulation and imaging approaches. *Neurosci. Biobehav. Rev.* 43, 100–117. doi: 10.1016/j.neubiorev.2014.04.001

Li, J. Y., Lai, P. H., and Chen, R. (2013). Transcallosal inhibition in patients with callosal infarction. *J. Neurophysiol.* 109, 659–665. doi: 10.1152/jn.01044.2011

Lulic, T., El-Sayes, J., Fassett, H. J., and Nelson, A. J. (2017). Physical activity levels determine exercise-induced changes in brain excitability. *PLoS ONE* 12:e0173672. doi: 10.1371/journal.pone.0173672

Maddock, R. J., Casazza, G. A., Fernandez, D. H., and Maddock, M. I. (2016). Acute modulation of cortical glutamate and GABA content by physical activity. *J. Neurosci.* 36, 2449–2457. doi: 10.1523/JNEUROSCI.3455-15.2016

Mathiowetz, V., Weber, K., Kashman, N., and Volland, G. (1985). Adult norms for the nine hole peg test of finger dexterity. *Occup. Ther. J. Res.* 5, 24–38. doi: 10.1177/153944928500500102

McDonnell, M. N., Orekhov, Y., and Ziemann, U. (2007). Suppression of LTP-like plasticity in human motor cortex by the GABAB receptor agonist baclofen. *Exp. Brain Res.* 180, 181–186. doi: 10.1007/s00221-006-0849-0

McGregor, K., Heilman, K., Nocera, J., Patten, C., Manini, T., Crosson, B., et al. (2012). Aging, aerobic activity and interhemispheric communication. *Brain Sci.* 2, 634–648. doi: 10.3390/brainsci2040634

McGregor, K. M., Nocera, J. R., Sudhyadhom, A., Patten, C., Manini, T. M., Kleim, J. A., et al. (2013). Effects of aerobic fitness on aging-related changes of interhemispheric inhibition and motor performance. *Front. Aging Neurosci.* 5:66. doi: 10.3389/fnagi.2013.00066

McGregor, K. M., Zlatar, Z., Kleim, E., Sudhyadhom, A., Bauer, A., Phan, S., et al. (2011). Physical activity and neural correlates of aging: a combined TMS/fMRI study. *Behav. Brain Res.* 222, 158–168. doi: 10.1016/j.bbr.2011.03.042

Meyer, B. U., Röricht, S., Von Einsiedel, H. G., Kruggel, F., and Weindl, A. (1995). Inhibitory and excitatory interhemispheric transfers between motor cortical areas in normal humans and patients with abnormalities of the corpus callosum. *Brain* 118, 429–440. doi: 10.1093/brain/118.2.429

Mooney, R. A., Cirillo, J., and Byblow, W. D. (2017). GABA and primary motor cortex inhibition in young and older adults: a multimodal reliability study. *J. Neurophysiol.* 118, 425–433. doi: 10.1152/jn.00199.2017

Nathan, P. W., Smith, M., and Deacon, P. (1996). Vestibulospinal, reticulospinal and descending propriospinal nerve fibres in man. *Brain* 119, 1809–1833. doi: 10.1093/brain/119.6.1809

Nocera, J. R., McGregor, K. M., Hass, C. J., and Crosson, B. (2015). Spin exercise improves semantic fluency in previously sedentary older adults. *J. Aging Phys. Act.* 23, 90–94. doi: 10.1123/JAPA.2013-0107

Oldfield, R. C. (1971). The assessment and analysis of handedness: the Edinburgh inventory. *Neuropsychologia* 9, 97–113. doi: 10.1016/0028-3932(71)90067-4

Opie, G. M., Ridding, M. C., and Semmler, J. G. (2015). Age-related differences in pre- and post-synaptic motor cortex inhibition are task dependent. *Brain Stimul.* 8, 926–936. doi: 10.1016/j.brs.2015.04.001

Petitjean, M., and Ko, J. Y. L. (2013). An age-related change in the ipsilateral silent period of a small hand muscle. *Clin. Neurophysiol.* 124, 346–353. doi: 10.1016/j.clinph.2012.07.006

Phillips, C., Baktir, M. A., Srivatsan, M., and Salehi, A. (2014). Neuroprotective effects of physical activity on the brain: a closer look at trophic factor signaling. *Front. Cell Neurosci.* 20:170. doi: 10.3389/fncel.2014.00170

Reitan, R. M., and Wolfson, D. (2013). "Theoretical, methodological, and validational bases of the halstead-reitan neuropsychological test battery," in *Comprehensive Handbook of Psychological Assessment: Intellectual and Neuropsychological Assessment, Vol. 1* eds G. Goldstein, S. R. Beers, and M. Hersen (Hoboken, NJ: John Wiley & Sons, Inc.). doi: 10.1002/9780471726753.ch8

Roig, M., Skriver, K., Lundbye-Jensen, J., Kiens, B., and Nielsen, J. B. (2012). A single bout of exercise improves motor memory. *PLoS ONE* 7:e44594. doi: 10.1371/journal.pone.0044594

Rozycka, A., and Liguz-Lecznar, M. (2017). The space where aging acts: focus on the GABAergic synapse. *Aging Cell.* 16, 634–643. doi: 10.1111/acel.12605

Sale, M. V., and Semmler, J. G. (2005). Age-related differences in corticospinal control during functional isometric contractions in left and right hands. *J. Appl. Physiol.* 99, 1483–1493. doi: 10.1152/japplphysiol.00371.2005

Salthouse, T. A. (1996). The processing-speed theory of adult age differences in cognition. *Psychol. Rev.* 103, 403–428. doi: 10.1037/0033-295X.103.3.403

Schmolesky, M. T., Webb, D. L., and Hansen, R. A. (2013). The effects of aerobic exercise intensity and duration on levels of brain-derived neurotrophic factor in healthy men. *J. Sports Sci. Med.* 12, 502–511.

Siebner, H. R., Dressnandt, J., Auer, C., and Conrad, B. (1998). Continuous intrathecal baclofen infusions induced a marked increase of the transcranially evoked silent period in a patient with generalized dystonia. *Muscle Nerve* 21, 1209–1212. doi: 10.1002/(SICI)1097-4598(199809)21:9<1209::AIDMUS15>3.0.CO;2-M

Singh, A. M., Duncan, R. E., Neva, J. L., and Staines, W. R. (2014). Aerobic exercise modulates intracortical inhibition and facilitation in a nonexercised upper limb muscle. *BMC Sports Sci. Med. Rehabil.* 6:23. doi: 10.1186/2052-1847-6-23

Spirduso, W. W. (1975). Reaction and movement time as a function of age and physical activity level. *J. Gerontol.* 30, 435–440. doi: 10.1093/geronj/30.4.435

Stagg, C. J., Bachtiar, V., and Johansen-Berg, H. (2011). The role of GABA in human motor learning. *Curr. Biol.* 21, 480–484. doi: 10.1016/j.cub.2011.01.069

Szuhany, K. L., Bugatti, M., and Otto, M. W. (2015). A meta-analytic review of the effects of exercise on brain-derived neurotrophic factor. *J. Psychiatr. Res.* 60, 56–64. doi: 10.1016/j.jpsychires.2014.10.003

Talelli, P., Waddingham, W., Ewas, A., Rothwell, J. C., and Ward, N. S. (2008). The effect of age on task-related modulation of interhemispheric balance. *Exp. Brain Res.* 186, 59–66. doi: 10.1007/s00221-007-1205-8

Tang, S. W., Chu, E., Hui, T., Helmeste, D., and Law, C. (2008). Influence of exercise on serum brain-derived neurotrophic factor concentrations in healthy human subjects. *Neurosci. Lett.* 431, 62–65. doi: 10.1016/j.neulet.2007.11.019

Taubert, M., Villringer, A., and Lehmann, N. (2015). Endurance exercise as an "Endogenous" neuro-enhancement strategy to facilitate motor learning. *Front. Hum. Neurosci.* 9:692. doi: 10.3389/fnhum.2015.00692

Tiffin, J., and Asher, E. J. (1948). The Purdue pegboard; norms and studies of reliability and validity. *J. Appl. Psychol.* 32, 234–247. doi: 10.1037/h0061266

Udupa, K., Ni, Z., Gunraj, C., and Chen, R. (2010). Effect of long interval interhemispheric inhibition on intracortical inhibitory and facilitatory circuits. *J. Physiol.* 588(Pt 14), 2633–2641. doi: 10.1113/jphysiol.2010.189548

Voelcker-Rehage, C., Godde, B., and Staudinger, U. M. (2010). Physical and motor fitness are both related to cognition in old age. *Eur. J. Neurosci.* 31, 167–176. doi: 10.1111/j.1460-9568.2009.07014.x

Wischnewski, M., Kowalski, G. M., Rink, F., Belagaje, S. R., Haut, M. W., Hobbs, G., et al. (2016). Demand on skillfulness modulates interhemispheric inhibition of motor cortices. *J. Neurophysiol.* 115, 2803–2813. doi: 10.1152/jn.01076.2015

Ziemann, U., Ishii, K., Borgheresi, A., Yaseen, Z., Battaglia, F., Hallett, M., et al. (1999). Dissociation of the pathways mediating ipsilateral and contralateral motor-evoked potentials in human hand and arm muscles. *J. Physiol.* 518, 895–906. doi: 10.1111/j.1469-7793.1999.0895p.x

Ziemann, U., Reis, J., Schwenkreis, P., Rosanova, M., Strafella, A., Badawy, R., et al. (2015). TMS and drugs revisited 2014. *Clin. Neurophysiol.* 126, 1847–1868. doi: 10.1016/j.clinph.2014.08.028

11

Balance Training Enhances Vestibular Function and Reduces Overactive Proprioceptive Feedback in Elderly

Isabella K. Wiesmeier [1], Daniela Dalin [1], Anja Wehrle [2, 3], Urs Granacher [4], Thomas Muehlbauer [5], Joerg Dietterle [1], Cornelius Weiller [1], Albert Gollhofer [2] and Christoph Maurer [1]*

[1] Department of Neurology and Neurophysiology, University Hospital Freiburg, Freiburg, Germany, [2] Institute for Sports and Sport Science, University of Freiburg, Freiburg, Germany, [3] Department of Internal Medicine, Institute for Exercise and Occupational Medicine, University Hospital Freiburg, Freiburg, Germany, [4] Division of Training and Movement Science, University of Potsdam, Potsdam, Germany, [5] Division of Movement and Training Sciences, Biomechanics of Sport, Institute of Sport and Movement Sciences, University Duisburg-Essen, Essen, Germany

*Correspondence:
Christoph Maurer
christoph.maurer@uniklinik-freiburg.de

Objectives: Postural control in elderly people is impaired by degradations of sensory, motor, and higher-level adaptive mechanisms. Here, we characterize the effects of a progressive balance training program on these postural control impairments using a brain network model based on system identification techniques.

Methods and Material: We analyzed postural control of 35 healthy elderly subjects and compared findings to data from 35 healthy young volunteers. Eighteen elderly subjects performed a 10 week balance training conducted twice per week. Balance training was carried out in static and dynamic movement states, on support surfaces with different elastic compliances, under different visual conditions and motor tasks. Postural control was characterized by spontaneous sway and postural reactions to pseudorandom anterior-posterior tilts of the support surface. Data were interpreted using a parameter identification procedure based on a brain network model.

Results: With balance training, the elderly subjects significantly reduced their overly large postural reactions and approximated those of younger subjects. Less significant differences between elderly and young subjects' postural control, namely larger spontaneous sway amplitudes, velocities, and frequencies, larger overall time delays and a weaker motor feedback compared to young subjects were not significantly affected by the balance training.

Conclusion: Balance training reduced overactive proprioceptive feedback and restored vestibular orientation in elderly. Based on the assumption of a linear deterioration of postural control across the life span, the training effect can be extrapolated as a juvenescence of 10 years. This study points to a considerable benefit of a continuous balance training in elderly, even without any sensorimotor deficits.

Keywords: age, balance, vestibular, proprioception, training

INTRODUCTION

Impairments of postural control result in increased rates of unintentional falls. In fact, falls are the leading cause of injuries and subsequent deaths among people 65 years and older, and generate a fundamental financial burden to the healthcare system (Burns et al., 2016). There is general consensus that altered postural control in elderly people is determined by degradations of the sensory channels, i.e., vestibular, visual, and proprioceptive cues (Rauch et al., 2001; Goble et al., 2009; Grossniklaus et al., 2013), of the motor system (Macaluso and De Vito, 2004), and by deficits in higher-level adaptive systems (Shumway-Cook and Woollacott, 2001). It is still under debate whether, in addition, elderly's central weighting of sensory signals is affected. While some authors reported an impaired sensory weighting (Teasdale and Simoneau, 2001; Eikema et al., 2014), others found it to be unimpaired (e.g., Allison et al., 2006; Jeka et al., 2006). This controversy is possibly caused by different experimental strategies to assess sensory weighting. For example, it is well known that sensory weighting is modified by e.g., type and size of external disturbances, available sensory information, training status etc. (Oie et al., 2002; Peterka, 2002; Maurer et al., 2006). In general, it is unclear which subsystem mainly determines the degradation of postural control, given the fact that many subsystems are altered during aging.

From a diagnostic side, postural control is often monitored via spontaneous sway measures and, more rarely, challenged by external perturbations leading to motor reactions. Some authors reported age-related changes in spontaneous sway in terms of increased mean velocity, or increased sway frequencies (Prieto et al., 1996; Qu et al., 2009). However, the diagnostic value of spontaneous sway measures has been questioned (Maurer and Peterka, 2005; Pasma et al., 2014). For a more detailed analysis of postural control, the application of external perturbations has frequently been suggested. Interestingly, postural reactions to external perturbations (proprioceptive, vestibular, or visual) have been reported to be altered in the elderly (e.g., Ghulyan et al., 2005; Maitre et al., 2013; Eikema et al., 2014). More recently, the relationship between stimulus and subsequent body motion was systematically evaluated using model simulations (e.g., Peterka, 2002; Davidson et al., 2011; Nishihori et al., 2011; van der Kooij and Peterka, 2011). Models are usually based on simple feedback mechanisms, involving inverted pendulum bodies, stiffness, damping, feedback time delay, and sensory weighting (Maurer et al., 2006; van der Kooij and Peterka, 2011; Engelhart et al., 2014; Wiesmeier et al., 2015). They have already been applied to elderly people's postural control (Maurer and Peterka, 2005; Cenciarini et al., 2010; Davidson et al., 2011; Nishihori et al., 2011). Some authors reported increased damping of the system in the elderly (Cenciarini et al., 2010; Davidson et al., 2011). Stiffness findings are inconsistent (Maurer and Peterka, 2005; Cenciarini et al., 2010; Davidson et al., 2011; Nishihori et al., 2011). Surprisingly, systematic evaluations of intervention programs like balance training are completely lacking.

The improvement of elderly people's postural control via balance training is well documented (see e.g., Nagy et al., 2007; Gillespie et al., 2012). However, evidence for an optimal training program of healthy elderly people is scarce (Lesinski et al., 2015). Recently, Lesinski et al. (2015) concluded from a systematic review and metaanalysis of numerous training studies that an optimal training should last 11–12 weeks with a training frequency of three sessions per week resulting in a total number of 36–40 training sessions. A single training session should take 31–45 min. Over the last few years, balance training has been further diversified into traditional, perturbation-based, and multitask balance training approaches (see e.g., Granacher et al., 2011). A growing body of literature deals with the specific neurophysiological effects of balance training. Balance training may be able to reduce coactivation of antagonist muscles, to shorten onset latency of muscle activation, to augment reflex activity, to increase maximal and explosive force production capacity, increase the length of recovery steps subsequent to external perturbations (see Granacher et al., 2011). On a functional level, gait speed and step length, with or without external perturbations, have been reported to be increased, while step time variability seems to be reduced. Performance in clinical tests like Berg Balance Scale (BBS) and Timed Up and Go (TUG) test appears to be improved. This improvement was backed up by electrophysiological correlates, such as, the reduction of the Hoffmann reflex (Granacher et al., 2011; Nagai et al., 2012). However, it is unclear as yet, how balance training affects physiological subsystems of postural control, such as, use of sensory input, central processing, and motor output.

In the current study, we aimed to assess the main subsystems of elderly people's altered postural control with a focus on their sensitivity to balance training using parameter identification techniques based on brain network model simulations. We expected that balance training could change elderly subjects' postural control so that it resembles postural control of younger subjects, similar to a "juvenescence."

METHODS

Forty elderly subjects between 65 and 80 years who lived independently in the community, were randomly allocated either into a balance training or into a control group that did not receive balance training. Allocation followed a matched-pair protocol on the basis of age and sex (see **Figure 1**). Each subject was examined by a senior consultant neurologist in order to identify sensory deficits or neurodegenerative diseases. In addition, we asked for the amount of physical activity, fear of falling and number of falls during the last 3 years prior to the study (for questionnaire, see Supplementary Material). As part of the neurological examination, vestibular function was specifically tested using Frenzel goggles on a turning chair (vestibulo-ocular reflex, VOR). Proprioceptive function was evaluated by testing position sense and by measuring vibration sense with a tuning fork. Elderly subjects with relevant sensory deficits were excluded from the study. Moreover, subjects suffering from any other acute or chronic disease that may interact with the postural control were excluded. Finally, 35 elderly subjects [73 ± 3.3 years (mean age ± SD)] contributed to the study.

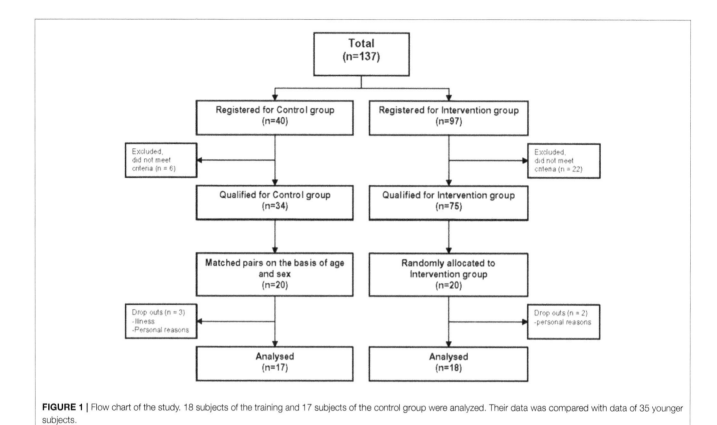

FIGURE 1 | Flow chart of the study. 18 subjects of the training and 17 subjects of the control group were analyzed. Their data was compared with data of 35 younger subjects.

In order to identify age-related changes in elderly subjects' postural control, we used younger subjects' data [$n = 35$, 37 ± 11.2 years (mean age $\pm$ SD)] generated with a similar experimental set in our laboratory, as a reference group. The study was approved by the ethics committee of the University of Freiburg and performed according to the ethical standards of the Declaration of Helsinki. Written informed consent was obtained from all subjects prior to study participation.

For evaluating postural control we used a dynamic posturography approach. Subjects were standing on a custom-built motion platform (**Figure 2B**) with eyes open (eo) and with eyes closed (ec). Spontaneous sway was recorded with the platform fixed while postural reactions were measured during continuous platform perturbations. Posturographic assessments were composed of 20 trials divided into two sessions: During the first 10 trials subjects were told to close their eyes while the other 10 trials were carried out with eyes open. The first and last trial of each ten-trial sequence (eyes closed or eyes open) was a 'spontaneous sway' trial. The other eight trials were conducted while the platform tilted. Each trial took 1 min. Breaks of about 10 s were taken between trials, according to the subject's needs. Subjects were told to stand comfortably in an upright position. They were asked not to talk.

Spontaneous sway was quantified by center-of-pressure (COP) sway paths detected with the help of a force transducing platform (Kistler platform type 9286, Winterthur, Switzerland). Extracted measures consisted of sway amplitude (Root Mean Square, RMS), sway velocity (Mean Velocity, MV), and the

frequency content of sway (Mean Frequency, MF). Postural reactions were measured on a tilting platform. The tilts consisted of platform rotations in the sagittal plane with the axis running through subjects' ankle joints. Platform tilts were designed as pseudorandom stimuli (PRTS, pseudorandom ternary sequence, **Figure 2A**) with two peak angular displacements (0.5 and 1°) and analyzed at 11 frequencies (0.05, 0.15, 0.3, 0.4, 0.55, 0.7, 0.9, 1.1, 1.35, 1.75, and 2.2 Hz).

Angular excursions of the platform and the body (hip-to-ankle, shoulder-to-hip) in space were quantified with an optoelectronic device using markers attached to shoulder, hip, and a rigid bar on the platform (Optotrak 3020, Waterloo, Canada). Each marker contained three light-emitting diodes (LEDs). 3-D LED positions were used to calculate marker movements (**Figures 2A,B**). Kistler® and Optotrak® output as well as the stimulus signals were sampled at 100 Hz using an analog-digital converter and stored on a PC via LabView® (National Instruments, Austin, Texas, USA) for offline analysis. Data was analyzed using custom-made software programmed in MATLAB® (The MathWorks Inc., Natick, MA, USA).

The relationship between the postural reactions and platform stimuli were represented by "transfer functions" in the frequency domain. Transfer functions were calculated using discrete Fourier transforms. From transfer functions, GAIN, PHASE, and Coherence values were extracted as a function of stimulus frequencies. GAIN represents the size of the postural reaction, i.e., lower body or upper body response in terms of angular excursion, as a function of stimulus size (platform angle). A

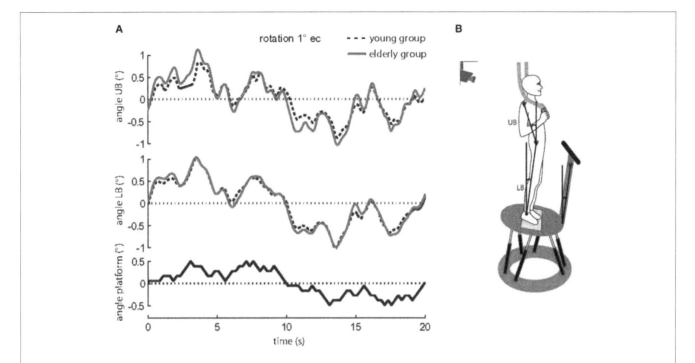

FIGURE 2 | (A) Motor reactions of the mean body excursions of young and elderly subjects in relation to platform tilts. Shown are motor reactions in degrees of the upper body (angle UB), lower body (angle LB), and platform movements (sample stimulus, black bottom line). The traces of the young and elderly groups represent means across all subjects at 1° stimulus amplitude with eyes closed (s, seconds). **(B)** Experimental setup. Picture of a subject standing on the platform. For safety reasons subjects held ropes in their hands which hung loosely from the ceiling. The six linear motors created platform tilts with the axis running through the ankle joints. Angular excursions of the platform, the upper body (UB) and the lower body (LB) in space were quantified with an optoelectronic device using markers attached to shoulder, hip, and a rigid bar on the platform.

GAIN of 1 would indicate a perfect match between body and platform excursion. PHASE is related to the relative timing between postural reaction and stimulus. Negative PHASE values (PHASE lag) represent delays. Coherence is a measure for reproducibility of postural reactions across stimulus cycles. Coherence values of 1 signify perfectly reproduced postural reactions; zero would indicate no similarity between subsequent postural reactions.

Findings in the elderly were compared with data of a young reference group. In addition, data of the elderly group before (first assessment, A1) was compared to data after balance training (second assessment, A2). The second assessment was conducted between 4 and 10 days following the last training session.

In addition, the TUG and the Functional Reach Test (FRT) were assessed twice (A1 and A2) in elderly subjects. The TUG quantifies the time (in seconds), a subject needs to do the following motor task: standing up from a chair, walking 3 m straight, turning around, walking back, and sitting down. The FRT measures the maximum distance in centimeters before and after reaching the arm forward at shoulder level without losing balance (Enkelaar et al., 2013). Mean FRT was calculated across three attempts.

Parameter Identification

Transfer functions served as a basis for simulating postural control using well-established models of upright stance to extract relevant parameters (Peterka, 2002; Engelhart et al., 2014). The

model includes a body defined by mass and height, a Neural Controller containing stiffness and damping, a feedback time delay, and a sensory feedback mechanism. A negative feedback loop links body excursions perceived by visual, vestibular, and proprioceptive channels to a corrective torque through a Neural Controller with proportional [P], derivative [D] and integral [I] contributions (PDI-controller, **Figure 3**). The external stimuli, i.e., anterior-posterior platform tilt angles, serve as an input of the model. Body sway, represented by the center of mass (COM) angle, is the model output. Since Neural Controller values depend on mass and height of the individual subjects (see Peterka, 2002; Cenciarini et al., 2010), these values are corrected by (mgh), which corresponds to the gravitational pull (body mass) × (gravitational constant) × (height of the COM from the ankle joint), leading to [P/mgh], [D/mgh], and [I/mgh]. Other parts of the model were: a lumped time delay [Td], representing the time interval between the postural reaction and the stimulus, and a sensory weighting mechanism. The sensory weighting mechanism specifies the reference frame for body orientation (space coordinates vs. platform coordinates), represented by [Wp]. The value [Wp] stands for the proprioceptive share of the sensory feedback. A value of 1 corresponds to 100 % proprioceptive control, i.e., stabilization in platform coordinates, a value of 0 relates to 0% proprioceptive control and 100% stabilization in space. Moreover, the model includes a biomechanics part that represents torque related to passive elasticity [Ppas] and damping [Dpas] of muscles and tendons, in

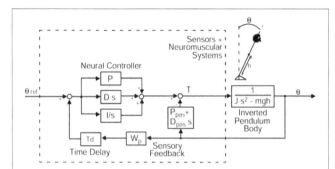

FIGURE 3 | Model simulation describing perturbed stance. The model
includes a body in terms of an inverted pendulum with the sensory and
neuromuscular systems including a Neural Controller. The mass is
concentrated at the center of mass (COM) of the body. Θ, body sway angle;
h, height of the COM above the ankle joints; Θ ref, external stimulus;
P, proportional gain (stiffness factor), D, derivative gain (damping factor),
I, integral gain of the Neural Controller; Ppas, passive stiffness factor; Dpas,
passive damping factor; Wp, proprioceptive sensory weight; Td, feedback
time delay; T, control torque; J, moment of inertia of the body; mgh, body
mass·gravitational constant·height of the COM from the ankle joint; s, Laplace
transform variable.

parallel to the active corrective torque, which is determined by the
Neural Controller (**Figure 3**). With the help of an optimization
procedure (fmincon/ Matlab, Mathworks), model simulations
were fitted to the experimental transfer functions under different
stimulus amplitudes and visual conditions. Similar to the model
provided by Peterka (2002), we assume that all sensory feedback
signals add up to a feedback gain of unity. For example, if the
proprioceptive gain is 0.6 (60%) in the eyes-closed condition, the
vestibular gain would be 0.4 (40%). In the eyes-open condition,
vestibular and visual gains both contribute to the space reference.
The strength of the visual feedback could be estimated by
subtracting the gain of the space reference in the eyes-closed
condition from the space reference in the eyes-open condition.
Another assumption refers to the allowed range of all gains
([P/mgh], [D/mgh], [I/mgh], [Wp], [Ppas], [Dpas]), and time
delay [Td], which were constrained to positive values. Goodness-
of-fit measures, limitations of the model, and comparisons to
simulations of datasets from other studies are provided as
Supplementary Material.

Balance Training Program

The balance training group received a balance training twice
a week over a period of 10 weeks (one session 60 min,
20 sessions in total). It was developed and conducted by
professional instructors from the Institute for Sports and Sport
Science (University of Freiburg) and the Institute for Exercise-
and Occupational Medicine (Department of Internal Medicine,
University Hospital Freiburg) on the basis of previous research
(Granacher et al., 2010). The training group was divided into two
smaller exercise groups which were supervised by two instructors
in order to guarantee a small participant-to-instructor ratio (1
instructor vs. 5 subjects). Each session included 10 min warm-up
and 10 min cool-down. Exercises were carried out under static
(standing) and dynamic (walking) conditions and were modified

by using either a stable or an unstable support surface (e.g., foam
mats), by closing or opening the eyes and by performing the
exercises in bipedal, semi-tandem, tandem and monopedal stance
with an additional motor task like catching and throwing a ball.
One set of exercises consisted of 4 periods of 20 s exercise and 40 s
rest. The number of sets was increased over time. Many exercises
were performed in pairs or as circuit training.

Statistical Analysis

Statistical analyses were performed using Microsoft Excel and
statistic programs (JMP® and Statview by SAS Institute Inc.,
Cary, NC, USA). Statistical significance of the difference
between healthy young and elderly subjects before training
was tested with the help of an analysis of variance (ANOVA).
The between-subject variable was group (young, elderly). For
spontaneous sway, the within-subject variables were: visual
condition (eyes open, eyes closed), sway direction (mediolateral,
anteroposterior), and body segment (COP, hip, shoulder). For
the perturbed stance experiments, the within-subject variables
were: visual condition, stimulus amplitude (0.5 and 1°) and body
segment (hip, shoulder). Intervention effects in the two groups
of elderly subjects before (A1) and after (A2) balance training
including FRT and TUG was tested by multivariate analyses
of variance (MANOVA) with time (A1, A2) as an additional
degree of freedom. Statistical significance was assumed at $p \leq$
0.05. Moreover, the relationships between parameters related to
platform measures and clinical test parameters were examined
with a Pearson Correlation Test. A matrix of correlation
coefficients was created, which illustrates the strength of linear
relationships between each pair of parameters.

RESULTS
Baseline Characteristics

Thirty-five healthy elderly [73 ± 3.3 years (mean age ± SD),
17 female, 18 male] and 35 young subjects [37 ± 11.2 years
(mean age ± SD), 19 female, 16 male] were included in the
analysis. None of the subjects reported any training or test-related
injuries. For detailed information see **Tables 1, 2**. Three subjects
of the control group dropped out due to failure to attend the
second assessment for personal reasons and illness. Two subjects
of the training group dropped out during the training period due
to personal reasons not associated with balance training. Both,
the training and control groups were well balanced at baseline
concerning age, sex, body mass, and physical activity (**Table 2**).
In total, 11 subjects claimed to have fallen during the last 3 years
prior to the study (training group: 6, control group: 5). The
number of falls was similar in both groups (training group: 10
falls, control group: 7 falls). Reasons for falling were e.g., tripping
or leisure time activities. Seven subjects reported fear of falling
(training group: 4, control group: 3) which was always associated
with particular situations such as, clear ice or standing on a
ladder.

Spontaneous Sway

Root Mean Square (0.51 vs. 0.42 cm; $F = 23.4$, $p < 0.001$),
MV (1.03 vs. 0.70 cm/s; $F = 60.9$, $p < 0.001$), and MF (0.49

TABLE 1 | Information about the young group.

Subject number	Age [ys]	Body mass [kg]	Body height [m]
1	20–25	#	1.67
2	25–30	40.5	1.63
3	25–30	97.0	1.69
4	30–35	90.3	1.80
5	20–25	#	1.58
6	25–30	#	1.63
7	30–35	73.5	1.79
8	25–30	72.5	1.82
9	20–25	66.0	1.80
10	20–25	43.0	1.60
11	30–35	79.8	1.78
12	25–30	79.3	#
13	25–30	72.5	1.78
14	30–35	#	1.90
15	25–30	82.0	1.84
16	30–35	76.0	1.83
17	25–30	92.0	2.03
18	20–25	74.5	1.64
19	20–25	66.0	1.79
20	45–50	#	1.67
21	40–45	77.0	1.75
22	40–45	58.5	1.80
23	55–60	83.3	1.72
24	40–45	88.8	1.90
25	50–55	67.8	#
26	45–50	60.3	1.60
27	55–60	82.8	1.70
28	45–50	#	1.76
29	45–50	50.3	1.68
30	45–50	#	1.56
31	45–50	97.0	1.78
32	45–50	50.8	1.72
33	45–50	53.8	1.66
34	50–55	65.0	1.66
35	35–40	#	1.69

35 subjects; 19 female; 16 male. m, masculine; f, feminine; ys, years; kg, kilogram; m, meters; #, no data available.

TABLE 2 | Information about the training and control group.

Subject number	Group	Age [ys]	Body mass [kg]	Body height [m]	Physical activity [h/week]	Fear of falling	Number of falls in the last 3 years
1	Control	70–75	56.0	1.58	8.5	No	
2	Control	70–75	79.0	1.76	1.0	No	
3	Control	65–70	98.0	1.91	6.0	No	
4	Control	70–75	68.0	1.61	2.5	Yes	1
5	Control	75–80	71.5	1.71	0	No	
6	Control	70–75	55.0	1.52	14.0	No	2
9	Control	70–75	75.0	1.61	2.5	No	1
10	Control	75–80	61.5	1.57	5.0	Yes	
11	Control	65–70	95.0	1.72	4.0	No	
12	Control	70–75	94.5	1.86	8.5	No	
13	Control	75–80	73.0	1.67	12.5	No	
14	Control	70–75	80.5	1.83	5.0	No	1
15	Control	70–75	98.5	1.80	0.0	No	
16	Control	75–80	64.0	1.56	7.0	No	2
17	Control	65–70	80.0	1.76	2.0	No	
18	Control	75–80	67.0	1.58	2.0	No	
19	Control	75–80	60.5	1.62	4.0	Yes	
21	Training	80–85	68.0	1.63	1.0	Yes	3
23	Training	65–70	90.0	1.76	0.0	No	1
25	Training	65–70	64.5	1.51	9.0	No	
26	Training	70–75	79.0	1.74	6.0	Yes	
27	Training	65–70	90.5	1.77	10.0	No	2
28	Training	70–75	71.5	1.67	2.0	No	
29	Training	75–80	65.0	1.51	1.5	No	
30	Training	65–70	89.0	1.76	0	Yes	
31	Training	70–75	75.0	1.65	4.5	No	
32	Training	75–80	65.5	1.70	6.5	No	
33	Training	70–75	65.0	1.68	3.5	No	
34	Training	70–75	81.5	1.78	4.0	No	
35	Training	70–75	64.5	1.67	0	No	
36	Training	75–80	86.0	1.71	4.5	No	
37	Training	70–75	70.0	1.66	10.5	No	1
38	Training	70–75	88.5	1.75	4.0	Yes	
39	Training	75–80	70.0	1.52	1.0	No	1
40	Training	75–80	71.0	1.73	6.5	No	2

35 subjects; 17 female; 18 male. m, masculine; f, feminine; control, control group; training, training group; ys, years; kg, kilogram; m, meters; h, hours.

vs. 0.41 Hz; $F = 20.5$, $p < 0.001$) were significantly larger in elderly before training (A1) compared to younger subjects (see **Figure 4**). We found no significant interactions between age and visual condition ($F = 0.8$, $p = 0.39$), sway direction (mediolateral, anteroposterior; $F = 1.8$, $p = 0.18$), and body segments ($F = 1.9$, $p = 0.16$). None of the measures significantly interacted with balance training for the elderly (RMS: $F = 2.6$, $p = 0.11$, MV: $F = 1.7$, $p = 0.20$, MF: $F = 0.05$, $p = 0.83$).

Externally Perturbed Stance
GAIN

In elderly subjects before training, GAIN was significantly larger (2.31; $F = 553.7$, $p < 0.001$) than in young subjects (1.77). Across the age groups, GAIN was significantly larger with eyes closed than with eyes open (eyes closed, ec: 2.36, eyes open, eo: 1.72; $F = 766.7$, $p < 0.001$). Stimulus amplitudes ($0.5°$: 2.24, $1°$: 1.84; $F = 307.4$, $p < 0.001$), stimulus frequencies ($F = 4954.3$, $p < 0.001$), and body segments (hip: 1.60, shoulder: 2.48, $F = 1482.5$, $p < 0.001$) significantly influenced GAIN. Age group significantly interacted with frequency ($F = 12.7$, $p < 0.001$), with the most prominent GAIN difference between age groups in the lower frequency range (see GAIN plots in **Figure 5A1**). Moreover, we found a significant interaction between age group and body segments ($F = 379.1$, $p < 0.001$). This exemplifies that elderly

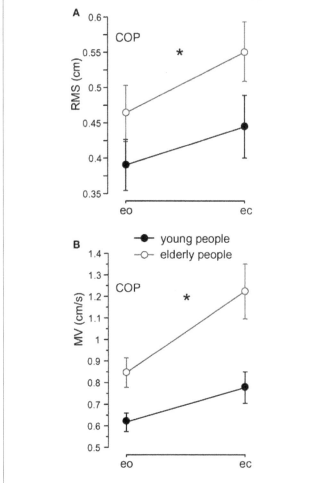

FIGURE 4 | Spontaneous sway measures computed from center of pressure (COP) traces. **(A)** Root Mean Square (RMS). **(B)** Mean Velocity (MV) of the two age groups; eo, eyes open; ec, eyes closed. * Statistically significant difference ($p < 0.05$).

subjects' shoulder GAIN (2.98) was almost twice as large as hip GAIN (1.64), whereas, young subjects' shoulder GAIN (1.99) was 20% larger than hip GAIN (1.55, **Figure 5B1**). Lastly, age group did not significantly interact with visual condition ($F = 3.3$, $p = 0.07$) or stimulus amplitude ($F = 0.7$, $p = 0.41$).

GAIN as a function of time (A1/A2) significantly interacted with balance training ($F = 25.4$, $p < 0.001$, **Figure 5C1**). While GAIN of the training group significantly decreased from 2.36 to 2.23 ($p < 0.05$), GAIN of the control group slightly increased (A1: 2.26, A2: 2.31, $p > 0.05$). Frequency did not interact significantly with GAIN as a function of time ($F = 0.4$, $p = 0.95$). However, GAIN as a function of time significantly interacted with body segments ($F = 5.2$, $p = 0.02$): Whereas GAIN of the shoulder decreased over time (2.97 to 2.90), GAIN of the hip hardly changed as a function of time (1.64 to 1.65). The decrease in shoulder GAIN is an effect of balance training. Shoulder GAIN of the training group decreased from 3.0 to 2.8, whereas shoulder GAIN of the control group slightly increased from 2.9 to 3.0 ($F = 17.9$,

$p < 0.001$). In both groups, GAIN of the hip was nearly equal as a function of time (training group A1: 1.70, A2: 1.71; control group A1: 1.57, A2: 1.59). There were no significant interactions between time and visual condition ($F = 0.4$, $p = 0.54$), and between time and stimulus amplitude ($F = 0.08$, $p = 0.78$).

Phase
PHASE, indicating the temporal relationship between response and stimulus, differed significantly between the age groups (young subjects: $-127.27°$, elderly subjects: $-122.34°$; $F = 8.9$, $p = 0.003$). Across the age groups, PHASE was mainly determined by frequency, showing a PHASE lead in the low frequency range ($F = 1035.9$, $p < 0.0001$). In general, the significant interaction between age and frequency ($F = 4.1$, $p < 0.001$) showed the effect of age on PHASE as a function of frequency. The young group showed a moderate slope of PHASE as a function of stimulus frequencies, whereas the elderly group displayed a steeper relationship between PHASE and frequencies (see **Figure 5A2**). PHASE lag was found to be significantly smaller with eyes closed ($-120.63°$) than with eyes open ($-128.99°$, $F = 25.7$, $p < 0.001$), significantly smaller at the hip ($-101.07°$) than at the shoulder level ($-148.54°$, $F = 828.6$, $p < 0.001$) across all age groups. It did not significantly vary with different stimulus amplitudes ($F = 0.009$, $p = 0.9$). We found a significant interaction between age group and body segment ($F = 45.2$, $p < 0.001$) representing the fact that PHASE difference between shoulder and hip decreases with age (**Figure 5B2**). Age group did not significantly interact with visual condition ($F = 1.6$, $p = 0.2$) or stimulus amplitude ($F = 0.6$, $p = 0.5$).

PHASE lag as a function of time significantly interacted with balance training ($F = 5.3$, $p = 0.02$, **Figure 5C2**). Both, PHASE lag of the training group ($-123.67°$ to $-126.69°$, $p > 0.05$) and PHASE lag of the control group ($-120.94°$ to $-131.70°$, $p < 0.05$) increased as a function of time, with the increase being more pronounced in the control group. Time did not interact significantly with frequency ($F = 0.1$, $p = 1.00$). In addition, PHASE as a function of time significantly interacted with body segments ($F = 22.1$, $p < 0.001$). Whereas, PHASE lag of the hip was nearly stationary over time (-104.1 to -103.1), PHASE lag of the shoulder increased as a function of time (-140.5 to -155.3). However, we found no significant interaction between balance training and body segments as a function of time ($F = 1.0$, $p = 0.3$).

Coherence
In both, young and elderly subjects, coherence significantly depended on frequency (higher coherence with lower frequencies, $F = 931.9$, $p < 0.001$, **Figure 5A3**), stimulus amplitude (higher coherence with larger stimulus amplitude, $F = 908.6$, $p < 0.001$), on body segments (hip 0.49, shoulder 0.48; $F = 7.5$, $p = 0.006$), but not on visual condition ($F = 0.6$, $p = 0.4$). The coherence of the elderly group (0.52) was significantly higher than the coherence of the young group (0.46; $F = 217.2$, $p < 0.001$). There were significant interactions between age group and frequency (larger coherence differences between groups with lower frequencies, $F = 5.8$, $p < 0.001$),

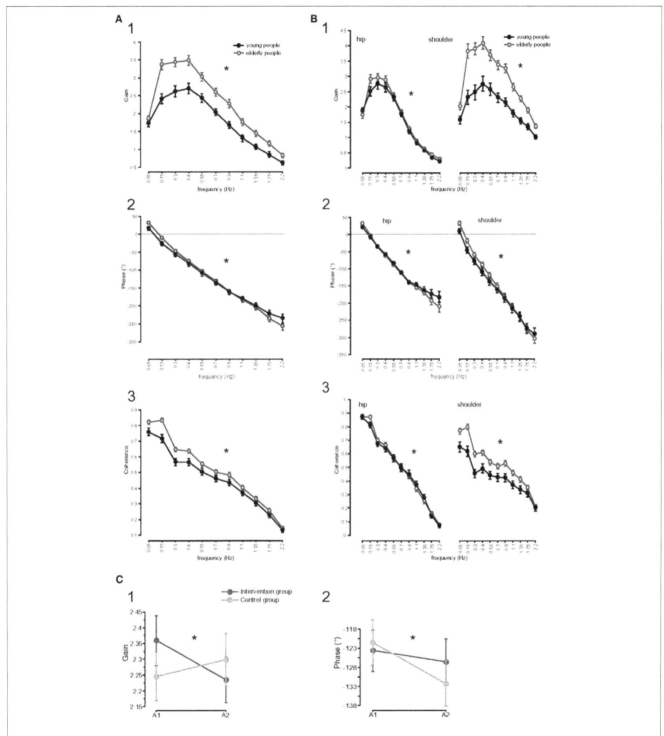

FIGURE 5 | Parameters of perturbed stance analyzed at 11 frequencies. **(A)** GAIN (1), PHASE (2), and Coherence (3) of the two age groups across all stimulus amplitudes, body segments, and visual conditions. * Statistically significant difference ($p < 0.05$). °Degree; Hz, Hertz. **(B)** GAIN, PHASE, and Coherence, interactions between age and body segments. GAIN (1), PHASE (2), and Coherence (3) of the two age groups across all stimulus amplitudes and visual conditions separated by body segments. * Statistically significant difference ($p < 0.05$). °Degree; Hz, Hertz. **(C)** Influence of balance training on parameters of perturbed stance. GAIN (1) and PHASE (2) curves of the training and control group before (A1) and after (A2) training. *Statistically significant difference ($p < 0.05$). °Degree.

between age group and body segment (larger shoulder than hip coherence in elderly, smaller shoulder than hip coherence in young subjects, $F = 142.9$, $p < 0.001$, **Figure 5B3**). Age group did not significantly interact with stimulus amplitude ($F = 0.4$, $p = 0.5$) and coherence did not significantly interact with balance training ($F = 0.1$, $p = 0.77$).

Model Parameters (see Figures 6A–C)

The integral gain, [I/mgh], was significantly higher in the young group (0.12 $s^{-1}\cdot rad^{-1}$) than in the elderly group (0.10 $s^{-1}\cdot rad^{-1}$; $F = 35.0$, $p < 0.001$). It was significantly higher with eyes open (0.12 $s^{-1}\cdot rad^{-1}$) than with eyes closed (0.10 $s^{-1}\cdot rad^{-1}$; $F = 20.5$, $p < 0.001$). In addition, [Td] was significantly larger in elderly (0.17 s) compared to young subjects (0.16 s; $F = 19.4$, $p < 0.001$). Moreover, [Wp] was significantly larger in elderly compared to young subjects (0.71 vs. 0.67; $F = 5.8$, $p = 0.016$, **Figure 6B**). It was significantly larger with eyes closed than with eyes open (0.79 vs. 0.58; $F = 143.3$, $p < 0.001$) and it was larger at a stimulus amplitude of 0.5° (0.74) than at 1° (0.64; $F = 34.5$, $p < 0.001$). Age group significantly interacted with visual condition ($F = 4.3$, $p = 0.04$). The difference of [Wp] between the eyes-open and eyes-closed condition was greater in young (0.24) than in elderly subjects (0.17). We found no significant interaction between age group and stimulus amplitude. The derivative gain, [D/mgh], was not significantly different between the age groups (elderly subjects: 0.376 $s\cdot rad^{-1}$, young subjects: 0.378 $s\cdot rad^{-1}$; $F = 0.06$, $p = 0.8$). The proportional gain, [P/mgh], was significantly lower in elderly subjects (1.33 vs. 1.44 rad^{-1} in young subjects; $F = 10.7$, $p = 0.001$) and significantly lower at a stimulus amplitude of 0.5° (1.35 vs. 1.43 rad^{-1} at 1°; $F = 6.3$, $p = 0.013$). Passive stiffness, [Ppas], and passive damping, [Dpas], were significantly larger in young subjects compared to elderly subjects ([Ppas], young: 89.4, elderly: 84.4; $F = 15.1$, $p = 0.001$; [Dpas], young: 60.3, elderly: 57.4; $F = 8.5$, $p = 0.004$). In general, [Ppas] und [Dpas] were larger with eyes open ([Ppas], eo: 92.9, ec: 80.9; $F = 78.1$, $p < 0.001$; [Dpas], eo: 61.6, ec 56.1; $F = 32.5$, $p < 0.001$). Visual condition and age group significantly interacted ($F = 4.1$, $p = 0.042$). The difference in [Ppas] between eyes-open and eyes-closed was greater in young (14.5) than in elderly subjects (10.7). Stimulus amplitude did not have a significant effect on [Ppas] ($F = 2.6$, $p = 0.1$).

Balance training did not have a significant effect on most model parameters ([I/mgh]: $F = 0.004$, $p = 0.5$, [P/mgh]: $F = 0.8$, $p = 0.4$, [D/mgh]: $F = 1.3$, $p = 0.3$, [Ppas]: $F = 1.3$, $p = 0.3$, [Dpas]: $F = 0.3$, $p = 0.6$, [Td]: $F = 0.0$, $p = 1.0$). However, the proprioceptive sensory weight, [Wp], changed significantly as a function of time ($F = 4.0$, $p = 0.048$, **Figure 6C**). [Wp] of the training group decreased from 0.73 to 0.70 ($p < 0.05$), [Wp] of the control group increased from 0.69 at the first assessment to 0.70 at the second assessment ($p > 0.05$).

Clinical Tests

The average reach distance of the training group increased significantly from 28.24 cm before to 32.08 cm after training ($F = 7.4$, $p = 0.01$). The reach distance of the control group decreased from 31.40 cm (A1) to 29.92 cm (A2) without being significant ($F = 0.9$, $p = 0.4$). Data of the TUG of the training group decreased during training but was not significant (A1: 8.48 s, A2: 8.34 s; $F = 0.2$, $p = 0.7$). Similar to the training group, there was no significant change in the TUG of the control group as a function of time (A1: 8.27 s, A2: 8.02 s; $F = 0.2$, $p = 0.6$).

Correlations

A correlation matrix was computed between measures (spontaneous sway and perturbed stance measures) and parameters that differed significantly between young and elderly subjects. Spontaneous sway measures RMS ($r = 0.56$, $p = 0.0005$) and MV ($r = 0.42$, $p = 0.013$), significantly correlated with GAIN. RMS also correlated with [Wp] ($r = 0.36$, $p = 0.03$). GAIN correlated with [Wp] ($r = 0.37$, $p = 0.03$) and [Td] ($r = 0.45$, $p = 0.008$, see **Figure 6D**).

DISCUSSION

Here, the effect of balance training on postural control in elderly people was analyzed using a disturbance-related reactive motor approach. Postural control was assessed by spontaneous sway measures and measures of externally perturbed stance. Stimulus-response data were interpreted using a systems analysis approach (Engelhart et al., 2014; Pasma et al., 2014; Wiesmeier et al., 2015). We hypothesized that elderly subjects' postural control differed from that of young subjects, and that it was modified by balance training toward young subjects' postural control. In fact, elderly subjects displayed larger spontaneous sway amplitudes, velocities, and larger postural reactions than young subjects. Balance training reduced postural reaction sizes, which approached the range of values of young subjects. Using parameter identification techniques based on brain network model simulations, we found that balance training reduced overactive proprioceptive feedback and restored vestibular orientation in elderly. In the next paragraphs, we discuss the main findings sorted by the parameters analyzed, starting with age effects and followed by training effects, respectively.

Spontaneous sway was assessed using amplitude-related (RMS), velocity-related (MV), and frequency-related (MF) measures. All these measures have been reported to be higher in elderly than in young people (e.g., Prieto et al., 1996; Maurer and Peterka, 2005). In the present study, these differences were reproduced consistently.

While some authors reported effects of elderly's balance training on spontaneous sway (Judge, 2003; Hue et al., 2004; Nagy et al., 2007), we did not find significant effects. Some researchers interpreted smaller postural sway as improved balance (Judge, 2003; Hue et al., 2004). Others interpreted increased sway after balance training as an improved balance due to increased confidence (Nagy et al., 2007). As discussed in recent papers, different postural control deficits might lead to similar abnormalities in spontaneous sway measures reducing its usability for specific assessments of balance (Ghulyan et al., 2005; Wiesmeier et al., 2015).

Subjects' postural reactions as a function of external perturbations, i.e., anterior-posterior platform tilts, were characterized using GAIN and PHASE curves. Similar to reports in earlier papers, elderly subjects' postural reactions, i.e., GAIN values, were larger than in young subjects. This effect was more pronounced at the shoulder than at the hip level (Ghulyan et al., 2005; Wiesmeier et al., 2015). In other words, elderly subjects were dragged with the platform, while young subjects were more stable in space.

Balance training significantly reduced GAIN values toward the values of young subjects. The benefit of training amounted

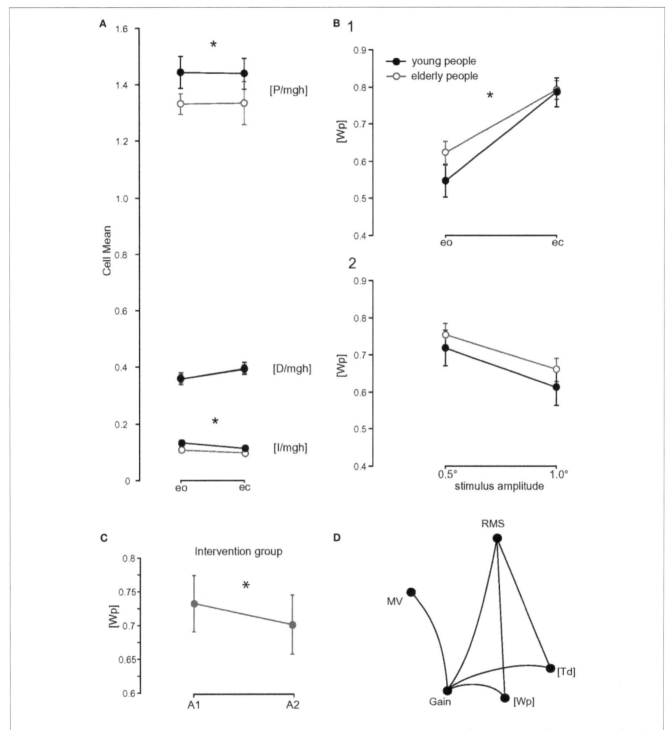

FIGURE 6 | Model parameters and correlation matrix. **(A)** Model parameters of the two age groups ([P/mgh] in rad^{-1}, [D/mgh] in s·rad^{-1}, and [I/mgh] in s^{-1}·rad^{-1}); eo, eyes open; ec, eyes closed. * Statistically significant difference ($p < 0.05$). **(B)** [Wp] (proprioceptive sensory weight) of the two age groups with respect to visual condition (1) and stimulus amplitude (2); eo, eyes open; ec, eyes closed. * Statistically significant difference ($p < 0.05$). **(C)** Influence of balance training on [Wp]. [Wp] of the training group before (A1) and after (A2) balance training. **(D)** Correlation matrix of measures (spontaneous sway and perturbed stance measures) and parameters that differed significantly between young and elderly subjects. Only significant correlations are shown. RMS, Root Mean Square; MV, Mean Velocity; MF, Mean Frequency; [Wp], proprioceptive sensory weight; [Td], time delay.

to about 30% of the GAIN difference between elderly and young subjects. If we assume a linear relationship between deterioration of postural control and age, based on former studies (Era et al., 2006; Wiesmeier et al., 2015), the training effect could be extrapolated as a juvenescence of about 10 years given the average age difference of 36 years between the two age groups.

In general, larger postural reactions in elderly could be due to an intensified use of ankle proprioception and a reduced use of vestibular information. Vestibular information would be used to stabilize the body in space. Other reasons for large postural reactions might include general muscle weakness, or an increased time delay between stimulus and response. In order to separate the different possible subsystems responsible for increased postural reactions, we applied a systems analysis approach based on a well-known postural control model (Engelhart et al., 2014; Pasma et al., 2014).

Using model simulations, we were in fact able to identify larger contributions of proprioception to sensory feedback in elderly as compared to young subjects. The higher the proprioceptive feedback, the lower the contributions of space cues, i.e., the vestibular information, when eyes were closed, and vestibular and visual information with eyes open. With a decreased vestibular feedback, elderly people are closer to vestibular loss patients (see in Maurer et al., 2006) than to patients suffering from polyneuropathy (unpublished data). As we showed before (Maurer et al., 2006), vestibular loss patients, who are forced to rely 100% on proprioception, tend to fall on tilting platforms, signifying the problems with a pure proprioceptive strategy.

After training, the proprioceptive feedback was significantly reduced with both eyes open and eyes closed. The decrease of proprioceptive feedback in the eyes-closed condition can only be explained by an increase of the vestibular feedback. This indicates that elderly subjects learned to weigh vestibular information higher. Because the increase of the weight for space cues is similar in the eyes-open condition, we assume that this, again, is caused by an increase of the vestibular feedback. Interestingly, proprioceptive feedback was not only the most prominent difference between elderly and young subjects, but also the only parameter that was affected by training. The other parameters, that differed between young and elderly subjects (larger time delay [Td], smaller integral gain [I/mgh], smaller proportional gain [P/mgh], smaller passive stiffness factor [Ppas], and smaller passive damping factor [Dpas] in elderly), were not significantly affected by balance training. This could be due to the fact that the parameters not affected by training represent those physiological constituents of postural control that may be closely related to anatomical features of the subject (Peterka, 2002), such as, height of the COM, mass distribution, patterns of muscle recruitment, or nerve conduction time. While balance training could principally affect plastic central weighting processes, it is less likely that they directly influence anatomical constraints of the body.

Additional differences between young and elderly subjects' postural reactions were related to a more pronounced PHASE slope and a smaller PHASE lag (Ghulyan et al., 2005; Wiesmeier et al., 2015). More specifically, PHASE difference between shoulder and hip decreased with age, pointing to a different coordination of body segments. We interpreted this as a change in reactive balance strategy using more hip flexion and extension. This effect might be in accordance to a hypothesis presented by Kuo et al. (1998) that the use of hip flexion/extension may be enhanced in conditions where the support surface is not reliable, i.e., in unstable platform conditions. All these additional differences were not significantly affected by balance training.

Experimental results were compared with known clinical tests for the assessment of postural deficits, namely the FRT and the TUG TEST (Enkelaar et al., 2013). The FRT was significantly ameliorated by balance training. This is in accordance with the expected effects of balance training, as FRT clinically stands for the ability to balance. FRT values of our elderly group were similar to the ones reported by Duncan et al. (1990) who assessed 128 volunteers between 21 and 87 years. The TUG was improved after balance training (not significantly). The TUG scores of the training and control groups corresponded to scores reported by Nagy et al. (2007; 8.9–10.3 s) and Enkelaar et al. (2013; 9.3 s).

The correlation analysis of elderly's data before and after training revealed that the significant effect of balance training, represented by the larger postural reactions (GAIN) significantly correlated with the strength of proprioceptive feedback [Wp], with RMS, with MV, and with time delay [Td]. This correlation pattern indicates that there is a certain tendency that the elderly ameliorated spontaneous sway measures and time delay with training, which is correlated with the main training effect of the recovery of vestibular function.

CONCLUSION

Balance training reduced elderly subjects' overactive proprioceptive feedback and enhanced vestibular orientation. The modified use of sensory information can be interpreted as a change in postural control strategies representing a higher level adaptive mechanism. Based on the assumption of a linear deterioration of postural control across the life span, the training effect can be extrapolated as a juvenescence of about 10 years. This is even more surprising, given the fact that the elderly subjects evaluated here were in a healthy and active state prior to the study. We hold that this study points to a considerable benefit of a continuous balance training in elderly, even without any sensorimotor deficits.

AUTHOR CONTRIBUTIONS

IW and CM: substantial contributions to the conception and design of the study, data acquisition, analysis, and interpretation, drafted and revised manuscript, DD: substantial contributions to the conception and design of the study, acquisition, analysis, and interpretation of data, AW and JD: conception and design of the study, data acquisition, revised manuscript, UG, TM, CW, and AG: substantial contributions to the conception and design of the study, data acquisition and interpretation, revised manuscript.

FUNDING

CM was partially funded by a European Union FP7 grant (EMBALANCE: Grant Agreement no 610454), the Brainlinks-Braintools Cluster of Excellence funded by the German Research foundation (DFG, grant no ADV139) and by DFG (MA 2543/3-1).

REFERENCES

Allison, L. K., Kiemel, T., and Jeka, J. J. (2006). Multisensory reweighting of vision and touch is intact in healthy and fall-prone older adults. *Exp. Brain Res.* 175, 342–352. doi: 10.1007/s00221-006-0559-7

Burns, E. R., Stevens, J. A., and Lee, R. (2016). The direct costs of fatal and non-fatal falls among older adults - United States. *J. Safety Res.* 58, 99–103. doi: 10.1016/j.jsr.2016.05.001

Cenciarini, M., Loughlin, P. J., Sparto, P. J., and Redfern, M. S. (2010). Stiffness and damping in postural control increase with age. *IEEE Trans. Biomed. Eng.* 57, 267–275. doi: 10.1109/TBME.2009.2031874

Davidson, B. S., Madigan, M. L., Southward, S. C., and Nussbaum, M. A. (2011). Neural control of posture during small magnitude perturbations: effects of aging and localized muscle fatigue. *IEEE Trans. Biomed. Eng.* 58, 1546–1554. doi: 10.1109/TBME.2010.2095500

Duncan, P. W., Weiner, D. K., Chandler, J., and Studenski, S. (1990). Functional reach: a new clinical measure of balance. *J. Gerontol.* 45, M192–M197. doi: 10.1093/geronj/45.6.M192

Eikema, D. J., Hatziataki, V., Tzovaras, D., and Papaxanthis, C. (2014). Application of intermittent galvanic vestibular stimulation reveals age-related constraints in the multisensory reweighting of posture. *Neurosci. Lett.* 561, 112–117. doi: 10.1016/j.neulet.2013.12.048

Engelhart, D., Pasma, J. H., Schouten, A. C., Meskers, C. G., Maier, A. B., Mergner, T., et al. (2014). Impaired standing balance in elderly: a new engineering method helps to unravel causes and effects. *J. Am. Med. Dir. Assoc.* 15, 227.e1-6. doi: 10.1016/j.jamda.2013.09.009

Enkelaar, L., Smulders, E., van Schrojenstein Lantman-de Valk, H., Weerdesteyn, V., and Geurts, A. C. (2013). Clinical measures are feasible and sensitive to assess balance and gait capacities in older persons with mild to moderate intellectual disabilities. *Res. Dev. Disabil.* 34, 276–285. doi: 10.1016/j.ridd.2012.08.014

Era, P., Sainio, P., Koskinen, S., Haavisto, P., Vaara, M., and Aromaa, A. (2006). Postural balance in a random sample of 7,979 subjects aged 30 years and over. *Gerontology* 52, 204–213. doi: 10.1159/000093652

Ghulyan, V., Paolino, M., Lopez, C., Dumitrescu, M., and Lacour, M. (2005). A new translational platform for evaluating aging or pathology-related postural disorders. *Acta Otolaryngol.* 125, 607–617. doi: 10.1080/00016480510026908

Gillespie, L. D., Robertson, M. C., Gillespie, W. J., Sherrington, C., Gates, S., Clemson, L. M., et al. (2012). Interventions for preventing falls in older people living in the community. *Cochrane Database Syst. Rev.* 9:CD007146. doi: 10.1002/14651858.CD007146.pub3

Goble, D. J., Coxon, J. P., Wenderoth, N., van Impe, A., and Swinnen, S. P. (2009). Proprioceptive sensibility in the elderly: degeneration, functional consequences and plastic-adaptive processes. *Neurosci. Biobehav. Rev.* 33, 271–278. doi: 10.1016/j.neubiorev.2008.08.012

Granacher, U., Muehlbauer, T., Bridenbaugh, S., Bleiker, E., Wehrle, A., and Kressig, R. W. (2010). Balance training and multi-task performance in seniors. *Int. J. Sports Med.* 31, 353–358. doi: 10.1055/s-0030-1248322

Granacher, U., Muehlbauer, T., Zahner, L., Gollhofer, A., and Kressig, R. W. (2011). Comparison of traditional and recent approaches in the promotion of balance and strength in older adults. *Sports Med.* 41, 377–400 doi: 10.2165/11539920-000000000-00000

Grossniklaus, H. E., Nickerson, J. M., Edelhauser, H. F., Bergman, L. A., and Berglin, L. (2013). Anatomic alterations in aging and age-related diseases of the eye. *Invest. Ophthalmol. Vis. Sci.* 54, ORSF23–27. doi: 10.1167/iovs.13-12711

Hue, O. A., Seynnes, O., Ledrole, D., Colson, S. S., and Bernard, P. L. (2004). Effects of a physical activity program on postural stability in older people. *Aging Clin. Exp. Res.* 16, 356–362. doi: 10.1007/BF03324564

Jeka, J., Allison, L., Saffer, M., Zhang, Y., Carver, S., and Kiemel, T. (2006). Sensory reweighting with translational visual stimuli in young and elderly adults: the role of state-dependent noise. *Exp. Brain Res.* 174, 517–527. doi: 10.1007/s00221-006-0502-y

Judge, J. O. (2003). Balance training to maintain mobility and prevent disability. *Am. J. Prev. Med.* 25(3 Suppl. 2), 150–156. doi: 10.1016/S0749-3797(03)00178-8

Kuo, A., Speers, R., Peterka, R., and Horak, F. (1998). Effect of altered sensory conditions on multivariate descriptors of human postural sway. *Exp. Brain Res.* 122, 185–195. doi: 10.1007/s002210050506

Lesinski, M., Hortobagyi, T., Muehlbauer, T., Gollhofer, A., and Granacher, U. (2015). Effects of balance training on balance performance in healthy older adults: a systematic review and meta-analysis. *Sports Med.* 45, 1721–1738. doi: 10.1007/s40279-015-0375-y

Macaluso, A., and De Vito, G. (2004). Muscle strength, power and adaptations to resistance training in older people. *Eur. J. Appl. Physiol.* 91, 450–472. doi: 10.1007/s00421-003-0991-3

Maitre, J., Gasnier, Y., Bru, N., Jully, J. L., and Paillard, T. (2013). Discrepancy in the involution of the different neural loops with age. *Eur. J. Appl. Physiol.* 113, 1821–1831. doi: 10.1007/s00421-013-2608-9

Maurer, C., Mergner, T., and Peterka, R. J. (2006). Multisensory control of human upright stance. *Exp. Brain Res.* 171, 231–250. doi: 10.1007/s00221-005-0256-y

Maurer, C., and Peterka, R. J. (2005). A new interpretation of spontaneous sway measures based on a simple model of human postural control. *J. Neurophysiol.* 93, 189–200. doi: 10.1152/jn.00221.2004

Nagai, K., Yamada, M., Tanaka, B., Uemura, K., Mori, S, Aoyama, T. et al. (2012). Effects of balance training on muscle coactivation during postural control in older adults, a randomized controlled trial. *J. Gerontol. A Biol. Sci. Med. Sci.* 67, 882–889. doi: 10.1093/gerona/glr252

Nagy, E., Feher-Kiss, A., Barnai, M., Domján-Preszner, A., Angyan, L., and Horvath, G. (2007). Postural control in elderly subjects participating in balance training. *Eur. J. Appl. Physiol.* 100, 97–104. doi: 10.1007/s00421-007-0407-x

Nishihori, T., Aoki, M., Jian, Y., Nagasaki, S., Furuta, Y., and Ito, Y. (2011). Effects of aging on lateral stability in quiet stance. *Aging Clin. Exp. Res.* 24, 162–170. doi: 10.3275/7626

Oie, K. S., Kiemel, T., and Jeka, J. J. (2002). Multisensory fusion: simultaneous reweighting of vision and touch for the control of human posture. *Cogn. Brain Res.* 14, 164–176. doi: 10.1016/S0926-6410(02)00071-X

Pasma, J. H., Engelhart, D., Schouten, A. C., van der Kooij, H., Maier, A. B., and Meskers, C. G. (2014). Impaired standing balance: the clinical need for closing the loop. *Neuroscience* 267, 157–165. doi: 10.1016/j.neuroscience.2014.02.030

Peterka, R. J. (2002). Sensorimotor integration in human postural control. *J. Neurophysiol.* 88, 1097–1118. doi: 10.1152/jn.00605.2001

Prieto, T. E., Myklebust, J. B., Hoffmann, R. G., Lovett, E. G., and Myklebust, B. M. (1996). Measures of postural steadiness: differences between healthy young and elderly adults. *IEEE Trans. Biomed. Eng.* 43, 956–966. doi: 10.1109/10.532130

Qu, X., Nussbaum, M. A., and Madigan, M. L. (2009). Model-based assessments of the effects of age and ankle fatigue on the control of upright posture in humans. *Gait Posture* 30, 518–522. doi: 10.1016/j.gaitpost.2009.07.127

Rauch, S. D., Velázquez-Villaseñor, L., Dimitri, P. S., and Merchant, S. N. (2001). Decreasing hair cell counts in aging humans. *Ann. N.Y. Acad. Sci.* 942, 220–227. doi: 10.1111/j.1749-6632.2001.tb03748.x

Shumway-Cook, A., and Woollacott, M. (2001). "Chapter 9: Aging and postural control," in *Motor Control: Theory and Practical Applications, 2nd Edn* ed M. Biblis (Philadelphia, PA: Lippincott Williams & Wilkins), 222–247.

Teasdale, N., and Simoneau, M. (2001). Attentional demands for postural control: the effects of aging and sensory reintegration. *Gait Posture* 14, 203–210. doi: 10.1016/S0966-6362(01)00134-5

van der Kooij, H., and Peterka, R. J. (2011). Non-linear stimulus-response behavior of the human stance control system is predicted by optimization of a system with sensory and motor noise. *J. Comput. Neurosci.* 30, 759–778. doi: 10.1007/s10827-010-0291-y

Wiesmeier, I. K., Dalin, D., and Maurer, C. (2015). Elderly use proprioception rather than visual and vestibular cues for postural motor control. *Front. Aging Neurosci.* 7:97. doi: 10.3389/fnagi.2015.00097

12

Age-Related Differences in Reorganization of Functional Connectivity for a Dual Task with Increasing Postural Destabilization

Cheng-Ya Huang [1, 2], Linda L. Lin [3] and Ing-Shiou Hwang [4, 5]*

[1] School and Graduate Institute of Physical Therapy, College of Medicine, National Taiwan University, Taipei, Taiwan,
[2] Physical Therapy Center, National Taiwan University Hospital, Taipei, Taiwan, [3] Institute of Physical Education, Health and Leisure Studies, National Cheng Kung University, Tainan, Taiwan, [4] Institute of Allied Health Sciences, College of Medicine, National Cheng Kung University, Tainan, Taiwan, [5] Department of Physical Therapy, College of Medicine, National Cheng Kung University, Tainan, Taiwan

*Correspondence:
Ing-Shiou Hwang
ishwang@mail.ncku.edu.tw

The aged brain may not make good use of central resources, so dual task performance may be degraded. From the brain connectome perspective, this study investigated dual task deficits of older adults that lead to task failure of a suprapostural motor task with increasing postural destabilization. Twelve younger (mean age: 25.3 years) and 12 older (mean age: 65.8 years) adults executed a designated force-matching task from a level-surface or a stabilometer board. Force-matching error, stance sway, and event-related potential (ERP) in the preparatory period were measured. The force-matching accuracy and the size of postural sway of the older adults tended to be more vulnerable to stance configuration than that of the young adults, although both groups consistently showed greater attentional investment on the postural task as sway regularity increased in the stabilometer condition. In terms of the synchronization likelihood (SL) of the ERP, both younger and older adults had net increases in the strengths of the functional connectivity in the whole brain and in the fronto-sensorimotor network in the stabilometer condition. Also, the SL in the fronto-sensorimotor network of the older adults was greater than that of the young adults for both stance conditions. However, unlike the young adults, the older adults did not exhibit concurrent deactivation of the functional connectivity of the left temporal-parietal-occipital network for postural-suprapostural task with increasing postural load. In addition, the older adults potentiated functional connectivity of the right prefrontal area to cope with concurrent force-matching with increasing postural load. In conclusion, despite a universal negative effect on brain volume conduction, our preliminary results showed that the older adults were still capable of increasing allocation of neural sources, particularly via compensatory recruitment of the right prefrontal loop, for concurrent force-matching under the challenging postural condition. Nevertheless, dual-task performance of the older adults tended to be more vulnerable to postural load than that of the younger adults, in relation to inferior neural economy or a slow adaptation process to stance destabilization for scant dissociation of control hubs in the temporal-parietal-occipital cortex.

Keywords: aging, EEG, dual task, functional connectivity, balance control

INTRODUCTION

Maintenance of postural balance requires attentional resources corresponding to the degree of postural threat (Remaud et al., 2012). Postural response requires complexity and numerous micro-adjustments, and stable bilateral stance is principally regulated by an automatic process using brainstem synergy (Honeycutt et al., 2009). Increasing postural destabilization shifts postural control to a more controlled process involving the frontal and cortical-basal ganglia loop (Jacobs and Horak, 2007; Boisgontier et al., 2013). Due to the additional attentional investment, postural response becomes more regular in the controlled process (Donker et al., 2007; Stins et al., 2009). Central resource allocation of a postural-suprapostural dual-task is an elaborate trade-off, flexibly depending on response compatibility of the two subtasks. Addition of a secondary task (or suprapostural task; Mitra and Fraizer, 2004) to a postural task does not necessarily result in dual-task degradation due to resource competition (Chen and Stoffregen, 2012; Stoffregen, 2016); instead, postural response can be integrated with suprapostural activity to facilitate suprapostural performance (Stoffregen et al., 1999; Prado et al., 2007). On the other hand, although a great number of the studies conducted on dual tasks have employed two cognitive tasks, very few neuroimaging studies have focused on postural-suprapostural dual tasks because of methodological constraints. With the event-related potential (ERP) of scalp electroencephalogram (EEG), Huang and Hwang (2013) reported that the amplitudes of the N1 and P2 waves in the preparation period prior to executing a secondary motor task varied with task loads of the postural and suprapostural tasks, respectively. The N1 amplitude reflected anticipatory arousal and postural response preceding the force-matching (Adkin et al., 2008; Mochizuki et al., 2008; Sibley et al., 2010; Huang et al., 2014). An increasing N1 amplitude in the sensorimotor and parietal areas implies more attentive control required for postural destabilization (Huang and Hwang, 2013; Little and Woollacott, 2015). On the other hand, P2 amplitude related to neural resource for visuomotor processing of the subsequent force-matching event, with a greater P2 amplitude associated with a less task load of force-matching (Huang and Hwang, 2013; Hwang and Huang, 2016).

In older adults, the shrinkage of a wide range of cortical areas causes evolving dysfunction of a dual task (Fernandes et al., 2006; Hartley et al., 2011). Degeneration of the frontal-parietal network specifically impairs executive processes keyed to dual tasking, such as response inhibition, task switching (Cole et al., 2013), and selective attention to relevant information (Mozolic et al., 2011). Age-related dual task deficits also manifest with a resource ceiling (Geerligs et al., 2014) and compensatory recruitment of additional brain resources (Hartley et al., 2011; Boisgontier et al.,

2013), especially when the dual task places high demands on those resources. Behavioral studies have shown that postural destabilization can multiply the dual task cost for the elderly of a postural-suprapostural task. Past researches employing a choice reaction time task (Shumway-Cook and Woollacott, 2000) and digit 2-back task (Rapp et al., 2006; Doumas et al., 2008) highlighted age-related differences in suprapostural performance by increasing stance instability rather than degrading visual stimulation of the suprapostural task. In effect, the brain's residual capacity wanes with aging, which causes negative postural penetrability to suprapostural processing. Hence, older adults often adopt a postural prioritization strategy to keep attentional resources on the postural task (Lacour et al., 2008; Liston et al., 2014). However, behavioral data that elucidate the neural correlates of resource allocation in older adults during a postural-suprapostural task are very limited. Although, neural evidence of age-related deficits has been extensively sought using classic dual tasks, the findings up to date cannot be directly applied to postural-suprapostural dual tasks on account of issues of response compatibility (Salo et al., 2015). For instance, the task quality of a suprapostural motor task such as juggling or tray-carrying takes advantage of stance stability (Balasubramaniam et al., 2000; Wulf et al., 2004; McNevin et al., 2013), whereas parallel loading of two cognitive tasks always causes mutual interference. To our knowledge, no studies have investigated alterations in information transfer for a postural-suprapostural task performed by older adults, despite the degeneration of the white matter integrity of the brain with aging (Furst and Fellgiebel, 2011; de Groot et al., 2016). Hence, it is worthwhile to characterize the differences in the functional connectivity of the frontal/prefrontal areas to other cortical regions [such as the parietal (Gontier et al., 2007) and premotor areas (Marois et al., 2006)] of young and older adults during a postural-suprapostural task.

A challenging postural set-up is a sensitive way to highlight age-related differences in a postural-suprapostural task. To explore the underlying neural mechanisms of dual-task interference of a postural-suprapostural task, we investigated age effect on ERP dynamics for force-matching from the level-surface to stabilometer stances during the preparatory period of the particular dual task. Defined as the time window between the execution beep and onset of the force-matching act, the preparatory period consists of posture-dependent N1 and suprapostural-dependent P2 waves that encrypt cognitive processing of pre-movement stance regulation, task switching from the posture subtask to supraposture subtask, and planning of the subsequent force-matching act (Huang and Hwang, 2013; Huang et al., 2014; Hwang and Huang, 2016). For the young healthy adults, a postural-suprapostural task with increasing postural instability caused reorganization of functional connectivity in the preparatory period with anterior shift of processing resources and dissociation of control hubs in the parietal-occipital cortex (Huang et al., 2016). Within the brain connectome context, this study aimed to extend on previous work by exploring differences in the component amplitudes (N1 and P2) and functional connectivity of the ERP in young and older adults during the performance of a

---

Abbreviations: NFE, normalized force error; RT, reaction time; SampEn, sample entropy; AMF_RMS, root mean square value of ankle fluctuation movements; AMF_SampEn, sample entropy of ankle fluctuation movements; GF, global frontal; SM, sensorimotor; PO, parietal-occipital; SL, synchronization likelihood; NBS, network-based statistics; FSM, fronto-sensorimotor; TPO, temporal-parietal-occipital.

suprapostural motor task with increasing postural challenge. This study hypothesized that, with increasing postural load, young adults would exhibit smaller changes than older adults in the component amplitudes of ERP (N1 and P2) and functional connectivity, especially those for the fronto-parietal network in the preparatory period. We also hypothesized that topological reorganization of functional connectivity due to increasing postural load would differ in the two populations.

MATERIALS AND METHODS

Subjects

Twelve young healthy adults (5 female and 7 male, age: 25.25 ± 1.25 years, range 21–33 years) and 12 older healthy adults (5 female and 7 male, age: 65.83 ± 1.01 years, range: 61–73 years) participated in this study. Subjects were volunteers from the local community and university campus who responded to a poster or a network advertisement. All of the participants were right-handed and had no history of neurological or musculoskeletal diagnoses. The older adults in this study, who had regular exercise habits, had experienced no falls in the previous 6 months. They participated in the postural-suprapostural experiment after signing personal consent forms approved by the local ethics committee (University Hospital, National Cheng Kung University, Taiwan).

Procedures

Before the main experiment, each participant was instructed to stand on a stabilometer in a shoulder-width stance with their arms hanging by their sides. The stabilometer was a wooden platform (50 × 69 cm) with a curved base (height: 18.5 cm). When the platform of the stabilometer was in the horizontal position, the midline of the platform (34.5 cm from the front/rear edge) passed through the anterior aspect of the participant's bilateral lateral malleolus. The positions of the participant's feet were used in the following experiment. Then the maximal angle of anterior tilt was determined from the readings of an electrogoniometer (Model SG110, Biometrics Ltd., UK; output accuracy: 1 mv = 0.09 degrees) on the ankle joint as the participants tilted the stabilometer with maximum plantarflexion of the ankle joint. In addition, we determined the force of each participant's maximum voluntary contraction (MVC) from three attempts of the right thumb-index precision grip during quiet upright stance. The stabilometer is commonly used to train balance in clinics and provides postural challenge for single postural task (Wulf et al., 2001; McNevin et al., 2003; Chiviacowsky et al., 2010) and postural-suprapostural dual-task in the laboratories (Wulf et al., 2003; Huang et al., 2014, 2016; Hwang and Huang, 2016). Therefore, we used the stabilometer to produce postural destabilization in this study.

The formal experiment required the participants to conduct a dual task (suprapostural force-matching and postural tasks) with on-line visual feedback under two different randomized stance conditions (level-surface vs. stabilometer). A monitor that displayed force output, ankle movement, and the target signals was placed 60 cm in front of the subject at eye-level. The subject conducted a thumb-index precision grip to couple a target line of 50% MVC force (pre-determined in the experiment) and concurrently maintained a stable upright stance with minimal ankle movement on a wooden level surface or a tilted stabilometer. Participants were not told to prioritize either task, and they were instructed to perform both postural and force-matching tasks as well as possible. The stabilometer produced less postural disturbance than was used in our previous studies (Hwang and Huang, 2016) because the balance capacity of the elderly participants was poorer than that of the young adults. The postural task in the level-surface and stabilometer conditions required the participants to couple the ankle joint angle derived from the readings of the electrogoniometer to the target line, based on visual feedback. The target lines for the postural task in the level-surface and stabilometer conditions were set at the horizontal surface and 50% of the maximal anterior tilt, respectively (**Figure 1A**). The postural tasks are known as postural tasks of visual internal focus (Huang et al., 2014), with which the participants should control upright stance with ankle angular displacement (or an internal aspect of body movement). Utilization of an internal focus for a postural task will interfere with postural automatic processes, especially when difficulty is added to stance control in a dual task condition for the elderly (Chiviacowsky et al., 2010). To minimize the potential visual load during the concurrent tasking, the target signals for posture and force-matching were carefully scaled at the same vertical position of the monitor for each participant (**Figure 1A**). We fully understood that the relative task difficulty of the postural and suprapostural tasks was a critical determinant of the reciprocal effect of the postural-suprapostural task. An earlier pilot experiment had shown that the present dual task setup would not significantly degrade the force-matching accuracy of the young adults between the level-surface and stabilometer conditions (Hung et al., 2016). In this particular dual task design, stance destabilization was expected to produce a decline in force-matching performance due to increasing postural threat (stabilometer vs. level-surface) in the older participants (Boisgontier et al., 2013). With this design, we were able to examine the age effect on the compensatory mechanisms underlying perseverance of quality of the secondary motor task when balance contexts varied.

Execution of the suprapostural force-matching in an experimental trial was first cued by a warning signal (an 800 Hz tone lasting for 100 ms). Upon hearing an executive tone (a 500 Hz tone lasting for 100 ms), the participants then started a quick thumb-index precision grip (force impulse duration <0.5 s) to couple instantaneously the peak precision-grip force with the force target on the monitor. The warning-executive signal pairs were randomly presented at different intervals of 1.5, 1.75, 2, 2.25, 2.5, 2.75, or 3 s (**Figure 1B**). The interval between the end of the executive tone and the beginning of the next warning tone was 3.5 s. There were a total of 14 warning-executive signal pairs in an experimental trial (80 s per trial) and six experimental trials of the postural-motor dual task for each stance condition. Both young and older subjects were allowed for a fixed rest duration between trials (1 min) to minimize fatigue effect.

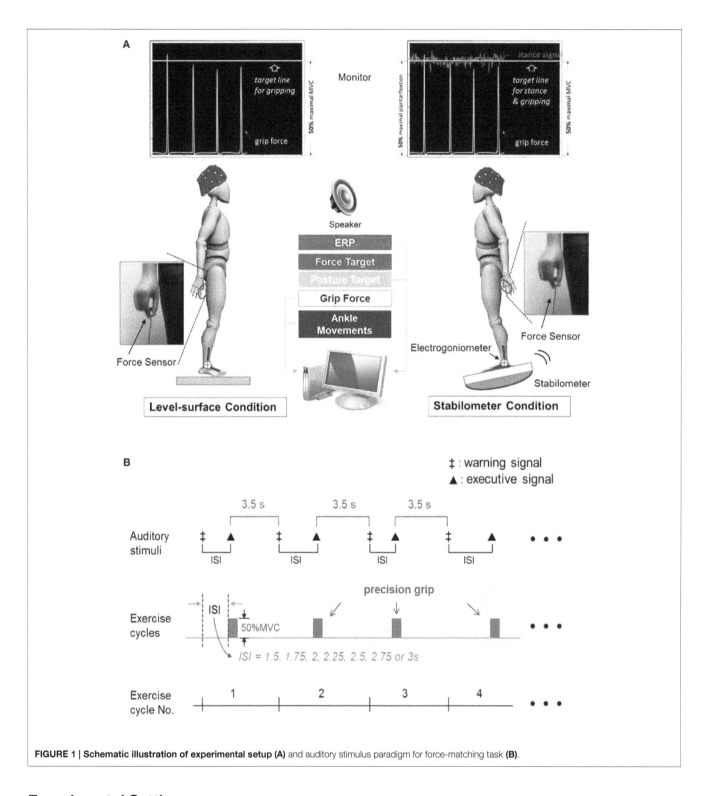

FIGURE 1 | Schematic illustration of experimental setup (A) and auditory stimulus paradigm for force-matching task (B).

Experimental Setting

A 40-channel NuAmps amplifier (NeuroScan Inc., EI Paso, TX, USA) with Ag-AgCl scalp electrodes was used to record scalp voltage fluctuations from different 30 EEG channels (Fp$_{1/2}$, F$_z$, F$_{3/4}$, F$_{7/8}$, FT$_{7/8}$, FC$_z$, FC$_{3/4}$, C$_z$, C$_{3/4}$, CP$_z$, CP$_{3/4}$, P$_z$, P$_{3/4}$, T$_{3/4}$, T$_{5/6}$, TP$_{7/8}$, O$_z$, and O$_{1/2}$). The ground electrode was placed

along the midline ahead of F$_z$. Electrodes placed above the arch of the left eyebrow and below the eye were used to monitor eye movements and blinks. The impedances of all the electrodes were below 5 kΩ and were referenced to linked mastoids of both sides. The EEG data was recorded with a band-pass filter set at 0.1–100 Hz and with a sampling rate of 1 kHz. The electrogoniometer was attached to the dominant ankle joint to record the angular motion of the ankle joint. The electrogoniometer consisted of two sensors. One sensor was placed at the dorsum of the right foot between the second and third metatarsal heads, and the other sensor was fastened along the midline of the middle third of the anterior aspect of lower leg. A load cell (15-mm diameter × 10-mm thickness, net weight = 7 g; Model: LCS, Nippon Tokushu Sokki Co., Japan) on the right thumb was used to record the level of force-matching. All physiological data were synchronized and digitized at a sampling rate of 1 kHz in LabVIEW software (National Instruments, Austin, TX, USA).

Data Analyses
Behavior Data
Normalized force error (NFE) of force-matching was used to represent suprapostural performance in the present study. Force-matching error was represented in terms of NFE, or $\frac{|TF-PGF|}{TF} \times 100\%$ (PGF: peak grip force; TF: target force; **Figure 2**). The NFEs of all force-matching events were averaged across trials for each subject in the level-surface and stabilometer conditions. The reaction time (RT) of force-matching was denoted as the timing interval between the executive tone and the onset of grip force. Postural performance was characterized with the fluctuation properties of ankle movement during the interval between the warning signal and the onset of force pulse. We applied root mean square (RMS) and sample entropy (SampEn) to assess the amplitude and complexity of the ankle movement fluctuations (AMF_RMS and AMF_SampEn) after resampling the kinematic data to 125 Hz. SampEn is an appropriate entropy measure for reliably quantifying the variability structure of biological data with a short

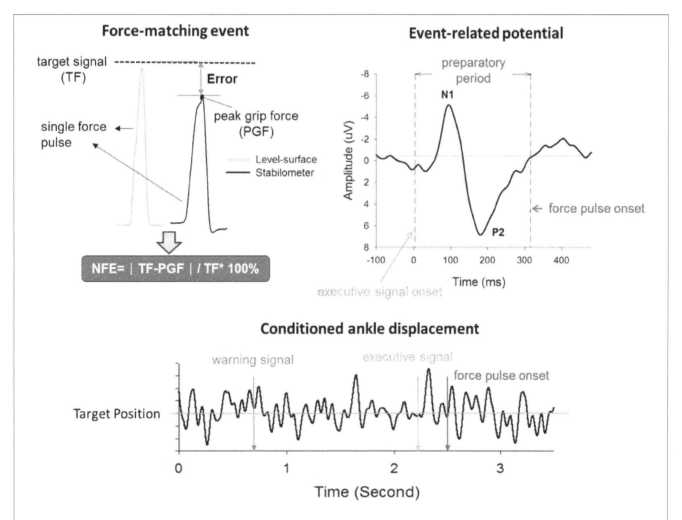

FIGURE 2 | Real-time display of precision grip force, ankle displacement, and target signals for concurrent force-matching and postural tasks. To reduce the visual load during the experiment, the target signals of both postural and force-matching tasks were displayed in an identical position on the monitor, by separate scale-tuning of the manual force target and postural target. Force-matching performance was assessed with normalized force error (NFE). The event-related potential (ERP) associated with force-matching was registered with scalp electroencephalography. ERP between the executive tone and the onset of the force-impulse profile was denoted as the preparatory period. ERP in this period primarily contained N1 and P2 components. The ankle displacement after conditioning with a low-pass filter is labeled by three critical events (warning signal, executive tone, and force-impulse onset). TF, target force; PGF, peak grip force.

length (Yentes et al., 2013). The mathematical formula for SampEn was

$$SampEn\,(m, r, N) = -\log(\frac{\sum_{i=1}^{N-m} A_i}{\sum_{i=1}^{N-m} B_i})$$

where $r = 15\%$ of the standard deviation of the ankle movement fluctuations, m is the length of the template ($m = 3$), and N is the number of data points in the time series. Ai is the number of matches of the ith template of length $m + 1$ data points, and Bi is the number of matches of the ith template of length m data points. A SampEn close to 0 represents greater periodicity (or regularity), while a value near 2 represents higher complexity (or irregularity). Higher regularity (or lower SampEn value) of postural sway represents the more attentional focus being paid to postural control, and vice versa (Donker et al., 2007; Borg and Laxåback, 2010; Kuczyński et al., 2011).

Component Amplitudes and Functional Connectivity of Multi-Channel ERP

ERP data was analyzed off-line with the NeuroScan 4.3 software program (NeuroScan Inc., EI Paso, TX, USA). Prior to ERP quantitative analysis, third-order trend correction and eye movement correction protocols were applied to the entire set of recorded data to remove the DC shift and eye movement artifacts. The eye movement artifacts were removed from the EEG using regression analysis (Semlitsch et al., 1986), and the number of eye blinks in each trial was roughly 10–15 across subjects. After eye movement was removed, the EEG data were conditioned with a low-pass filter (40 Hz/48 dB roll-off), and then the conditioned EEG data were segmented into epochs of 700 ms, including 100 ms before the onset of each execution signal. Epochs were all baseline-corrected at the pre-stimulus interval. Poor epochs, such as those affected by excessive drift or eye blinks, were discarded by visual inspection (rejection rate of inappropriate trials: <8%). The remaining artifact-free epochs were averaged for an experimental trial in the level-surface and stabilometer conditions, and then the ERP data were also grouped according to a two-factor design (population: the young and older adults; postural task: level-surface and stabilometer stances).

As postural-suprapostural behaviors involve information mastery dependent upon the fronto-motor-parietal network (Huang and Hwang, 2013), we expected age-related differences in regional activity of ERP due to increasing difficulty of the postural subtask of the dual task in the global frontal (GF: Fp_1, Fp_2, F_3, F_z, F_4, F_7, and F_8), sensorimotor (SM: C_3, C_z, C_4, CP_3, CP_z, and CP_4), and parietal-occipital (PO: P_3, P_z, P_4, O_1, O_z, and O_2) areas for the level-surface and stabilometer conditions. The N1 and P2 amplitudes were quantified as the peak amplitude in two separate time windows (80–150 ms, 150–240 ms after executive signal onset). The ERP of each electrode contained N1 and P2 components, which were selectively averaged to obtain amplitudes of the N1 and N2 of the above-mentioned areas. For instance, amplitudes of N1 and P2 recorded from the electrodes of the Fp_1, Fp_2, F_3, F_z, F_4, F_7, and F_8 were averaged to represent the size of N1 and P2 of the global frontal area.

Based on multi-channel ERP signal, we also quantified statistical interdependencies of non-stationary ERP in the preparatory period with one of the most popular approaches, synchronization likelihood (SL). The SL measures the degrees of linear and non-linear dimensions of EEG/MEG coupling within cortical networks (Leistedt et al., 2009; Boersma et al., 2011). Theoretically, SL takes into account the recurrences of state space vectors occurring at the same moment that are converted from two time-series of interest (Stam et al., 2005). SL can sensitively detect slight variations in the coupling strength for a fine time scale (Stam and van Dijk, 2002), which is appropriate for resolve ERP synchronization patterns in a short period. An SL close to 0 indicates no coupling; an SL of 1 indicates complete coupling. For brevity, detailed descriptions of SL calculation (Stam and van Dijk, 2002; Stam et al., 2003) and parameter settings (Montez et al., 2006) can be found in previous works. Computation of the SL across all pairs of ERP data of the channels in the preparatory phase (the time interval between the executive tone and the force-matching onset) produced a square 30×30 SL adjacent matrix. Each entry in the SL adjacent matrix represented the connectivity strength within the functional networks. For each participant, the overall SL adjacent matrix from all experimental trials in the level-surface or stabilometer condition was averaged. SL thresholds from 0.1 to 0.9 were selected to build functional connectomes of different connection strengths. The SL adjacent matrix was rescaled with the proportion of strongest weights, such that all other weights below a given threshold (including SL on the main diagonal) were set to 0. Namely, the selection of the SL threshold of 0.1 merely accounted for the strongest 10% of the weights in the SL adjacent matrix (or functional connectivity in the functional connectome). SL was calculated with the functions of HERMES for Matlab (Niso et al., 2013). The mean value of SL for all the electrode pairs was defined as SL_All. The mean values of SL that connected to the specified areas, the fronto-sensorimotor (SL_FSM), and parietal-occipital (SL_PO) areas, were determined for the level-surface and stabilometer conditions.

Statistical Analyses

The purpose of this study was to examine the neural mechanisms underlying age and stance effects on postural-suprapostural performance. The current experimental design focused on the neural mechanisms responsible for differential stance effects on force-matching accuracy between young and older adults. Two way repeated measures ANOVA with population (young and older) and postural load (level-surface and stabilometer) were used to examine the significance of differences in behavior parameters (NFE, RT, AMF_RMS, and AMF_SampEn), and the mean SL of the areas of interest (SL_All, SL_FSM, and SL_PO) across different threshold values. The level of significance of the above-mentioned statistical analyses was set at $p = 0.05$. The significance of the *post-hoc* test for stance and age effects was $p = 0.0125$ using the Bonferroni correction. Moreover, network-based statistics (NBS) were performed to vigorously identify stance-related changes in the functional connectivity of all the node pairs for the young and older groups. For each group, paired *t*-tests were independently performed at each synchronization value, and t-statistics larger than an uncorrected threshold of $t_{(13)}$ = 3.012 ($p = 0.005$) were extracted into a set of supra-threshold connections. Then we identified all connected components in the adjacency matrix of supra-threshold links and saved the number of links. A permutation test was performed 5,000 times to estimate the null distribution of the maximal component size, and the corrected p-value was calculated as the proportion of permutations for which the most connected components consisted of two or more links. Methodological details of NBS are documented in Zalesky et al. (2010). The age effect on the topological distribution of significant stance-related differences in synchronization value were examined with visual inspection. Statistical analyses were performed in Matlab (Mathworks Inc. Natick, MA, USA) and SPSS v.19.0 (SPSS Inc. Chicago, IL, USA). All data are presented as mean ± standard error.

RESULTS

Behavior Performance

Figure 3 shows means and standard errors of task performance of force-matching and postural response for young and older groups under the level-surface and stabilometer conditions. The ANOVA results revealed that NFE was subject to both stance and age effects [stance: $F_{(1, 22)} = 10.36$, $p = 0.004$; age: $F_{(1, 22)} = 4.60$, $p = 0.043$; stance × age: $F_{(1, 22)} = 3.04$, $p = 0.095$]. On account of a marginal interaction effect, we continued the *post-hoc* analysis which indicated that NFE of the older group was more susceptible to stance configuration and the older adults performed worse force-matching in the stabilometer condition than in the level-surface condition ($p = 0.002$). In contrast, NFE of the young group was not affected by stance configuration ($p = 0.307$). The

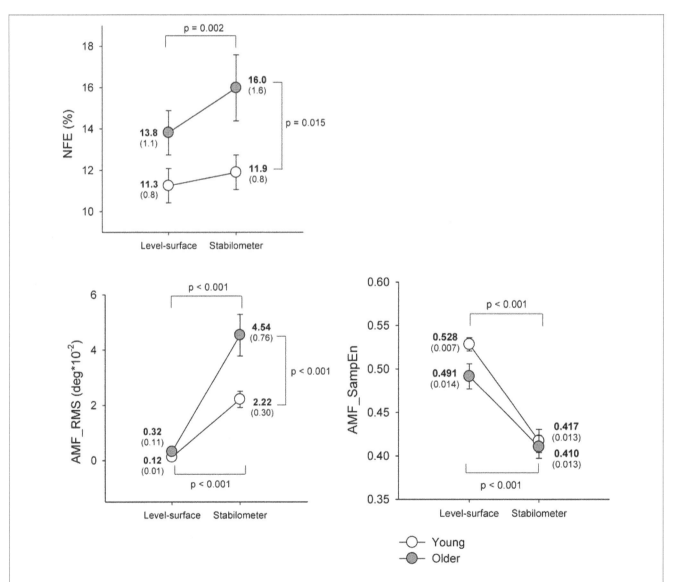

FIGURE 3 | Means and standard errors of force-matching and postural variables for the concurrent force-matching and postural tasks under the level-surface and stabilometer conditions for young and older populations. NFE, normalized force error; AMF_RMS, root mean square value of ankle fluctuation movements; AMF_SampEn, sample entropy of ankle fluctuation movements.

RT of the force-matching was not age dependent [$F_{(1, 22)} = 1.57$, $p = 0.223$], but varied with stance pattern [$F_{(1, 22)} = 4.55$, $p = 0.044$] without a significant interaction [$F_{(1, 22)} = 1.06$, $p = 0.315$; Young: level-surface $= 307.2 \pm 7.8$ ms, stabilometer: 326.4 ± 5.6 ms; Older: level-surface $= 303.0 \pm 8.3$ ms, stabilometer: 308.9 ± 4.5 ms]. In terms of RMS, the magnitude of ankle movement fluctuations was also a function of age and stance configuration [stance: $F_{(1, 22)} = 67.22$, $p < 0.001$; age: $F_{(1, 22)} = 8.50$, $p = 0.008$; stance $\times$ age: $F_{(1, 22)} = 7.63$, $p = 0.011$]. Post-hoc analysis revealed that both the young and the older adults exhibited greater ankle movement fluctuations during the stabilometer stance than during surface stance ($p < 0.001$). In particular, the ankle movement fluctuations of the older adults were greater than those of the young adults in the stabilometer condition ($p < 0.001$). In addition, irregularity of the ankle movement fluctuations was subject to stance configuration rather than to age effect [stance: $F_{(1, 22)} = 73.46$, $p < 0.001$; age: $F_{(1, 22)} = 2.62$, $p = 0.120$; stance $\times$ age: $F_{(1, 22)} = 1.79$, $p = 0.125$]. Increases in stance difficulty resulted in a consistently lower AMF_SampEn (more regularity) of the ankle movement fluctuations in the young and older groups ($p < 0.001$).

ERP Component Amplitude

Figure 4 show pooled ERP profiles of the each electrode of the young and older adults in the level-surface and stabilometer conditions. Stance-related differences in the ERP profiles were evident in the anterior portions of the cortex, irrespective of the populations. The N1 amplitude in the GF and SM areas varied significantly with age [GF: $F_{(1, 22)} = 8.14$, $p = 0.009$; SM: $F_{(1, 22)} = 5.54$, $p = 0.028$], but not with stance [GF: $F_{(1, 22)} = 2.74$, $p = 0.112$; SM: $F_{(1, 22)} = 0.31$, $p = 0.582$] or interaction effects [GF: $F_{(1, 22)} = 0.01$, $p = 0.919$; SM: $F_{(1, 22)} = 0.15$, $p = 0.699$]. However, N1 amplitude of the PO areas did not significantly vary with stance and age effects [stance: $F_{(1, 22)} = 0.03$, $p = 0.860$; age: $F_{(1, 22)} = 1.66$, $p = 0.211$; stance $\times$ age: $F_{(1, 22)} = 0.44$, $p = 0.513$]. In contrast, the P2 amplitudes in the GF, SM, and PO areas were all dependent on stance configuration [GF: $F_{(1, 22)} = 12.32$, $p = 0.002$; SM: $F_{(1, 22)} = 13.37$, $p = 0.001$; PO: $F_{(1, 22)} = 6.03$, $p = 0.022$], rather than on age [GF: $F_{(1, 22)} = 0.17$, $p = 0.683$; SM: $F_{(1, 22)} = 0.71$, $p = 0.408$; PO: $F_{(1, 22)} = 2.30$, $p = 0.143$] or interaction effects [GF: $F_{(1, 22)} = 0.79$, $p = 0.382$; SM: $F_{(1, 22)} = 0.34$, $p = 0.566$; PO: $F_{(1, 22)} = 0.05$, $p = 0.818$; **Figure 5**].

Functional Connectivity of ERP in the Preparatory Phase

Figure 6 presents the mean SL (SL_All) of all electrode pairs in the level-surface and stabilometer conditions and stance-related change in SL (ΔSL_All) as a function of threshold value. For the both groups, SL_All tended to be larger in the stabilometer condition than in the level-surface condition. **Table 1** shows the detailed results of ANOVA for age and stance effects on SL_All across different thresholds. For thresholds of 0.1 and 0.2, main effects of stance and age on SL_All were not significant ($p > 0.05$). For thresholds of 0.3–0.9, SL_All was subject to a main effect of stance, and SL was significantly larger in stabilometer condition than in the level-surface condition ($p < 0.05$). **Figure 7A** presents the mean SL of the electrode pairs

in the fronto-sensorimotor network (SL_FSM) for the level-surface and stabilometer conditions and stance-related change in SL (ΔSL_FSM) as a function of threshold value. **Table 2** summarizes the ANOVA results for age and stance effects on SL_FSM across different thresholds. For all threshold values, SL_FSM varied with age and stance configuration ($p < 0.05$), except for a marginal effect of age for a threshold setting of 0.2. That was, the SL_FSM of the young and older adults increased in the stabilometer condition for all threshold values ($p < 0.006$), and the older adults exhibited a larger SL_FSM than the young adults in the level-surface and stabilometer conditions ($p < 0.05$). The most remarkable difference in SL modulation for stance difficulty increment between the young and older groups was in the PO area (**Figure 7B**). **Table 3** summarizes the ANOVA results for age and stance effects on SL_PO across different thresholds. For threshold values of 0.2–0.4, SL_PO was significantly subject to the interaction effect of age and stance configuration ($p < 0.05$). For the young adults, post-hoc analysis further showed that SL_PO in the stabilometer condition was smaller than that in the level-surface condition ($p < 0.0125$). Notably, such a stance-dependent decline in SL_PO at lower threshold value was not present in the older group ($p > 0.0125$). Interaction effect of age and stance configuration on SL_PO for the threshold values of 0.8 and 0.9 was also significant ($p < 0.05$). Particularly at the threshold value of 0.9, post-hoc analysis revealed that the SL_PO for the older adults potentiated with increasing postural load ($p = 0.009$), but not the SL_PO of the young adults ($p > 0.05$). The stance-related modulations of the SL_PO between the young and older adults were opposite for the selection of threshold value (**Figure 7B**).

The significance of spatial distribution change in SL (threshold value = 0.3) with respect to stance configuration was examined with NBS. The threshold was selected to contrast the alterations in the brain wiring diagram at relatively stronger functional connectivity. For the strongest SL with thresholds set at 0.1 and 0.2, the stance-dependent difference in SL variables was not always evident between the young and older adults (**Tables 1–3**). **Figure 8** presents the pooled adjacent matrix of SL of preparatory ERP in the level-surface and stabilometer conditions for the young and older groups (threshold value = 0.3). The SL difference of all electrode pairs between the level-surface and stabilometer conditions was labeled with the adjacent matrix of t-values ($t > 1.771$: stabilometer SL > level-surface SL, $p < 0.05$; $t < -1.771$: level-surface SL > stabilometer SL, $p < 0.05$; **Figure 9**, upper row). The results of NBS indicated that changes in stance configuration significantly altered the brain functional connectivity in both groups ($p = 0.0002$, corrected; **Figure 9**, lower row). In addition, there were notable topological differences in dual task organization of supra-threshold connectivity for the young and older adults to cope with increasing postural load. The young adults in the stabilometer condition exhibited a global potentiation of supra-threshold connectivity in the fronto-sensorimotor cortex and reduction in supra-threshold connectivity between the left temporal area and the parietal-occipital cortex, as compared with the level-surface condition. In contrast, when postural load increased, the older adults enhanced supra-threshold

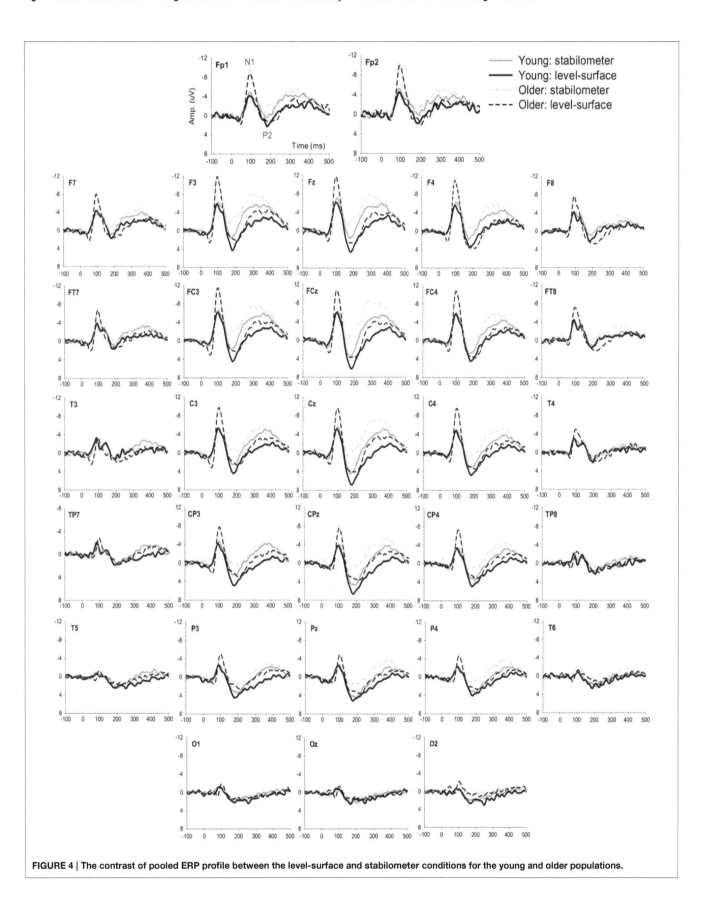

FIGURE 4 | The contrast of pooled ERP profile between the level-surface and stabilometer conditions for the young and older populations.

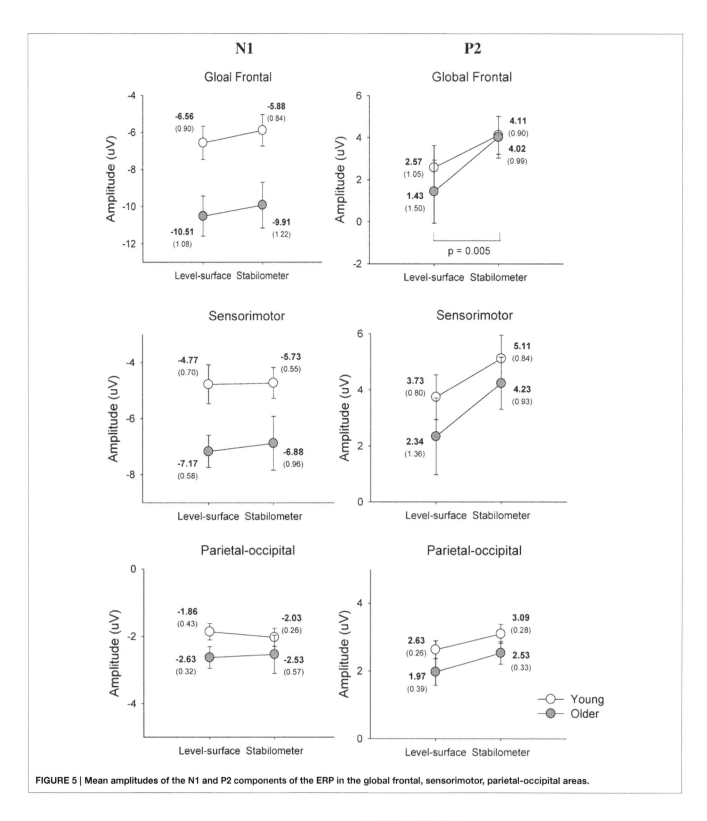

FIGURE 5 | Mean amplitudes of the N1 and P2 components of the ERP in the global frontal, sensorimotor, parietal-occipital areas.

connectivity in the fronto-sensorimotor cortex of the bilateral hemispheres and between the frontal and right prefrontal cortex. No significant suppression of supra-threshold connectivity was noted for conducting force-matching with increasing postural load in the older group.

DISCUSSION

The present postural-supraposatural task produced an expected outcome: the suprapostural performance and the size of postural sway of the older adults were more vulnerable to increasing

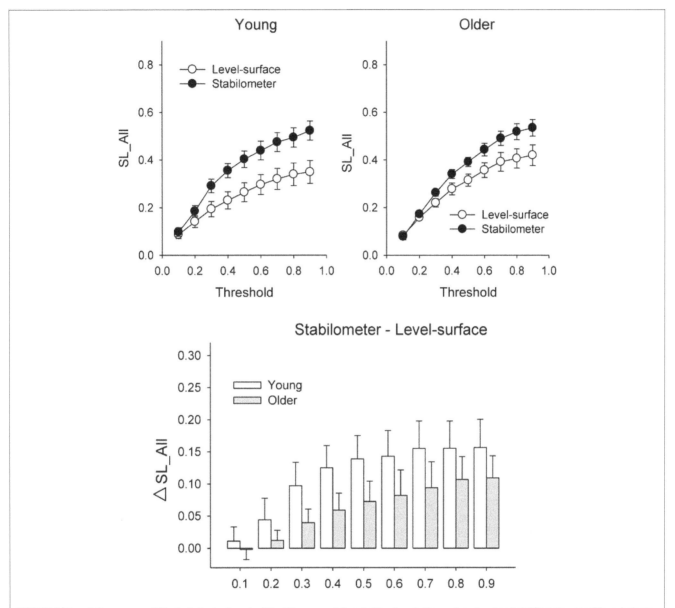

FIGURE 6 | Population means of SL of all electrode pairs (SL_All) across all threshold values in the surface-level and stabilometer conditions (refer to Table 1). The stance-related differences in SL (stabilometer—level-surface) across various threshold values are highlighted for the young and older groups in the lower plot. At the threshold values of 0.3–0.9, there was a significant stance effect on SL_All, with increasing SL_All for the stabilometer condition for young and older adults.

postural load than those of the young adults (**Figure 3**). Contrary to the idea of attention withdrawal from the postural task to facilitate supraposture performance (Donker et al., 2007; Kuczyński et al., 2011), additional investment of neural resource on the postural task was necessary to prepare for concurrent force-matching with increasing postural load, in light of increased AMF_RMS and decreased AMF_SampEn for the young and older adults in the stabilometer condition. Our behavior results imply distinct brain mechanisms to cope with posture destabilization in young and older adults during a postural-suprapostural dual task. In terms of ERP connectivity analysis, the aged brain exhibited compensatory recruitment of the right prefrontal network and lack of sufficient neural

economy for task switching from a postural task to a secondary force-matching act, when postural load multiplied during the stabilometer stance.

Increase in the Strength of Functional Connectivity for Postural Destabilization

The primary finding of this study was that the increase in postural load from level-surface to stabilometer stances is associated with a marked increase in global functional connectivity (SL_All) for the young and older adults (**Figure 6**, **Table 1**). Generally speaking, our data revealed the feasibility of utilizing central residual capacity for the healthy elderly to deal with stance instability during a postural-suprapostural task.

TABLE 1 | Summary of ANOVA results for age and stance effects on synchronization likelihood of all the electrode pairs (SL_All).

Threshold	ANOVA statistics	Post-hoc analysis (Stance effect)
0.1	Stance: $F_{(1, 22)} = 0.10$, $p = 0.756$; Age: $F_{(1, 22)} = 0.37$, $p = 0.551$; Stance × Age: $F_{(1, 22)} = 0.20$, $p = 0.659$	N.S.
0.2	Stance: $F_{(1, 22)} = 2.64$, $p = 0.118$; Age: $F_{(1, 22)} = 0.08$, $p = 0.784$; Stance × Age: $F_{(1, 22)} = 0.32$, $p = 0.575$	N.S.
0.3	Stance: $F_{(1, 22)} = 11.04$, $p = 0.003$; Age: $F_{(1, 22)} = 0.02$, $p = 0.892$; Stance × Age: $F_{(1,22)} = 0.93$, $p = 0.332$	–
0.4	Stance: $F_{(1, 22)} = 18.40$, $p < 0.001$; Age: $F_{(1, 22)} = 0.44$, $p = 0.515$; Stance × Age: $F_{(1, 22)} = 1.05$, $p = 0.317$	–
0.5	Stance: $F_{(1, 22)} = 18.19$, $p < 0.001$; Age: $F_{(1, 22)} = 0.32$, $p = 0.579$; Stance × Age: $F_{(1, 22)} = 0.38$, $p = 0.544$	–
0.6	Stance: $F_{(1, 22)} = 16.69$, $p < 0.001$; Age: $F_{(1, 22)} = 0.85$, $p = 0.366$; Stance × Age: $F_{(1, 22)} = 0.00$, $p = 0.974$	–
0.7	Stance: $F_{(1, 22)} = 18.31$, $p < 0.001$; Age: $F_{(1, 22)} = 1.16$, $p = 0.294$; Stance × Age: $F_{(1, 22)} = 0.31$, $p = 0.584$	–
0.8	Stance: $F_{(1, 22)} = 23.16$, $p < 0.001$; Age: $F_{(1, 22)} = 0.13$, $p = 0.727$; Stance × Age: $F_{(1, 22)} = 1.05$, $p = 0.316$	–
0.9	Stance: $F_{(1, 22)} = 23.73$, $p < 0.001$; Age: $F_{(1, 22)} = 1.14$, $p = 0.296$; Stance × Age: $F_{(1, 22)} = 0.10$, $p = 0.753$	–

N.S., non-significance.
–, post-hoc analysis should not be processed due to non-significant interaction effect.

The whole fronto-parietal network is integrated to coordinate a postural-suprapostural task (Karim et al., 2013; Ferraye et al., 2014). On account of a stance-related increase in functional connectivity of the fronto-sensorimotor network (SL_FSM) for both the young and older adults (**Figure 7A**, **Table 2**), it was plausible that force-matching from stabilometer stance caused a shift to a state in which the frontal control predominated, linking to increase in attentional demand to posture stabilization. In fact, several previous studies reported a parallel enhancement of cortical recording from the frontal cortex and supplementary motor area following posture perturbation (Mihara et al., 2008; Fujita et al., 2016). Also, the stabilometer fluctuation movements aggravated externally-induced retinal image motion, so as to hampered precise visual target location (Sipp et al., 2013; Hülsdünker et al., 2015) and then enhance mid-frontal activity for action monitoring and error processing prior to force-matching (Mihara et al., 2008). The stance-dependent increases in SL_FSM also accounted for the unexpected lack of an increase in N1 amplitude in the stabilometer condition. Our previous work on a posture-motor task revealed that force-matching from unipedal stance led to a greater N1 amplitude than force-matching from bipedal stance (Huang and Hwang, 2013). Originated in the fronto-central region (Adkin et al., 2008), N1 amplitude reflects monitoring of the attentional states (Huang and Hwang, 2013; Huang et al., 2014) and sensory processing (Sibley et al., 2010) of postural perturbation in a postural-suprapostural task. The insignificant variation in N1 amplitude in this study may partly due to the use of a stabilometer of low curvature that did not produce as much stance instability as unipedal stance would have. Moreover, the most appealing explanation to reconcile the paradoxical finding is that a dual task may not necessarily alter regional activation, instead altering the interactions of the frontal/prefrontal areas with other cortical regions [such as parietal (Gontier et al., 2007) and premotor areas (Marois et al., 2006)]. Of note, the older adults exhibited a stronger SL_FSM than the young adults (**Figure 7A**, **Table 2**). Although, the older adults seemingly recruited more central resource in the fronto-sensorimotor network in the both stance conditions, yet it could not nicely explain why dual-task performance of the older adults tended to be more vulnerable to higher postural load.

Lack of Neural Economy in the Elderly

The interaction effect of age and stance configuration of SL_PO plays a critical role in age-dependent differences in dual-task performance with increasing postural load. The young adults showed surprising desynchronization of the PO network, in view of the decline in SL_PO with increasing postural load at the threshold values of 0.2, 0.3, and 0.4 (**Figure 7B**, **Table 3**). During concurrent execution of force-matching in the stabilometer condition, the young adults appeared to avoid division of attentional resources toward multisensory information by dissociating the neuro-anatomical implementation in the PO network. As stabilometer stance did not cause inferior force-matching performance in the young adults (**Figure 3**), the scenario suggests neural economy (Schubert, 2008) or adaptive resource sharing (Mitra and Fraizer, 2004), with which the young adults could minimize the dual-task cost to facilitate task switching for the subsequent force-matching event (Huang et al., 2016). In contrast, the older adults increased the weak functional connectivity (threshold value = 0.9) of the PO network in the stabilometer condition (**Figure 7B**, **Table 3**). The genesis of the relatively weak connectivity simply taxed a limited central resource from the aged brain, because there was no significant performance benefits associated with increasing postural load for the older adults (**Figure 3**).

Further supporting the notion of age-related deficits in neural economy for a postural-suprapostural task is the topology of the wiring diagram (**Figure 9**). The left temporal lobe is known to handle the timing of complex movements with auditory cues (Nakai et al., 2005). Previous fMRI studies revealed that the superior temporal sulcus and posterior middle temporal gyrus of the left hemisphere are more selective to body actions and actions performed on other objects, respectively (Jellema and Perrett, 2006; Assmus et al., 2007). Studies of the macaque monkey (Perrett et al., 1989; Jellema and Perrett, 2003) have shown the superior temporal sulcus to be modulated by body posture during target reaching. Hence, the functional connectivity of the left temporal-parietal-occipital network (TPO network) in a postural-suprapostural task might serve to identify the execution beep (distinguishing the tone from the warning signal) and integration of sensory information from the parietal cortex regarding body schema representation (Pellijeff et al.,

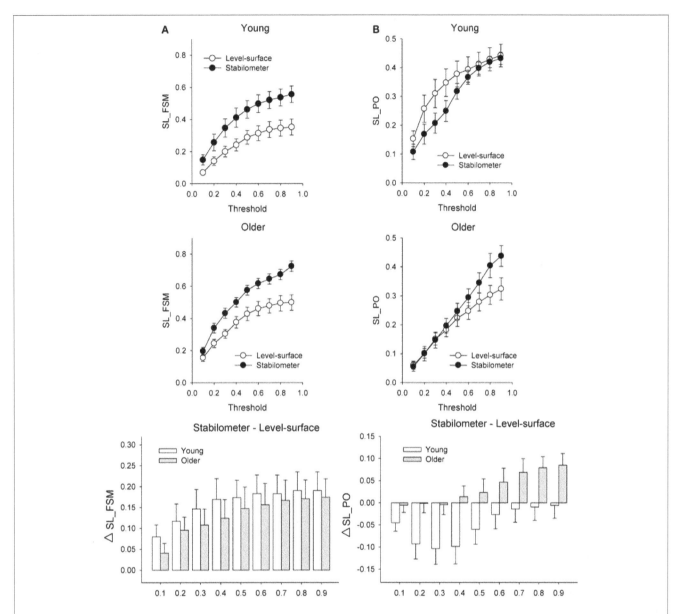

FIGURE 7 | Population means of SL of all electrode pairs in the fronto-sensorimotor (FSM, refer to Table 2) (A) and parietal-occipital (PO, refer to **Table 3**) **(B)** networks across all threshold values in the surface-level and stabilometer conditions. The stance-related differences in SL (stabilometer−level-surface) across various threshold values are highlighted for the young and older groups in the lowest plots. With increasing stance difficulty from level-surface to stabilometer, there were significant age and stance effects on SL_FSM for all threshold values, except that age effect on SL_FSM was marginally significant at the threshold value of 0.2.

2006) as well as stance fluctuations (Noppeney et al., 2005; Vangeneugden et al., 2011). For the young adults, multimodal sensory integration to detect postural instability using the TPO network was conditionally disengaged before force-matching. In that brief moment, postural control could be temporarily regulated by automatic responses using postural synergy in the midbrain (Jacobs and Horak, 2007). The suppression of information transfer in the left TPO network would augment resource availability upon retrieval of spatial information of the visual target for force-matching (Chelazzi et al., 1993; Kastner and Ungerleider, 2001), such as occurs in solving task conflicts (Schall et al., 2002; Schulz et al., 2011) and

facilitating task-switching from stabilometer stance to force-matching (Hwang and Huang, 2016) using frontal executive function. In fact, changes in P2 amplitude with respect to stance configuration also support the argument that the elderly paid less attention to force-matching preparation. In experiments of force-matching to couple a static or a dynamic target, P2 amplitude is inversely related to attentional focus on the visual target of the force-matching task (Huang and Hwang, 2013; Huang et al., 2014). Hence, greater P2 amplitude in the stabilometer condition (**Figure 5**, the right column) might indicate that the participants did not focus well on the force-matching event during posture challenge, especially in older adults.

TABLE 2 | Summary of ANOVA results for age and stance effects on synchronization likelihood of the electrode pairs in the fronto-sensorimotor area (SL_FSM).

Threshold	ANOVA statistics	Post-hoc analysis (stance effect)
0.1	Stance: $F_{(1, 22)} = 9.24$, $p = 0.006$; Age: $F_{(1, 22)} = 4.69$, $p = 0.041$; Stance × Age: $F_{(1, 22)} = 0.96$, $p = 0.338$	–
0.2	Stance: $F_{(1, 22)} = 14.19$, $p = 0.001$; Age: $F_{(1, 22)} = 4.09$, $p = 0.056$; Stance × Age: $F_{(1, 22)} = 0.14$, $p = 0.709$	–
0.3	Stance: $F_{(1, 22)} = 16.73$, $p < 0.001$; Age: $F_{(1, 22)} = 4.34$, $p = 0.049$; Stance × Age: $F_{(1, 22)} = 0.40$, $p = 0.532$	–
0.4	Stance: $F_{(1, 22)} = 17.92$, $p < 0.001$; Age: $F_{(1, 22)} = 5.49$, $p = 0.029$; Stance × Age: $F_{(1, 22)} = 0.00$, $p = 0.974$	–
0.5	Stance: $F_{(1, 22)} = 20.18$, $p < 0.001$; Age: $F_{(1, 22)} = 5.31$, $p = 0.031$; Stance × Age: $F_{(1, 22)} = 0.13$, $p = 0.719$	–
0.6	Stance: $F_{(1, 22)} = 21.57$, $p < 0.001$; Age: $F_{(1, 22)} = 5.17$, $p = 0.033$; Stance × Age: $F_{(1, 22)} = 0.00$, $p = 0.974$	–
0.7	Stance: $F_{(1, 22)} = 24.15$, $p < 0.001$; Age: $F_{(1, 22)} = 4.92$, $p = 0.037$; Stance × Age: $F_{(1, 22)} = 0.05$, $p = 0.823$	–
0.8	Stance: $F_{(1, 22)} = 28.09$, $p < 0.001$; Age: $F_{(1, 22)} = 5.49$, $p = 0.029$; Stance × Age: $F_{(1, 22)} = 0.08$, $p = 0.778$	–
0.9	Stance: $F_{(1, 22)} = 29.23$, $p < 0.001$; Age: $F_{(1, 22)} = 5.03$, $p = 0.035$; Stance × Age: $F_{(1, 22)} = 0.06$, $p = 0.813$	–

–, post-hoc analysis should not be processed due to non-significant interaction effect.

TABLE 3 | Summary of ANOVA results for age and stance effects on synchronization likelihood of the electrode pairs in the parietal-occipital area (SL_PO).

Threshold	ANOVA statistics	Post-hoc analysis (stance effect)
0.1	Stance: $F_{(1, 22)} = 3.40$, $p = 0.079$; Age: $F_{(1, 22)} = 5.70$, $p = 0.026$; Stance × Age: $F_{(1, 22)} = 2.16$, $p = 0.156$	–
0.2	Stance: $F_{(1, 22)} = 4.61$, $p = 0.043$; Age: $F_{(1, 22)} = 6.07$, $p = 0.022$; Stance × Age: $F_{(1, 22)} = 4.38$, $p = 0.048$	Young: $F_{(1, 22)} = 8.99$, $p = 0.007$ Older: $F_{(1, 22)} = 0.00$, $p = 0.971$
0.3	Stance: $F_{(1, 22)} = 3.70$, $p = 0.068$; Age: $F_{(1, 22)} = 2.09$, $p = 0.162$; Stance × Age: $F_{(1, 22)} = 6.38$, $p = 0.019$	Young: $F_{(1, 22)} = 9.89$, $p = 0.005$ Older: $F_{(1, 22)} = 0.18$, $p = 0.674$
0.4	Stance: $F_{(1, 22)} = 2.88$, $p = 0.104$; Age: $F_{(1, 22)} = 5.36$, $p = 0.030$; Stance × Age: $F_{(1, 22)} = 5.11$, $p = 0.034$	Young: $F_{(1, 22)} = 7.83$, $p = 0.010$ Older: $F_{(1, 22)} = 0.16$, $p = 0.695$
0.5	Stance: $F_{(1, 22)} = 0.56$, $p = 0.463$; Age: $F_{(1, 22)} = 6.58$, $p = 0.018$; Stance × Age: $F_{(1, 22)} = 2.91$, $p = 0.102$	–
0.6	Stance: $F_{(1, 22)} = 0.17$, $p = 0.683$; Age: $F_{(1, 22)} = 6.38$, $p = 0.019$; Stance × Age: $F_{(1, 22)} = 2.28$, $p = 0.145$	–
0.7	Stance: $F_{(1, 22)} = 1.38$, $p = 0.253$; Age: $F_{(1, 22)} = 4.43$, $p = 0.047$; Stance × Age: $F_{(1, 22)} = 3.19$, $p = 0.088$	–
0.8	Stance: $F_{(1, 22)} = 2.72$, $p = 0.113$; Age: $F_{(1, 22)} = 3.09$, $p = 0.093$; Stance × Age: $F_{(1, 22)} = 4.35$, $p = 0.049$	Young: $F_{(1, 22)} = 0.10$, $p = 0.760$ Older: $F_{(1, 22)} = 6.98$, $p = 0.015$
0.9	Stance: $F_{(1, 22)} = 3.49$, $p = 0.075$; Age: $F_{(1, 22)} = 2.42$, $p = 0.134$; Stance × Age: $F_{(1, 22)} = 4.55$, $p = 0.044$	Young: $F_{(1, 22)} = 0.04$, $p = 0.853$ Older: $F_{(1, 22)} = 8.07$, $p = 0.009$

–, post-hoc analysis should not be processed due to non-significant interaction effect.

A slower adaptive process for the aged brain is an alternative explanation for why control hubs in the TPO network of the older adults was not dissociated with high postural load. According to the free energy principle (Friston et al., 2006; Friston, 2010), the predictive coding is generated by communication with actual sensory feedback connections to update cortical representations on a trial-by-trial basis (Panichello et al., 2013). When the incoming sensory information coincides with the predictive coding, free energy is minimized. Instead, the brain keeps estimating most-likely likelihood from the information changes in the sensory feedback with environment contexts. For those young adults who could more quickly adapt to stabilometer stance before force-matching, the left TPO network was less activated for a small prediction error when descending prediction efficiency interpreted the actual sensory input. A natural consequence of aging causes slow adaptation and deviance detection of environmental changes. For our older cohort, the TPO network in the stabilometer condition was not suppressed, because they still kept reinforcing internal generative model by comparing of predictions and actual sensory inputs (primarily the ventral visual sources) till free energy was optimally minimized (Panichello et al., 2013).

Compensatory Recruitment of the Right Prefrontal Network in the Elderly

Unlike the young adults, the older adults revealed stance-related enhancements of functional connectivity between the right pre-frontal and frontal areas (**Figure 9**, right). In contrast to the level-surface condition, the associated force-matching with the stabilometer stance recruited more attentional resources to deal with increases in postural sway and stance-induced difficulty in target detection prior to force-matching. Recently, the prefrontal area has been linked to balance control, especially when unexpected external postural perturbation is provided (Maki and McIlroy, 2007; Mihara et al., 2008). In healthy adults and stroke patients, the right prefrontal lobe plays a greater role than the left prefrontal lobe in stance control during postural perturbation (Ugur et al., 2000; Fujita et al., 2016). Prefrontal lateralization is related to resetting eye positions in accordance with using spatial working memory processes

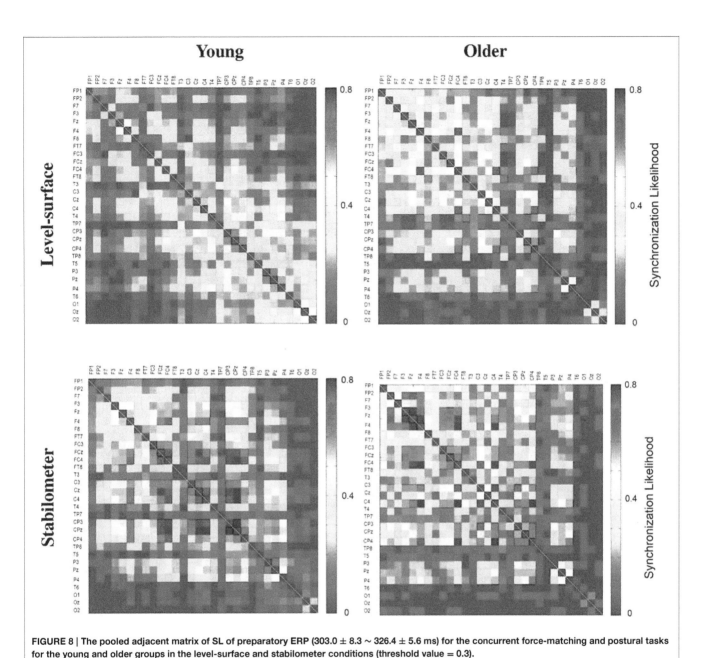

FIGURE 8 | The pooled adjacent matrix of SL of preparatory ERP (303.0 ± 8.3 ∼ 326.4 ± 5.6 ms) for the concurrent force-matching and postural tasks for the young and older groups in the level-surface and stabilometer conditions (threshold value = 0.3).

(Mihara et al., 2008; Fujita et al., 2016). The dorsolateral prefrontal cortex was also found to play a critical role in goal-directed behavior (de Wit et al., 2009), integrating environmental contexts with information on body positioning of the elderly (Wang et al., 2016). The prefrontal area, which receives cerebellum influences via the thalamus (Middleton and Strick, 2001), has dense projections to the pontine nuclei (Ramnani et al., 2006) for reflexive control of postural balance following external stance perturbation (Hartmann-von Monakow et al., 1981; Mihara et al., 2008). Previous behavioral studies have shown that the elderly often prioritize attentional allocation to posture maintenance above supraposture performance with increasing stance destabilization, known as a "posture-first

strategy" (Shumway-Cook and Woollacott, 2000; Doumas et al., 2008). Hence, the age-dependent compensatory recruitment of the right prefrontal lobe is in a good agreement with the greater need for spatial attention of the elderly adults in the postural-suprapostural task with increasing postural load. The prevailing attentional focus on the posture subtask of the elderly added to the difficulty in task-switching at the cost of inferior force-matching performance. In fact, for healthy cognitive aging, additional recruitment of cognitive processes mediated by the prefrontal cortex and its vast interconnections were found to increase with task demand (Allali et al., 2014; Toepper et al., 2014), in accordance with the compensation-related utilization of neural circuits hypothesis (Reuter-Lorenz and Cappell, 2008).

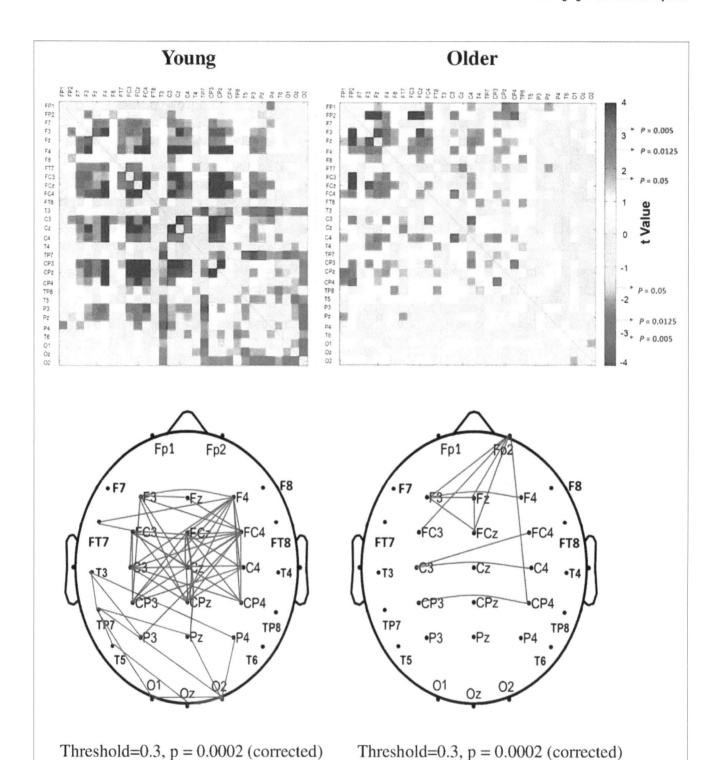

FIGURE 9 | The adjacent matrix of *t*-values that contrasts SL between the level-surface and stabilometer conditions for the young and older groups (upper plot). The adjacent matrix of *t*-values clearly shows a different trend of stance-related modulation of SL across all electrode pairs for the young and older groups, (*t* > 1.771: stabilometer SL > level-surface SL, *p* < 0.05; *t* < −1.771: level-surface SL > stabilometer SL, *p* < 0.05). The lower plots display the results of connectivity analysis with network-based statistics (threshold value = 0.3). A contrasting wiring diagram shows topological distributions of the suprathreshold connectivity that vary with stance difficulty increase for the young and older groups. Red line: stabilometer connectivity of supra-threshold > level-surface connectivity of supra-threshold, *p* < 0.005; blue line: level-surface connectivity of supra-threshold > stabilometer connectivity of supra-threshold, *p* < 0.005.

Methodology Issues

To date, SL has most commonly been used to characterize multiple synchronized neural sources in the brain (Stam and van Dijk, 2002) using low-density (Smit et al., 2012; Herrera-Díaz et al., 2016) or high-density EEG (Polanía et al., 2011). The major methodological advantage of using SL is that it can sensibly detect slight and intricate variations in the coupling strength (Koenis et al., 2013), resolving rapid synchronization patterns in the non-stationary ERP profile at a short time scale (Stam and van Dijk, 2002; Betzel et al., 2012). Some simulation studies have argued that SL could bring about spurious coupling due to a volume conduction effect (Stam et al., 2005; Tognoli and Kelso, 2009). The authors agree that an increase in postural challenge probably led to enhanced volume conduction for the recruitment of more neurons in the stabilometer condition, especially for those functional connectivity grouped with neighboring regions. If the physical synchronization did exist, we could not completely deny overestimation of the functional connectivity within neighboring electrodes. However, physical synchronization does not rationally explain our major finding of age-related differences in connectivity reorganization with increasing postural load. In contrast to the young adults, the older adults did not exhibited a polarization modulation of spatially-distributed communities for the FSM and TPO networks with increasing postural load (**Figure 9**). Particularly for the stronger functional connectivity, the stance-related modulations of the two distinct networks in young adults and lack of the paralleling connectivity change in the elderly were hard to reconcile with the global rise or fall of state transition to intermittent activity of a single common-source volume conduction. Moreover, we did not intend to specify any age-related differences in functional connectivity of neighboring electrodes or small-range excitability of a recording electrode, as we did accentuate age-dependent parametric changes on a network basis (**Figures 5–7**). Although, some measures of functional connectivity, such as phase lag index, have been proposed to minimize common sources (Stam et al., 2007), phase-based approaches that can be more sensitive to noise measure temporal-spatial properties of functional connectivity that are quite different from SL (Vinck et al., 2011). Phase-based approaches are not appropriate for accessing the inter-dependences of two short-length ERP profiles in the presence of non-stationarities (Cohen, 2015). As no quantification of functional connectivity is perfect, future work may consider a combination of local cerebral hemodynamic properties and spontaneous neural activity. However, it is not feasible to fully rule out potential common sources with the present setup.

CONCLUSION

At the neural level, the present work first reveals neural underpinnings which are associated with (but not necessarily causal to) why dual-task performance of the older adults is tended to be more easily affected by postural load increment. In comparison with the young adults, high postural load produced more dual-task cost of the older adults, pertaining to lack of neural economy to timely deactivate the left TPO network. In addition, the age-dependent compensatory recruitment of the right prefrontal lobe indicates that the older adults may need a greater spatial attention for dual-task control against fluctuating stabilometer movements.

AUTHOR CONTRIBUTIONS

Substantial contributions to the conception or design of the work or the acquisition: CH, LL, and IH. Analysis or interpretation of data for the work: CH and IH. Drafting the work or revising it critically for important intellectual content: CH and IH. Final approval of the version to be published and agreement to be accountable for all aspects of the work in ensuring that questions related to the accuracy or integrity of any part of the work are appropriately investigated and resolved: CH, LL, and IH.

FUNDING

This research was supported by a grant from the Ministry of Science and Technology, Taiwan, ROC, under grant no. MOST 103-2314-B-002-007-MY3 and MOST 104-2314-B-006-016-MY3.

REFERENCES

Adkin, A. L., Campbell, A. D., Chua, R., and Carpenter, M. G. (2008). The influence of postural threat on the cortical response to unpredictable and predictable postural perturbations. *Neurosci. Lett.* 435, 120–125. doi: 10.1016/j.neulet.2008.02.018

Allali, G., van der Meulen, M., Beauchet, O., Rieger, S. W., Vuilleumier, P., and Assal, F. (2014). The neural basis of age-related changes in motor imagery of gait: an fMRI study. *J. Gerontol. A Biol. Sci. Med. Sci.* 69, 1389–1398. doi: 10.1093/gerona/glt207

Assmus, A., Giessing, C., Weiss, P. H., and Fink, G. R. (2007). Functional interactions during the retrieval of conceptual action knowledge: an fMRI study. *J. Cogn. Neurosci.* 19, 1004–1012. doi: 10.1162/jocn.2007.19.6.1004

Balasubramaniam, R., Riley, M. A., and Turvey, M. T. (2000). Specificity of postural sway to the demands of a precision task. *Gait Posture* 11, 12–24. doi: 10.1016/S0966-6362(99)00051-X

Betzel, R. F., Erickson, M. A., Abell, M., O'Donnell, B. F., Hetrick, W. P., and Sporns, O. (2012). Synchronization dynamics and evidence for a repertoire of network states in resting EEG. *Front. Comput. Neurosci.* 6:74. doi: 10.3389/fncom.2012.00074

Boersma, M., Smit, D. J., de Bie, H. M., Van Baal, G. C., Boomsma, D. I., de Geus, E. J., et al. (2011). Network analysis of resting state EEG in the developing young brain: structure comes with maturation. *Hum. Brain Mapp.* 32, 413–425. doi: 10.1002/hbm.21030

Boisgontier, M. P., Beets, I. A., Duysens, J., Nieuwboer, A., Krampe, R. T., and Swinnen, S. P. (2013). Age-related differences in attentional cost associated with postural dual tasks: increased recruitment of generic cognitive resources in older adults. *Neurosci. Biobehav. Rev.* 37, 1824–1837. doi: 10.1016/j.neubiorev.2013.07.014

Borg, F. G., and Laxåback, G. (2010). Entropy of balance–some recent results. *J. Neuroeng. Rehabil.* 7:38. doi: 10.1186/1743-0003-7-38

Chelazzi, L., Miller, E. K., Duncan, J., and Desimone, R. (1993). A neural basis for visual search in inferior temporal cortex. *Nature* 363, 345–347.

Chen, F. C., and Stoffregen, T. A. (2012). Specificity of postural sway to the demands of a precision task at sea. *J. Exp. Psychol. Appl.* 18, 203–212. doi: 10.1037/a0026661

Chiviacowsky, S., Wulf, G., and Wally, R. (2010). An external focus of attention enhances balance learning in older adults. *Gait Posture* 32, 572–575. doi: 10.1016/j.gaitpost.2010.08.004

Cohen, M. X. (2015). Effects of time lag and frequency matching on phase-based connectivity. *J. Neurosci. Methods* 250, 137–146. doi: 10.1016/j.jneumeth.2014.09.005

Cole, M. W., Reynolds, J. R., Power, J. D., Repovs, G., Anticevic, A., and Braver, T. S. (2013). Multi-task connectivity reveals flexible hubs for adaptive task control. *Nat. Neurosci.* 16, 1348–1355. doi: 10.1038/nn.3470

de Groot, M., Cremers, L. G., Ikram, M. A., Hofman, A., Krestin, G. P., van der Lugt, A., et al. (2016). White matter degeneration with aging: longitudinal diffusion MR imaging analysis. *Radiology* 279, 532–541. doi: 10.1148/radiol.2015150103

de Wit, S., Corlett, P. R., Aitken, M. R., Dickinson, A., and Fletcher, P. C. (2009). Differential engagement of the ventromedial prefrontal cortex by goal-directed and habitual behavior toward food pictures in humans. *J. Neurosci.* 29, 1130–1138. doi: 10.1523/JNEUROSCI.1639-09.2009

Donker, S. F., Roerdink, M., Greven, A. J., and Beek, P. J. (2007). Regularity of center-of-pressure trajectories depends on the amount of attention invested in postural control. *Exp. Brain Res.* 181, 1–11. doi: 10.1007/s00221-007-0905-4

Doumas, M., Smolders, C., and Krampe, R. T. (2008). Task prioritization in aging: effects of sensory information on concurrent posture and memory performance. *Exp. Brain Res.* 187, 275–281. doi: 10.1007/s00221-008-1302-3

Fernandes, M. A., Pacurar, A., Moscovitch, M., and Grady, C. (2006). Neural correlates of auditory recognition under full and divided attention in younger and older adults. *Neuropsychologia* 44, 2452–2464. doi: 10.1016/j.neuropsychologia.2006.04.020

Ferraye, M. U., Debû, B., Heil, L., Carpenter, M., Bloem, B. R., and Toni, I. (2014). Using motor imagery to study the neural substrates of dynamic balance. *PLoS ONE* 9:e91183. doi: 10.1371/journal.pone.0091183

Friston, K. (2010). The free-energy principle: a unified brain theory? *Nat. Rev. Neurosci.* 11, 127–138. doi: 10.1038/nrn2787

Friston, K., Kilner, J., and Harrison, L. (2006). A free energy principle for the brain. *J. Physiol. Paris* 100, 70–87. doi: 10.1016/j.jphysparis.2006.10.001

Fujita, H., Kasubuchi, K., Wakata, S., Hiyamizu, M., and Morioka, S. (2016). Role of the frontal cortex in standing postural sway tasks while dual-tasking: a functional near-infrared spectroscopy study examining working memory Capacity. *Biomed. Res. Int.* 2016:7053867. doi: 10.1155/2016/7053867

Furst, A. J., and Fellgiebel, A. (2011). White matter degeneration in normal and pathologic aging: the pattern matters. *Neurology* 77, 14–15. doi: 10.1212/WNL.0b013e3182231455

Geerligs, L., Saliasi, E., Renken, R. J., Maurits, N. M., and Lorist, M. M. (2014). Flexible connectivity in the aging brain revealed by task modulations. *Hum. Brain Mapp.* 35, 3788–3804. doi: 10.1002/hbm.22437

Gontier, E., Le Dantec, C., Leleu, A., Paul, I., Charvin, H., Bernard, C., et al. (2007). Frontal and parietal ERPs associated with duration discriminations with or without task interference. *Brain Res.* 1170, 79–89. doi: 10.1016/j.brainres.2007.07.022

Hartley, A. A., Jonides, J., and Sylvester, C. Y. (2011). Dual-task processing in younger and older adults: similarities and differences revealed by fMRI. *Brain Cogn.* 75, 281–291. doi: 10.1016/j.bandc.2011.01.004

Hartmann-von Monakow, K., Akert, K., and Künzle, H. (1981). Projection of precentral, premotor and prefrontal cortex to the basilar pontine grey and to nucleus reticularis tegmenti pontis in the monkey. *Schweiz. Arch. Neurol. Neurochir. Psychiatr.* 129, 189–208.

Herrera-Díaz, A., Mendoza-Quiñones, R., Melie-Garcia, L., Martínez-Montes, E., Sanabria-Diaz, G., Romero-Quintana, Y., et al. (2016). Functional connectivity and quantitative EEG in women with alcohol use disorders: a resting-state study. *Brain Topogr.* 29, 368–381. doi: 10.1007/s10548-015-0467-x

Honeycutt, C. F., Gottschall, J. S., and Nichols, T. R. (2009). Electromyographic responses from the hindlimb muscles of the decerebrate cat to horizontal support surface perturbations. *J. Neurophysiol.* 101, 2751–2761. doi: 10.1152/jn.91040.2008

Huang, C. Y., Chang, G. C., Tsai, Y. Y., and Hwang, I. S. (2016). An increase in postural load facilitates an anterior shift of processing resources to frontal executive function in a postural-suprapostural task. *Front. Hum. Neurosci.* 10:420. doi: 10.3389/fnhum.2016.00420

Huang, C. Y., and Hwang, I. S. (2013). Behavioral data and neural correlates for postural prioritization and flexible resource allocation in concurrent postural and motor tasks. *Hum. Brain Mapp.* 34, 635–650. doi: 10.1002/hbm.21460

Huang, C. Y., Zhao, C. G., and Hwang, I. S. (2014). Neural basis of postural focus effect on concurrent postural and motor tasks: phase-locked electroencephalogram responses. *Behav. Brain Res.* 274, 95–107. doi: 10.1016/j.bbr.2014.07.054

Hülsdünker, T., Mierau, A., Neeb, C., Kleinöder, H., and Strüder, H. K. (2015). Cortical processes associated with continuous balance control as revealed by EEG spectral power. *Neurosci. Lett.* 592, 1–5. doi: 10.1016/j.neulet.2015.02.049

Hung, Y. T., Yu, S. H., Fang, J. H., and Huang, C. Y. (2016). Effects of precision-grip force on postural-suprapostural task. *Formosan J. Phys. Ther.* 41, 223–229. doi: 10.6215/FJPT.PTS1454119867

Hwang, I. S., and Huang, C. Y. (2016). Neural correlates of task cost for stance control with an additional motor task: phase-locked electroencephalogram responses. *PLoS ONE* 11:e0151906. doi: 10.1371/journal.pone.0151906

Jacobs, J. V., and Horak, F. B. (2007). Cortical control of postural responses. *J. Neural. Transm.* 114, 1339–1348. doi: 10.1007/s00702-007-0657-0

Jellema, T., and Perrett, D. I. (2003). Cells in monkey STS responsive to articulated body motions and consequent static posture: a case of implied motion? *Neuropsychologia* 41, 1728–1737. doi: 10.1016/S0028-3932(03)00175-1

Jellema, T., and Perrett, D. I. (2006). Neural representations of perceived bodily actions using a categorical frame of reference. *Neuropsychologia* 44, 1535–1546. doi: 10.1016/j.neuropsychologia.2006.01.020

Karim, H., Fuhrman, S. I., Sparto, P., Furman, J., and Huppert, T. (2013). Functional brain imaging of multi-sensory vestibular processing during computerized dynamic posturography using near-infrared spectroscopy. *Neuroimage* 74, 318–325. doi: 10.1016/j.neuroimage.2013.02.010

Kastner, S., and Ungerleider, L. G. (2001). The neural basis of biased competition in human visual cortex. *Neuropsychologia* 39, 1263–1276. doi: 10.1016/S0028-3932(01)00116-6

Koenis, M. M., Romeijn, N., Piantoni, G., Verweij, I., Van der Werf, Y. D., Van Someren, E. J., et al. (2013). Does sleep restore the topology of functional brain networks? *Hum. Brain Mapp.* 34, 487–500. doi: 10.1002/hbm.21455

Kuczynski, M., Szymanska, M., and Biec, E. (2011). Dual-task effect on postural control in high-level competitive dancers. *J. Sports Sci.* 29, 539–545. doi: 10.1080/02640414.2010.544046

Lacour, M., Bernard-Demanze, L., and Dumitrescu, M. (2008). Posture control, aging, and attention resources: models and posture-analysis methods. *Neurophysiol. Clin.* 38, 411–421. doi: 10.1016/j.neucli.2008.09.005

Leistedt, S. J., Coumans, N., Dumont, M., Lanquart, J. P., Stam, C. J., and Linkowski, P. (2009). Altered sleep brain functional connectivity in acutely depressed patients. *Hum. Brain Mapp.* 30, 2207–2219. doi: 10.1002/hbm.20662

Liston, M. B., Bergmann, J. H., Keating, N., Green, D. A., and Pavlou, M. (2014). Postural prioritization is differentially altered in healthy older compared to younger adults during visual and auditory coded spatial multitasking. *Gait Posture* 39, 198–204. doi: 10.1016/j.gaitpost.2013.07.004

Little, C. E., and Woollacott, M. (2015). EEG measures reveal dual-task interference in postural performance in young adults. *Exp. Brain Res.* 233, 27–37. doi: 10.1007/s00221-014-4111-x

Maki, B. E., and McIlroy, W. E. (2007). Cognitive demands and cortical control of human balance-recovery reactions. *J. Neural. Transm.* 114, 1279–1296. doi: 10.1007/s00702-007-0764-y

Marois, R., Larson, J. M., Chun, M. M., and Shima, D. (2006). Response-specific sources of dual-task interference in human pre-motor cortex. *Psychol. Res.* 70, 436–447. doi: 10.1007/s00426-005-0022-6

McNevin, N., Weir, P., and Quinn, T. (2013). Effects of attentional focus and age on suprapostural task performance and postural control. *Res. Q. Exerc. Sport* 84, 96–103. doi: 10.1080/02701367.2013.762321

McNevin, N. H., Shea, C. H., and Wulf, G. (2003). Increasing the distance of an external focus of attention enhances learning. *Psychol. Res.* 67, 22–29. doi: 10.1007/s00426-002-0093-6

Middleton, F. A., and Strick, P. L. (2001). Cerebellar projections to the prefrontal cortex of the primate. *J. Neurosci.* 21, 700–712. Available online at: http://www.jneurosci.org/content/21/2/700.long

Mihara, M., Miyai, I., Hatakenaka, M., Kubota, K., and Sakoda, S. (2008). Role of the prefrontal cortex in human balance control. *Neuroimage* 43, 329–336. doi: 10.1016/j.neuroimage.2008.07.029

Mitra, S., and Fraizer, E. V. (2004). Effects of explicit sway-minimization on postural-suprapostural dual-task performance. *Hum. Mov. Sci.* 23, 1–20. doi: 10.1016/j.humov.2004.03.003

Mochizuki, G., Sibley, K. M., Esposito, J. G., Camilleri, J. M., and McIlroy, W. E. (2008). Cortical responses associated with the preparation and reaction to full-body perturbations to upright stability. *Clin. Neurophysiol.* 119, 1626–1637. doi: 10.1016/j.clinph.2008.03.020

Montez, T., Linkenkaer-Hansen, K., van Dijk, B. W., and Stam, C. J. (2006). Synchronization likelihood with explicit time-frequency priors. *Neuroimage* 33, 1117–1125. doi: 10.1016/j.neuroimage.2006.06.066

Mozolic, J. L., Long, A. B., Morgan, A. R., Rawley-Payne, M., and Laurienti, P. J. (2011). A cognitive training intervention improves modality-specific attention in a randomized controlled trial of healthy older adults. *Neurobiol. Aging* 32, 655–668. doi: 10.1016/j.neurobiolaging.2009.04.013

Nakai, T., Matsuo, K., Ohgami, Y., Oishi, K., and Kato, C. (2005). An fMRI study of temporal sequencing of motor regulation guided by an auditory cue–a comparison with visual guidance. *Cogn. Process.* 6, 128–135. doi: 10.1007/s10339-005-0051-5

Niso, G., Bruña, R., Pereda, E., Gutiérrez, R., Bajo, R., Maestú, F., et al. (2013). HERMES: towards an integrated toolbox to characterize functional and effective brain connectivity. *Neuroinformatics* 11, 405–434. doi: 10.1007/s12021-013-9186-1

Noppeney, U., Josephs, O., Kiebel, S., Friston, K. J., and Price, C. J. (2005). Action selectivity in parietal and temporal cortex. *Brain Res. Cogn. Brain Res.* 25, 641–649. doi: 10.1016/j.cogbrainres.2005.08.017

Panichello, M. F., Cheung, O. S., and Bar, M. (2013). Predictive feedback and conscious visual experience. *Front. Psychol.* 3:620. doi: 10.3389/fpsyg.2012.00620

Pellijeff, A., Bonilha, L., Morgan, P. S., McKenzie, K., and Jackson, S. R. (2006). Parietal updating of limb posture: an event-related fMRI study. *Neuropsychologia* 44, 2685–2690. doi: 10.1016/j.neuropsychologia.2006.01.009

Perrett, D. I., Harries, M. H., Bevan, R., Thomas, S., Benson, P. J., Mistlin, A. J., et al. (1989). Frameworks of analysis for the neural representation of animate objects and actions. *J. Exp. Biol.* 146, 87–113.

Polanía, R., Nitsche, M. A., and Paulus, W. (2011). Modulating functional connectivity patterns and topological functional organization of the human brain with transcranial direct current stimulation. *Hum. Brain Mapp.* 32, 1236–1249. doi: 10.1002/hbm.21104

Prado, J. M., Stoffregen, T. A., and Duarte, M. (2007). Postural sway during dual tasks in young and elderly adults. *Gerontology* 53, 274–281. doi: 10.1159/000102938

Ramnani, N., Behrens, T. E., Johansen-Berg, H., Richter, M. C., Pinsk, M. A., Andersson, J. L., et al. (2006). The evolution of prefrontal inputs to the cortico-pontine system: diffusion imaging evidence from Macaque monkeys and humans. *Cereb. Cortex* 16, 811–818. doi: 10.1093/cercor/bhj024

Rapp, M. A., Krampe, R. T., and Baltes, P. B. (2006). Adaptive task prioritization in aging: selective resource allocation to postural control

is preserved in Alzheimer disease. *Am. J. Geriatr. Psychiatry* 14, 52–61. doi: 10.1097/01.JGP.0000192490.43179.e7

Remaud, A., Boyas, S., Caron, G. A., and Bilodeau, M. (2012). Attentional demands associated with postural control depend on task difficulty and visual condition. *J. Mot. Behav.* 44, 329–340. doi: 10.1080/00222895.2012.708680

Reuter-Lorenz, P. A., and Cappell, K. A. (2008). Neurocognitive aging and the compensation hypothesis. *Curr. Direct. Psychol. Sci.* 17, 177–182. doi: 10.1111/j.1467-8721.2008.00570.x

Salo, E., Rinne, T., Salonen, O., and Alho, K. (2015). Brain activations during bimodal dual tasks depend on the nature and combination of component tasks. *Front. Hum. Neurosci.* 9:102. doi: 10.3389/fnhum.2015.00102

Schall, J. D., Stuphorn, V., and Brown, J. W. (2002). Monitoring and control of action by the frontal lobes. *Neuron* 36, 309–322. doi: 10.1016/S0896-6273(02)00964-9

Schubert, T. (2008). The central attentional limitation and executive control. *Front. Biosci.* 13, 3569–3580. doi: 10.2741/2950

Schulz, K. P., Bédard, A. C., Czarnecki, R., and Fan, J. (2011). Preparatory activity and connectivity in dorsal anterior cingulate cortex for cognitive control. *Neuroimage* 57, 242–250. doi: 10.1016/j.neuroimage.2011.04.023

Semlitsch, H. V., Anderer, P., Schuster, P., and Presslich, O. (1986). A solution for reliable and valid reduction of ocular artifacts, applied to the P300 ERP. *Psychophysiology* 23, 695–703. doi: 10.1111/j.1469-8986.1986.tb00696.x

Shumway-Cook, A., and Woollacott, M. (2000). Attentional demands and postural control: the effect of sensory context. *J. Gerontol. A Biol. Sci. Med. Sci.* 55, M10–M16. doi: 10.1093/gerona/55.1.M10

Sibley, K. M., Mochizuki, G., Frank, J. S., and McIlroy, W. E. (2010). The relationship between physiological arousal and cortical and autonomic responses to postural instability. *Exp. Brain Res.* 203, 533–540. doi: 10.1007/s00221-010-2257-8

Sipp, A. R., Gwin, J. T., Makeig, S., and Ferris, D. P. (2013). Loss of balance during balance beam walking elicits a multifocal theta band electrocortical response. *J. Neurophysiol.* 110, 2050–2060. doi: 10.1152/jn.00744.2012

Smit, D. J., Boersma, M., Schnack, H. G., Micheloyannis, S., Boomsma, D. I., Hulshoff Pol, H. E., et al. (2012). The brain matures with stronger functional connectivity and decreased randomness of its network. *PLoS ONE* 7:e36896. doi: 10.1371/journal.pone.0036896

Stam, C. J., Breakspear, M., van Cappellen van Walsum, A. M., and van Dijk, B. W. (2003). Nonlinear synchronization in EEG and whole-head MEG recordings of healthy subjects. *Hum. Brain Mapp.* 19, 63–78. doi: 10.1002/hbm.10106

Stam, C. J., Montez, T., Jones, B. F., Rombouts, S. A., van der Made, Y., Pijnenburg, Y. A., et al. (2005). Disturbed fluctuations of resting state EEG synchronization in Alzheimer's disease. *Clin. Neurophysiol.* 116, 708–715. doi: 10.1016/j.clinph.2004.09.022

Stam, C. J., Nolte, G., and Daffertshofer, A. (2007). Phase lag index: assessment of functional connectivity from multi-channel EEG and MEG with diminished bias from common sources. *Hum. Brain Mapp.* 28, 1178–1193. doi: 10.1002/hbm.20346

Stam, C. J., and van Dijk, B. W. (2002). Synchronization likelihood: an unbiased measure of generalized synchronization in multivariate data sets. *Phys. D* 163, 236–251. doi: 10.1016/S0167-2789(01)00386-4

Stins, J. F., Michielsen, M. E., Roerdink, M., and Beek, P. J. (2009). Sway regularity reflects attentional involvement in postural control: effects of expertise, vision and cognition. *Gait Posture* 30, 106–109. doi: 10.1016/j.gaitpost.2009.04.001

Stoffregen, T. A. (2016). Functional control of stance in older adults. *Kinesiol. Rev.* 5, 23–29. doi: 10.1123/kr.2015-0049

Stoffregen, T. A., Smart, L. J., Bardy, B. G., and Pagulayan, R. J. (1999). Postural stabilization of looking. *J. Exp. Psychol. Hum. Percept. Perform.* 25, 1641–1658. doi: 10.1037/0096-1523.25.6.1641

Toepper, M., Gebhardt, H., Bauer, E., Haberkamp, A., Beblo, T., Gallhofer, B., et al. (2014). The impact of age on load-related dorsolateral prefrontal cortex activation. *Front. Aging Neurosci.* 6:9. doi: 10.3389/fnagi.2014.00009

Tognoli, E., and Kelso, J. A. (2009). Brain coordination dynamics: true and false faces of phase synchrony and metastability. *Prog. Neurobiol.* 87, 31–40. doi: 10.1016/j.pneurobio.2008.09.014

Ugur, C., Gücüyener, D., Uzuner, N., Ozkan, S., and Ozdemir, G. (2000). Characteristics of falling in patients with stroke. *J. Neurol. Neurosurg. Psychiatry* 69, 649–651. doi: 10.1136/jnnp.69.5.649

Vangeneugden, J., De Mazière, P. A., Van Hulle, M. M., Jaeggli, T., Van Gool, L., and Vogels, R. (2011). Distinct mechanisms for coding of visual actions in macaque temporal cortex. *J. Neurosci.* 31, 385–401. doi: 10.1523/JNEUROSCI.2703-10.2011

Vinck, M., Oostenveld, R., van Wingerden, M., Battaglia, F., and Pennartz, C. M. (2011). An improved index of phase-synchronization for electrophysiological data in the presence of volume-conduction, noise and sample-size bias. *Neuroimage* 55, 1548–1565. doi: 10.1016/j.neuroimage.2011.01.055

Wang, B., Zhang, M., Bu, L., Xu, L., Wang, W., and Li, Z. (2016). Posture-related changes in brain functional connectivity as assessed by wavelet phase coherence of NIRS signals in elderly subjects. *Behav. Brain Res.* 312, 238–245. doi: 10.1016/j.bbr.2016.06.037

Wulf, G., McNevin, N., and Shea, C. H. (2001). The automaticity of complex motor skill learning as a function of attentional focus. *Q. J. Exp. Psychol. A* 54,

1143–1154. doi: 10.1080/713756012

Wulf, G., Mercer, J., McNevin, N., and Guadagnoli, M. A. (2004). Reciprocal influences of attentional focus on postural and suprapostural task performance. *J. Mot. Behav.* 36, 189–199. doi: 10.3200/JMBR.36.2.189-199

Wulf, G., Weigelt, M., Poulter, D., and McNevin, N. (2003). Attentional focus on suprapostural tasks affects balance learning. *Q. J. Exp. Psychol. A.* 56, 1191–1211. doi: 10.1080/02724980343000062

Yentes, J. M., Hunt, N., Schmid, K. K., Kaipust, J. P., McGrath, D., and Stergiou, N. (2013). The appropriate use of approximate entropy and sample entropy with short data sets. *Ann. Biomed. Eng.* 41, 349–365. doi: 10.1007/s10439-012-0668-3

Zalesky, A., Fornito, A., and Bullmore, E. T. (2010). Network-based statistic: identifying differences in brain networks. *Neuroimage* 53, 1197–1207. doi: 10.1016/j.neuroimage.2010.06.041

13

Age-Dependent Modulations of Resting State Connectivity Following Motor Practice

Elena Solesio-Jofre[1,2]*, Iseult A. M. Beets[1], Daniel G. Woolley[1], Lisa Pauwels[1], Sima Chalavi[1], Dante Mantini[1,3,4] and Stephan P. Swinnen[1,5]

[1] Movement Control and Neuroplasticity Research Group, Department of Movement Sciences, KU Leuven, Leuven, Belgium, [2] Department of Biological and Health Psychology, Autonomous University of Madrid, Madrid, Spain, [3] Department of Health Sciences and Technology, ETH Zurich, Zurich, Switzerland, [4] Department of Experimental Psychology, University of Oxford, Oxford, United Kingdom, [5] Leuven Research Institute for Neuroscience and Disease, KU Leuven, Leuven, Belgium

*Correspondence:
Elena Solesio-Jofre
elena.solesio@uam.es

Recent work in young adults has demonstrated that motor learning can modulate resting state functional connectivity. However, evidence for older adults is scarce. Here, we investigated whether learning a bimanual tracking task modulates resting state functional connectivity of both inter- and intra-hemispheric regions differentially in young and older individuals, and whether this has behavioral relevance. Both age groups learned a set of complex bimanual tracking task variants over a 2-week training period. Resting-state and task-related functional magnetic resonance imaging scans were collected before and after training. Our analyses revealed that both young and older adults reached considerable performance gains. Older adults even obtained larger training-induced improvements relative to baseline, but their overall performance levels were lower than in young adults. Short-term practice resulted in a modulation of resting state functional connectivity, leading to connectivity increases in young adults, but connectivity decreases in older adults. This pattern of age differences occurred for both inter- and intra-hemispheric connections related to the motor network. Additionally, long-term training-induced increases were observed in intra-hemispheric connectivity in the right hemisphere across both age groups. Overall, at the individual level, the long-term changes in inter-hemispheric connectivity correlated with training-induced motor improvement. Our findings confirm that short-term task practice shapes spontaneous brain activity differentially in young and older individuals. Importantly, the association between changes in resting state functional connectivity and improvements in motor performance at the individual level may be indicative of how training shapes the short-term functional reorganization of the resting state motor network for improvement of behavioral performance.

Keywords: aging, resting state functional connectivity, motor learning, motor network, bimanual coordination

INTRODUCTION

A large body of research has shown reduced abilities in motor skill performance and learning with age (Swinnen, 1998; Serrien et al., 2000; Bangert et al., 2010; Seidler et al., 2010; Solesio-Jofre et al., 2014; Pauwels et al., 2015; Serbruyns et al., 2015). As almost every motor skill used in daily life requires practice before being efficiently implemented, it is crucial to understand the neural mechanisms by which motor skills are learned and how they are modified with age. Behavioral research has shown that the motor learning process follows different stages. First, during an early acquisition stage considerable improvement in performance is achieved within a relatively short time, i.e., within a session. Second, in a later phase, performance becomes stable, with subtler training-induced improvement that involves consolidation processes. This is achieved over a longer period of time, i.e., between sessions spread over a period of several weeks (Ungerleider et al., 2002; Floyer-Lea and Matthews, 2005).

Converging evidence suggests that, although older adults are still able to acquire new motor skills, they may experience difficulties with the consolidation of acquired representations that occur in the later phase of learning (Voelcker-Rehage and Alberts, 2007; Brown et al., 2009; Wilson et al., 2012; Fogel et al., 2014; Pauwels et al., 2015; Mary et al., 2017). Neuroimaging research has shown a functional reorganization of different neural networks subtending motor performance in young individuals, involving neural plasticity mechanisms (Ma et al., 2010; Albouy et al., 2015). Among other regions, these networks include both inter- and intra-hemispheric connections between the supplementary motor area (SMA), the premotor cortex (PM), and the primary motor cortex (M1) (Donchin et al., 1998; Byblow et al., 2007; O'Shea et al., 2007; Talelli et al., 2008; Hinder et al., 2011). However, a reduced motor plasticity with progressing age may be responsible for the observed deficits in consolidation processes (Todd et al., 2010; Freitas et al., 2011; May and Zwaan, 2017).

Besides task training-induced functional activation changes, recent research has devoted increasing attention to resting state functional connectivity (rs-FC) as a reliable indicator of functional reorganization of brain networks supporting different mental processes (Biswal et al., 1995; Fox and Raichle, 2007; Greicius, 2008; van den Heuvel and Hulshoff Pol, 2010; Ma et al., 2011; van Dijk et al., 2017). Resting state functional magnetic resonance imaging (rs-fMRI) measures the large-scale covariance of low frequency spontaneous fluctuations in the blood oxygen level-dependent (BOLD) signal during rest. The strength of the correlation reflects the degree of functional connectivity between two or more brain regions.

Resting state functional magnetic resonance imaging studies investigating changes in functional connectivity following motor learning, have demonstrated that rs-FC can be modulated within and between training sessions in young individuals (Woolley et al., 2015). In one of the earliest studies, Albert et al. (2009) found that initial learning modulated both a fronto-parietal and a cerebellar resting state network. In a more confined motor network, Tung et al. (2013) showed that initial motor learning modulated functional connectivity between the right and left motor cortices, exhibiting increases in post-task compared to pre-task periods. Looking into a later phase of learning, increases in rs-FC in the superior parietal cortex (Daselaar et al., 2010) and in the postcentral and supramarginal gyrus (Ma et al., 2011) were observed. In short, these and other studies have shown that both short-term (Waites et al., 2005; Barnes et al., 2009;

Stevens et al., 2010; Gregory et al., 2014; Sami et al., 2014; Mary et al., 2017) and long-term (Buchel et al., 1999; Voss et al., 2008; Tambini et al., 2010; Taubert et al., 2011; Yoo et al., 2013; Hardwick et al., 2015; Sampaio-Baptista et al., 2015; Woolley et al., 2015; Mehrkanoon et al., 2016; Amad et al., 2017; May and Zwaan, 2017) learning effects can modulate rs-FC in young individuals.

Importantly, rs-FC has also been shown to correlate with motor improvement in young adults (Ma et al., 2011; Vahdat et al., 2011; Wu et al., 2014; Zhang et al., 2014), indicating that functional network reorganization can, to some extent, predict behavioral changes (Tambini et al., 2010; Deco and Corbetta, 2011; Wu et al., 2014). However, results about motor training-induced modulation of resting state networks in older adults are very scarce, with only one study to date showing age-related rs-FC changes following motor sequence learning (Mary et al., 2017).

Here, we investigated whether and how motor skill acquisition and consolidation of a bimanual tracking task (BTT) (Solesio-Jofre et al., 2014; Serbruyns et al., 2015; Santos Monteiro et al., 2017) modulates rs-FC within a task-related motor network in young and older adults. Resting state activity was obtained across four scans (**Figure 1A**): two scans before a motor training protocol conducted over the course of 2 (one scan before a task-related fMRI scan and the other after the task-related fMRI scan), and two scans following completion of the motor training protocol (again, one scan before a task-related fMRI scan and the other after the task-related fMRI scan). The motor network was selected based on the results of a task-related fMRI study in which the same tracking task was used (Santos Monteiro et al., 2017). Due to the bimanual nature of the task, both inter- and intra-hemispheric functional connectivity were examined. It is well established that bimanual coordination relies on coupling between motor areas of both cerebral hemispheres (Serrien, 2008) through the corpus callosum (Gooijers et al., 2013; Gooijers and Swinnen, 2014). Moreover, learning a new bimanual coordination pattern results in changes in both intra- and inter-hemispheric coherence between pairs of motor regions, as shown by EEG studies (Andres et al., 1999; Gerloff and Andres, 2002; Serrien, 2009). In the current study, we specifically considered both homotopic (i.e., geometrically corresponding regions in each hemisphere) and non-homotopic inter-hemispheric, as well as right and left intra-hemispheric connectivity patterns. To the best of our knowledge, this is the first study examining motor training-induced modulations in both inter-and intra-hemispheric rs-FC as a function of aging during the early and late learning phase. Based on the study from Mary et al. (2017), we predicted an age-dependent reorganization of the motor network, not only immediately but also weeks after initial practice, with more prominent changes anticipated after the former.

Finally, to investigate the behavioral relevance of training-induced changes in functional connectivity, we correlated changes in rs-FC with bimanual task improvement over the course of learning. In accordance with previous studies (Ma et al., 2011; Taubert et al., 2011; Vahdat et al., 2011; Zhang et al., 2011, 2014; Wu et al., 2014), we expected both inter- and

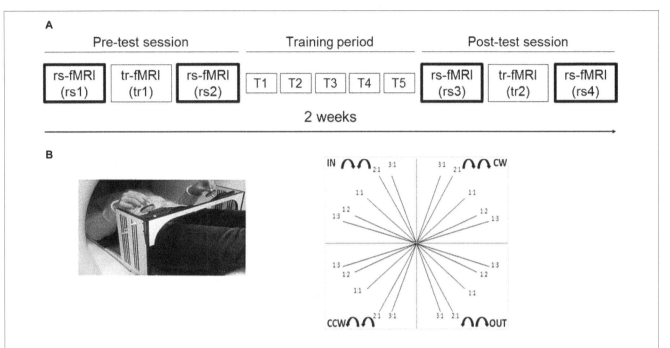

FIGURE 1 | Experimental setup and task. **(A)** Schematic representation of the experimental setup. Two scan sessions occurred before (pre-test session) and after (post-test session) five training sessions (training period), distributed across 2 weeks. Each scan session included a rest scan (rs1 and rs3, respectively) before a task-related scan, a task-related scan (tr1 and tr2, respectively) and a rest scan after the task-related scan (rs2 and rs4, respectively). We mainly focused on rest scans (i.e., two runs within each scan session, four runs in total: rs1, rs2, rs3, and rs4); **(B)** The goal of the bimanual tracking task was to track a white target dot over a blue target line, presented on a screen, by rotating two dials with both hands simultaneously in one of four directional patterns: inward (IN), outward (OUT), clockwise (CW), and counter-clockwise manner (CCW); at five different relative frequency ratios: 1:1, 1:2, 1:3, 2:1, and 3:1 (left: right). This resulted in 20 different bimanual patterns and target line directions.

intra-hemispheric connectivity increases to be associated with improvements on the bimanual task.

MATERIALS AND METHODS

Participants

Twenty-six healthy young adults (YA) and 25 older adults (OA) participated in the study. All participants had normal or corrected-to-normal vision, and were right-handed according to the Edinburgh Handedness Inventory (Oldfield, 1971). They were naive with respect to the experimental paradigm. None of the participants reported a history of neurological, psychiatric, or vascular disease. Older participants above 60 years old ($N = 25$) were screened for cognitive impairments with the Montreal Cognitive Assessment test (MoCA) using the standard cutoff score of 26 (Nasreddine et al., 2005). All participants obtained a score within normal limits (≥ 26, mean = 28.02, $SD = 1.18$, range = 26–30). Three YA were excluded from the analysis due to technical problems with the scanner. Four OA were excluded due to either brain atrophy/lesions, or inability to comply with task instructions. As a result, our final sample included 23 YA (age range = 17–26 years, mean age = 21.19, $SD = 1.99$, 12 females) and 21 OA (age range = 61–81 years, mean age = 68.85, $SD = 5.89$, 12 females). Informed consent was obtained before testing and participants were financially compensated for participation. The experiment was approved

by the local ethics committee for biomedical research of KU Leuven (Belgium), and was performed in accordance with the Declaration of Helsinki (1964).

Experimental Setup

Magnetic resonance imaging (MRI) occurred twice: before (pre-test session) and after (post-test session) five training sessions (training period), distributed across 2 weeks (see **Figure 1A**). Each training session had a total duration of 1 h. The rest-task-rest fMRI design of both scan sessions was identical with a total duration of 1.5 h. Therefore, the overall experimental procedure was as follows: the pre-test session included a rest scan (rs1), followed by a task-related scan (tr1), after which another rest scan (rs2) was obtained. Hence, rs1 and rs2 referred to the within pre-test session rest scans corresponding to the early phase of learning. The pre-test session was followed by a bimanual task training period of 2 weeks (T1, T2, T3, T4, T5). Following completion of 2 weeks of task training, the post-test session included a rest scan (rs3), followed by a task-related scan (tr2), and subsequently another rest scan (rs4). Hence, rs3 and rs4 referred to the within post-test session rest scans corresponding to the late phase of learning. The present study mainly focused on rest scans (i.e., two runs within each scan session, four runs in total: rs1, rs2, rs3, and rs4). All rest scans had the same protocol and lasted 8 min, in which participants were instructed to keep their eyes open and to fixate a target point. Results regarding the task-related fMRI study are published elsewhere (Santos Monteiro et al., 2017).

Bimanual Tracking Task (BTT)

The BTT task was performed during the task-related scans. It enables the evaluation of bimanual coordination accuracy, relying on the execution of complex bimanual patterns (Sisti et al., 2011). This task requires intensive practice to successfully integrate the two separate limb movements into one common spatiotemporal pattern. Learning such a task involves breaking away from the natural tendency to move both limbs in phase with the same velocity, i.e., a 1:1 frequency ratio (Swinnen et al., 1997; Swinnen, 2002).

The goal of the BTT was to track a white target dot over a blue target line, presented on a screen, by rotating two dials with both hands simultaneously in one of four directional patterns: both hands rotated inward (IN) or outward (OUT) together, or in a clockwise (CW) or counter-clockwise manner (CCW) (Sisti et al., 2011, 2012; Gooijers et al., 2013). The left (L) and right (R) hands controlled movements on the ordinate and abscissa, respectively. To increase complexity of the task, each directional combination was performed at five different relative frequency ratios: 1:1, 1:2, 1:3, 2:1, and 3:1 (L:R). For example, a 1:2 ratio indicated that the left hand was required to rotate twice as slow as the right hand. This resulted in 20 different bimanual patterns and target line directions (**Figure 1B**).

Each trial started with the presentation of the single blue target line with a distinct orientation. At the origin of this line, in the center of the PC display, the white target dot was presented, after which it began to move along the blue target line, toward the peripheral endpoint. The target dot moved at a constant rate and for a total duration of 9 s. The beginning and end of the trajectory were marked with an auditory cue (126 ms, begin: 525 Hz, end: 442 Hz). The inter-trial interval was 3 s. The goal was to match the target trajectory as closely as possible.

Each BTT fMRI session consisted of 144 trials, divided equally across six runs, each of which lasted 6 min, with an inter-run interval of approximately 3 min. A run consisted of 24 target lines, presented in a pseudorandom order. The required frequency ratio was randomly distributed such that one third of trials required a 1:1 ratio, one-third required a 1:2 or 2:1 ratio and one-third required a 1:3 or 3:1 ratio. There were 96 "move" trials in which bimanual tracking was actively performed. The remaining trials were "no move" trials, containing the same information as the "move" trials but required no movement. They provided the baseline measure for the BOLD contrasts conducted in the task-related fMRI analysis (Santos Monteiro et al., 2017). Prior to the first MRI session, participants practiced the task briefly in a dummy scanner until the task was fully understood (~10 min).

Training Sessions

In the training sessions, participants were seated in front of a PC-screen (distance approximately 0.5 m) and performed the BTT. For each of the five training days, 10 blocks of 20 randomized trials corresponding to 20 bimanual patterns, i.e., five different frequency ratios in four directions, were performed.

Kinematic Analyses

Data were recorded and analyzed with the Labview software (version 8.5, National Instruments, Austin, TX, United States). Offline analysis was carried out using Matlab R2011b. The x and y positions of the target dot and the cursor were sampled at 100 Hz. For each trial, we calculated the target deviation as a measure of accuracy, using the following multistep procedure: (a) Every 10 ms, the difference between the target position and the cursor position, d, was calculated, using the Euclidean distance:

$$d = \sqrt{(x_2 - x_1)^2 + (y_2 - y_1)^2}$$

Where x_2 and y_2 refer to the position of the participant's cursor on the x- and y-axis, respectively, and x_1 and y_1 correspond to the position of the target dot on the x- and y-axis, respectively. (b) At the end of each trial, the average of these distances was computed and defined as the trial's target deviation, expressed in units (U). A target deviation equal to 0 U would indicate that during the whole trial, the cursor was precisely on top of the white target dot, representing perfect performance. Accordingly, greater target deviation scores reflect greater error and, hence, poorer performance.

To determine whether participants generally met the task requirements, all data were transformed into z-scores [(X-MEAN/SD)]. Trials were discarded from the analysis when $z > 3$ (outlier) and/or when only one hand moved (2.7 and 1.1% of all trials during BTT fMRI 1 and BTT fMRI 2, respectively). For each participant, the average error scores were computed for both scan sessions with and without augmented visual feedback, and these error scores were used as an indicator of bimanual performance accuracy.

Statistical Analyses

Statistical analyses were performed using SPSS Version 22.0 (Armonk, NY, United States).

In accordance with previous results from our own group using the BTT task (Gooijers et al., 2013, 2016; Solesio-Jofre et al., 2014; Beets et al., 2015), movement directions (IN, OUT, CW, and CCW) were fully counterbalanced in the design and of no interest for the present analyses. Additionally, we collapsed trials into two levels: trials with the same (ISO, 1:1) and trials with different (N-ISO, 1:2, 1:3, 2:1, 3:1 collapsed) cycling frequency ratios.

Behavioral data acquired during both the pre- and post-test session were subjected to a 2 × 2 × 2 (age × scan session × frequency ratio) repeated measures ANOVA. Here, age (young, older) was the between-subject factor, and scan session (pre-test session and post-test session) and frequency ratio (ISO, N-ISO) were the within-subject factors.

The level of significance was set at $p < 0.05$. Significant effects were further explored using *post hoc* paired t-tests using Bonferroni correction for multiple comparisons. The partial eta squared statistic (η_p^2) was calculated as the effect size measure for main and interaction effects in the repeated measures ANOVA. According to Cohen (1992), η_p^2 values of 0.01, 0.06 and 0.13 represent small, medium and large effects, respectively.

MRI Data Acquisition

Data acquisition, pre-processing, and analyses followed the same steps for the four resting state runs (rs1, rs2, rs3, and rs4). A Siemens 3-T Magnetom Trio MRI scanner (Siemens, Erlangen, Germany) with a 12 channel head coil was used. For anatomical details, a 3D high-resolution T1-weighted image was obtained first (magnetization prepared rapid gradient echo, time repetition/time echo = 2300/2.98 ms, 1 mm × 1 mm × 1.1 mm voxels, field of view (FOV) = 240 × 256, 160 sagittal slices), lasting 8 min. Then a field map was acquired to address local distortions.

Functional resting state data were acquired with a descending gradient echo planar imaging (EPI) pulse sequence for $T_2{}^*$ − weighted images (repetition time = 3,000 ms; echo time = 30 ms; flip angle = 90°; 50 oblique axial slices each 2.8 mm thick; inter-slice gap = 0.028 mm; in-plane resolution 2.5 mm × 2.5 mm; 80 × 80 matrix, 160 volumes).

MRI Data Pre-processing

Standard preprocessing procedures were performed using SPM8 (Statistical Parametric Mapping software, SPM: Wellcome Department of Imaging Neuroscience, London, United Kingdom[1]), which is implemented in Matlab 7.7 (The Mathworks, Natick, MA, United States).

Functional images were slice-time corrected to the middle slice (reference slice = 25), spatially realigned to the first image in the time series, normalized to the standard EPI template in Montreal Neurological Institute (MNI) space, and resampled into 3 mm isotropic voxels (Friston et al., 1995). Spatial smoothing was not applied in order to avoid introducing artificial local spatial correlations (Salvador et al., 2005; Achard et al., 2006; Achard and Bullmore, 2007).

We took additional preprocessing steps to remove spurious sources of variance. We defined a small, bilateral region of interest in the ventricles, a region of interest in the deep white matter, and one covering the whole brain; we then calculated the average signals in these three regions, which are typically referred to as cerebrospinal fluid, white matter and global signals (Fox et al., 2005, 2009). Next, we performed a regression analysis on the fMRI time-courses, modeling the three aforementioned signals and the parameters obtained by rigid body head motion realignment (Fox et al., 2005, 2009), as well as their temporal derivatives, as regressors.

Recently, there has been considerable discussion over the impact of head motion on rs-FC connectivity analyses. In addition to regressing out the three-dimensional motion parameters and their first derivatives, we also included regressors to deweight scans with a framewise displacement greater than 0.5 mm. A separate regressor was included for each outlier scan, with a 1 at the outlier time point and a zero at all other time points. Framewise displacement was calculated as the sum of the absolute scan to scan difference of the six translational and rotational realignment parameters (Power et al., 2014). Only 0.9% of all scans exceeded this threshold, and there was no significant difference in mean framewise displacement between the four resting state scans [one-way ANOVA: $F(3,172) = 1.90$, $p = 0.14$)].

The BOLD time course in each voxel was then temporally band-pass filtered (0.01–0.08 Hz) to reduce low-frequency drift and high-frequency noise.

Region Definition

Candidate ROIs were generated from task-related fMRI scans (Santos Monteiro et al., 2017), in which the main aim was to explore the effects of aging on brain plasticity associated with motor learning while subjects performed the BTT. The main BOLD contrast of interest was bimanual visuomotor task performance (movement) vs. baseline condition (no movement) in young and older adults. Young and old z-score maps from the task-based fMRI study were combined to find overlapping ROIs by means of a conjunction analysis [young (bimanual visuomotor task > baseline) ∩ old (bimanual visuomotor task > baseline)] (Nichols et al., 2005). The statistical threshold was set to $p < 0.05$, FWE corrected for multiple comparisons and a minimal cluster size of 20 voxels.

To define regions for our resting state connectivity analysis, we chose the peak voxel with the highest z-score ($z \geq 4.10$) in the positive group analysis. Our ROIs were composed of 6-mm radius spheres centered on these peak voxels and were created using the MarsBAR toolbox[2]. The size of the spheres was selected to ensure that they contained voxels that were significantly activated in all cases. We defined the following a priori ROIs: SMA (R, L); dorsal premotor area (PMd: R, L); ventral premotor area (PMv: R, L); primary motor cortex (M1: R, L); and primary somatosensory area (S1: R, L). ROI coordinates are listed in **Table 1**, and are illustrated in **Figure 2**.

Functional Connectivity Analysis

For each subject and within each of the four resting state scans, regional mean time series were extracted by averaging the functional MRI time series across all voxels within each ROI. Then, the correlation strength between every pair of ROIs was calculated using Pearson correlation coefficients creating a functional network captured by a 10 × 10 correlation matrix. These Pearson correlation values were converted to Z-scores by Fischer's r-to-z transformation (Zar, 1998), correcting the degrees of freedom for the autocorrelation in the time series (Shumway and Stoffer, 2006). Group-level correlation matrices were created by using a random-effects analysis across subjects (Ebisch et al., 2011; Pravata et al., 2011).

Next, we calculated the average connectivity score for a group of ROI pairs, which is the average of the component Fisher Z-scores for the corresponding ROI pairs. Specifically, we report four kinds of average functional connectivity (FC) scores, including homotopic inter-hemispheric FC, heterotopic inter-hemispheric FC, right intra-hemispheric FC and left intra-hemispheric FC. Average connectivity scores were subjected to repeated measures ANOVAs. We conducted a 2 × 2 × 2 × 2 (age × inter-hemispheric FC × scan session × scan location) repeated measures ANOVA, with age (young, older) as the between-subject factor and inter-hemispheric FC (homotopic, heterotopic), scan session (pre-test session, post-test session)

---

[1]http://www.fil.ion.ucl.ac.uk/spm/

[2]http://marsbar.sourceforge.net

TABLE 1 | Regions defined for the resting state motor network.

Area	Hemisphere	x	y	z	z-score
Movement > baseline					
Supplementary motor area (SMA)	R	10	4	68	4.12
	L	−10	4	68	4.88
Dorsal premotor area (PMd)	R	28	−4	68	5.56
	L	−28	−4	68	6.63
Ventral premotor area (PMv)	R	54	8	34	6.06
	L	−54	8	34	4.31
Primary motor cortex (M1)	R	37	−21	58	8.02
	L	−37	−21	58	8.05
Primary somatosensory area (S1)	R	28	−40	52	4.64
	L	−28	−40	52	7.58

Regions obtained after a conjunction analysis (young ∩ old) from a task-based fMRI study, $p_{FWE} < 0.05$, $z \geq 4.10$. Six-mm radius spheres centered on z-peak voxels. R, right; L, left; SMA, supplementary motor area; PMd, dorsal premotor area; M1, primary motor cortex; S1, primary somatosensory area; PMv, ventral premotor area.

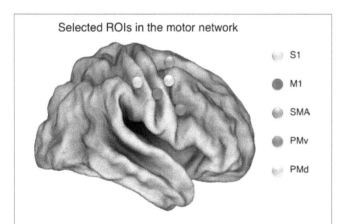

FIGURE 2 | Selected ROIs in the motor network. Spherical ROIs were defined bilaterally for the following areas: SMA, supplementary motor area; PMd, dorsal premotor area; M1, primary motor cortex; S1, primary somatosensory area; PMv, ventral premotor area. The ROIs are illustrated over a cortical representation for the right hemisphere only.

and scan location (before task-related scan, after task-related scan) as the within-subject factors. Additionally, we conducted a $2 \times 2 \times 2 \times 2$ (age × intra-hemispheric FC × scan session × scan location) repeated measures ANOVA, with age (young, older) as the between-subject factor and intra-hemispheric FC (right, left), scan session (pre-test session, post-test session) and scan location (before task-related scan, after task-related scan) as the within-subject factors. All statistical tests were completed with alpha set at 0.05, and significant interaction effects were further explored by *post hoc* paired *t*-tests using Bonferroni correction for each repeated measures ANOVA conducted. The partial eta squared statistic (η_p^2) was calculated as the effect size measure for main and interaction effects in the repeated measures ANOVA and the size of the effects was interpreted according to Cohen (1992).

Finally, we calculated brain-behavior correlations to determine the extent to which training-induced changes in inter- and intra-hemispheric connectivity corresponded with the subsequent gain in behavioral performance, considering the entire sample of participants. We used two different calculations to quantify training-induced changes in inter- and intra-hemispheric connectivity during the early phase of learning and the overall learning process: (1) the difference in the average rs-FC between the second (rs2) and the first (rs1) resting state scans to study the effect of task learning during the early phase of learning; and (2) the difference in the average rs-FC between the last (rs4) and the first (rs1) resting state scans to investigate the effect of long-term practice.

Similarly, we used two different calculations to quantify the behavioral gain during the early phase of learning and the overall learning process: (a) the difference in the average target deviation between the last block of trials (15 trials in total) and the first block of trials (15 trials in total) in the first task-related fMRI scan (tr1) to study the effect of task practice during the early phase of learning; (b) the difference between the average target deviation in the last block of trials (15 in total) of the second task-related fMRI scan (tr2) and the first block of trials (15 in total) in tr1 to investigate the effect of long-term practice.

Hence, we performed brain-behavior correlations between the following functional connectivity measures: (A) Homotopic connections extracted from rs2 minus rs1 (Hm FC short-term learning) difference 1; (B) Heterotopic connections extracted from rs2 minus rs1 (Ht FC short-term learning); (C) Homotopic connections extracted from rs4 minus rs1 (Hm FC long-term learning); (D) Heterotopic connections extracted from rs4 minus rs1 (Ht FC long-term learning); (E) Right hemispheric connections extracted from rs2 minus rs1 (R FC short-term learning); (F) Left hemispheric connections extracted from rs2 minus rs1 (L FC short-term learning); (G) Right hemispheric connections extracted from rs4 minus rs1 (R FC long-term learning); (H) Left hemispheric connections extracted from rs4 minus rs1 (L FC long-term learning),

BTT gain measures were defined as follows:

(A) The last 15 trials of tr1 minus first 15 trials of tr1 for N-ISO condition (BTT Gain 1); (B) The last 15 trials of tr2 minus the first 15 trials of tr1 for N-ISO condition (BTT Gain 2). We focused on the N-ISO conditions as these represented new unfamiliar patterns requiring practice to improve proficiency whereas the

ISO conditions reflected familiar patterns that constitute the default coordination modes (not requiring elaborate practice) (Sisti et al., 2011). Greater BTT gains reflect larger improvements in performance. **Figure 3** illustrates the correlations computed. Correlations surviving Bonferroni correction ($p < 0.025$) were considered significant.

RESULTS

Kinematic Data

Scan Sessions

Motor performance during the scan sessions was assessed with a $2 \times 2 \times 2$ (age $\times$ scan session $\times$ frequency ratio) repeated measures ANOVA for average target deviation. There was a main effect of age [$F(1,42) = 49.59$, $p < 0.0001$, $\eta_p^2 = 0.54$], with YA performing better than OA.

There was also a strong learning effect from pre- to post-training period, reflected by the main effect of scan session [$F(1,42) = 109.8$, $p < 0.0001$, $\eta_p^2 = 0.72$], indicating that performance improved as a result of training.

We also observed a main effect of frequency ratio [$F(1,42) = 197.50$, $p < 0.0001$, $\eta_p^2 = 0.83$], suggesting that subjects had more difficulty in performing the most difficult (N-ISO) as compared with the easiest (ISO) frequency ratios.

A significant age $\times$ scan session interaction effect [$F(1,42) = 20.71$, $p < 0.001$, $\eta_p^2 = 0.33$] indicated that, although both age groups were able to significantly improve their performance as a result of training [YA: $t(22) = 8.95$, $p < 0.0001$: OA: $t(20) = 7.65$, $p < 0.0001$], OA improved their performance to a higher degree as compared to YA from pre-test to post-test session. Furthermore, a significant age $\times$ frequency ratio interaction effect was observed [$F(1,42) = 10.25$, $p = 0.003$, $\eta_p^2 = 0.20$], reflecting that OA, but not YA, had more difficulty

in performing the most difficult (N-ISO) relative to the easiest (ISO) condition [$t(42) = -9.03$, $p < 0.0001$].

Training Sessions

A $2 \times 5 \times 2$ (age $\times$ training session $\times$ frequency ratio) repeated measures ANOVA was conducted for the average target deviation scores obtained across training days.

There was a main effect of age [$F(1,42) = 33.94$, $p < 0.0001$, $\eta_p^2 = 0.48$], indicating that the overall performance level of YA was better than the one of OA.

The main effect of training session was also significant [$F(4,168) = 99.90$, $p < 0.0001$, $\eta_p^2 = 0.70$], suggesting a strong practice effect. *Post hoc* t-tests revealed that the five sessions differed from each other (all $p < 0.001$). However, greater differences were observed for the first two sessions as compared to sessions 3, 4, and 5, suggesting that the practice effect was strongest at the first training sessions and a plateau effect was reached toward the final two sessions.

A significant main effect of frequency ratio [$F(1,42) = 120.57$, $p < 0.0001$, $\eta_p^2 = 0.74$] reflected greater error rates for N-ISO as compared to ISO ratio.

We observed a significant age $\times$ training session interaction effect [$F(4,168) = 7.85$, $p < 0.0001$, $\eta_p^2 = 0.16$]. *Post hoc* t-tests revealed that, although YA had a better performance than OA in all the five training sessions, these age differences were statistically greater during training session 1 compared to sessions 4 [$t(42) = -3.29$, $p < 0.004$] and 5 [$t(42) = -3.76$, $p < 0.001$], suggesting that as training progressed, the differences in performance between YA and OA decreased.

As not much learning was required for the ISO condition, **Figure 4** focuses on the behavioral performance during both the scan and training sessions for the N-ISO condition.

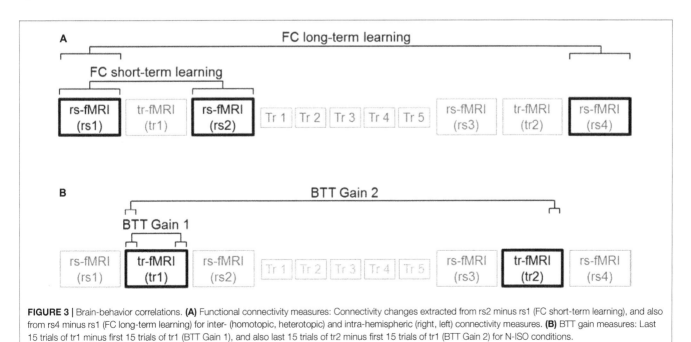

FIGURE 3 | Brain-behavior correlations. **(A)** Functional connectivity measures: Connectivity changes extracted from rs2 minus rs1 (FC short-term learning), and also from rs4 minus rs1 (FC long-term learning) for inter- (homotopic, heterotopic) and intra-hemispheric (right, left) connectivity measures. **(B)** BTT gain measures: Last 15 trials of tr1 minus first 15 trials of tr1 (BTT Gain 1), and also last 15 trials of tr2 minus first 15 trials of tr1 (BTT Gain 2) for N-ISO conditions.

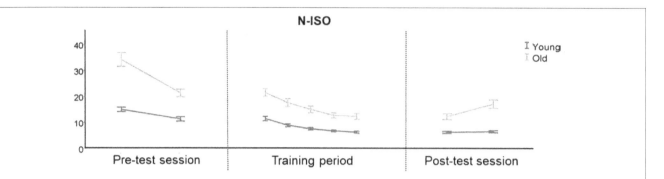

FIGURE 4 | Behavioral performance during the scan and training sessions for the N-ISO condition. There was an initial reduction in target deviation error during the pre-test session, indicative of initial learning. During the training period, BTT performance became more stable, particularly during the last two training days. YA showed a more stable performance during the post-test session than OA, especially in the most difficult task condition (N-ISO). Error bars represent the standard error of the mean (SEM). N-ISO, non-isofrequency.

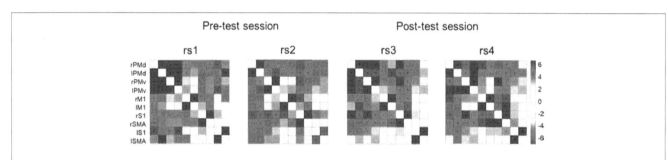

FIGURE 5 | Correlation matrices across all participants showing the strength of functional connectivity between each pair of regions from the motor network for the four rest scans collected in the present study. Significant correlations (Bonferroni corrected probability, $p < 0.001$) are indicated with a black dot. Color bar on the right indicates t-values.

Imaging Data

We studied low-frequency functional correlations associated with a task-specific motor network composed of 10 ROIs: left and right SMA, PMd, PMv, M1, and S1. We calculated Pearson correlation coefficients between each pair of ROIs across subjects, and within each of the four resting state scans. **Figure 5** shows the resulting 10×10 correlation matrix for each resting state scan, which reflects the strength of functional connectivity between each pair of regions. Next, we calculated average functional connectivity scores regarding four different groups of ROI pairs, including homotopic inter-hemispheric FC, heterotopic inter-hemispheric FC, right intra-hemispheric FC and left intra-hemispheric FC.

Modulations of Resting State Inter-Hemispheric Connectivity in Young and Older Adults throughout the Learning Process

The $2 \times 2 \times 2 \times 2$ (age $\times$ inter-hemispheric FC $\times$ scan session $\times$ scan location) repeated measures ANOVAs revealed a main effect of inter-hemispheric functional connectivity [$F(1,42) = 247.26, p < 0.0001, \eta_p^2 = 0.86$], with greater homotopic than heterotopic connectivity values (Hm: 6.68 ± 0.29, Ht: 2.52 ± 0.18) (**Figure 6**). Main effects of age group, scan session and phase were not significant.

A significant age $\times$ scan location interaction indicated that young and older adults showed a different pattern of rs-FC

change as a function of performance of the BTT both during the pre- and post-test sessions [$F(1,42) = 9.01, p = 0.005, \eta_p^2 = 0.18$]. Subsequent *post hoc* unpaired t-tests demonstrated that rs-FC increased after practicing the BTT, that is from rs1 to rs2 and from rs3 to rs4, in YA, whereas OA showed the opposite pattern [$t(42) = -2.21, p = 0.002$. YA, pre-task rs: 4.48 ± 0.41, post-task rs: 4.71 ± 0.28; OA, pre-task rs: 5.03 ± 0.33, post-task rs: 4.16 ± 0.30)]. This effect was true for both homotopic and heterotopic connections. **Figure 6** depicts the age $\times$ scan location interaction. None of the remaining interactions reached significance.

Modulations of Resting State Intra-Hemispheric Connectivity in Young and Older Adults throughout the Learning Process

The $2 \times 2 \times 2 \times 2$ (age $\times$ intra-hemispheric FC $\times$ scan session $\times$ scan location) repeated measures ANOVAs revealed no significant main effects of age, intra-hemispheric FC, scan session and learning phase.

There was a significant age $\times$ scan location interaction, in which young and older adults showed different patterns of rs-FC change as a function of task practice [$F(1,42) = 6.21, p = 0.017, \eta_p^2 = 0.13$]. Subsequent *post hoc* unpaired t-tests demonstrated that rs-FC increased after BTT performance in YA, that is from rs1 to rs2 and from rs3 to rs4, whereas OA exhibited the opposite pattern [$t(42) = -2.56, p = 0.003$.

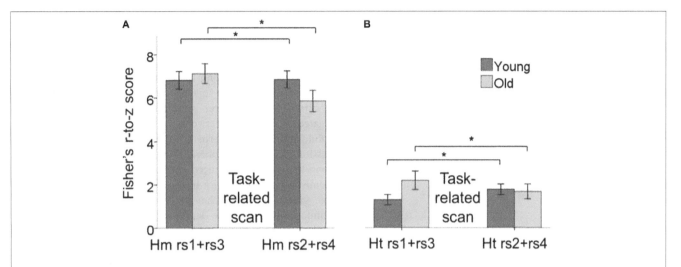

FIGURE 6 | Bar plots showing the age × scan location interaction effect for inter-hemispheric functional connectivity. **(A)** Changes in connectivity in homotopic pairs of regions. **(B)** Changes in connectivity in heterotopic pairs of regions. In both cases, functional connectivity increased after task performance in YA, whereas it decreased in OA and we observed this pattern of results within both the pre- and post-test sessions. Moreover, homotopic functional connectivity was greater than heterotopic functional connectivity. Error bars represent SEM. Hm rs1+rs3, homotopic rest scans before task-related scans; Hm rs2+rs4, homotopic rest scans after task-related scans; Ht rs1+rs3, heterotopic rest scans before task-related scans; Ht rs2+rs4, heterotopic rest scans after task-related scans.

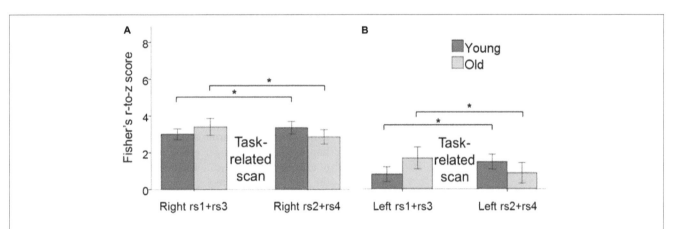

FIGURE 7 | Bar plots show the age × scan location interaction effect for intra-hemispheric functional connectivity. **(A)** Changes in connectivity in right hemisphere pairs of regions. **(B)** Changes in connectivity in left hemisphere pairs of regions. In both cases, functional connectivity increased after task performance in YA, whereas it decreased after task performance in OA within pre- and post-test sessions. Error bars represent SEM.

YA, pre-task rs: 2.75 ± 0.22, post-task rs: 3.15 ± 0.23; OA, pre-task rs: 3.23 ± 0.39, post-task rs: 2.70 ± 0.32)]. Of note, this is the same pattern as previously observed for inter-hemispheric functional connectivity. Moreover, this age-related difference in the pattern of functional connectivity occurred for both left and right hemisphere connections. **Figure 7** depicts the age × scan location interaction.

We also observed a significant intra-hemispheric functional connectivity × scan session interaction effect, indicating that functional connectivity within the right and left hemisphere showed a differential change from pre- to post-test session. [$F(1,42)$ = 4.55, p = 0.04, η_p^2 = 0.10]. Subsequent *post hoc* paired *t*-tests revealed training-related increases in functional connectivity in the right hemisphere, but not in the left hemisphere, after the training period [$t(43)$ = 2.62, p = 0.004;

Right post-test session: 3.41 ± 0.32; Right pre-test session: 2.89 ± 0.24]. None of the remaining main and interaction effects reached significance.

Correlation between Resting State Functional Connectivity and Behavior

We tested whether changes in rs-FC corresponded with gains in behavioral performance as a general tendency across both age groups.

Increases in inter-hemispheric connectivity for both homotopic (Hm FC long-term learning) and heterotopic (Ht FC long-term learning) connections correlated with greater gains in BTT performance (BTT Gain 2 N-ISO) (Hm: r = 0.40, p = 0.010; Ht: r = 0.30, p = 0.04). Of note, the first result survived Bonferroni correction (p < 0.013), whereas the second did not. None of the remaining correlations

TABLE 2 | Correlations between inter- and intra-hemispheric rs-FC changes and BTT gains.

	Gain 1 N-ISO	Gain 2 N-ISO
Hm FC short-term learning	$r = 0.23$	$r = 0.19$
	$p = 0.13$	$p = 0.21$
Ht FC short-term learning	$r = 0.02$	$r = 0.15$
	$p = 0.90$	$p = 0.34$
Hm FC long-term learning	$r = 0.21$	$\boldsymbol{r = 0.40}$
	$p = 0.16$	$\boldsymbol{p = 0.01}$
Ht FC long-term learning	$r = -0.06$	$r = 0.30$
	$p = 0.68$	$p = 0.04$
R FC short-term learning	$r = 0.03$	$r = 0.12$
	$p = 0.85$	$p = 0.44$
L FC short-term learning	$r = 0.12$	$r = 0.19$
	$p = 0.45$	$p = 0.22$
R FC long-term learning	$r = 0.04$	$r = 0.26$
	$p = 0.81$	$p = 0.09$
L FC long-term learning	$r = -0.07$	$r = 0.18$
	$p = 0.66$	$p = 0.25$

Increases in inter-hemispheric connectivity from the first to the last resting state scan for both homotopic and heterotopic connections (Hm FC long-term learning, Ht FC long-term learning) correlated significantly with greater gains in BTT performance from the first 15 trials of the first task-related scan to the last 15 trials of the second task-related scan in the N-ISO condition (Gain 2). Only the bolded values corresponding to the correlation between homotopic rs-FC change and Gain 2 survived Bonferroni correction (p < 0.025). r, Pearson coefficient; p, probability value.

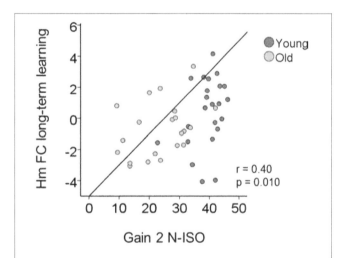

FIGURE 8 | Brain connectivity-behavior correlation. Scatter plot representing the significant correlation surviving Bonferroni correction (p < 0.025) between rs-FC change (y-axis) and bimanual coordination gain (x-axis). r, Pearson coefficient.

reached significance. See **Table 2** and **Figure 8** for further details.

DISCUSSION

We investigated whether learning a bimanual tracking task modulates rs-FC in the early and late phase of practice and

whether this has behavioral relevance. Compared with YA, OA showed a lower motor performance in general, but a larger improvement relative to baseline after 2 weeks of training. Short-term practice effects achieved within pre- and post-test sessions modulated rs-FC, leading to connectivity increases in YA, but connectivity decreases in OA. This pattern of age differences occurred for both inter- and intra-hemispheric connections related to the motor network. We did not observe age-related modulations of long-term practice (i.e., from pre- to post-test session) on interhemispheric rs-FC at the group level. However, long-term training-induced increases were observed in intra-hemispheric connectivity in the right hemisphere (across both age groups). Finally, changes in inter-hemispheric functional connectivity from the start to end of practice correlated with training-induced motor improvement, underscoring the behavioral significance of rs-fMRI for prediction of motor skill learning. We discuss these findings in detail below.

Aging Effects on Bimanual Coordination Learning

Kinematic analyses revealed that older individuals encountered particular difficulties with performing the bimanual tasks with different frequency ratios. This is a consequence of the higher complexity of these tasks. Strikingly, we observed greater performance improvement in older compared to young adults, which is in accordance with previous studies (Wishart et al., 2002; Voelcker-Rehage and Willimczik, 2006). This may be a consequence of the lower performance levels of older adults at baseline, giving rise to a larger window for improvement. However, both age groups showed a similar overall pattern of improvement: a stronger practice effect during the initial phase of learning (pre-test scan session), followed by a plateau toward the final phase (post-test scan session), reflecting relatively stable performance.

Functional Connectivity Changes in Young and Older Adults as a Result of Short-Term Practice

We consistently observed an age-related change in rs-FC after short-term practice both during the early and later stages of learning (pre- and post-test sessions, respectively). Specifically, we observed increases in functional connectivity in young adults but decreases in older adults after task performance. Hence, task practice induced a differential short-term functional reorganization within the resting brain in young and older individuals. However, we did not observe an age-related functional reorganization of our motor network over the longer course of training across 2 weeks (from pre- to post-test session). This implies that the involvement in the training protocol did not induce long-term changes in rs-FC, at least not significantly different between both age groups. Hence, our pattern of results does not support our initial hypothesis of an age-dependent reorganization of the motor network that is more pronounced during the early (pre-test session) compared to the later stage of learning (post-test session), with the most dramatic changes in motor performance occurring in the former stage (Mary et al., 2017).

The findings observed in young adults are generally in accordance with previous research showing short-term effects on rs-FC after task practice (Peltier et al., 2005; Waites et al., 2005; Boonstra et al., 2007; Houweling et al., 2008; Barnes et al., 2009; Stevens et al., 2010; Klingner et al., 2012; Tung et al., 2013). In this regard, it seems reasonable to suggest that the short-term rs-FC increases following the execution of the motor task observed in young adults may reflect tighter communication between motor network areas. Although speculative, these processes may entail sensorimotor integration (Loayza et al., 2011; Ma et al., 2011; Wu et al., 2014) and short-term storage of visuomotor skills (Johnson-Frey et al., 2005; Ma et al., 2011).

The rs-FC decreases due to short-term practice, as observed in older adults, are more difficult to understand. In an attempt to come to grips with this finding, it is important to bear in mind that network organization differs between young and older adults and this pertains to within-network as well as between-network rs-FC. Previous work has shown that rs-FC within the motor network is higher in older as compared to younger adults and this is negatively associated with motor performance (Solesio-Jofre et al., 2014). Furthermore, FC among the different resting state networks is also increased in older adults, pointing to reduced overall network segregation (Geerlings et al., 2014; Chan et al., 2017; King et al., 2017), associated with poorer cognitive performance or no performance benefits at all (Nashiro et al., 2017). This is supportive of a dedifferentiation process, referring to an age-related diminished specificity in the cortical response to some stimulus categories and a reduction in the fidelity of neural representations (Grady et al., 1992; Park et al., 2004; Voss et al., 2008). Against the backdrop of these age-related changes, it is conceivable that training led to a reorganization of the motor network by strengthening interactions with other networks that have functional relevance for the task (such as attention or executive networks) and reducing interactions with other networks that are less or not relevant for task performance (such as the default mode network). This process of increasing efficiency of brain activity may be associated with a temporary reduction in FC between areas of the motor network, as observed in our findings. However, this is a hypothetical account that requires confirmation in future research.

Age-Related Modulations of Inter- and Intra-Hemispheric Functional Connectivity

Interestingly, we observed the same pattern of age group differences for both inter- and intra-hemispheric connections. Regarding the former, it is important to remark that we observed greater homotopic relative to heterotopic functional connectivity values. Increased functional and structural homotopic connections have been commonly reported during the acquisition of bimanual coordination skills. On the basis of other studies employing rs-fMRI, this tendency for homotopic regions to exhibit stronger functional connectivity relative to heterotopic regions is more prevalent for regions of the

adult human brain, such as motor, somatosensory, visual and subcortical regions (Zuo et al., 2010; Ruddy et al., 2017). In the same vein, previous research in non-human primates (Rouiller et al., 1994; Dancause et al., 2007) and humans (Ruddy et al., 2017) has reported that the largest proportions of interhemispheric fibers connecting to M1, SMA and PM originate in their homologous region in the contralateral hemisphere.

Finally, we observed that the strength of rs-FC within the right hemisphere increased after 2 weeks of training in both age groups, highlighting the importance of increased interregional interactions in the right hemisphere during motor skill learning in general and bimanual skill learning in particular (Halsband and Lange, 2006; Ma et al., 2011). This finding may reflect increased functional interactions among the right hemisphere motor areas to control the less skilled non-dominant hand as part of the unified bimanual kinematic chain. Successful coordination is contingent on the cooperation between both hemispheres/hands and this requires elevation of non-dominant hand function to better interact with the dominant hand.

Behavioral Relevance for Learning-Related Modulations in Functional Connectivity

Even though neither of the groups exhibited a change in interhemispheric rs-FC across long-term practice, we observed an association between FC change and behavioral change across long-term practice at the individual level. Increases in the strength of inter-hemispheric connections across the 2-week period were associated with higher motor improvement in both young and older individuals, also across the 2-week period, suggesting that the resting state motor network may support the functional reorganization of the motor system in order to improve behavioral performance and ultimately, motor consolidation. This is in accordance with previous studies suggesting a role for resting state networks in terms of keeping active relevant functional systems to improve behavioral performance (Raichle et al., 2001; Miall and Robertson, 2006; van den Heuvel and Hulshoff Pol, 2010). Specifically, resting state networks become relevant functional units that may be recruited whenever a task needs extra support to be successfully performed.

In the light of these results, we suggest that resting state networks do not simply reflect physiological markers of anatomical pathways, but represent highly efficient modules of brain organization, somehow capable of predicting behavioral performance and improvement following motor learning.

CONCLUSION

In this study, we provided behavioral evidence that motor learning capacity is preserved in aging. Furthermore, we demonstrated that shorter-term practice modulates the resting state differentially in young and older individuals. On the one hand, increased within-network connectivity after task practice observed in young adults may be indicative of enhanced interactions between motor network areas that are engaged in motor learning. On the other hand, an age-related reduction in within-network connectivity after task practice may be an indirect consequence of how the motor network interacts with other networks to optimize overall brain activity for task performance. Older adults may necessitate extra resources to learn the motor task, becoming more dependent on cognitive processes embodied in motor learning. Hence, further research is warranted to shed light on the behavioral relevance of functional interactions across the motor, memory and attentional networks during the resting state.

AUTHOR CONTRIBUTIONS

ES-J performed the data analyses and wrote the manuscript. IB conducted the data collection. DW helped with data analyses and language check. LP helped with behavioral analysis. SC helped with behavioral analysis. DM developed the pipeline for data analysis and helped with the writing of the manuscript. SS is the principal investigator of this project and helped with the writing of the manuscript.

FUNDING

This work was supported by the Research Program of the Research Foundation – Flanders (FWO) [G.0708.14, G.0898.18N], the Wellcome Trust [101253/Z/13/Z], the Interuniversity Attraction Poles Program of the Belgian Federal Government [P7/11], the Special Research Fund KU Leuven [C16/15/070], and Excellence of Science grant (EOS, 30446199, MEMODYN).

REFERENCES

Achard, S., and Bullmore, E. (2007). Efficiency and cost of economical brain functional networks. *PLOS Comput. Biol.* 3:e17. doi: 10.1371/journal.pcbi. 0030017

Achard, S., Salvador, R., Whitcher, B., Suckling, J., and Bullmore, E. (2006). A resilient, low-frequency, small-world human brain functional network with highly connected association cortical hubs. *J. Neurosci.* 26, 63–72. doi: 10.1523/JNEUROSCI.3874-05.2006

Albert, N. B., Robertson, E. M., and Miall, R. C. (2009). The resting human brain and motor learning. *Curr. Biol.* 19, 1023–1027. doi: 10.1016/j.cub.2009.04.028

Albouy, G., Fogel, S., King, B. R., Laventure, S., Benali, H., Karni, A., et al. (2015). Maintaining vs. enhancing motor sequence memories: respective roles of striatal and hippocampal systems. *Neuroimage* 108, 423–434. doi: 10.1016/j.neuroimage.2014.12.049

Amad, A., Seidman, J., Draper, S. B., Bruchhage, M. M. K., Lowry, R. G., Wheeler, J., et al. (2017). Motor learning induces plasticity in the resting brain-drumming up a connection. *Cereb. Cortex* 27, 2010–2021. doi: 10.1093/cercor/bhw048

Andres, F. G., Mima, T., Schulman, A. E., Dichgans, J., Hallett, M., and Gerloff, C. (1999). Functional coupling of human cortical sensorimotor areas during bimanual skill acquisition. *Brain* 122, 855–870. doi: 10.1093/brain/122.5.855

Bangert, A. S., Reuter-Lorenz, P. A., Walsh, C. M., Schachter, A. B., and Seidler, R. D. (2010). Bimanual coordination and aging: neurobehavioral implications. *Neuropsychologia* 48, 1165–1170. doi: 10.1016/j.neuropsychologia.2009.11.013

Barnes, A., Bullmore, E. T., and Suckling, J. (2009). Endogenous human brain dynamics recover slowly following cognitive effort. *PLOS ONE* 4:e6626. doi: 10.1371/journal.pone.0006626

Beets, I. A., Gooijers, J., Boisgontier, M. P., Pauwels, L., Coxon, J. P., Wittenberg, G., et al. (2015). Reduced neural differentiation between feedback conditions after bimanual coordination training with and without augmented visual feedback. *Cereb. Cortex* 25, 1958–1969. doi: 10.1093/cercor/bhu005

Biswal, B., Yetkin, F. Z., Haughton, V. M., and Hyde, J. S. (1995). Functional connectivity in the motor cortex of resting human brain using echo-planar MRI. *Magn. Reson. Med.* 34, 537–541. doi: 10.1002/mrm.1910340409

Boonstra, T. W., Daffertshofer, A., Breakspear, M., and Beek, P. J. (2007). Multivariate time-frequency analysis of electromagnetic brain activity during bimanual motor learning. *Neuroimage* 36, 370–377. doi: 10.1016/j.neuroimage. 2007.03.012

Brown, L. E., Wilson, E. T., and Gribble, P. L. (2009). Repetitive transcranial magnetic stimulation to the primary motor cortex interferes with motor learning by observing. *J. Cogn. Neurosci.* 21, 1013–1022. doi: 10.1162/jocn.2009. 21079

Buchel, C., Coull, J. T., and Friston, K. J. (1999). The predictive value of changes in effective connectivity for human learning. *Science* 283, 1538–1541. doi: 10. 1126/science.283.5407.1538

Byblow, W. D., Coxon, J. P., Stinear, C. M., Fleming, M. K., Williams, G., Muller, J. F., et al. (2007). Functional connectivity between secondary and primary motor areas underlying hand-foot coordination. *J. Neurophysiol.* 98, 414–422. doi: 10.1152/jn.00325.2007

Chan, M. Y., Alhazmi, F. H., Park, D. C., Savalia, N. K., and Wig, G. S. (2017). Resting-state network topology differentiates task signals across the adult life span. *J. Neurosci.* 37, 2734–2745. doi: 10.1523/JNEUROSCI.2406-16.2017

Cohen, J. (1992). A power primer. *Psychol. Bull.* 112, 155–159. doi: 10.1037/0033-2909.112.1.155

Dancause, N., Barbay, S., Frost, S. B., Mahnken, J. D., and Nudo, R. J. (2007). Interhemispheric connections of the ventral premotor cortex in a new world primate. *J. Comp. Neurol.* 505, 701–715. doi: 10.1002/cne.21531

Daselaar, S. M., Huijbers, W., de Jonge, M., Goltstein, P. M., and Pennartz, C. M. (2010). Experience-dependent alterations in conscious resting state activity following perceptuomotor learning. *Neurobiol. Learn. Mem.* 93, 422–427. doi: 10.1016/j.nlm.2009.12.009

Deco, G., and Corbetta, M. (2011). The dynamical balance of the brain at rest. *Neuroscientist* 17, 107–123. doi: 10.1177/1073858409354384

Donchin, O., Gribova, A., Steinberg, O., Bergman, H., and Vaadia, E. (1998). Primary motor cortex is involved in bimanual coordination. *Nature* 395, 274–278. doi: 10.1038/26220

Ebisch, S. J., Gallese, V., Willems, R. M., Mantini, D., Groen, W. B., Romani, G. L., et al. (2011). Altered intrinsic functional connectivity of anterior and posterior insula regions in high-functioning participants with autism spectrum disorder. *Hum. Brain Mapp.* 32, 1013–1028. doi: 10.1002/hbm.21085

Floyer-Lea, A., and Matthews, P. M. (2005). Distinguishable brain activation networks for short- and long-term motor skill learning. *J. Neurophysiol.* 94, 512–518. doi: 10.1152/jn.00717.2004

Fogel, S. M., Albouy, G., Vien, C., Popovicci, R., King, B. R., Hoge, R., et al. (2014). fMRI and sleep correlates of the age-related impairment in motor memory consolidation. *Hum. Brain Mapp.* 35, 3625–3645. doi: 10.1002/hbm.22426

Fox, M. D., and Raichle, M. E. (2007). Spontaneous fluctuations in brain activity observed with functional magnetic resonance imaging. *Nat. Rev. Neurosci.* 8, 700–711. doi: 10.1038/nrn2201

Fox, M. D., Snyder, A. Z., Vincent, J. L., Corbetta, M., Van Essen, D. C., and Raichle, M. E. (2005). The human brain is intrinsically organized into dynamic, anticorrelated functional networks. *Proc. Natl. Acad. Sci. U.S.A.* 102, 9673–9678. doi: 10.1073/pnas.0504136102

Fox, M. D., Zhang, D., Snyder, A. Z., and Raichle, M. E. (2009). The global signal and observed anticorrelated resting state brain networks. *J. Neurophysiol.* 101, 3270–3283. doi: 10.1152/jn.90777.2008

Freitas, C., Perez, J., Knobel, M., Tormos, J. M., Oberman, L., Eldaief, M., et al. (2011). Changes in cortical plasticity across the lifespan. *Front. Aging Neurosci.* 3:5. doi: 10.3389/fnagi.2011.00005

Friston, K. J., Frith, C. D., Frackowiak, R. S., and Turner, R. (1995). Characterizing dynamic brain responses with fMRI: a multivariate approach. *Neuroimage* 2, 166–172. doi: 10.1006/nimg.1995.1019

Geerligs, L., Maurits, N. M., Renken, R. J., and Lorist, M. M. (2014). Reduced specificity of functional connectivity in the aging brain during task performance. *Hum. Brain Mapp.* 35, 319–330. doi: 10.1002/hbm.22175

Gerloff, C., and Andres, F. G. (2002). Bimanual coordination and interhemispheric interaction. *Acta Psychol.* 110, 161–186. doi: 10.1016/S0001-6918(02)00032-X

Gooijers, J., Beets, I. A., Albouy, G., Beeckmans, K., Michiels, K., Sunaert, S., et al. (2016). Movement preparation and execution: differential functional activation patterns after traumatic brain injury. *Brain* 139(Pt 9), 2469–2485. doi: 10.1093/brain/aww177

Gooijers, J., Caeyenberghs, K., Sisti, H. M., Geurts, M., Heitger, M. H., Leemans, A., et al. (2013). Diffusion tensor imaging metrics of the corpus callosum in relation to bimanual coordination: effect of task complexity and sensory feedback. *Hum. Brain Mapp.* 34, 241–252. doi: 10.1002/hbm.21429

Gooijers, J., and Swinnen, S. P. (2014). Interactions between brain structure and behavior: the corpus callosum and bimanual coordination. *Neurosci. Biobehav. Rev.* 43, 1–19. doi: 10.1016/j.neubiorev.2014.03.008

Grady, C. L., Haxby, J. V., Horwitz, B., Schapiro, M. B., Rapoport, S. I., Ungerleider, L. G., et al. (1992). Dissociation of object and spatial vision in human extrastriate cortex: age-related changes in activation of regional cerebral blood flow measured with [(15) o]water and positron emission tomography. *J. Cogn. Neurosci.* 4, 23–34. doi: 10.1162/jocn.1992.4.1.23

Gregory, M. D., Agam, Y., Selvadurai, C., Nagy, A., Vangel, M., Tucker, M., et al. (2014). Resting state connectivity immediately following learning correlates with subsequent sleep-dependent enhancement of motor task performance. *Neuroimage* 102(Pt 2), 666–673. doi: 10.1016/j.neuroimage.2014.08.044

Greicius, M. (2008). Resting-state functional connectivity in neuropsychiatric disorders. *Curr. Opin. Neurol.* 21, 424–430. doi: 10.1097/WCO.0b013e328306f2c5

Halsband, U., and Lange, R. K. (2006). Motor learning in man: a review of functional and clinical studies. *J. Physiol. Paris* 99, 414–424. doi: 10.1016/j.jphysparis.2006.03.007

Hardwick, R. M., Lesage, E., Eickhoff, C. R., Clos, M., Fox, P., and Eickhoff, S. B. (2015). Multimodal connectivity of motor learning-related dorsal premotor cortex. *Neuroimage* 123, 114–128. doi: 10.1016/j.neuroimage.2015.08.024

Hinder, M. R., Schmidt, M. W., Garry, M. I., Carroll, T. J., and Summers, J. J. (2011). Absence of cross-limb transfer of performance gains following ballistic motor practice in older adults. *J. Appl. Physiol.* 110, 166–175. doi: 10.1152/japplphysiol.00958.2010

Houweling, S., Daffertshofer, A., van Dijk, B. W., and Beek, P. J. (2008). Neural changes induced by learning a challenging perceptual-motor task. *Neuroimage* 41, 1395–1407. doi: 10.1016/j.neuroimage.2008.03.023

Johnson-Frey, S. H., Newman-Norlund, R., and Grafton, S. T. (2005). A distributed left hemisphere network active during planning of everyday tool use skills. *Cereb. Cortex* 15, 681–695. doi: 10.1093/cercor/bhh169

King, B. R., van Ruitenbeek, P., Leunissen, I., Cuypers, K., Heise, K. F., Santos Monteiro, T., et al. (2017). Age-related declines in motor performance are associated with decreased segregation of large-scale resting state brain networks. *Cereb. Cortex* 9, 1–13. doi: 10.1093/cercor/bhx297

Klingner, C. M., Volk, G. F., Brodoehl, S., Burmeister, H. P., Witte, O. W., and Guntinas-Lichius, O. (2012). Time course of cortical plasticity after facial nerve palsy: a single-case study. *Neurorehabil. Neural Repair* 26, 197–203. doi: 10.1177/1545968311418674

Loayza, F. R., Fernandez-Seara, M. A., Aznarez-Sanado, M., and Pastor, M. A. (2011). Right parietal dominance in spatial egocentric discrimination. *Neuroimage* 55, 635–643. doi: 10.1016/j.neuroimage.2010.12.011

Ma, L., Narayana, S., Robin, D. A., Fox, P. T., and Xiong, J. (2011). Changes occur in resting state network of motor system during 4 weeks of motor skill learning. *Neuroimage* 58, 226–233. doi: 10.1016/j.neuroimage.2011.06.014

Ma, L., Wang, B., Narayana, S., Hazeltine, E., Chen, X., Robin, D. A., et al. (2010). Changes in regional activity are accompanied with changes in inter-regional connectivity during 4 weeks motor learning. *Brain Res.* 1318, 64–76. doi: 10.1016/j.brainres.2009.12.073

Mary, A., Wens, V., Op de Beeck, M., Leproult, R., De Tiege, X., and Peigneux, P. (2017). Age-related differences in practice-dependent resting-state functional connectivity related to motor sequence learning. *Hum. Brain Mapp.* 38, 923–937. doi: 10.1002/hbm.23428

May, C. M., and Zwaan, B. J. (2017). Relating past and present diet to phenotypic and transcriptomic variation in the fruit fly. *BMC Genomics* 18:640. doi: 10.1186/s12864-017-3968-z

Mehrkanoon, S., Boonstra, T. W., Breakspear, M., Hinder, M., and Summers, J. J. (2016). Upregulation of cortico-cerebellar functional connectivity after motor learning. *Neuroimage* 128, 252–263. doi: 10.1016/j.neuroimage.2015.12.052

Miall, R. C., and Robertson, E. M. (2006). Functional imaging: is the resting brain resting? *Curr. Biol.* 16, R998–R1000. doi: 10.1016/j.cub.2006.10.041

Nashiro, K., Sakaki, M., Braskie, M. N., and Mather, M. (2017). Resting-state networks associated with cognitive processing show more age-related decline than those associated with emotional processing. *Neurobiol. Aging* 54, 152–162. doi: 10.1016/j.neurobiolaging.2017.03.003

Nasreddine, Z. S., Phillips, N. A., Bedirian, V., Charbonneau, S., Whitehead, V., Collin, I., et al. (2005). The Montreal cognitive assessment, MoCA: a brief screening tool for mild cognitive impairment. *J. Am. Geriatr. Soc.* 53, 695–699. doi: 10.1111/j.1532-5415.2005.53221.x

Nichols, T., Brett, M., Andersson, J., Wager, T., and Poline, J. B. (2005). Valid conjunction inference with the minimum statistic. *Neuroimage* 25, 653–660. doi: 10.1016/j.neuroimage.2004.12.005

Oldfield, R. C. (1971). The assessment and analysis of handedness: the Edinburgh inventory. *Neuropsychologia* 9, 97–113. doi: 10.1016/0028-3932(71)90067-4

O'Shea, J., Sebastian, C., Boorman, E. D., Johansen-Berg, H., and Rushworth, M. F. (2007). Functional specificity of human premotor-motor cortical interactions during action selection. *Eur. J. Neurosci.* 26, 2085–2095. doi: 10.1111/j.1460-9568.2007.05795.x

Park, D. C., Polk, T. A., Park, R., Minear, M., Savage, A., and Smith, M. R. (2004). Aging reduces neural specialization in ventral visual cortex. *Proc. Natl. Acad. Sci. U.S.A.* 101, 13091–13095. doi: 10.1073/pnas.0405148101

Pauwels, L., Vancleef, K., Swinnen, S. P., and Beets, I. A. (2015). Challenge to promote change: both young and older adults benefit from contextual interference. *Front. Aging Neurosci.* 7:157. doi: 10.3389/fnagi.2015.00157

Peltier, S. J., LaConte, S. M., Niyazov, D. M., Liu, J. Z., Sahgal, V., Yue, G. H., et al. (2005). Reductions in interhemispheric motor cortex functional connectivity after muscle fatigue. *Brain Res.* 1057, 10–16. doi: 10.1016/j.brainres.2005.06.078

Power, J. D., Mitra, A., Laumann, T. O., Snyder, A. Z., Schlaggar, B. L., and Petersen, S. E. (2014). Methods to detect, characterize, and remove motion artifact in resting state fMRI. *Neuroimage* 84, 320–341. doi: 10.1016/j.neuroimage.2013.08.048

Pravata, E., Sestieri, C., Mantini, D., Briganti, C., Colicchio, G., Marra, C., et al. (2011). Functional connectivity MR imaging of the language network in patients with drug-resistant epilepsy. *AJNR Am. J. Neuroradiol.* 32, 532–540. doi: 10.3174/ajnr.A2311

Raichle, M. E., MacLeod, A. M., Snyder, A. Z., Powers, W. J., Gusnard, D. A., and Shulman, G. L. (2001). A default mode of brain function. *Proc. Natl. Acad. Sci. U.S.A.* 98, 676–682. doi: 10.1073/pnas.98.2.676

Rouiller, E. M., Babalian, A., Kazennikov, O., Moret, V., Yu, X. H., and Wiesendanger, M. (1994). Transcallosal connections of the distal forelimb representations of the primary and supplementary motor cortical areas in macaque monkeys. *Exp. Brain Res.* 102, 227–243. doi: 10.1007/BF00227511

Ruddy, K. L., Leemans, A., and Carson, R. G. (2017). Transcallosal connectivity of the human cortical motor network. *Brain Struct. Funct.* 222, 1243–1252. doi: 10.1007/s00429-016-1274-1

Salvador, R., Suckling, J., Coleman, M. R., Pickard, J. D., Menon, D., and Bullmore, E. (2005). Neurophysiological architecture of functional magnetic resonance images of human brain. *Cereb. Cortex* 15, 1332–1342. doi: 10.1093/cercor/bhi016

Sami, S., Robertson, E. M., and Miall, R. C. (2014). The time course of task-specific memory consolidation effects in resting state networks. *J. Neurosci.* 34, 3982–3992. doi: 10.1523/JNEUROSCI.4341-13.2014

Sampaio-Baptista, C., Filippini, N., Stagg, C. J., Near, J., Scholz, J., and Johansen-Berg, H. (2015). Changes in functional connectivity and GABA levels with long-term motor learning. *Neuroimage* 106, 15–20. doi: 10.1016/j.neuroimage.2014.11.032

Santos Monteiro, T., Beets, I. A. M., Boisgontier, M. P., Gooijers, J., Pauwels, L., Chalavi, S., et al. (2017). Relative cortico-subcortical shift in brain activity but preserved training-induced neural modulation in older adults during bimanual motor learning. *Neurobiol. Aging* 58, 54–67. doi: 10.1016/j.neurobiolaging.2017.06.004

Seidler, R. D., Bernard, J. A., Burutolu, T. B., Fling, B. W., Gordon, M. T., Gwin, J. T., et al. (2010). Motor control and aging: links to age-related brain structural, functional, and biochemical effects. *Neurosci. Biobehav. Rev.* 34, 721–733. doi: 10.1016/j.neubiorev.2009.10.005

Serbruyns, L., Gooijers, J., Caeyenberghs, K., Meesen, R. L., Cuypers, K., Sisti, H. M., et al. (2015). Bimanual motor deficits in older adults predicted by diffusion tensor imaging metrics of corpus callosum subregions. *Brain Struct. Funct.* 220, 273–290. doi: 10.1007/s00429-013-0654-z

Serrien, D. J. (2008). Coordination constraints during bimanual versus unimanual performance conditions. *Neuropsychologia* 46, 419–425. doi: 10.1016/j.neuropsychologia.2007.08.011

Serrien, D. J. (2009). Functional connectivity patterns during motor behaviour: the impact of past on present activity. *Hum. Brain Mapp.* 30, 523–531. doi: 10.1002/hbm.20518

Serrien, D. J., Swinnen, S. P., and Stelmach, G. E. (2000). Age-related deterioration of coordinated interlimb behavior. *J. Gerontol. B Psychol. Sci. Soc. Sci.* 55, 295–303. doi: 10.1093/geronb/55.5.P295

Shumway, R. H., and Stoffer, D. S. (2006). *Time Series Analysis and Its Applications*. New York, NY: Springer, 520.

Sisti, H. M., Geurts, M., Clerckx, R., Gooijers, J., Coxon, J. P., Heitger, M. H., et al. (2011). Testing multiple coordination constraints with a novel bimanual visuomotor task. *PLOS ONE* 6:e23619. doi: 10.1371/journal.pone.0023619

Sisti, H. M., Geurts, M., Gooijers, J., Heitger, M. H., Caeyenberghs, K., Beets, I. A., et al. (2012). Microstructural organization of corpus callosum projections to prefrontal cortex predicts bimanual motor learning. *Learn. Mem.* 19, 351–357. doi: 10.1101/lm.026534.112

Solesio-Jofre, E., Serbruyns, L., Woolley, D. G., Mantini, D., Beets, I. A., and Swinnen, S. P. (2014). Aging effects on the resting state motor network and interlimb coordination. *Hum. Brain Mapp.* 35, 3945–3961. doi: 10.1002/hbm.22450

Stevens, W. D., Buckner, R. L., and Schacter, D. L. (2010). Correlated low-frequency BOLD fluctuations in the resting human brain are modulated by recent experience in category-preferential visual regions. *Cereb. Cortex* 20, 1997–2006. doi: 10.1093/cercor/bhp270

Swinnen, S. P. (1998). Age-related deficits in motor learning and differences in feedback processing during the production of a bimanual coordination pattern. *Cogn. Neuropsychol.* 15, 439–466. doi: 10.1080/026432998381104

Swinnen, S. P. (2002). Intermanual coordination: from behavioural principles to neural-network interactions. *Nat. Rev. Neurosci.* 3, 348–359. doi: 10.1038/nrn807

Swinnen, S. P., Van Langendonk, L., Verschueren, S., Peeters, G., Dom, R., and De Weerdt, W. (1997). Interlimb coordination deficits in patients with Parkinson's disease during the production of two-joint oscillations in the sagittal plane. *Mov. Disord.* 12, 958–968. doi: 10.1002/mds.870120619

Talelli, P., Waddingham, W., Ewas, A., Rothwell, J. C., and Ward, N. S. (2008). The effect of age on task-related modulation of interhemispheric balance. *Exp. Brain Res.* 186, 59–66. doi: 10.1007/s00221-007-1205-8

Tambini, A., Ketz, N., and Davachi, L. (2010). Enhanced brain correlations during rest are related to memory for recent experiences. *Neuron* 65, 280–290. doi: 10.1016/j.neuron.2010.01.001

Taubert, M., Lohmann, G., Margulies, D. S., Villringer, A., and Ragert, P. (2011). Long-term effects of motor training on resting-state networks and underlying brain structure. *Neuroimage* 57, 1492–1498. doi: 10.1016/j.neuroimage.2011.05.078

Todd, G., Kimber, T. E., Ridding, M. C., and Semmler, J. G. (2010). Reduced motor cortex plasticity following inhibitory rTMS in older adults. *Clin. Neurophysiol.* 121, 441–447. doi: 10.1016/j.clinph.2009.11.089

Tung, K. C., Uh, J., Mao, D., Xu, F., Xiao, G., and Lu, H. (2013). Alterations in resting functional connectivity due to recent motor task. *Neuroimage* 78, 316–324. doi: 10.1016/j.neuroimage.2013.04.006

Ungerleider, L. G., Doyon, J., and Karni, A. (2002). Imaging brain plasticity during motor skill learning. *Neurobiol. Learn. Mem.* 78, 553–564.

Vahdat, S., Darainy, M., Milner, T. E., and Ostry, D. J. (2011). Functionally specific changes in resting-state sensorimotor networks after motor learning. *J. Neurosci.* 31, 16907–16915. doi: 10.1523/JNEUROSCI.2737-11.2011

van den Heuvel, M. P., and Hulshoff Pol, H. E. (2010). Exploring the brain network: a review on resting-state fMRI functional connectivity. *Eur. Neuropsychopharmacol.* 20, 519–534. doi: 10.1016/j.euroneuro.2010.03.008

van Dijk, V. F., Delnoy, P., Smit, J. J. J., Ramdat Misier, R. A., Elvan, A., van Es, H. W., et al. (2017). Preliminary findings on the safety of 1.5 and 3 Tesla magnetic resonance imaging in cardiac pacemaker patients. *J. Cardiovasc. Electrophysiol.* 28, 806–810. doi: 10.1111/jce.13231

Voelcker-Rehage, C., and Alberts, J. L. (2007). Effect of motor practice on dual-task performance in older adults. *J. Gerontol. B Psychol. Sci. Soc. Sci.* 62, 141–148.

Voelcker-Rehage, C., and Willimczik, K. (2006). Motor plasticity in a juggling task in older adults-a developmental study. *Age Ageing* 35, 422–427. doi: 10.1093/ageing/afl025

Voss, M. W., Erickson, K. I., Chaddock, L., Prakash, R. S., Colcombe, S. J., Morris, K. S., et al. (2008). Dedifferentiation in the visual cortex: an fMRI investigation of individual differences in older adults. *Brain Res.* 1244, 121–131. doi: 10.1016/j.brainres.2008.09.051

Waites, A. B., Stanislavsky, A., Abbott, D. F., and Jackson, G. D. (2005). Effect of prior cognitive state on resting state networks measured with functional connectivity. *Hum. Brain Mapp.* 24, 59–68. doi: 10.1002/hbm.20069

Wilson, J. K., Baran, B., Pace-Schott, E. F., Ivry, R. B., and Spencer, R. M. (2012). Sleep modulates word-pair learning but not motor sequence learning in healthy older adults. *Neurobiol. Aging* 33, 991–1000. doi: 10.1016/j.neurobiolaging.2011.06.029

Wishart, L. R., Lee, T. D., Cunningham, S. J., and Murdoch, J. E. (2002). Age-related differences and the role of augmented visual feedback in learning a bimanual coordination pattern. *Acta Psychol.* 110, 247–263.

Woolley, D. G., Mantini, D., Coxon, J. P., D'Hooge, R., Swinnen, S. P., and Wenderoth, N. (2015). Virtual water maze learning in human increases functional connectivity between posterior hippocampus and dorsal caudate. *Hum. Brain Mapp.* 36, 1265–1277. doi: 10.1002/hbm.22700

Wu, J., Srinivasan, R., Kaur, A., and Cramer, S. C. (2014). Resting-state cortical connectivity predicts motor skill acquisition. *Neuroimage* 91, 84–90. doi: 10.1016/j.neuroimage.2014.01.026

Yoo, K., Sohn, W. S., and Jeong, Y. (2013). Tool-use practice induces changes in intrinsic functional connectivity of parietal areas. *Front. Hum. Neurosci.* 7:49. doi: 10.3389/fnhum.2013.00049

Zar, J. H. (1998). *Biostatistical Analysis*. New York, NY: Prentice-Hall, 450.

Zhang, H., Long, Z., Ge, R., Xu, L., Jin, Z., Yao, L., et al. (2014). Motor imagery learning modulates functional connectivity of multiple brain systems in resting state. *PLOS ONE* 9:e85489. doi: 10.1371/journal.pone.0085489

Zhang, H., Zhang, Y. J., Duan, L., Ma, S. Y., Lu, C. M., and Zhu, C. Z. (2011). Is resting-state functional connectivity revealed by functional near-infrared spectroscopy test-retest reliable? *J. Biomed. Opt.* 16:067008. doi: 10.1117/1.3591020

Zuo, X. N., Kelly, C., Di Martino, A., Mennes, M., Margulies, D. S., Bangaru, S., et al. (2010). Growing together and growing apart: regional and sex differences in the lifespan developmental trajectories of functional homotopy. *J. Neurosci.* 30, 15034–15043. doi: 10.1523/JNEUROSCI.2612-10.2010

14

Beta-Band Functional Connectivity Influences Audiovisual Integration in Older Age: An EEG Study

Luyao Wang[1†], Wenhui Wang[2†], Tianyi Yan[2*], Jiayong Song[3], Weiping Yang[4], Bin Wang[5], Ritsu Go[1,6], Qiang Huang[1,7] and Jinglong Wu[1,6*]

[1] Intelligent Robotics Institute, School of Mechatronical Engineering, Beijing Institute of Technology, Beijing, China, [2] School of Life Science, Beijing Institute of Technology, Beijing, China, [3] The Affiliated High School of Peking University, Beijing, China, [4] Department of Psychology, Hubei University, Wuhan, China, [5] College of Computer Science and Technology, Taiyuan University of Technology, Shanxi, China, [6] International Joint Research Laboratory of Biomimetic Robots and Systems, Ministry of Education, Beijing, China, [7] Key Laboratory of Biomimetic Robots and Systems, Ministry of Education, Beijing, China

*Correspondence:
Tianyi Yan
yantianyi@bit.edu.cn
Jinglong Wu
wujl@bit.edu.cn

[†] These authors have contributed equally to this work.

Audiovisual integration occurs frequently and has been shown to exhibit age-related differences via behavior experiments or time-frequency analyses. In the present study, we examined whether functional connectivity influences audiovisual integration during normal aging. Visual, auditory, and audiovisual stimuli were randomly presented peripherally; during this time, participants were asked to respond immediately to the target stimulus. Electroencephalography recordings captured visual, auditory, and audiovisual processing in 12 old (60–78 years) and 12 young (22–28 years) male adults. For non-target stimuli, we focused on alpha (8–13 Hz), beta (13–30 Hz), and gamma (30–50 Hz) bands. We applied the Phase Lag Index to study the dynamics of functional connectivity. Then, the network topology parameters, which included the clustering coefficient, path length, small-worldness global efficiency, local efficiency and degree, were calculated for each condition. For the target stimulus, a race model was used to analyze the response time. Then, a Pearson correlation was used to test the relationship between each network topology parameters and response time. The results showed that old adults activated stronger connections during audiovisual processing in the beta band. The relationship between network topology parameters and the performance of audiovisual integration was detected only in old adults. Thus, we concluded that old adults who have a higher load during audiovisual integration need more cognitive resources. Furthermore, increased beta band functional connectivity influences the performance of audiovisual integration during normal aging.

Keywords: functional connectivity, EEG, audiovisual integration, aging, beta band

INTRODUCTION

In daily life, our brain must constantly combine all kinds of information in one or more cues from different sensory modalities. A large body of evidence from daily life has suggested that cognitive functions decline during normal aging. This decline brings trouble during elderly life. As auditory and visual information become more important, the study of age-related differences in audiovisual integration helps us understand the aging process.

Abbreviations: A, unimodal auditory stimulus; AUC, area under the curve of parameters; AV, bimodal audiovisual stimulus; CDFs, cumulative distribution functions; EEG, electroencephalography; PLI, phase lag index; V, unimodal visual stimulus.

To understand the processing of audiovisual stimuli, recent Event-related potentials (ERPs) studies analyzed the time course of visual, auditory and audiovisual stimuli (Fort et al., 2002; Stekelenburg et al., 2004). Furthermore, oscillatory responses in the alpha, beta, and gamma bands have been related to sensory processing. It may be related to harmonize activation of cell assemblies. Fu et al. (2001) showed that the alpha-suppression mechanism occurs during audiovisual stimulus with the use of auditory cues in an attention experiment. Studies with EEG and magnetoencephalogram (MEG) have suggested that the gamma band is also related to the integration of information (Basar, 2013). For the beta band, several groups discussed it during different cognitive processes. The results indicated that oscillatory beta forms an important substrate of human cognition processes, such as attention, working memory and audiovisual integration. Senkowski et al. (2006) investigated beta oscillatory facilitation behavior in an ERP study during visual, auditory and audiovisual stimuli. Sakowitz et al. (2005) found increased beta responses during audiovisual stimuli in comparison to unisensory stimuli on the basis of the intersensory component. Senkowski et al. (2008) used a sensory gating paradigm, which is an integration of meaningful semantic inputs, and they reported that crossmodal effects were related to evoked beta responses.

Recent studies have described age-related audiovisual integration. Some behavioral researches have reported enhanced audiovisual integration in older adults (Laurienti et al., 2006; Peiffer et al., 2007; Mahoney et al., 2011). However, most of the studies were behavioral studies and did not focus on different oscillatory frequency bands. There are many factors that influence the audiovisual integration, such as the location of the presented experimental (Molholm et al., 2004). When the audiovisual stimuli were presented peripherally, the integration could also be elicited. In addition, age-related differences were significant. The maximal behavioral enhancement in older adults occurred more delayer and the time window was longer than in younger adults (Wu et al., 2012). ERP and EEG studies have shown the deficits in attentional control affected the audiovisual integration (Mozolic et al., 2012). Some study using arrow as cue to investigate the age-related visuospatial attention. The results shown the performance for old and young adults is similar. In addition, old adults had slower ERP components and similarly amplitude compared to young adults (Curran et al., 2001). These findings indicate that there are some changes to audiovisual integration with aging, but the underlying neuronal mechanisms are still not fully understood.

Recent research has shown that functional interactions between brain areas are crucial for effective cognitive functioning (Wen et al., 2012), a concept referred to as "functional connectivity." Functional connections play an important role in multisensory processing. Connections not only between sensory related subcortical structures but also between cortical areas can mediate multisensory integration (Beer et al., 2011; Bishop et al., 2012; van den Brink et al., 2014). Some studies investigated the functional network affects audiovisual integration in different ways. The network could be reorganized due to long-term training

(Paraskevopoulos et al., 2015). In addition, functional connectivity could be reorganized by cognitive training (Bamidis et al., 2014; Klados et al., 2016). However, the age-related differences of functional connectivity during audiovisual integration is still unknown.

We used EEG to investigate age-related audiovisual integration; its high temporal resolution makes it rather suitable for the identification of synchronization across frequency bands. The EEG signals were recorded over brain to study the functional connectivity. The PLI, a synchronization measure, reflects the extent of inter-trial phase variability for a given frequency across time. PLI is defined as a period of phase locking between two events, and it can only be estimated in a statistical sense. It removes and attenuates the synchronization that occurs at or near the zero phase difference. From this way, we could reduce the interference of signals from common sources or volume conduction, which were regarded as spurious synchronization (Stam et al., 2007; Doesburg et al., 2013).

In this study, we sought to investigate the functional connectivity in different oscillatory frequency bands during audiovisual integration. We hypothesized that functional connection could influence the audiovisual integration and there are differences between old and young adults. To address this issue, we designed three stimuli: V, A, and bimodal audiovisual (AV) stimuli, which are presented peripherally. We combined the phase synchrony of electrode interactions and graph-theoretical metrics of network topography to investigate task-dependent functional connectivity derived from EEG data. The PLI computed for each pair of sensors was used to construct graphs in various frequency bands independently.

MATERIALS AND METHODS

Participants

Twelve old male adults (60–78 years, mean age ± SD, 68.6 ± 4.74) and 12 young male adults (22–28 years, mean age ± SD, 23.9 ± 1.73) participated in this study. To confirm their cognitive function, all of the participants did the mini-mental state exam to identify cognitive function. Participant who had a score more than 2.5 SD from the mean score that matched his age and level of education were excluded (Bravo and Hebert, 1997). In addition, participants were excluded if they self-reported any disease. Due to the experiment requirement, all of the participants had normal or corrected-to-normal vision (none of the participants were color blind) and normal hearing capabilities. The individuals provided written informed consent, which was previously approved by the ethics committee of Okayama University.

Stimuli and Task

The experiment was performed in a dimly lit, sound-attenuated, electrically shielded room (laboratory room; Okayama University, Japan). Stimuli presentation and response collection were determined using the Presentation software (Neurobehavioral Systems Inc., Albany, CA, United States). A 21-inch computer monitor with a black background was

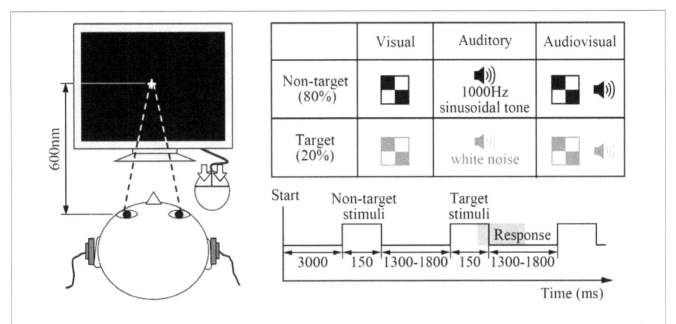

FIGURE 1 | Experimental design. The visual target stimulus was a red and white block, and the non-target visual stimulus was a black and white block. The auditory target stimulus was a white noise, and the non-target auditory stimulus was a 1000 Hz sinusoidal noise. The audiovisual stimulus consisted of the simultaneous presentation of both visual and auditory target or non-target stimuli. In addition, non-target stimuli were presented at a frequency of 80% of the total stimuli.

positioned 60 cm in the front of the participant's eyes and was used to present visual stimuli. The auditory stimuli were presented through an earphone. Each block consisted of 300 visual stimuli, 300 auditory stimuli and 300 audiovisual stimuli. All of the stimuli were randomly presented and had an equal probability of appearing to the left or right of the central fixation point.

The visual target stimulus was a red and white block, and the non-target visual stimulus was a black and white block (5.2 cm × 5.2 cm with a subtending visual angle of ∼5°). These visual stimuli were peripherally presented at an angle of ∼12° from a centrally presented fixation point in the lower visual fields (∼5° below the horizontal meridian) (He et al., 1996; Talsma and Woldorff, 2005). The auditory target stimulus was white noise, and the non-target auditory stimulus was a 1000 Hz sinusoidal tone (60 dB sound pressure level, 5 ms rise or fall time). The audiovisual stimulus consisted of the simultaneous presentation of both the visual and auditory target or non-target stimuli. In addition, non-target stimuli were presented at a frequency of 80% of the total stimuli (**Figure 1**).

At the beginning, each participant was required to complete five experimental blocks, and each block lasted ∼5 min. In formal experiment, each block had a 3000 ms fixation period, followed by the test stimulus. Each type of stimulus displayed 150 ms and continued with 1300 – 1800 ms interstimulus interval time. Within the interval time, participant responded to the target stimulus and the screen was cleared. The experiment continued regardless of whether the participant responded. Participants were instructed to click the left or right button with the forefinger or middle finger quickly and accurately when the target stimuli occurred. They were also

instructed to stare at the central white cross during the whole experiment.

EEG Data Collection

The EEG signals were recorded from 30 scalp electrodes mounted on an electrode cap (Easy cap, Germany), as specified by the International 10–20 System, and 2 electrooculogram electrodes that were referenced to the earlobes. Data were bandpass filtered from 0.05 to 100 Hz during the recordings and were digitized at a sampling rate of 500 Hz by BrainAmp amplifiers (BrainProducts, Munich, Germany).

DATA ANALYSIS

Interregional Phase Synchronization

Our data were pre-processed with Matlab R2013a (Mathworks Inc., Natick, MA, United States) with the following open source toolboxes: EEGLAB[1] (Swartz Center for Computational Neuroscience, La Jolla, CA, United States). An Independent Component Analysis was used to remove artifacts (e.g., eye artifacts, muscle artifacts and electrocardiographic activity) from the data within all channels. We also corrected the baseline for each epoch.

The non-target stimuli were filtered into alpha (8–13 Hz), beta (13–30 Hz), and gamma (30–50 Hz) frequency ranges. The network synchronization of all three bands was investigated. For each subject, the Hilbert transform was employed to obtain the time series of instantaneous phase measures for each trial, source

---

[1]http://sccn.ucsd.edu/eeglab/

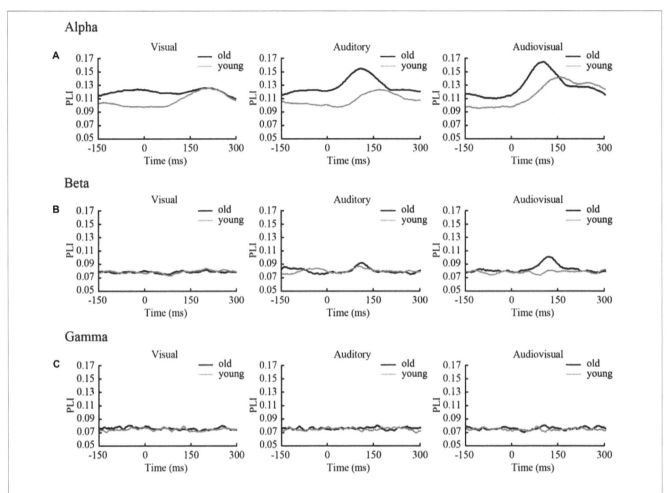

FIGURE 2 | Time courses of average PLI in three frequencies. **(A)** PLI of each time point (including 150 ms before stimulus onset and 300 ms after stimulus onset) in the alpha band. **(B)** PLI of each time point (the same as in the alpha band) in the beta band. **(C)** PLI of each time point (the same as in the alpha band) in the gamma band.

and frequency band. Phase locking was calculated for each EEG sensor pair and frequency with the PLI (Stam et al., 2007).

$$PLI = \left|\langle \text{sign}(\Delta\phi(t_n))\rangle\right| = \left|\frac{1}{M}\sum_{k=1}^{M}\text{sigh}(\Delta\phi(t_n))\right| \quad (1)$$

At a given time point, it measures the reliability of phase relations between two EEG sensors, which produces a sensor-by-sensor adjacency matrix. Epochs were extracted from 300 ms before stimulus onset until 500 ms after stimulus onset. We removed the first and last 150 ms (75 sample points) due to the distortions caused by Hilbert transform at the edges of the epochs (Doesburg et al., 2008). These were then averaged within each group (old adults and young adults) for each trial condition (auditory, visual and audiovisual, each condition includes two orientations). The average PLI values across EEG sensors for each time point reflect task-dependent dynamic network connectivity. For each participants, we calculated it at each frequency, respectively. An two-sample t-test (sample size of bootstrap is 1000) was performed at each time point to compare the differential PLI value of the old and young adults. Time points

with significant age differences were used to identify windows for further analyses.

Statistical Analysis of Network Dynamics

According to the results of the two-sample t-test above and previous studies, adjacency matrices for non-overlapping 150 ms time-windows after stimulus onset were extracted for each frequency: 0–150 ms for alpha and gamma bands and 50–200 ms for the beta band. To characterize task-dependent network connectivity dynamics, these adjacency matrices were averaged and represent the mean connectivity within this active window for each subject.

Task-dependent network synchronization was analyzed by Network Based Statistic (NBS), which is a data-driven approach. Statistical significance of group differences could be displayed, which was corrected for multiple comparisons. (Zalesky et al., 2010, 2012). In this study, the purpose of the NBS is to identify any connected structures that are significantly different between old adults and young adults. At first, we applied a univariate statistical threshold to each

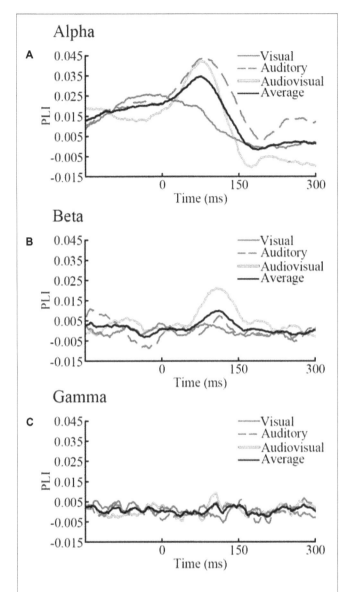

FIGURE 3 | Subtraction of PLI. We subtracted the PLI of young adults from the PLI of old adults for visual, auditory and audiovisual stimuli for each frequency band. The black solid line is the average of each stimuli condition. **(A)** Results in the alpha band **(B)** Results in the beta band **(C)** Results in the gamma band.

element in the compared adjacency matrix, and multiple comparisons was achieved regardless of this threshold. In this case, a *t*-test was performed in the 30 × 30 adjacency matrix ($p < 0.05$) (Zalesky et al., 2010, 2012). Then, data surrogation was repeated 5,000 times to establish statistical confidence.

Graph of Theoretical Analysis of Dynamic Network Topologies

Functional connectivity among sensors was measured by computing the PLI for every possible pair during the time window. The resulting non-linear correlation matrices were converted to weighted graphs. To characterize the task-dependent weighted network dynamics, we constructed network G (30 × 30) for each trial, frequency and subject by GRETNA (Wang et al., 2015) by using the time window identified in the above analysis.

For the constructed brain networks, we calculated brain network parameters (including the clustering coefficient, path length, small-worldness, global efficiency, local efficiency and degree) to examine both the global and regional topological characteristic variations. Each attribute was compared with those of 100 random networks. We applied a sparsity threshold ($0 < S < 1$), which normalized the networks, to examine the relative network organization. In addition, task-dependent areas under the curve (AUCs) of parameters were calculated for each network measure to provide a scalar that did not depend on the specific threshold selection.

Statistical Analysis

SPSS version 20.0 (SPSS, Inc., Chicago, IL, United States) was used for statistical analyses. For each frequency, repeated-measures ANOVAs were carried out separately for the averaged adjacency matrices of PLI and task-dependent AUC of eight network parameters. A 2 (age group: old, young) × 3 (sensory modality: A, V, or AV) × 2 (stimuli direction: left, right) repeated-measures ANOVA analysis was performed separately to examine the effects of audiovisual integration and age as well as their interaction. The Greenhouse-Geisser epsilon value was obtained in all cases in which the repeated-measures data failed the sphericity test (Greenhouse and Geisser, 1982). All statistical comparisons were two-tailed with $\alpha = 0.05$. We used the Bonferroni correction to correct for the effect of multiple comparisons in neural oscillations.

Relationship between Network Topology Parameters and Behavior Data

Trials with target stimuli were extracted for behavior analysis. A race model was used to identify whether audiovisual integration occurred (Miller, 1986). For each participant, the target stimuli were analyzed with CDFs for the V, A and AV stimuli. In addition, the CDFs for the V, A and AVstimuli were generated using 10 ms time bins. At each time bin, the distribution of race model was calculated by the following formula: [P (V) + P (A)] − [P (V) × P (A)]. Each participant's race model curve was then subtracted from their AV CDF. The peak time point of each probability difference curve was recorded, which represented the response time at that the audiovisual integration most likely occurred. A one-way ANOVA was performed to compare age differences (two-tailed with $\alpha = 0.05$, Bonferroni correction).

Furthermore, at each oscillatory frequency, a Pearson correlation was conducted to test the relationship between each network parameter and behavior peak time point.

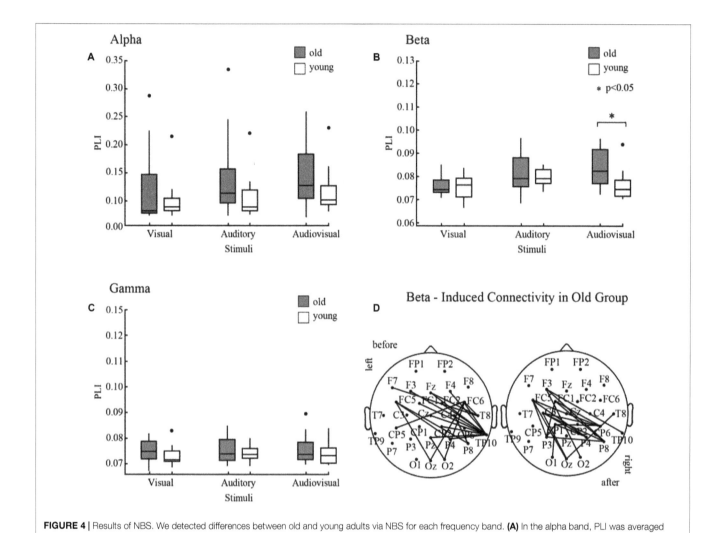

FIGURE 4 | Results of NBS. We detected differences between old and young adults via NBS for each frequency band. **(A)** In the alpha band, PLI was averaged 0–150 ms after stimulus onset. **(B)** In the beta band, PLI was averaged 50–200 ms after stimulus onset. **(C)** In the gamma band, PLI was averaged 0–150 ms after stimulus onset. **(D)** In the beta band, a significant induced connection in old adults during audiovisual processing was detected.

RESULTS

Time Courses of Average PLI

We filtered the EEG data into alpha (8–13 Hz), beta (13–30 Hz), and gamma (30–50 Hz) frequency ranges. The phase synchronization of these frequencies was calculated. For each time point, we averaged the PLI of each subject within groups (**Figure 2**). For subsequent analyses, no differences were found between the left and right hemi-spaces (see Supplementary Figure 1) in the strength of PLI and network topology parameters, and we averaged the results of the two orientations.

The results show that in both the alpha and beta band, there were clear dynamic changes after stimulus onset for all condition, especially for the audiovisual stimulus. There was a significant ($p < 0.05$) difference within 50–200 ms for the beta band. This finding indicates that the strength of functional connectivity in old adults is higher than in young adults. In alpha and gamma band, only a small part of the time point within 0–150 ms was different between groups. To compare the differences between groups, we performed a subtraction for each condition. The main results obtained from our studies are summarized in **Figure 3**.

Topographical Analysis between Groups

According to time courses of average PLI and previous ERP studies (Fort et al., 2002; Stekelenburg et al., 2004), we choose the 150 ms time window after stimulus onset (0–150 ms for alpha and gamma, 50–200 ms for beta) and averaged them to characterize the task-dependent weighted network connectivity. As presented in **Figure 2**, we averaged the results of the two orientations (**Figures 4A–C**). In beta band, results of repeated-measures ANOVA shown that there is significant interaction between group and stimuli type [$p = 0.02$, $F(2,44) = 4.800$]. The simple effect results showed that there are significant differences between old and young participants during the AV target stimulus task [$p = 0.03$, $F(1,22) = 5.39$] (**Figure 4B**). The results that contains two orientations are in Supplementary Figure 2.

A strict statistical analysis was performed with Network Based Statistics to investigate group differences in phase synchrony

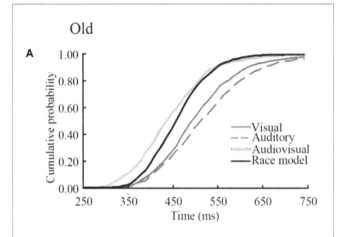

Old

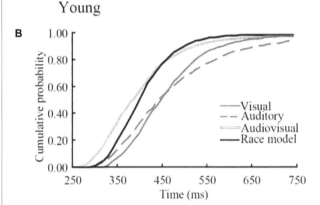

Young

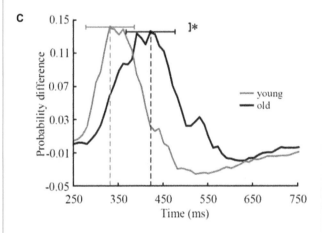

FIGURE 5 | Distributions of response time of old and young adults. **(A)** CDFs for response times to visual, auditory and audiovisual stimuli in young adults. The summed probability of visual and auditory responses is shown by the race model curve (race model). **(B)** CDFs in old adults. **(C)** The cumulative probability difference curve for old adults (solid line) and the young adults (gray line). The peak time point is significant difference between two groups.
* $p < 0.05$.

in a distributed network of EEG sensors only in the AV stimulus condition ($p < 0.05$, corrected, two-tailed) in **Figure 4B**. However, a left or right stimulus activated contralateral brain results in different pairwise connections of two orientations (**Figure 4D**). No significant group differences were observed for other stimulus trials.

However, NBS only reveals connected structures that are significantly different between groups. It does not reveal any statistically significant differences in topological properties.

Statistical Results in Task-Dependent Network Topology Parameters

To assess age differences in brain network connectivity during the task, the AUC of the clustering coefficient (Cp), path length (Lp), small-worldness (Gamma, Lambda, Sigma), global efficiency (Eg), local efficiency (Eloc), and degree was analyzed. For each frequency, a 2 (age group: old, young) × 3 (sensory modality: A, V, or AV) × 2 (stimuli direction: left, right) repeated-measures ANOVA was performed.

The detailed results are shown in **Table 1**. Differential parameters between groups are presented in larger fonts. In the alpha band, there are significant interactions for the Cp value [$p = 0.04$, $F(2,44) = 6.367$]. In the beta band, there are significant interactions for Cp [$p = 0.049$, $F(2,44) = 3.255$], Gamma [$p = 0.04$, $F(2,44) = 6.642$], Sigma [$p = 0.02$, $F(2,44) = 7.412$], Lp [$p = 0.013$, $F(2,44) = 4.820$], Eg [$p = 0.021$, $F(2,44) = 4.374$], Eloc [$p = 0035$, $F(2,44) = 3.739$], and Degree [$p = 0.014$, $F(2,44) = 4.721$] values. In the gamma band, there are significant interactions for Gamma [$p = 0.30$, $F(2,44) = 4.054$], and Sigma [$p = 0.036$, $F(2,44) = 3.781$] values.

The simple effect results showed that there are significant trends for old individuals to have lower Cp or Gamma (normalized value of Cp) values during the visual task than young individuals for the alpha band [$p = 0.045$, $F(1,22) = 4.53$], beta band [$p = 0.036$, $F(1,22) = 5.01$], and gamma band [$p = 0.02$, $F(1,22) = 12.60$]. In addition, for the beta band, all of the parameters showed significant differences between old and young participants during the AV target stimulus task for Cp [$p = 0.049$, $F(1,22) = 4.35$], Gamma [$p = 0.003$, $F(1,22) = 11.57$], Sigma [$p = 0.002$, $F(1,22) = 12.49$], Lp [$p = 0.008$, $F(1,22) = 8.42$], Eg [$p = 0.018$, $F(1,22) = 6.58$], Eloc [$p = 0.024$, $F(1,22) = 5.90$], and Degree [$p = 0.024$, $F(1,22) = 5.86$].

Relation to Behavior

The results of CDFs of V, A, AV and race model was shown in **Figure 5A** (old adults) and **Figure 5B** (young adults). The distribution of CDFs revealed that the responses to the AV stimuli were faster than the response to V or A stimuli in both age groups. Furthermore, to identify whether audiovisual integration occurred, we measured the response time to the AV stimuli by subtracting the race model for each age group independently (**Figure 5C**). The time window of behavioral

during each condition for each frequency range. In the beta band, NBS revealed induced connectivity in the old group facilitation in older adults was longer and more delayed than that in the younger adults. The peak time point of each probability difference curve was recorded for each participant in each age group. There was a significant difference between groups in terms of peak time point ($p = 0.02$). For the young adults, the average peak time point was 330 ms (SD: $\pm$ 56 ms), whereas the old adults had delayed response times at 420 ms (SD: $\pm$ 55 ms).

At each oscillatory frequency, a Pearson correlation was conducted to test the relationship between network parameters and behavior response. No significant relationships were observed for the alpha and gamma bands. For the beta band, only for the AV stimulus, the network topology parameters showed a significant relationship with the peak time point (**Figure 6**). It is interesting that only old adults showed a strong relationship.

DISCUSSION

Summary

Neuroanatomical changes have been recognized and are thought to account for the cognitive declines during aging. However, the underlying neuronal mechanisms in age-related audiovisual integration are still unclear. This study explored this question by analyzing phase synchronization and the graph-theoretical

network of EEG data. Studies have shown that EEG is rather suitable for the identification of synchronization across frequency bands in functional networks (Stam et al., 2007). Synchronous oscillatory neural activity is a possible candidate mechanism for the coordination of neural activity between functionally specialized brain regions.

The goal of the present study was to clarify the age-related functional connectivity in alpha, beta and gamma bands during visual, auditory and audiovisual stimuli. We found age differences within 200 ms after stimulus onset, which is consistent with previous studies (Fort et al., 2002; Stekelenburg et al., 2004). The results show that old adults have stronger functional connectivity while performing the same tasks, especially for audiovisual stimuli. Furthermore, beta oscillatory network connectivity influences the performance of audiovisual integration during normal aging.

Age-Related Beta Band Functional Connectivity in Audiovisual Integration

Oscillatory phenomena corresponding to the EEG frequency bands play a major role in functional communication in the brain during cognitive process. The present study is the first to analyze age-related oscillatory functional connectivity during audiovisual integration. We focused on the alpha, beta and gamma bands, which have been related to sensory processing (Fu et al., 2001;

TABLE 1 | Statistical results of network topology parameters for each condition.

		Visual		Auditory		Audiovisual	
		Old	Young	Old	Young	Old	Young
Alpha	Cp	0.0103 ± 0.0019	0.0119 ± 0.0024	0.0119 ± 0.0019	0.0108 ± 0.0029	0.0114 ± 0.0018	0.0115 ± 0.0020
	Lp	0.5006 ± 0.1513	0.5050 ± 0.1215	0.4196 ± 0.1305	0.4973 ± 0.1258	0.4007 ± 0.1237	0.4483 ± 0.1269
	Gamma	0.0451 ± 0.0048	0.0466 ± 0.0078	0.0449 ± 0.0057	0.0442 ± 0.0066	0.0434 ± 0.0060	0.0429 ± 0.0065
	Lambda	0.0508 ± 0.0008	0.0511 ± 0.0012	0.0510 ± 0.0007	0.0505 ± 0.0009	0.0514 ± 0.0012	0.0509 ± 0.0012
	Sigma	0.0444 ± 0.0048	0.0456 ± 0.0074	0.0439 ± 0.0054	0.0437 ± 0.0063	0.0423 ± 0.0058	0.0421 ± 0.0060
	Eg	0.0057 ± 0.0025	0.0054 ± 0.0019	0.0068 ± 0.0028	0.0055 ± 0.0021	0.0069 ± 0.0022	0.0062 ± 0.0023
	Eloc	0.0054 ± 0.0027	0.0056 ± 0.0023	0.0069 ± 0.0029	0.0055 ± 0.0026	0.0070 ± 0.0027	0.0061 ± 0.0023
	Degree	0.7425 ± 0.4244	0.6638 ± 0.2622	0.8799 ± 0.4435	0.6806 ± 0.2599	0.9258 ± 0.3597	0.7535 ± 0.2804
Beta	Cp	0.0259 ± 0.0040	0.0290 ± 0.0034	0.0284 ± 0.0040	0.0281 ± 0.0032	0.0271 ± 0.0035	0.0300 ± 0.0036
	Lp	1.2825 ± 0.1058	1.3105 ± 0.1332	1.2165 ± 0.1607	1.2419 ± 0.1071	1.1466 ± 0.1577	1.3038 ± 0.1188
	Gamma	0.0986 ± 0.0044	0.0978 ± 0.0039	0.0968 ± 0.0049	0.0975 ± 0.0039	0.0950 ± 0.0048	0.0999 ± 0.0047
	Lambda	0.1005 ± 0.0008	0.1004 ± 0.0006	0.1006 ± 0.0010	0.1008 ± 0.0007	0.1008 ± 0.0010	0.1005 ± 0.0006
	Sigma	0.0982 ± 0.0044	0.0974 ± 0.0037	0.0962 ± 0.0052	0.0968 ± 0.0038	0.0942 ± 0.0049	0.0944 ± 0.0039
	Eg	0.0078 ± 0.0007	0.0077 ± 0.0008	0.0084 ± 0.0012	0.0081 ± 0.0007	0.0089 ± 0.0015	0.0077 ± 0.0008
	Eloc	0.0080 ± 0.0007	0.0079 ± 0.0009	0.0086 ± 0.0013	0.0084 ± 0.0009	0.0092 ± 0.0017	0.0080 ± 0.0009
	Degree	0.4270 ± 0.0408	0.4200 ± 0.0434	0.4584 ± 0.0688	0.4455 ± 0.0408	0.5006 ± 0.1163	0.4231 ± 0.0479
Gamma	Cp	0.0110 ± 0.0025	0.0128 ± 0.0021	0.0118 ± 0.0019	0.0124 ± 0.0025	0.0114 ± 0.0026	0.0118 ± 0.0016
	Lp	0.7597 ± 0.0680	0.7981 ± 0.0546	0.7513 ± 0.0704	0.7921 ± 0.0475	0.7572 ± 0.0702	0.7923 ± 0.0627
	Gamma	0.0464 ± 0.0042	0.0503 ± 0.0039	0.0474 ± 0.0043	0.0485 ± 0.0043	0.0481 ± 0.0044	0.0473 ± 0.0045
	Lambda	0.0500 ± 0.0005	0.0502 ± 0.0003	0.0503 ± 0.0006	0.0501 ± 0.0003	0.0501 ± 0.0004	0.0501 ± 0.0004
	Sigma	0.0463 ± 0.0040	0.0501 ± 0.0039	0.0471 ± 0.0045	0.0483 ± 0.0043	0.0480 ± 0.0043	0.0472 ± 0.0045
	Eg	0.0033 ± 0.0003	0.0031 ± 0.0004	0.0034 ± 0.0003	0.0032 ± 0.0002	0.0033 ± 0.0003	0.0032 ± 0.0003
	Eloc	0.0030 ± 0.0005	0.0030 ± 0.0004	0.0033 ± 0.00060	0.0029 ± 0.0002	0.0032 ± 0.0006	0.0029 ± 0.0004
	Degree	0.3906 ± 0.0349	0.3742 ± 0.0291	0.3972 ± 0.0373	0.3797 ± 0.0238	0.3962 ± 0.0413	0.3787 ± 0.0305

The size of indexes that significantly different between groups was not larger.

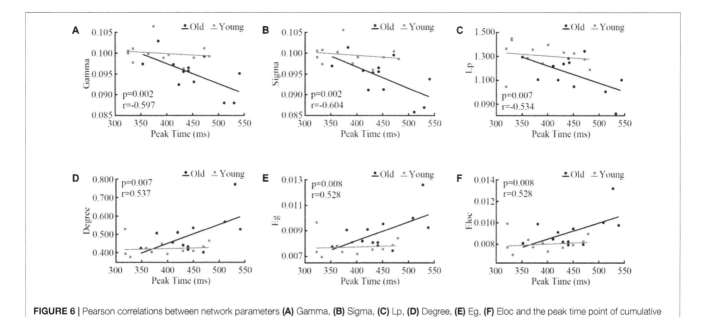

FIGURE 6 | Pearson correlations between network parameters **(A)** Gamma, **(B)** Sigma, **(C)** Lp, **(D)** Degree, **(E)** Eg, **(F)** Eloc and the peak time point of cumulative probability difference curves. We only detected significant correlations in the beta band during audiovisual stimuli.

Senkowski et al., 2006; Basar, 2013). The results indicated that age-related differences occurred during audiovisual stimuli only in the beta band. von Stein and Sarnthein (2000) showed that the beta band serves as a communication mechanism between distant cortical areas. These findings confirmed that the beta band connection plays an important role in visual, auditory and audiovisual processes during aging (Sakowitz et al., 2005; Senkowski et al., 2008).

Both old and young adults showed increased PLI in beta bands after stimulus onset. In addition, only in the beta band, old adults had a significantly higher PLI during audiovisual processing (**Figure 4B**), which indicates the presence of stronger phase locking while performing tasks. As presented in this study, we avoid effects of motor responses and analyzed only non-target stimuli. Some studies reported the same results in responses to both target and non-target stimulation (Missonnier et al., 2007; Kukleta et al., 2009). One explanation of our results is that the beta band connection increases with higher load during normal aging, which suggests that the amount of processing resources allocated to audiovisual tasks is larger for old than young adults. To achieve audiovisual tasks, old adults need to activate more beta band connection than young adults. Our result is in line with previous studies that old adults exhibit larger responses in the beta frequency range during cognitive processing (Sebastian et al., 2011; Sallard et al., 2016). Hong et al. (2016) used a Go/NoGo task to examine the effects of aging on brain networks, and showed increased phase synchrony in the beta band that was more robust in old adults. Zarahn et al. (2007) showed an increased beta response during the memory load task. In addition, researches have reported that lower cognitive reserve was related to higher functional connectivity (Lopez et al., 2014).

The NBS results shown the connected structures are significantly different between groups. Statistical results in task-dependent network topology parameters confirmed this

difference. Furthermore, the peak time point of each probability difference curve was different between old and young adults (**Figure 5C**). The peak time point represents the likely occurrence of audiovisual integration. In the beta band, network topology parameters of audiovisual processing showed strong correlations with peak time points in old adults but not in young adults (**Figure 6**). However, no age differences were detected for unimodal stimuli. This finding indicates that beta band functional connectivity influences the performance of audiovisual integration during normal aging. Old adults need more cognitive resources to perform highly demanding tasks (Sakowitz et al., 2005), which leads to changes in communication within the cortical system. Diaconescu et al. (2013) revealed that the engaged additional regions during audiovisual stimuli compared to younger adults. Audiovisual integration requires a higher level of cognition than visual or auditory processing and requires an old adult to think. However, young adults do not need to try to achieve tasks that lead to a low relationship with behavior results. Our results are supported by the study by Steffener et al. (2014), who revealed the relationship between cognitive performance and functional brain activity. These previous findings suggested that increased functional brain activity relates to worse (slower) task performance in old adults but not in young adults.

Therefore, our study is in good accordance with previous studies, which showed that audiovisual integration is different between old adults and young adults. Furthermore, the oscillatory beta network functional connectivity increased and graph characteristics changed during normal aging, which influence the reaction to audiovisual stimuli.

In the future, we will determine how to adjust beta band functional connectivity to benefit audiovisual integration during normal aging. Because our participants included old adults who are unable to adapt the long-term experiment, we chose 30 scalp electrode channels to construct the brain network. One main limitation of this study may be that the node of the network is relatively small.

AUTHOR CONTRIBUTIONS

LW analyzed and interpreted the data, wrote the paper. WW analyzed and interpreted the data. JS, WY, and QH performed the experiments. BW and RG conceived and designed the experiments. TY and JW revised the paper, approved the final version.

ACKNOWLEDGMENTS

We acknowledge and thank the subjects involved in the study. This study was financially supported by the National Natural Science Foundation of China (grant numbers 61473043 and 81671776), the Beijing Municipal Science & Technology Commission (grant number Z161100002616020), Beijing Nova Program (grant number Z171100001117057), and in part by the "111" Project under Grant B08043.

REFERENCES

Bamidis, P. D., Vivas, A. B., Styliadis, C., Frantzidis, C., Klados, M., Schlee, W., et al. (2014). A review of physical and cognitive interventions in aging. *Neurosci. Biobehav. Rev.* 44, 206–220. doi: 10.1016/j.neubiorev.2014.03.019

Basar, E. (2013). A review of gamma oscillations in healthy subjects and in cognitive impairment. *Int. J. Psychophysiol.* 90, 99–117. doi: 10.1016/j.ijpsycho.2013.07.005

Beer, A. L., Plank, T., and Greenlee, M. W. (2011). Diffusion tensor imaging shows white matter tracts between human auditory and visual cortex. *Exp. Brain Res.* 213, 299–308. doi: 10.1007/s00221-011-2715-y

Bishop, C. W., London, S., and Miller, L. M. (2012). Neural time course of visually enhanced echo suppression. *J. Neurophysiol.* 108, 1869–1883. doi: 10.1152/jn.00175.2012

Bravo, G., and Hebert, R. (1997). Age- and education-specific reference values for the mini-mental and modified mini-mental state examinations derived from a non-demented elderly population. *Int. J. Geriatr. Psychiatry* 12, 1008–1018. doi: 10.1002/(Sici)1099-1166(199710)12:10<1008::Aid-Gps676>3.0.Co;2-A

Curran, T., Hills, A., Patterson, M. B., and Strauss, M. E. (2001). Effects of aging on visuospatial attention: an ERP study. *Neuropsychologia* 39, 288–301. doi: 10.1016/S0028-3932(00)00112-3

Diaconescu, A. O., Hasher, L., and McIntosh, A. R. (2013). Visual dominance and multisensory integration changes with age. *Neuroimage* 65, 152–166. doi: 10.1016/j.neuroimage.2012.09.057

Doesburg, S. M., Roggeveen, A. B., Kitajo, K., and Ward, L. M. (2008). Large-scale gamma-band phase synchronization and selective attention. *Cereb. Cortex* 18, 386–396. doi: 10.1093/cercor/bhm073

Doesburg, S. M., Vidal, J., and Taylor, M. J. (2013). Reduced theta connectivity during set-shifting in children with autism. *Front. Hum. Neurosci.* 7:785. doi: 10.3389/Fnhum.2013.00785

Fort, A., Delpuech, C., Pemier, J., and Giard, M. H. (2002). Early auditory-visual interactions in human cortex during nonredundant target identification. *Cogn. Brain Res.* 14, 20–30. doi: 10.1016/S0926-6410(02)00058-7

Fu, K. M. G., Foxe, J. J., Murray, M. M., Higgins, B. A., Javitt, D. C., and Schroeder, C. E. (2001). Attention-dependent suppression of distracter visual input can be cross-modally cued as indexed by anticipatory parieto-occipital alpha-band oscillations. *Cogn. Brain Res.* 12, 145–152. doi: 10.1016/S0926-6410(01)00034-9

Greenhouse, S. W., and Geisser, S. (1982). On methods in the analysis of profile data. *Psychometrika* 24, 95–112. doi: 10.1007/BF02289823

He, S., Cavanagh, P., and Intriligator, J. (1996). Attentional resolution and the locus of visual awareness. *Nature* 383, 334–337. doi: 10.1038/383334a0

Hong, X. F., Liu, Y. L., Sun, J. F., and Tong, S. B. (2016). Age-related differences in the modulation of small-world brain networks during a go/NoGo task. *Front. Aging Neurosci.* 8:100. doi: 10.3389/Fnagi.2012.00100

Klados, M. A., Styliadis, C., Frantzidis, C. A., Paraskevopoulos, E., and Bamidis, P. D. (2016). Beta-band functional connectivity is reorganized in mild cognitive impairment after combined computerized physical and cognitive training. *Front. Neurosci.* 10:55. doi: 10.3389/Fnins.2016.00055

Kukleta, M., Bob, P., Brazdil, M., Roman, R., and Rektor, I. (2009). Beta 2-band synchronization during a visual oddball task. *Physiol. Res.* 58, 725–732.

Laurienti, P. J., Burdette, J. H., Maldjian, J. A., and Wallace, M. T. (2006). Enhanced multisensory integration in older adults. *Neurobiol. Aging* 27, 1155–1163. doi: 10.1016/j.neurobiolaging.2005.05.024

Lopez, M. E., Aurtenetxe, S., Pereda, E., Cuesta, P., Castellanos, N. P., Bruna, R., et al. (2014). Cognitive reserve is associated with the functional organization of the brain in healthy aging: a MEG study. *Front. Aging Neurosci.* 6:125. doi: 10.3389/Fnagi.2014.00125

Mahoney, J. R., Li, P. C. C., Oh-Park, M., Verghese, J., and Holtzer, R. (2011). Multisensory integration across the senses in young and old adults. *Brain Res.* 1426, 43–53. doi: 10.1016/j.brainres.2011.09.017

Miller, J. (1986). Timecourse of coactivation in bimodal divided attention. *Percept. Psychophys.* 40, 331–343. doi: 10.3758/Bf03203025

Missonnier, P., Deiber, M. P., Gold, G., Herrmann, F. R., Millet, P., Michon, A., et al. (2007). Working memory load-related electroencephalographic parameters can differentiate progressive from stable mild cognitive impairment. *Neuroscience* 150, 346–356. doi: 10.1016/j.neuroscience.2007.09.009

Molholm, S., Ritter, W., Javitt, D. C., and Foxe, J. J. (2004). Multisensory visual-auditory object recognition in humans: a high-density electrical mapping study. *Cereb. Cortex* 14, 452–465. doi: 10.1093/cercor/bhh007

Mozolic, J. L., Hugenschmidt, C. E., Peiffer, A. M., and Laurienti, P. J. (2012). "'Multisensory integration and aging," in *The Neural Bases of Multisensory Processes*, eds M. Murray and M. T. Wallace (Boca Raton, FL: CRC Press), 381–395.

Paraskevopoulos, E., Kraneburg, A., Herholz, S. C., Bamidis, P. D., and Pantev, C. (2015). Musical expertise is related to altered functional connectivity during audiovisual integration. *Proc. Natl. Acad. Sci. U.S.A.* 112, 12522–12527. doi: 10.1073/pnas.1510662112

Peiffer, A. M., Mozolic, J. L., Hugenschmidt, C. E., and Laurienti, P. J. (2007). Age-related multisensory enhancement in a simple audiovisual detection task. *Neuroreport* 18, 1077–1081. doi: 10.1097/Wnr.0b013e3281e72ae7

Sakowitz, O. W., Quiroga, R. Q., Schurmann, M., and Basar, E. (2005). Spatio-temporal frequency characteristics of intersensory components in audiovisually evoked potentials. *Cogn. Brain Res.* 23, 316–326. doi: 10.1016/j.cogbrainres.2004.10.012

Sallard, E., Tallet, J., Thut, G., Deiber, M. P., and Barral, J. (2016). Age-related changes in post-movement beta synchronization during a selective inhibition task. *Exp. Brain Res.* 234, 3543–3553. doi: 10.1007/s00221-016-4753-y

Sebastian, M., Reales, J. M., and Ballesteros, S. (2011). Ageing affects event-related potentials and brain oscillations: a behavioral and electrophysiological study using a haptic recognition memory task. *Neuropsychologia* 49, 3967–3980. doi: 10.1016/j.neuropsychologia.2011.10.013

Senkowski, D., Molholm, S., Gomez-Ramirez, M., and Foxe, J. J. (2006). Oscillatory beta activity predicts response speed during a multisensory audiovisual reaction time task: a high-density electrical mapping study. *Cereb. Cortex* 16, 1556–1565. doi: 10.1093/cercor/bhj091

Senkowski, D., Schneider, T. R., Foxe, J. J., and Engel, A. K. (2008). Crossmodal binding through neural coherence: implications for multisensory processing. *Trends Neurosci.* 31, 401–409. doi: 10.1016/j.tins.2008.05.002

Stam, C. J., Nolte, G., and Daffertshofer, A. (2007). Phase lag index: assessment of functional connectivity from multi channel EEG and MEG with diminished bias from common sources. *Hum. Brain Mapp.* 28, 1178–1193. doi: 10.1002/hbm.20346

Steffener, J., Barulli, D., Habeck, C., and Stern, Y. (2014). Neuroimaging explanations of age-related differences in task performance. *Front. Aging Neurosci.* 6:46. doi: 10.3389/Fnagi.2014.00046

Stekelenburg, J. J., Vroomen, J., and de Gelder, B. (2004). Illusory sound shifts induced by the ventriloquist illusion evoke the mismatch negativity. *Neurosci. Lett.* 357, 163–166. doi: 10.1016/j.neulet.2003.12.085

Talsma, D., and Woldorff, M. G. (2005). Selective attention and multisensory integration: multiple phases of effects on the evoked brain activity. *J. Cogn. Neurosci.* 17, 1098–1114. doi: 10.1162/0898929054475172

van den Brink, R. L., Cohen, M. X., van der Burg, E., Talsma, D., Vissers, M. E., and Slagter, H. A. (2014). Subcortical, modality-specific pathways contribute to multisensory processing in humans. *Cereb. Cortex* 24, 2169–2177. doi: 10.1093/cercor/bht069

von Stein, A., and Sarnthein, J. (2000). Different frequencies for different scales of cortical integration: from local gamma to long range alpha/theta synchronization. *Int. J. Psychophysiol.* 38, 301–313. doi: 10.1016/S0167-8760(00)00172-0

Wang, J. H., Wang, X. D., Xia, M. R., Liao, X. H., Evans, A., and He, Y. (2015). GRETNA: a graph theoretical network analysis toolbox for imaging connectomics. *Front. Hum. Neurosci.* 9:386. doi: 10.3389/Fnhum.2015.00458

Wen, X. T., Yao, L., Liu, Y. J., and Ding, M. Z. (2012). Causal interactions in attention networks predict behavioral performance. *J. Neurosci.* 32, 1284–1292. doi: 10.1523/Jneurosci.2817-11.2012

Wu, J. L., Yang, W. P., Gao, Y. L., and Kimura, T. (2012). Age-related multisensory integration elicited by peripherally presented audiovisual stimuli. *Neuroreport* 23, 616–620. doi: 10.1097/WNR.0b013e3283552b0f

Zalesky, A., Cocchi, L., Fornito, A., Murray, M. M., and Bullmore, E. T. (2012). Connectivity differences in brain networks. *Neuroimage* 60, 1055–1062. doi: 10.1016/j.neuroimage.2012.01.068

Zalesky, A., Fornito, A., and Bullmore, E. T. (2010). Network-based statistic: identifying differences in brain networks. *Neuroimage* 53, 1197–1207. doi: 10.1016/j.neuroimage.2010.06.041

Zarahn, E., Rakitin, B., Abela, D., Flynn, J., and Stern, Y. (2007). Age-related changes in brain activation during a delayed item recognition task. *Neurobiol. Aging* 28, 784–798. doi: 10.1016/j.neurobiolaging.2006.03.002

15

Aging and Network Properties: Stability Over Time and Links with Learning during Working Memory Training

Alexandru D. Iordan[1]*, Katherine A. Cooke[1], Kyle D. Moored[2], Benjamin Katz[3],
Martin Buschkuehl[4], Susanne M. Jaeggi[5], John Jonides[1], Scott J. Peltier[6], Thad A. Polk[1]
and Patricia A. Reuter-Lorenz[1]

[1] Department of Psychology, University of Michigan, Ann Arbor, MI, United States, [2] Department of Mental Health, Bloomberg
School of Public Health, Johns Hopkins University, Baltimore, MD, United States, [3] Department of Human Development and
Family Science, Virginia Tech, Blacksburg, VA, United States, [4] MIND Research Institute, Irvine, CA, United States, [5] School of
Education, University of California, Irvine, Irvine, CA, United States, [6] Functional MRI Laboratory, Department of Biomedical
Engineering, University of Michigan, Ann Arbor, MI, United States

*Correspondence:
Alexandru D. Iordan
adiordan@umich.edu

Growing evidence suggests that healthy aging affects the configuration of large-scale
functional brain networks. This includes reducing network modularity and local efficiency.
However, the stability of these effects over time and their potential role in learning
remain poorly understood. The goal of the present study was to further clarify previously
reported age effects on "resting-state" networks, to test their reliability over time, and
to assess their relation to subsequent learning during training. Resting-state fMRI data
from 23 young (YA) and 20 older adults (OA) were acquired in 2 sessions 2 weeks
apart. Graph-theoretic analyses identified both consistencies in network structure and
differences in module composition between YA and OA, suggesting topological changes
and less stability of functional network configuration with aging. Brain-wide, OA showed
lower modularity and local efficiency compared to YA, consistent with the idea of
age-related functional dedifferentiation, and these effects were replicable over time. At the
level of individual networks, OA consistently showed greater participation and lower local
efficiency and within-network connectivity in the cingulo-opercular network, as well as
lower intra-network connectivity in the default-mode network and greater participation of
the somato-sensorimotor network, suggesting age-related differential effects at the level
of specialized brain modules. Finally, brain-wide network properties showed associations,
albeit limited, with learning rates, as assessed with 10 days of computerized working
memory training administered after the resting-state sessions, suggesting that baseline
network configuration may influence subsequent learning outcomes. Identification of
neural mechanisms associated with learning-induced plasticity is important for further
clarifying whether and how such changes predict the magnitude and maintenance of
training gains, as well as the extent and limits of cognitive transfer in both younger and
older adults.

Keywords: intrinsic activity, functional connectivity, graph theory, reliability analysis, intraclass correlation

INTRODUCTION

Aging is associated with cognitive decline that may be linked in part to altered communication among various brain regions (Reuter-Lorenz and Park, 2014). Indeed, aging has been shown to affect the integration of information both within and between functional brain networks (Ferreira and Busatto, 2013; Dennis and Thompson, 2014; Damoiseaux, 2017), which may have implications for cognitive performance. Despite accumulating evidence suggesting age effects on the configuration of large-scale functional brain networks (Achard and Bullmore, 2007; Meunier et al., 2009a; Onoda and Yamaguchi, 2013; Betzel et al., 2014; Cao M. et al., 2014; Chan et al., 2014; Song et al., 2014; Geerligs et al., 2015; Ng et al., 2016), the stability of these effects over time remains poorly understood. One goal of the present study was to clarify this issue by assessing age differences in functional network properties at two different time points.

A substantial body of evidence suggests that aging influences the functional organization of the brain, both globally and at the level of individual brain networks (reviewed in Ferreira and Busatto, 2013; Dennis and Thompson, 2014; Sala-Llonch et al., 2015; Damoiseaux, 2017). The functional organization of the brain has traditionally been studied using fMRI-based "resting-state" functional connectivity (Greicius et al., 2003; Power et al., 2011) and more recently, with graph-theoretic analyses (Bullmore and Sporns, 2009; Rubinov and Sporns, 2010). The graph-theoretic approach enables characterization of the brain's connectivity structure and derives measures that assess global and local features that may be important for network function (Bullmore and Sporns, 2009; Rubinov and Sporns, 2010). One such measure is modularity (Newman and Girvan, 2004; Newman, 2006), which indexes the extent to which a graph is organized into separate modules with dense within- and sparse between-modules connections, a fundamental principle thought to support the brain's functional segregation and integration (Dehaene et al., 1998; Sporns and Betzel, 2015). A number of prior investigations have identified lower modularity in aging (Onoda and Yamaguchi, 2013; Betzel et al., 2014; Cao M. et al., 2014; Song et al., 2014; Geerligs et al., 2015; but see Meunier et al., 2009a), with networks becoming less distinct due to increased between- and decreased within-module integration. This evidence is consistent with the idea of functional dedifferentiation (Park et al., 2004, 2010; Grady, 2012). Another set of measures characterizes the efficiency of information flow across the graph. Global efficiency indexes graph-wide integration and has been linked with the capacity for rapid information exchange among distributed regions, whereas local efficiency indexes integration at a regional level and has been linked with fault tolerance within specialized regions (Latora and Marchiori, 2003; Achard and Bullmore, 2007). Previous investigations have associated aging with lower local efficiency (Achard and Bullmore, 2007; Cao M. et al., 2014; Song et al., 2014; Geerligs et al., 2015), while global efficiency was reported to be similar irrespective of age (Cao M. et al., 2014; Song et al., 2014; Geerligs et al., 2015; but see Achard and Bullmore, 2007).

Importantly, differences in connectivity structure observed at a brain-wide level may be related to specific patterns at the level of individual networks, and current evidence suggests differential effects of aging on particular brain networks (Ferreira and Busatto, 2013; Dennis and Thompson, 2014; Sala-Llonch et al., 2015; Damoiseaux, 2017). Although the majority of investigations have targeted the default-mode network (DMN), showing lower functional connectivity between its different sub-components with aging (Andrews-Hanna et al., 2007; Damoiseaux et al., 2008), recent evidence also points to age effects in other brain networks, such as the cingulo-opercular/salience and sensorimotor networks (Meier et al., 2012; Onoda et al., 2012; He et al., 2014; Geerligs et al., 2015; La Corte et al., 2016)[1]. Thus, to complement information provided by brain-wide network assessments, metrics applied at the level of individual networks can also be employed. This includes the participation coefficient, which indexes the relation between intra- and inter-network connectivity for each node (Guimerà and Amaral, 2005).

In sum, although there are some inconsistencies across studies, available evidence points to lower within- and higher between-network connectivity with aging. This is expressed topologically as lower modularity, and is associated with lower local efficiency and preserved global efficiency, compared to younger age (see Damoiseaux, 2017 for a recent discussion). The first main goal of the present study was to assess the replicability of these previously reported age effects on functional network configuration.

Inconsistencies across investigations of age differences in network properties may stem from methodological differences but also from variability of network measures over time (van Wijk et al., 2010; Zalesky et al., 2016; Ciric et al., 2017; Geerligs et al., 2017). One way to assess reliability is by measuring the same subjects at two or more time-points, while using the same methodology, and quantifying the level of agreement between measurements by calculating the intraclass correlation coefficient (ICC) (Shrout and Fleiss, 1979; McGraw and Wong, 1996). A meta-analysis of test-retest reliability of graph-theoretic brain-network metrics identified overall good reliability (Welton et al., 2015). However, the available evidence related to aging is very limited. Investigations of age differences in network properties have typically used singular assessments, and hence the reliability of such effects over time is not clear (but see Geerligs et al., 2017). Thus, the second main goal of the present investigation was to extend the assessment of age differences in network properties to multiple time points within the same individuals and to evaluate reliability.

Clarification of age differences in network properties and their stability over time is important for further assessment of changes associated with cognitive training in older adults. Specifically, if aging influences relations between functional network properties and training outcomes, then these effects

---

[1]While graph theory has been typically employed to assess global and local measures of connectivity, much evidence regarding aging effects on specific brain networks has been derived using complementary approaches, such as seed-based functional connectivity and independent component analysis. Although these approaches differ in important ways (see Ferreira and Busatto, 2013; Dennis and Thompson, 2014 for recent discussions), results have been overall convergent (see Geerligs et al., 2015 for a recent graph theory investigation at the level of individual networks).

need to be disentangled from variability of network measures in the absence of intervention. Recent evidence suggests potential links between baseline properties of functional brain organization and benefits accrued over the course of cognitive training in older adults (Gallen et al., 2016a), although at this point such evidence is only preliminary. Although a growing body of studies suggests that some working memory (WM) interventions may alter functional network organization and have beneficial, albeit limited, effects on cognitive functioning (Buschkuehl et al., 2008; Lustig et al., 2009; Brehmer et al., 2014; Karbach and Verhaeghen, 2014; Stepankova et al., 2014; Ballesteros et al., 2015; Bherer, 2015; Mewborn et al., 2017; Román et al., 2017), evidence linking baseline functional network characteristics with training is limited (Arnemann et al., 2015; Gallen et al., 2016a). In one investigation of this topic, Gallen et al. (2016a) showed that older adults displaying greater network modularity at baseline also showed greater improvements in gist reasoning, following a strategic memory and reasoning training intervention (Vas et al., 2011). However, the potential role of other network properties in learning remains largely unknown. Thus, the third main goal of this investigation was to assess relations between baseline network properties and subsequent learning during training in older adults.

These questions were investigated in a sample comprising both healthy younger and older adults, using resting-state fMRI data acquired in 2 different sessions, both preceding a WM training intervention. A complete treatment of training outcomes and other behavioral data will be reported separately. Based on the extant evidence, we expected to find lower modularity and local efficiency in older compared to younger adults, and similar global efficiency across groups. We also expected these differences to be stable over time. Finally, the limited evidence linking network properties with training effects suggests that modularity is beneficial (Gallen et al., 2016a); therefore, we expected that network properties, in particular modularity (i.e., as reflected in the modularity index), would be linked to learning rates.

METHODS

Participants

A sample of 23 younger (YA) and 23 healthy, cognitively normal older adults (OA) were recruited from the University of Michigan campus and community surrounding Ann Arbor, Michigan to participate in an adaptive verbal WM training study. All participants were right-handed, native English speakers with normal or corrected-to-normal hearing and vision and were screened for history of head injury, psychiatric illness, or alcohol/drug abuse. Data from 3 OA were excluded due to technical issues related to brain-imaging data acquisition. Thus, the sample for fMRI analyses consisted of 23 YA (age range: 18–28; 9 females) with a mean age (±S.D.) of 21.3 (±2.5) years and 20 OA (age range: 64–76; 9 females) with a mean age of 68.3 (±3.6) years. For analyses linking fMRI with behavioral results, 2 additional participants (1 OA) were excluded, due to technical issues related to behavioral task assessments, and thus these analyses were reported on 22 YA and 19 OA. Older

adult participants completed the Short Blessed Test (Katzman et al., 1983) over the phone prior to inclusion in the study to screen for potential mild cognitive impairment, and additional neuropsychological assessments using the Montreal Cognitive Assessment (Nasreddine et al., 2005) confirmed normal cognitive function for all participants (scores $\geq$ 26). Additionally, participants were screened for depressive symptoms that could affect cognitive functioning using the depression module of the Patient Health Questionnaire (Kroenke et al., 2001). The University of Michigan Institutional Review Board approved all procedures, and all participants provided informed consent prior to participating.

Imaging Protocol

Functional MRI data were acquired during 8 min of resting state, following completion of a verbal WM task, in 2 sessions 2 weeks apart (t_1, t_2) (see Supplementary Figure 1 for an illustration of the study timeline). Participants were instructed to view a fixation cross in the center of the screen while keeping their mind calm and relaxed. Imaging data were collected using a 3 T General Electric MR750 scanner with an eight-channel head coil. Functional images were acquired in ascending order using a spiral-in sequence, with MR parameters: TR = 2,000 ms; TE = 30 ms; flip angle = 90°; field of view = 220 × 220 mm^2; matrix size = 64 × 64; slice thickness = 3 mm, no gap; 43 slices; voxel size = 3.44 × 3.44 × 3 mm^3. After an initial 10 s of signal stabilization, 235 volumes were acquired. A high-resolution T_1-weighted anatomical image was also collected following the WM task and preceding resting-state acquisition, using spoiled-gradient-recalled acquisition (SPGR) in steady-state imaging (TR = 12.24 ms, TE = 5.18 ms; flip angle = 15°, field of view = 256 × 256 mm^2, matrix size = 256 × 256; slice thickness = 1 mm; 156 slices; voxel size = 1 × 1 × 1 mm^3). Images were de-spiked in k-space and reconstructed using an in-house iterative reconstruction algorithm with field-map correction (Sutton et al., 2003), which has superior reconstruction quality compared to non-iterative conjugate phase reconstruction.

Preprocessing

Preprocessing was performed using SPM12 (Wellcome Department of Cognitive Neurology, London). Functional images were slice-time corrected, realigned, and co-registered to the anatomical image using a mean functional image. A study-specific anatomical template was created (younger and older adults together; Geerligs et al., 2015), using Diffeomorphic Anatomical Registration Through Exponentiated Lie Algebra (DARTEL) (Ashburner, 2007), based on segmented gray matter and white matter tissue classes, to optimize inter-participant alignment (Klein et al., 2009). The DARTEL flowfields and MNI transformation were then applied to the functional images and to the segments, and the functional images were resampled to 3 × 3 × 3 mm^3 voxel size. To minimize artificial local spatial correlations, no additional spatial smoothing was applied (Salvador et al., 2005; Achard et al., 2006; Achard and Bullmore, 2007; Wang et al., 2010, 2011; Liao et al., 2011; Zalesky et al., 2012; Alakorkko et al., 2017).

Identification of outlier scans was performed using Artifact Detection Tools (ART; www.nitrc.org/projects/artifact_detect/), as follows. Scans were classified as outliers if frame-to-frame difference exceeded 0.5 mm in composite motion (combination of translational and rotational displacements) or 3 standard deviations in the global mean signal. On average, the proportion of outliers was below 5% in both YA (t_1: 4.42%; t_2: 2.72%) and OA (t_1: 3.68%; t_2: 3.74%). There were no significant differences between the two groups in the number of outlier scans (p's > 0.4), or in the average (p's > 0.1) or maximum (p's > 0.5) motion, either before or after correcting for outlier scans (see "scrubbing" below).

Graph Construction
Functional Connectivity Analysis

Brain-wide functional connectivity analyses were performed using the Connectivity Toolbox (CONN; Whitfield-Gabrieli and Nieto-Castanon, 2012). To construct a brain-wide graph, we employed a commonly used functional atlas (Power et al., 2011), which comprises 264 meta-analytically defined coordinates, including cortical and subcortical areas; a 5 mm-radius sphere was centered at each of these coordinates. To ensure that the graph comprised regions that were not susceptible to fMRI signal drop-out, each sphere was filtered through a sample-level signal intensity mask, calculated as follows: First, binary masks were calculated for each subject, at each time point, thresholded at >70% mean signal intensity (Geerligs et al., 2015), computed over all voxels, using ART. Then, a sample-level mask was calculated, across all subjects and time points, using logical conjunction (see Supplementary Figure 2 for an illustration of the mask). Regions with fewer than 8 voxels (~50% volume) overlap with the sample-level mask were excluded, leaving 234 regions of interest (ROIs).

To remove physiological and other sources of noise from the fMRI time series we used linear regression and the anatomical CompCor method (Behzadi et al., 2007; Chai et al., 2012; Muschelli et al., 2014), as implemented in CONN. Each participant's white matter and cerebrospinal fluid segments, eroded by 1 voxel to minimize partial volume effects, were used as noise ROIs. The following temporal covariates were added to the model: signal extracted from each participant's noise ROIs (5 principal component analysis parameters for each[2]), motion parameters (3 rotation and 3 translation parameters, plus their first-order temporal derivatives), regressors for each outlier scan (i.e., "scrubbing"; one covariate was added for each outlier scan, consisting of 0's everywhere but the outlier scan, coded as "1"), and a session-onset regressor (a delta function convolved with the hemodynamic response function plus its first-order temporal derivative). The residual fMRI time series were band-pass filtered ($0.01\,Hz < f < 0.1\,Hz$). Pearson correlation coefficients were computed between the

time courses of all pairs of functional ROIs, followed by Fisher-z transformation, and the diagonal of the connectivity matrix was set to zero. Graph construction and analyses were performed separately for each group and time point, using tools from the Brain Connectivity Toolbox (Rubinov and Sporns, 2010).

Group-Level Consensus Partitions

To achieve a community structure representative of each group, we used the Louvain community detection algorithm (Blondel et al., 2008), in conjunction with consensus clustering (Lancichinetti and Fortunato, 2012). This approach capitalizes on the consistency of each node's module affiliation across a set of partitions, to circumvent the known degeneracy of the Louvain algorithm (i.e., multiple partitioning solutions) (Good et al., 2010). To obtain a unique (i.e., threshold-independent) solution for each group, the Louvain algorithm was applied on weighted graph edges (positive only); see Cohen and D'Esposito (2016) for a similar approach. The group-level consensus partitions were employed to derive node–module assignments used for analyses at the level of individual modules/networks (see Network Measures sub-section below) and for display purposes (**Figure 1**).

Consensus clustering was applied first at the individual level, to generate a robust partition for each participant, and then at the group level, to generate a representative partition for each group and at each time point; see Dwyer et al. (2014) for a similar approach. First, to generate a robust partition for each participant, the Louvain algorithm was run 500 times. Because the algorithm is susceptible to local maxima, each initial partition was optimized using iterative community fine-tuning (Sun et al., 2009), which maximizes modularity by reassigning the nodes to modules and iterating the Louvain algorithm. For each participant, we constructed an agreement matrix representing the fraction of runs in which each pair of nodes was assigned to the same module. The Louvain algorithm was then iteratively run on the agreement matrix (500 Louvain runs at each step), to generate a consensus partition for each participant. For each iteration, the agreement matrix was recalculated and thresholded, until a single representative partition was obtained for each participant. Second, to generate a group-level representative partition, an agreement matrix was calculated based on the consensus partitions of all participants in one group. The Louvain algorithm was then run on the agreement matrix to obtain a consensus partition for each group, as described above. The resolution parameter of the Louvain community detection algorithm (γ) and the thresholding parameter for the agreement matrix (τ) were determined using a procedure that maximized modularity over all group-level partitions. Specifically, we ran the procedure described above for typical ranges of values for both parameters and chose those values that, on average, maximized modularity across all 4 group-level partitions (see below for a formal description of modularity). The value ranges were γ between 1 and 1.5 and τ between 0.2 and 0.5, with increments of 0.05 for each parameter. The maximum average modularity was $Q = 0.71$, achieved for $\gamma = 1.25$

---

[2]Regressing out multiple principal components from noise ROIs typically leads to better noise correction than regressing out the average noise signal because physiological noise (including motion) is not spatially homogeneous across the brain (Chai et al., 2012; Muschelli et al., 2014).

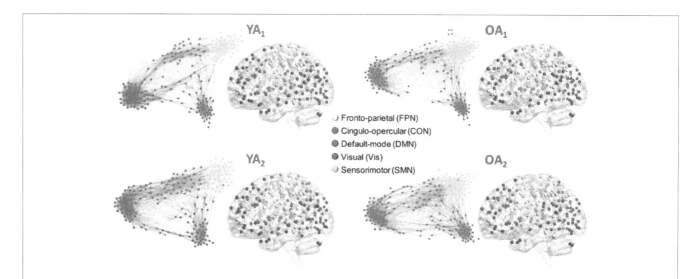

FIGURE 1 | Representative group-level partitions. Functional networks were identified separately for each group and time point, using consensus partitioning. Five main modules were identified in both YA and OA, consistent with the main functional networks described in the literature (see main text for details). Nodes are color-coded by module, and within-module connections are displayed in the same color as the nodes. Nodes not belonging to the five main modules are displayed in gray. For illustration purposes, the force-directed graph displays 20% of the strongest connections and the anatomical projection displays nodes that form 2% of the strongest connections. The force-direct graph and anatomical projection were displayed using Gephi (http://gephi.org) and BrainNet Viewer (http://www.nitrc.org/projects/bnv/), respectively.

and $\tau = 0.5$, and these parameters were used for subsequent analyses.

Connection Density Thresholding

We used density-based thresholding, which equates the number of edges across graphs and allows proper between-groups comparisons (van Wijk et al., 2010; Garrison et al., 2015). To ensure that results were not due to any specific threshold, calculations were performed for a range comprising 2–10% of the strongest connections, in 1% increments. This threshold range is similar to that used in generating the Power et al. (2011) functional atlas and matches the range previously employed by Geerligs et al. (2015), thus enabling comparison of results. In general, stringent threshold ranges are preferable because inclusion of false-positive connections is more detrimental to network measures computation than exclusion of false-negative connections (Zalesky et al., 2016). The average number of disconnected nodes at each threshold in the 2–10% range was as follows: 47, 27, 17, 10, 7, 4, 3, 2, and 1. Because average connectivity was similar across groups (as assessed by permutation testing on positive edges; $t_{1, 2}$: p's > 0.2), density-based thresholding was likely unbiased across groups (Zalesky et al., 2016; van den Heuvel et al., 2017). To calculate network measures, connectivity values were binarized for each threshold (i.e., 1 if above, 0 if below threshold). Between-groups comparisons of graph-theoretic measures used binarized graphs and reported graph metrics are values averaged across all thresholds, unless specified otherwise.

Network Measures

To assess the strength of module segregation, we calculated the modularity index (Q) (Newman and Girvan, 2004; Newman,

2006), which compares the observed intra-module connectivity with that which is expected by chance. Higher modularity values indicate stronger separation of the graph's modules. The modularity index is formally defined as follows:

$$Q = \frac{1}{2E} \sum_{ij} [A_{ij} - \gamma e_{ij}] \delta(m_i, m_j)$$

where E is the number of graph edges, A is the adjacency matrix, γ is the resolution parameter, e is the null model [$e = k_i k_j / 2E$, where k_i and k_j are the degrees (i.e., number of connections) of the nodes i and j], and δ is an indicator that equals 1 if nodes i and j belong to the same module and 0 otherwise. The modularity score for each participant was calculated as the average over 500 runs of the Louvain algorithm with iterative community fine-tuning. For consistency with the consensus clustering procedure described above, the same resolution parameter ($\gamma = 1.25$) was used.

To assess the integration of information, we calculated global and local efficiency (Latora and Marchiori, 2003). Global efficiency indexes integration at the level of the entire graph and it is defined as follows:

$$E_{glob} = \frac{1}{N(N-1)} \sum_{i \neq j} \frac{1}{L_{ij}}$$

where N is the number of nodes in the graph and L_{ij} is the shortest path length between nodes i and j. By contrast, local efficiency is a node-specific measure, and is defined relative to the sub-graph comprising the immediate neighbors of a node. Local efficiencies for all nodes were averaged to provide an estimate of the mean local efficiency of the entire graph or of a module. Local efficiency of a node i is defined as follows:

$$E_{loc}(i) = \frac{1}{N_{G_i}(N_{G_i}-1)} \sum_{j,h \in G_i} \frac{1}{L_{jh}}$$

where G_i is the sub-graph comprising all the immediate neighbors of the node i.

Another node-specific measure is the participation coefficient (Guimerà and Amaral, 2005), which indexes inter-network connectivity by quantifying the distribution of each node's connections across different modules. Participation coefficients of all nodes within a module were averaged to provide an estimate of mean participation for a module. Participation coefficient of a node i is defined as follows:

$$P(i) = 1 - \sum_{m=1}^{M} \left[\frac{k_i(m)}{k_i} \right]^2$$

where M is the number of modules in the graph, and $k_i(m)$ is the degree of node i within its own module m, and k_i is the degree of node i regardless of module membership.

Finally, to assess the convergence of results based on the graph-theoretic measures described above with simpler connectivity analyses, we calculated within- and between-module connectivity using an approach similar to Geerligs et al. (2015). For completeness, this procedure was performed separately for positive and negative connectivity values. First, the initial connectivity matrices were thresholded by retaining values that survived a false discovery rate (FDR) correction ($q < 0.05$) (Benjamini and Hochberg, 1995) and setting all the other values to zero. Then, for each module and pair of modules, we computed the sum of all connectivity values and divided by the number of possible connections to estimate within- and between-modules connectivity. Of note, this procedure was used only for the analysis of within- and between-networks connectivity, and it did not influence the previously introduced graph-theoretic measures, which were all calculated on unweighted (i.e., binary) graphs.

Statistical Methods

As a general strategy, assessments were performed on metrics averaged across all thresholds, and significant results were followed-up with tests for each threshold, to assess consistency across the threshold range.

Age Differences in Community Structure

To assess age differences in community structure, we compared module composition between groups using normalized mutual information (NMI) (Kuncheva and Hadjitodorov, 2004) and permutation testing. NMI measures how much information about the structure of one partition reduces uncertainty about the structure of another partition, and is a relative measure that varies from 0 (completely independent) to 1 (identical partitions). Because individual similarity measures are not independent, we used an unbiased procedure that compared the average between-groups similarity in the actual data with a null distribution

based on randomizing group memberships; see Alexander-Bloch et al. (2012) for a similar approach. Between-groups similarity in the actual data was calculated for each density threshold, by averaging the pair-wise partition similarity for all subjects across the two groups, separately at each time point. For each subject, we used the partition with the highest modularity for each threshold, calculated over 500 Louvain repetitions with community fine-tuning and resolution $\gamma = 1.25$. The null distribution was calculated in a similar way, using the randomly divided groups over 5,000 permutations, while retaining original group sizes. If the actual between-groups NMI was smaller than the 5th percentile of the null distribution, the difference was considered significant. Furthermore, to determine whether one group showed more similar partitions than the other, we examined within-group partition similarity. This analysis was performed in a similar way, by averaging pair-wise partition similarity separately for subjects in each group. Finally, to examine differences in the stability of partitions over time, we calculated within-subject partition similarity over the two sessions. A between-group difference in partition similarity over time was tested directly, using permutation testing (Groppe et al., 2011).

Age Differences in Network Measures

Age differences in network measures were first assessed brain-wide (modularity, global efficiency, and local efficiency) and then significant results were followed-up by analyses at the level of each module or network (participation coefficient and local efficiency). To ensure comparability at the level of individual networks, each module was represented only by those nodes that were consistently assigned to the same module, both across groups and time points, based on the group-level consensus partitions; see Geerligs et al. (2015) for a similar approach. Between-groups differences in network properties were assessed using permutation testing, and a family-wise error (FWE) correction for multiple comparisons based on the "max statistic" method (Blair and Karniski, 1993; Groppe et al., 2011) was applied to account for simultaneous testing of the five main modules identified (see Results section). As mentioned above, an ancillary analysis of within- and between-modules connectivity was also performed and the same FWE correction for multiple comparisons was applied for this analysis as well.

Reliability Analysis

The intraclass correlation coefficient (ICC) was employed to measure the absolute agreement for each graph metric between the two sessions (McGraw and Wong, 1996; Welton et al., 2015). We used a mixed model[3] $ICC_{(A,\ k)}$ to estimate the degree of absolute agreement of measurements that are averages of $k = 2$ independent measurements on randomly selected subjects.

---

[3]We made no assumption of interchangeability of t_1 and t_2 assessments because the resting-state data were acquired following completion of a verbal WM task inside the scanner, and thus potential differences in task performance at the two time points might have differentially influenced resting-state recordings. We also expected, however, that these effects would be mitigated by a ~6 min break (recording the T_1-weighted anatomical image) following the WM task and preceding the resting-state acquisition (Breckel et al., 2013).

ICC was calculated as follows: $ICC = (MS_R - MS_E)/[MS_R + (MS_C - MS_E)/n]$, where MS_R is mean square for rows/subjects, MS_E is mean square error, and MS_C is mean square for columns/assessments (Shrout and Fleiss, 1979; McGraw and Wong, 1996). We used the following guidelines for ICC interpretation: <0.20, poor; 0.21–0.40, fair; 0.41–0.60 moderate; 0.61–0.80 strong; >0.8, almost perfect (Montgomery et al., 2002; Telesford et al., 2010).

Links with Learning during WM Training

The second scanning session was followed by 10 days of computerized verbal WM training (Supplementary Figure 1). The adaptive training task consisted of a modified WM item-recognition task that required participants to encode and retain consonant letters of variable set size for several seconds (Sternberg, 1966; see also Stepankova et al., 2014); set size changed adaptively depending on participants' performance. Participants completed 6 blocks of 14 trials during each training session. Here, we focus on training-related improvements in WM performance specifically, as measured by mean set size achieved during each training session for each participant, to evaluate their relationship with network properties. Furthermore, we focused on early and late learning rates, defined as the performance change between training sessions 1 and 2 (*early* learning rate), and as the performance change across training sessions 2–10 (*late* learning rate), respectively, modeled for each individual using a linear spline term with a knot at the second training session (see Appendix for details). YA had a higher mean early slope than OA [$t_{(39)} = 3.59, p = 0.001$], but late slope did not differ by age group [$t_{(39)} = 1.64, p = 0.109$].

To assess links between network measures and learning rates, we calculated correlations between brain-wide network measures and early learning slopes, separately for each group and at each time point. We focused on early learning rates because age differences were identified in early but not in late learning slopes. Due to relatively small sample sizes, we employed Spearman's rank correlation coefficient (ρ) to minimize influence from extreme values. Significant brain-wide results were followed by assessments at the level of each module/network, corrected for multiple comparisons using the permutation-based "max statistic" method (Groppe et al., 2011). We took multiple steps to assess the robustness of our findings, using a procedure similar to Gallen et al. (2016a). First, to assess whether the relations between network measures and learning rates were constantly present over the threshold range, we tested these relations separately for each threshold. Second, given the absence of differences in motion across groups and time points (see Preprocessing subsection above), we performed partial Spearman correlations (ρ_p) to examine whether controlling for motion altered the relations between brain-wide network measures and learning rates.

RESULTS

Age Differences in Community Structure

Functional networks were identified separately for each group and time point, using consensus partitioning (see Methods section for details). Similar modules were identified in both YA and OA, consistent with the main functional networks described in the literature (Power et al., 2011; Yeo et al., 2011): fronto-parietal (FPN), cingulo-opercular/salience (CON), default-mode (DMN), visual (Vis) and somato-sensorimotor (SMN) (**Figure 1**). The community structure of the partitions for each age group was examined using normalized mutual information (NMI). Results showed differences in node-module assignment between YA and OA, at both time points (**Figure 2**). First, analysis of *between-groups* partition similarity showed that similarity of community structure between YA and OA was significantly lower than expected based on the permuted data ($t_{1, 2}$: p's < 0.001; **Figure 2A**). Second, analysis of *within-group* partition similarity showed less similarity for OA as a group. Specifically, partition similarity for YA was higher (t_1: $p = 0.003$; t_2: $p < 0.001$) whereas for OA was lower (t_1: $p = 0.007$; t_2: $p = 0.003$) than expected based on the permuted data (Supplementary Figure 3). This indicates that there is greater heterogeneity in OA's partitions, i.e., their partitions are less similar to one another than YA's partitions. Finally, analysis of *within-subject* similarity across time showed less within-subject consistency for OA ($p = 0.001$; **Figure 2B**), indicating more variability in node-module assignment in OA across time. In summary, although similar functional networks were identified in both YA and OA, their composition differed between groups, and OA showed less similarity, both as a group and across time, compared to YA.

Age Differences in Network Measures and Reliability Analysis

To complement the comparisons of community structure presented above, we assessed age differences in several network measures. Network measures were first calculated brain-wide, followed by an assessment of their reliability over time. Then, significant brain-wide differences were followed-up by assessments at the level of each of the five modules/networks.

Brain-Wide Network Measures

At a brain-wide level, OA showed lower modularity indices at both time points (t_1: $p = 0.046$, t_2: $p < 0.001$), indicating lower intra-module connectivity compared to YA. Furthermore, OA consistently showed lower local efficiency ($t_{1, 2}$: p's < 0.001), while global efficiency was not significantly different across groups ($t_{1, 2}$: p's > 0.1), suggesting age differences in local but not global integration of information (**Figure 3**). Ancillary correlation analyses between age and brain-wide network measures within the OA group revealed no significant results (p's > 0.05).

Reliability Analysis of Brain-Wide Network Measures

Reliability of brain-wide network measures was assessed using intraclass correlation (ICC), by calculating the absolute agreement of each graph metric across sessions. Brain-wide measures showed overall moderate to strong ICC over time (range 0.51–0.74), with the highest agreement for local efficiency (**Figure 4**). For each group, the agreement ranged from fair (>0.2) to strong (>0.6), with YA showing lowest agreement for global efficiency. Examination of the profiles of ICC values

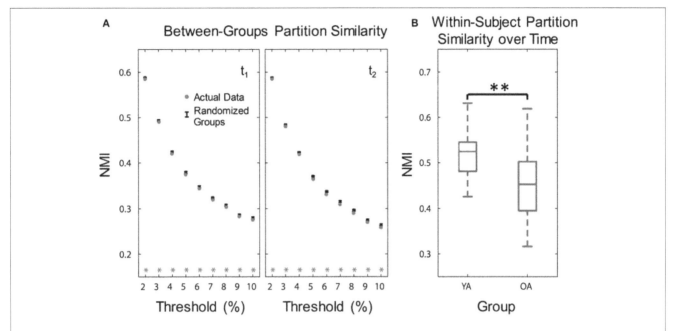

FIGURE 2 | Age differences in community structure. Similarity of community structure between YA and OA was significantly lower than expected based on the permuted data, at both time points and consistently across all thresholds **(A)**. Also, OA showed less within-subject partition similarity across time **(B)**. Boxplots in the right panel depict values averaged across all thresholds. NMI, normalized mutual information; t_1, time point 1; t_2, time point 2; YA, younger adults (blue color); OA, older adults (red color). Magenta asterisks indicate $p < 0.05$ for each threshold. **$p < 0.01$, across all thresholds.

across the range of thresholds indicated that the reproducibility of network measures was generally stable across thresholds, with the exception of global efficiency for YA.

Individual Network Measures

Network properties were also assessed at the level of each individual network (**Figure 5**). To ensure comparability across groups and time points, each network was represented by only those nodes that were consistently assigned to the same network, both across groups and time points (see Methods section for details). OA showed greater participation coefficient for CON (t_1: $p_{FWE} < 0.001$; t_2: $p_{FWE} = 0.002$) and SMN (t_1, $_2$: p_{FWE}'s < 0.001), indicating that, compared to YA, a larger proportion of the nodes in these networks had connections outside the networks they belonged to. OA also showed lower local efficiency for CON (t_1: $p_{FWE} = 0.014$; t_2: $p_{FWE} = 0.008$) at both time points, and for DMN ($p_{FWE} = 0.029$) and SMN ($p_{FWE} = 0.01$) at t_2. We also examined within- and between-network connectivity, using a procedure similar to Geerligs et al. (2015). Regarding *within*-networks connectivity, OA showed lower connectivity within DMN (t_1: $p_{FWE} = 0.04$; t_2: $p_{FWE} = 0.018$) and within CON ($p_{FWE} = 0.035$) at t_1, compared to YA. Regarding *between*-networks connectivity, OA showed greater positive connectivity between FPN and SMN ($p_{FWE} = 0.005$) and between CON and SMN ($p_{FWE} = 0.048$), as well as lower negative connectivity (anticorrelation) between CON and SMN ($p_{FWE} = 0.043$), at t_2. No other age differences in between-networks connectivity survived FWE correction for multiple comparisons. Ancillary correlation analyses between age and individual network measures within the OA group identified

a significant negative correlation between age and within-DMN connectivity at t_1 ($\rho = -0.65, p_{FWE} = 0.015$).

In summary, OA showed lower brain-wide modularity and local efficiency compared to YA, with the difference in local efficiency showing most consistency across time. At the level of individual networks, CON showed substantial differences between groups, reflected in all examined properties. Additionally, DMN and SMN were characterized by lower intra-network connectivity and greater participation, respectively, in OA.

Links with Learning during WM Training

To assess links between network measures and performance during cognitive training, we calculated Spearman correlation coefficients, separately for each group and at each time point. Similar to the assessment of age differences in network measures, significant brain-wide results were followed by analyses of robustness and assessments at the level of individual networks.

Brain-Wide Network Measures

Interestingly, significant relations between network measures and learning rates were detected only for OA and only at t_1. Specifically, modularity ($\rho = 0.51, p = 0.028$) and local efficiency ($\rho = 0.59, p = 0.01$) were positively correlated with early learning rates, whereas global efficiency ($\rho = -0.61, p = 0.007$) was negatively correlated with early learning rates (**Figure 6**, top panel). Ancillary analyses were performed to test for influences of educational level and sex on these results. There were no significant correlations between the number of years of education and networks measures (p's > 0.5), and controlling for the

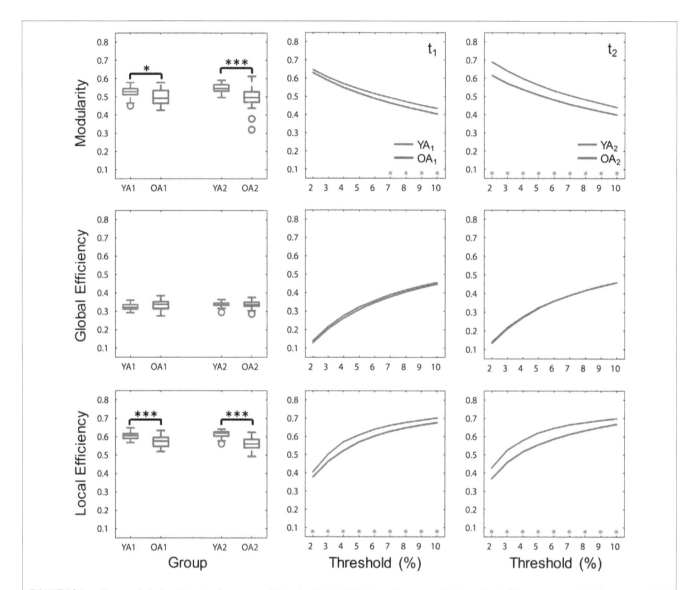

FIGURE 3 | Age differences in brain-wide network measures. At a brain-wide level, OA showed lower modularity and local efficiency compared to YA, whereas global efficiency was not significantly different across groups. Boxplots in the left panel depict values averaged across all thresholds. YA, younger adults (blue color); OA, older adults (red color); t_1, time point 1; t_2, time point 2. Magenta asterisks indicate $p < 0.05$ for each threshold. $^*p < 0.05$, $^{***}p < 0.001$, across all thresholds.

number of years of education did not substantially influence the relations between network measures and learning rates. Also, Spearman correlations performed separately by sex showed similar trends in both males and females, and there were no sex differences in correlation strengths (p's > 0.6).

Robustness Analysis

We took multiple steps to assess the robustness of our findings, using a procedure similar to Gallen et al. (2016a). First, we assessed whether the relations between network measures and learning rates were constantly present over the threshold range, and the results confirmed that all these relations were fairly consistent across thresholds (**Figure 6**, bottom panel). Second, given the absence of differences in motion across groups and time points (see Methods section), controlling for motion (i.e., partial

correlations) did not substantially alter the relations between any of the brain-wide network measures and learning rates (modularity: $\rho_p = 0.49$, $p = 0.04$; local efficiency: $\rho_p = 0.55$, $p = 0.019$; global efficiency: $\rho_p = -0.59$, $p = 0.01$).

Individual Network Measures

To further elucidate the relations between network characteristics and early learning rates, significant results at the brain-wide level were followed-up by analyses at the level of individual networks. The results showed that participation of CON at t_1 was negatively correlated with learning rates in OA ($\rho = -0.81$, $p_{FWE} < 0.001$), consistent with the brain-wide results. No other correlations survived FWE correction for multiple comparisons.

In summary, brain-wide network measures at t_1 were linked to learning rates during training in OA but not in YA. At the

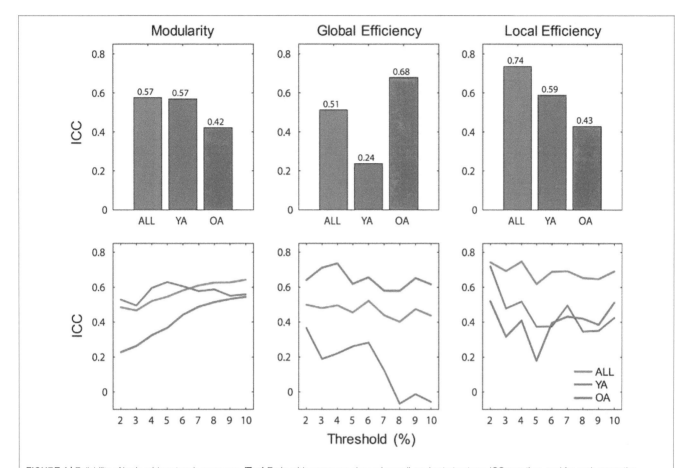

FIGURE 4 | Reliability of brain-wide network measures. **(Top)** Brain-wide measures showed overall moderate to strong ICC over time, and for each group the agreement ranged from fair (>0.2) to strong (>0.6); bar graphs depict ICC values calculated across all thresholds. **(Bottom)** Reliability of network measures was generally stable across thresholds, with the exception of global efficiency for YA; line graphs depict ICC values calculated for each threshold. ICC, intraclass correlation coefficient; ALL, all subjects (magenta color); YA, younger adults (blue color); OA, older adults (red color).

level of individual networks, participation of CON showed links with training effects consistent with the patterns identified by the brain-wide analyses.

DISCUSSION

The goals of the present investigation were to assess the replicability of previously reported age effects on resting-state networks, to examine their reliability over time, and to assess their relation to behavioral outcomes (namely learning rates during a cognitive training intervention). Similar to previous investigations, we identified both consistencies in network structure and differences in module composition between groups. Notably, OA showed less similarity of their network partitions compared to YA, both as a group and across time. Regarding brain-wide network measures, OA showed lower modularity and local efficiency compared to YA, with the difference in local efficiency showing most consistency across time. At the level of individual networks, OA showed substantial differences in CON, reflected in all examined metrics, as well as lower intra-network connectivity in DMN and greater participation of SMN. Finally, baseline brain-wide network

measures were linked to early learning rates in OA but not in YA, and the participation of CON showed links with early learning rates consistent with the patterns identified by the brain-wide analyses. The main findings are discussed, in turn, below.

The present results replicate previously reported age differences in functional network properties (Achard and Bullmore, 2007; Meunier et al., 2009a; Onoda and Yamaguchi, 2013; Betzel et al., 2014; Cao M. et al., 2014; Song et al., 2014; Geerligs et al., 2015) and extend these findings to multiple time points (Welton et al., 2015). Regarding community structure, the present results showing age differences in module composition, but overall similar modules are consistent with previous evidence (Geerligs et al., 2015) and suggest age-related topological changes in the context of overall similar functional configuration, irrespective of age. Furthermore, the results showing less similarity of network partitions in OA, both as a group and across time, are in line with recent evidence suggesting reduced baseline stability of network activity with aging (Tsvetanov et al., 2016).

Regarding age differences in network measures, we identified reliable age differences in brain-wide modularity and local efficiency, consistent with previous investigations (Achard and

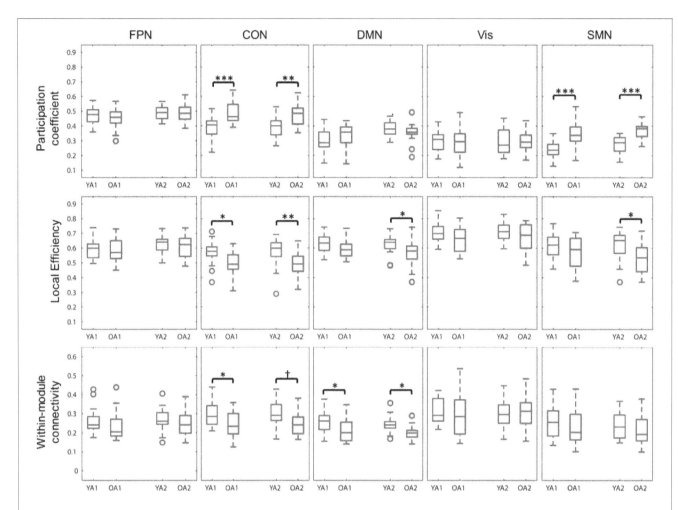

FIGURE 5 | Age differences in individual network measures. OA showed greater participation coefficients for CON and SMN, lower local efficiency for CON, and for DMN and SMN only at t_2, and lower within-module connectivity within DMN and within CON, compared to YA. FPN, fronto-parietal network; CON, cingulo-opercular network; DMN, default-mode network; Vis, visual network, SMN, somato-sensorimotor network; YA, younger adults (blue color); OA, older adults (red color). $^*p < 0.05$, $^{**}p < 0.01$, $^{***}p < 0.001$, across all thresholds and corrected for multiple comparisons. $^†p = 0.016$, across all thresholds, uncorrected.

Bullmore, 2007; Onoda and Yamaguchi, 2013; Betzel et al., 2014; Cao M. et al., 2014; Song et al., 2014; Geerligs et al., 2015). Modularity indexes the degree to which a graph can be partitioned into multiple communities, and is considered a central principle of brain organization, supporting functional segregation and integration through communication within- and between-modules, respectively (Dehaene et al., 1998; Sporns et al., 2000; Meunier et al., 2009b; Sporns and Betzel, 2015). Thus, results showing lower modularity in OA compared to YA suggest loss of functional specificity of the brain networks with aging (Ferreira and Busatto, 2013; Damoiseaux, 2017; Naik et al., 2017). Global efficiency indexes graph-wide integration and has been linked with information exchange among distributed regions, whereas local efficiency indexes regional-level integration and has been linked with fault tolerance within specialized areas (Latora and Marchiori, 2003; Achard and Bullmore, 2007). In general, the argument is that brains maximize cost-efficiency by favoring dense short-range connections and sparse long-range connections, because the latter are more costly (Achard

and Bullmore, 2007; Bullmore and Sporns, 2012). Thus, results showing lower local efficiency in OA compared to YA suggest a reduction of cost-efficiency in aging; under conditions of similar connection density, which is considered a proxy for wiring cost, efficiency is lower in OA compared to YA (Achard and Bullmore, 2007; Geerligs et al., 2015). It should be noted, however, that wiring costs can only be approximated in functional networks, because two functionally connected regions do not necessarily share a direct structural link (Rubinov and Sporns, 2010; Zalesky et al., 2012). In fact, modularity and local efficiency are related measures, such that a system with denser local connections also tends to be more modular (Bullmore and Sporns, 2012). On the other hand, similar global efficiency irrespective of age has been explained by a greater number of inter-module connections in OA; specifically, more inter-module connections may counterbalance less intra-module connections, resulting in similar amounts of shortest path lengths between distant nodes (Song et al., 2014; Geerligs et al., 2015). In sum, these findings are consistent with overall patterns of decreased within- and

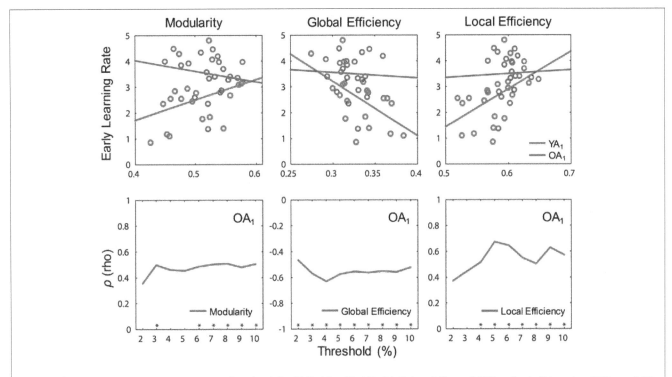

FIGURE 6 | Relations between network measures and learning during WM training. **(Top)** Modularity ($\rho = 0.51$, $p = 0.028$) and local efficiency ($\rho = 0.59$, $p = 0.01$) were positively correlated, whereas global efficiency ($\rho = -0.61$, $p = 0.007$) was negatively correlated with early learning rates in OA (red color), only at t_1; blue and red lines show least squares lines. **(Bottom)** Relations between network measures and learning rates (Spearman correlation) were fairly constant across thresholds. t_1, time point 1; YA, younger adults (blue color); OA, older adults (red color). *$p < 0.05$, for each threshold.

increased between-system connectivity, suggesting decreased "system segregation" in aging (Betzel et al., 2014; Chan et al., 2014; Ferreira et al., 2016).

The present findings may also be relevant for better understanding task-related neural over-activation in OA relative to YA, which has been linked with both compensation and dedifferentiation (Cabeza, 2002; Park et al., 2004, 2010; Davis et al., 2008; Grady, 2008; Reuter-Lorenz and Cappell, 2008; Reuter-Lorenz and Park, 2014). Task-related over-activation in OA may be related to altered intrinsic network dynamics, reflected in differences in modularity and local efficiency "at rest." Whereas the loss of functional specificity in aging (reflected by the decline in modularity) is consistent with the idea of dedifferentiation, reduced cost-efficiency (reflected by the decline in local efficiency) may be linked to compensatory processes that are overall less efficient than the primary computations (Reuter-Lorenz and Park, 2014). Thus, dedifferentiation and compensation may both be expressions of the same process of functional recalibration due to declining structure with aging (Naik et al., 2017). This also highlights the critical need for better integrating resting-state and task-related approaches, in order to develop a practical understanding of neurocognitive function and age-related change (Iordan and Reuter-Lorenz, 2016; see also Gallen et al., 2016b).

To assess the reliability of age differences in network properties, in the present study we measured the same participants over 2 sessions 2 weeks apart and calculated ICC of network properties between the 2 sessions (McGraw and Wong, 1996). Results showed consistent age differences in network properties over time, with overall strong to moderate ICCs, comparable to previous investigations (Telesford et al., 2010; Wang et al., 2011; Braun et al., 2012; Park et al., 2012; Cao H. et al., 2014; Welton et al., 2015), thus suggesting that the observed age differences are reliable. Interestingly, results showed relatively higher reliability for local compared to global efficiency (see also Park et al., 2012). This effect was driven by YA, who showed more global efficiency variability between the 2 sessions, and it might have been linked to residual effects from the WM tasks performed prior to the resting-state recordings (Barnes et al., 2009; Breckel et al., 2013; Gordon et al., 2014). In line with our findings, a study by Park et al. (2012) also identified low reliability of global efficiency in a test-retest investigation of resting-state data in YA, assessed over a 24-h period. The authors concluded that this was likely due to high variability of long-range connections (given the dependence of global efficiency on this topological feature), and may reflect greater influence of cognitive control on this measure, compared to local efficiency (Honey et al., 2009).

The results showing age differences in network properties at the level of individual modules complement and further elucidate the patterns of brain-wide results. Although DMN has traditionally been the most investigated resting-state network (Ferreira and Busatto, 2013; Damoiseaux, 2017), recent investigations also point to CON changes as prominent features of healthy aging (Meier et al., 2012; Onoda et al., 2012; He et al., 2014; La Corte et al., 2016). The cingulo-opercular network (or salience network, in alternative taxonomies) is anchored in the anterior cingulate and frontal operculum/anterior insula regions, and has been implicated both in stable set-maintenance (Dosenbach et al., 2006, 2007, 2008; Power and Petersen, 2013) and multimodal sensory integration (Seeley et al., 2007; Bressler and Menon, 2010; Menon, 2011). The present results, showing both higher participation coefficients and lower local efficiency and intra-module connectivity for CON in OA, suggest age-related dedifferentiation of this network and support the idea of changes in CON functionality as a hallmark of healthy aging (Meier et al., 2012; Onoda et al., 2012; He et al., 2014; La Corte et al., 2016). Greater participation coefficients for CON and SMN in OA indicate greater propensity of the nodes within these two networks to form links outside their own modules, and suggest that CON and SMN may drive the observed age differences in brain-wide modularity. Furthermore, local efficiency in CON was also consistently lower in OA, suggesting an age-related decline in local integration of information at the level of this network. In addition to CON, DMN showed consistent lower intra-module connectivity in OA relative to YA, in line with previous evidence (Andrews-Hanna et al., 2007; Damoiseaux et al., 2008; Ferreira and Busatto, 2013; Geerligs et al., 2015; Grady et al., 2016; Damoiseaux, 2017). Interestingly, our results did not show greater FPN-DMN inter-network connectivity in OA relative to YA (Geerligs et al., 2015; Turner and Spreng, 2015), which might have been related to the inclusion of relatively younger, high-functioning OA in our sample. Supporting this interpretation, a recent longitudinal study in OA (Ng et al., 2016) identified a u-shaped trajectory in which FPN-DMN inter-network connectivity initially *decreased* and then *increased* with age, with a turning point around 65–70 years of age. An alternative interpretation is that the functional interactions between FPN and DMN in OA might have been influenced by residual task-effects, as outlined above.

Regarding links between network measures and learning rates during training, the present results showed that higher resting-state modularity and local efficiency, as well as lower global efficiency prior to training, were associated with better early learning in OA. Early learning rates are thought to reflect the initial attainment of peak performance within an individual's baseline performance range, rather than plasticity *per se* (Lövden et al., 2010). Notably, associations between network properties and early learning rates were observed only for OA and only at t_1. While the presence of these associations only in OA could be interpreted in line with evidence pointing to age-related dissociations in the relations between network efficiency and cognitive performance (Stanley et al., 2015), the lack of consistency of these relations across time might be attributable to differences in residual task-effects related to the phenomenon of task exposure which may have, in turn, influenced the reliability of network measures across time. Specifically, if task exposure altered strategies for WM task performance across the two sessions for older but not for younger adults, the resting-state activity, which was always recorded subsequent to task performance, may have been differentially affected. Future analyses comparing the effects of task exposure on differences

between task-related and subsequently recorded resting-state network configurations are needed to further clarify this aspect of the results.

Although evidence linking network properties with benefits accrued over the course of cognitive training is scarce, the present results are in line with previous findings showing positive relations for modularity in OA (Gallen et al., 2016a) and in patients with traumatic brain injury (Arnemann et al., 2015). Consistent with the idea that modularity supports both functional segregation and integration, previous evidence has positively linked modularity with cognitive performance (Stevens et al., 2012; Sadaghiani et al., 2015), and thus greater modularity during resting-state may reflect a more "optimal" functional organization that promotes cognitive improvements with training (Gallen et al., 2016a). Results at the level of individual networks add specificity to this interpretation, by associating lower CON participation coefficients with higher learning rates in OA. Combined with evidence showing greater participation coefficients for this network in OA as a group, the present findings provide preliminary evidence for a link between preserved CON segregation and better learning in OA.

The present results linking network properties at rest with learning rates can be interpreted in the light of evidence from investigations of task-related performance (Stanley et al., 2015; Cohen and D'Esposito, 2016; Bolt et al., 2017). Specifically, investigations comparing network properties across resting and task contexts have shown that cognitive task states are characterized by overall *lower* modularity and local efficiency, as well as *greater* global efficiency, and that such levels are positively associated with cognitive performance at the individual level in YA (Cohen and D'Esposito, 2016; Bolt et al., 2017). Consistent with this evidence, age-related investigations have linked lower local efficiency during task performance with better WM performance irrespective of age, whereas greater global efficiency was associated with better WM performance in YA but relatively worse WM performance in OA (Stanley et al., 2015). By contrast, prior investigations (Gallen et al., 2016a), as well as the present results, point to a seemingly inverse pattern characterizing the relationship between modularity "at rest" and learning rates in OA, whereby *greater* modularity and local efficiency, as well as *lower* global efficiency "at rest", are associated with better learning. Although relations between resting and task-related network configurations are still not well understood, the present evidence suggests that the potential for dynamic network reconfiguration across different states might play an important role for understanding cognition and its plasticity in aging (Cole et al., 2014, 2016; Krienen et al., 2014; Iordan and Reuter-Lorenz, 2016). However, the exploratory nature of these findings advises their interpretation with caution.

Limitations and Future Directions

Reliance on extreme groups to understand effects of aging has clear limitations, and thus future work assessing a broader age range (e.g., Chan et al., 2014), as well as longitudinal assessments of the same individuals over periods of years (e.g., Ng et al., 2016), are necessary to provide more comprehensive insights. Regarding the timing of resting-state acquisition, whereas a 6-min break from a preceding task can be a sufficient "wash-out" period for certain individuals under certain task conditions (Breckel et al., 2013), it is not as efficient as longer breaks, and thus resting-state recording before any task should be preferred. Finally, our investigations at the level of individual modules have been partly exploratory. Future studies with strong a priori hypotheses are needed to further elucidate effects of aging on specific within- and between-networks interactions.

CONCLUSIONS

In conclusion, we successfully replicated previously reported age effects on resting-state networks, demonstrated their reliability over time, and identified links with initial learning during WM training. We identified both consistencies in network structure and differences in module composition between YA and OA, suggesting topological changes and less stability of functional network structure with aging. Lower modularity and local efficiency in OA suggests age effects on both functional segregation and integration of brain networks, consistent with the idea of age-related functional dedifferentiation. Importantly, these differences were replicable over time, with the difference in local efficiency showing most consistency. On the other hand, global efficiency did not differ between the two age groups and showed low reliability in YA. At the level of individual networks, specific differences were identified for CON, DMN, and SMN, suggesting age-related differential effects at the level of specialized brain modules. Finally, associations between

network properties and early learning rates were identified for OA only at t1, suggesting that baseline network configuration may be informative in predicting aspects of learning in OA, albeit with some limitations. The present findings advance our understanding of the effects of aging on the brain's large-scale functional organization and provide preliminary evidence for network characteristics associated with learning during training. Continued identification of neural mechanisms associated with training-induced plasticity is important for further clarifying whether and how such changes predict the magnitude and maintenance of training gains, as well as the extent and limits of cognitive transfer in both younger and older adults.

AUTHOR CONTRIBUTIONS

PR-L, JJ, TP, MB, SJ, BK, KC, KM, and SP designed the study. KC and KM collected the behavioral and brain imaging data, and analyzed the behavioral data. AI analyzed the resting-state brain imaging data and wrote the original draft. All authors reviewed and edited the final manuscript.

ACKNOWLEDGMENTS

This research was supported by National Institute on Aging [R21-AG-045460] grant to PR-L. The authors thank Sneha Rajen and KyungJun Kim for assistance with data analysis.

REFERENCES

Achard, S., and Bullmore, E. (2007). Efficiency and cost of economical brain functional networks. *PLoS Comput. Biol.* 3:e17. doi: 10.1371/journal.pcbi.0030017

Achard, S., Salvador, R., Whitcher, B., Suckling, J., and Bullmore, E. (2006). A resilient, low-frequency, small-world human brain functional network with highly connected association cortical hubs. *J. Neurosci.* 26, 63–72. doi: 10.1523/JNEUROSCI.3874-05.2006

Alakörkkö, T., Saarimäki, H., Glerean, E., Saramäki, J., and Korhonen, O. (2017). Effects of spatial smoothing on functional brain networks. *Eur. J. Neurosci.* 46, 2471–2480. doi: 10.1111/ejn.13717

Alexander-Bloch, A., Lambiotte, R., Roberts, B., Giedd, J., Gogtay, N., and Bullmore, E. (2012). The discovery of population differences in network community structure: new methods and applications to brain functional networks in schizophrenia. *Neuroimage* 59, 3889–3900. doi: 10.1016/j.neuroimage.2011.11.035

Andrews-Hanna, J. R., Snyder, A. Z., Vincent, J. L., Lustig, C., Head, D., Raichle, M. E., et al. (2007). Disruption of large-scale brain systems in advanced aging. *Neuron* 56, 924–935. doi: 10.1016/j.neuron.2007.10.038

Arnemann, K. L., Chen, A. J., Novakovic-Agopian, T., Gratton, C., Nomura, E. M., and D'Esposito, M. (2015). Functional brain network modularity predicts response to cognitive training after brain injury. *Neurology* 84, 1568–1574. doi: 10.1212/WNL.0000000000001476

Ashburner, J. (2007). A fast diffeomorphic image registration algorithm. *Neuroimage* 38, 95–113. doi: 10.1016/j.neuroimage.2007.07.007

Ballesteros, S., Kraft, E., Santana, S., and Tziraki, C. (2015). Maintaining older brain functionality: a targeted review. *Neurosci. Biobehav. Rev.* 55, 453–477. doi: 10.1016/j.neubiorev.2015.06.008

Barnes, A., Bullmore, E. T., and Suckling, J. (2009). Endogenous human brain dynamics recover slowly following cognitive effort. *PLoS ONE* 4:e6626. doi: 10.1371/journal.pone.0006626

Behzadi, Y., Restom, K., Liau, J., and Liu, T. T. (2007). A component based noise correction method (CompCor) for BOLD and perfusion based fMRI. *Neuroimage* 37, 90–101. doi: 10.1016/j.neuroimage.2007.04.042

Benjamini, Y., and Hochberg, Y. (1995). Controlling the false discovery rate: a practical and powerful approach to multiple testing. *J. R. Stat. Soc. Series B Stat. Methodol.* 57, 289–300.

Betzel, R. F., Byrge, L., He, Y., Goñi, J., Zuo, X.-N., and Sporns, O. (2014). Changes in structural and functional connectivity among resting-state networks across the human lifespan. *Neuroimage* 102, 345–357. doi: 10.1016/j.neuroimage.2014.07.067

Bherer, L. (2015). Cognitive plasticity in older adults: effects of cognitive training and physical exercise. *Ann. N.Y. Acad. Sci.* 1337, 1–6. doi: 10.1111/nyas.12682

Blair, R. C., and Karniski, W. (1993). An alternative method for significance testing of waveform difference potentials. *Psychophysiology* 30, 518–524. doi: 10.1111/j.1469-8986.1993.tb02075.x

Blondel, V. D., Guillaume, J.-L., Lambiotte, R., and Lefebvre, E. (2008). Fast unfolding of communities in large networks. *J. Stat. Mech.* 2008:P10008. doi: 10.1088/1742-5468/2008/10/P10008

Bolt, T., Nomi, J. S., Rubinov, M., and Uddin, L. Q. (2017). Correspondence between evoked and intrinsic functional brain network configurations. *Hum. Brain Mapp.* 38, 1992–2007. doi: 10.1002/hbm.23500

Braun, U., Plichta, M. M., Esslinger, C., Sauer, C., Haddad, L., Grimm, O., et al. (2012). Test-retest reliability of resting-state connectivity network characteristics using fMRI and graph theoretical measures. *Neuroimage* 59, 1404–1412. doi: 10.1016/j.neuroimage.2011.08.044

Breckel, T. P. K., Thiel, C. M., Bullmore, E. T., Zalesky, A., Patel, A. X., and Giessing, C. (2013). Long-term effects of attentional performance on functional brain network topology. *PLoS ONE* 8:e74125. doi: 10.1371/journal.pone.0074125

Brehmer, Y., Kalpouzos, G., Wenger, E., and Lövdén, M. (2014). Plasticity of brain and cognition in older adults. *Psychol. Res.* 78, 790–802. doi: 10.1007/s00426-014-0587-z

Bressler, S. L., and Menon, V. (2010). Large-scale brain networks in cognition: emerging methods and principles. *Trends Cogn. Sci.* 14, 277–290. doi: 10.1016/j.tics.2010.04.004

Bullmore, E., and Sporns, O. (2009). Complex brain networks: graph theoretical analysis of structural and functional systems. *Nat. Rev. Neurosci.* 10, 186–198. doi: 10.1038/nrn2575

Bullmore, E., and Sporns, O. (2012). The economy of brain network organization. *Nat. Rev. Neurosci.* 13, 336–349. doi: 10.1038/nrn3214

Buschkuehl, M., Jaeggi, S. M., Hutchison, S., Perrig-Chiello, P., Däpp, C., Müller, M., et al. (2008). Impact of working memory training on memory performance in old-old adults. *Psychol. Aging* 23, 743–753. doi: 10.1037/a0014342

Cabeza, R. (2002). Hemispheric asymmetry reduction in older adults: the HAROLD model. *Psychol. Aging* 17, 85–100. doi: 10.1037/0882-7974.17.1.85

Cao, H., Plichta, M. M., Schäfer, A., Haddad, L., Grimm, O., Schneider, M., et al. (2014). Test-retest reliability of fMRI-based graph theoretical properties during working memory, emotion processing, and resting state. *Neuroimage* 84, 888–900. doi: 10.1016/j.neuroimage.2013.09.013

Cao, M., Wang, J.-H., Dai, Z.-J., Cao, X.-Y., Jiang, L.-L., Fan, F.-M., et al. (2014). Topological organization of the human brain functional connectome across the lifespan. *Dev. Cogn. Neurosci.* 7, 76–93. doi: 10.1016/j.dcn.2013.11.004

Chai, X. J., Castanon, A. N., Ongur, D., and Whitfield-Gabrieli, S. (2012). Anticorrelations in resting state networks without global signal regression. *Neuroimage* 59, 1420–1428. doi: 10.1016/j.neuroimage.2011.08.048

Chan, M. Y., Park, D. C., Savalia, N. K., Petersen, S. E., and Wig, G. S. (2014). Decreased segregation of brain systems across the healthy adult lifespan. *Proc. Natl. Acad. Sci. U. S. A.* 111, E4997–E5006. doi: 10.1073/pnas.1415122111

Ciric, R., Wolf, D. H., Power, J. D., Roalf, D. R., Baum, G. L., Ruparel, K., et al. (2017). Benchmarking of participant-level confound regression strategies for the control of motion artifact in studies of functional connectivity. *Neuroimage* 154, 174–187. doi: 10.1016/j.neuroimage.2017.03.020

Cohen, J. R., and D'Esposito, M. (2016). The segregation and integration of distinct brain networks and their relationship to cognition. *J. Neurosci.* 36, 12083–12094. doi: 10.1523/JNEUROSCI.2965-15.2016

Cole, M. W., Bassett, D. S., Power, J. D., Braver, T. S., and Petersen, S. E. (2014). Intrinsic and task-evoked network architectures of the human brain. *Neuron* 83, 238–251. doi: 10.1016/j.neuron.2014.05.014

Cole, M. W., Ito, T., Bassett, D. S., and Schultz, D. H. (2016). Activity flow over resting-state networks shapes cognitive task activations. *Nat. Neurosci.* 19, 1718–1726. doi: 10.1038/nn.4406

Damoiseaux, J. S. (2017). Effects of aging on functional and structural brain connectivity. *Neuroimage* 160, 32–40. doi: 10.1016/j.neuroimage.2017.01.077

Damoiseaux, J. S., Beckmann, C. F., Arigita, E. J. S., Barkhof, F., Scheltens, P., Stam, C. J., et al. (2008). Reduced resting-state brain activity in the "default network" in normal aging. *Cereb. Cortex* 18, 1856–1864. doi: 10.1093/cercor/bhm207

Davis, S. W., Dennis, N. A., Daselaar, S. M., Fleck, M. S., and Cabeza, R. (2008). Que PASA? The posterior-anterior shift in aging. *Cereb. Cortex* 18, 1201–1209. doi: 10.1093/cercor/bhm155

Dehaene, S., Kerszberg, M., and Changeux, J.-P. (1998). A neuronal model of a global workspace in effortful cognitive tasks. *Proc. Natl Acad. Sci. U.S.A.* 95, 14529–14534. doi: 10.1073/pnas.95.24.14529

Dennis, E. L., and Thompson, P. M. (2014). Functional brain connectivity using fMRI in aging and Alzheimer's disease. *Neuropsychol. Rev.* 24, 49–62. doi: 10.1007/s11065-014-9249-6

Dosenbach, N. U. F., Fair, D. A., Cohen, A. L., Schlaggar, B. L., and Petersen, S. E. (2008). A dual-networks architecture of top-down control. *Trends Cogn. Sci.* 12, 99–105. doi: 10.1016/j.tics.2008.01.001

Dosenbach, N. U. F., Fair, D. A., Miezin, F. M., Cohen, A. L., Wenger, K. K., Dosenbach, R. A. T., et al. (2007). Distinct brain networks for adaptive and stable task control in humans. *Proc. Natl. Acad. Sci. U.S.A.* 104, 11073–11078. doi: 10.1073/pnas.0704320104

Dosenbach, N. U. F., Visscher, K. M., Palmer, E. D., Miezin, F. M., Wenger, K. K., Kang, H. C., et al. (2006). A core system for the implementation of task sets. *Neuron* 50, 799–812. doi: 10.1016/j.neuron.2006.04.031

Dwyer, D. B., Harrison, B. J., Yucel, M., Whittle, S., Zalesky, A., Pantelis, C., et al. (2014). Large-scale brain network dynamics supporting adolescent cognitive control. *J. Neurosci.* 34, 14096–14107. doi: 10.1523/JNEUROSCI.1634-14.2014

Ferreira, L. K., and Busatto, G. F. (2013). Resting-state functional connectivity in normal brain aging. *Neurosci. Biobehav. Rev.* 37, 384–400. doi: 10.1016/j.neubiorev.2013.01.017

Ferreira, L. K., Regina, A. C., Kovacevic, N., Martin Mda, G., Santos, P. P., Carneiro Cde, G., et al. (2016). Aging effects on whole-brain functional connectivity in adults free of cognitive and psychiatric disorders. *Cereb. Cortex* 26, 3851–3865. doi: 10.1093/cercor/bhv190

Gallen, C. L., Baniqued, P. L., Chapman, S. B., Aslan, S., Keebler, M., Didehbani, N., et al. (2016a). Modular brain network organization predicts response to cognitive training in older adults. *PLoS ONE* 11:e0169015. doi: 10.1371/journal.pone.0169015

Gallen, C. L., Turner, G. R., Adnan, A., and D'Esposito, M. (2016b). Reconfiguration of brain network architecture to support executive control in aging. *Neurobiol. Aging* 44, 42–52. doi: 10.1016/j.neurobiolaging.2016.04.003

Garrison, K. A., Scheinost, D., Finn, E. S., Shen, X., and Constable, R. T. (2015). The (in)stability of functional brain network measures across thresholds. *Neuroimage* 118, 651–661. doi: 10.1016/j.neuroimage.2015.05.046

Geerligs, L., Renken, R. J., Saliasi, E., Maurits, N. M., and Lorist, M. M. (2015). A brain-wide study of age-related changes in functional connectivity. *Cereb. Cortex* 25, 1987–1999. doi: 10.1093/cercor/bhu012

Geerligs, L., Tsvetanov, K. A., and Henson, R. N. (2017). Challenges in measuring individual differences in functional connectivity using fMRI: the case of healthy aging. *Hum. Brain Mapp.* 38, 4125–4156. doi: 10.1002/hbm.23653

Good, B. H., de Montjoye, Y.-A., and Clauset, A. (2010). Performance of modularity maximization in practical contexts. *Phys. Rev. E* 81:046106. doi: 10.1103/PhysRevE.81.046106

Gordon, E. M., Breeden, A. L., Bean, S. E., and Vaidya, C. J. (2014). Working memory-related changes in functional connectivity persist beyond task disengagement. *Hum. Brain Mapp.* 35, 1004–1017. doi: 10.1002/hbm.22230

Grady, C. (2012). The cognitive neuroscience of ageing. *Nat. Rev. Neurosci.* 13, 491–505. doi: 10.1038/nrn3256

Grady, C., Sarraf, S., Saverino, C., and Campbell, K. (2016). Age differences in the functional interactions among the default, frontoparietal control, and dorsal attention networks. *Neurobiol. Aging* 41, 159–172. doi: 10.1016/j.neurobiolaging.2016.02.020

Grady, C. L. (2008). Cognitive neuroscience of aging. *Ann. N.Y. Acad. Sci.* 1124, 127–144. doi: 10.1196/annals.1440.009

Greicius, M. D., Krasnow, B., Reiss, A. L., and Menon, V. (2003). Functional connectivity in the resting brain: a network analysis of the default mode hypothesis. *Proc. Natl. Acad. Sci. U.S.A.* 100, 253–258. doi: 10.1073/pnas.0135058100

Groppe, D. M., Urbach, T. P., and Kutas, M. (2011). Mass univariate analysis of event-related brain potentials/fields I: a critical tutorial review. *Psychophysiology* 48, 1711–1725. doi: 10.1111/j.1469-8986.2011.01273.x

Guimerà, R., and Amaral, L. A. N. (2005). Cartography of complex networks: modules and universal roles. *J. Stat. Mech.* 2005:P02001. doi: 10.1088/1742-5468/2005/02/P02001

He, X., Qin, W., Liu, Y., Zhang, X., Duan, Y., Song, J., et al. (2014). Abnormal salience network in normal aging and in amnestic mild cognitive impairment and Alzheimer's disease. *Hum. Brain Mapp.* 35, 3446–3464. doi: 10.1002/hbm.22414

Honey, C. J., Sporns, O., Cammoun, L., Gigandet, X., Thiran, J. P., Meuli, R., et al. (2009). Predicting human resting-state functional connectivity from structural connectivity. *Proc. Natl. Acad. Sci. U.S.A.* 106, 2035–2040. doi: 10.1073/pnas.0811168106

Iordan, A. D., and Reuter-Lorenz, P. A. (2016). Age-related change and the predictive value of the "resting state": a commentary on

Campbell and Schacter (2016). *Lang. Cogn. Neurosci.* 32, 674–677. doi: 10.1080/23273798.2016.1242759

Karbach, J., and Verhaeghen, P. (2014). Making working memory work: a meta-analysis of executive control and working memory training in younger and older adults. *Psychol. Sci.* 25, 2027–2037. doi: 10.1177/0956797614548725

Katzman, R., Brown, T., Fuld, P., Peck, A., Schechter, R., and Schimmel, H. (1983). Validation of a short orientation-memory-concentration test of cognitive impairment. *Am. J. Psychiatry* 140, 734–739. doi: 10.1176/ajp.140.6.734

Klein, A., Andersson, J., Ardekani, B. A., Ashburner, J., Avants, B., Chiang, M. C., et al. (2009). Evaluation of 14 nonlinear deformation algorithms applied to human brain MRI registration. *Neuroimage* 46, 786–802. doi: 10.1016/j.neuroimage.2008.12.037

Krienen, F. M., Yeo, B. T. T., and Buckner, R. L. (2014). Reconfigurable task-dependent functional coupling modes cluster around a core functional architecture. *Philos. Trans. R. Soc. Lond. B Biol. Sci.* 369:20130526. doi: 10.1098/rstb.2013.0526

Kroenke, K., Spitzer, R. L., and Williams, J. B. (2001). The PHQ-9: validity of a brief depression severity measure. *J. Gen. Intern. Med.* 16, 606–613. doi: 10.1046/j.1525-1497.2001.016009606.x

Kuncheva, L. I., and Hadjitodorov, S. T. (2004). Kuncheva, L. I., and Hadjitodorov, S. T. (2004). "Using diversity in cluster ensembles," in *2004 IEEE International Conference on Systems, Man and Cybernetics*, Vol. 2 (IEEE Cat. No. 04CH37583) (Hague), 1214–1219. doi: 10.1109/ICSMC.2004.1399790

Lancichinetti, A., and Fortunato, S. (2012). Consensus clustering in complex networks. *Sci. Rep.* 2:336. doi: 10.1038/srep00336

La Corte, V., Sperduti, M., Malherbe, C., Vialatte, F., Lion, S., Gallarda, T., et al. (2016). Cognitive decline and reorganization of functional connectivity in healthy aging: the pivotal role of the salience network in the prediction of age and cognitive performances. *Front. Aging Neurosci.* 8:204. doi: 10.3389/fnagi.2016.00204

Latora, V., and Marchiori, M. (2003). Economic small-world behavior in weighted networks. *Eur. Phys. J. B Condens. Matter* 32, 249–263. doi: 10.1140/epjb/e2003-00095-5

Liao, W., Ding, J., Marinazzo, D., Xu, Q., Wang, Z., Yuan, C., et al. (2011). Small-world directed networks in the human brain: multivariate Granger causality analysis of resting-state fMRI. *Neuroimage* 54, 2683–2694. doi: 10.1016/j.neuroimage.2010.11.007

Lövden, M., Backman, L., Lindenberger, U., Schaefer, S., and Schmiedek, F. (2010). A theoretical framework for the study of adult cognitive plasticity. *Psychol. Bull.* 136, 659–676. doi: 10.1037/a0020080

Lustig, C., Shah, P., Seidler, R., and Reuter-Lorenz, P. A. (2009). Aging, training, and the brain: a review and future directions. *Neuropsychol. Rev.* 19, 504–522. doi: 10.1007/s11065-009-9119-9

McGraw, K. O., and Wong, S. P. (1996). Forming inferences about some intraclass correlation coefficients. *Psychol. Methods* 1:30. doi: 10.1037/1082-989X.1.1.30

Meier, T. B., Desphande, A. S., Vergun, S., Nair, V. A., Song, J., Biswal, B. B., et al. (2012). Support vector machine classification and characterization of age-related reorganization of functional brain networks. *Neuroimage* 60, 601–613. doi: 10.1016/j.neuroimage.2011.12.052

Menon, V. (2011). Large-scale brain networks and psychopathology: a unifying triple network model. *Trends Cogn. Sci.* 15, 483–506. doi: 10.1016/j.tics.2011.08.003

Meunier, D., Achard, S., Morcom, A., and Bullmore, E. (2009a). Age-related changes in modular organization of human brain functional networks. *Neuroimage* 44, 715–723. doi: 10.1016/j.neuroimage.2008.09.062

Meunier, D., Lambiotte, R., Fornito, A., Ersche, K., and Bullmore, E. T. (2009b). Hierarchical modularity in human brain functional networks. *Front. Neuroinformatics* 3:37. doi: 10.3389/neuro.11.037.2009

Mewborn, C. M., Lindbergh, C. A., and Miller, L. S. (2017). Cognitive interventions for cognitively healthy, mildly impaired, and mixed samples of older adults: a systematic review and meta-analysis of randomized-controlled trials. *Neuropsychol. Rev.* doi: 10.1007/s11065-017-9350-8. [Epub ahead of print].

Montgomery, A. A., Graham, A., Evans, P. H., and Fahey, T. (2002). Inter-rater agreement in the scoring of abstracts submitted to a primary care research conference. *BMC Health Serv. Res.* 2:8. doi: 10.1186/1472-6963-2-8

Muschelli, J., Nebel, M. B., Caffo, B. S., Barber, A. D., Pekar, J. J., and Mostofsky, S. H. (2014). Reduction of motion-related artifacts in resting state fMRI using aCompCor. *Neuroimage* 96, 22–35. doi: 10.1016/j.neuroimage.2014.03.028

Naik, S., Banerjee, A., Bapi, R. S., Deco, G., and Roy, D. (2017). Metastability in senescence. *Trends Cogn. Sci.* 21, 509–521. doi: 10.1016/j.tics.2017.04.007

Nasreddine, Z. S., Phillips, N. A., Bedirian, V., Charbonneau, S., Whitehead, V., Collin, I., et al. (2005). The montreal cognitive assessment, moca: a brief screening tool for mild cognitive impairment. *J. Am. Geriatr. Soc.* 53, 695–699. doi: 10.1111/j.1532-5415.2005.53221.x

Newman, M. E. J. (2006). Modularity and community structure in networks. *Proc. Natl. Acad. Sci. U.S.A.* 103, 8577–8582. doi: 10.1073/pnas.0601602103

Newman, M. E. J., and Girvan, M. (2004). Finding and evaluating community structure in networks. *Phys. Rev. E* 69:026113. doi: 10.1103/PhysRevE.69.026113

Ng, K. K., Lo, J. C., Lim, J. K. W., Chee, M. W. L., and Zhou, J. (2016). Reduced functional segregation between the default mode network and the executive control network in healthy older adults: a longitudinal study. *Neuroimage* 133, 321–330. doi: 10.1016/j.neuroimage.2016.03.029

Onoda, K., Ishihara, M., and Yamaguchi, S. (2012). Decreased functional connectivity by aging is associated with cognitive decline. *J. Cogn. Neurosci.* 24, 2186–2198. doi: 10.1162/jocn_a_00269

Onoda, K., and Yamaguchi, S. (2013). Small-worldness and modularity of the resting-state functional brain network decrease with aging. *Neurosci. Lett.* 556, 104–108. doi: 10.1016/j.neulet.2013.10.023

Park, B., Kim, J. I., Lee, D., Jeong, S.-O., Lee, J. D., and Park, H.-J. (2012). Are brain networks stable during a 24-hour period? *Neuroimage* 59, 456–466. doi: 10.1016/j.neuroimage.2011.07.049

Park, D. C., Polk, T. A., Park, R., Minear, M., Savage, A., and Smith, M. R. (2004). Aging reduces neural specialization in ventral visual cortex. *Proc. Natl. Acad. Sci. U.S.A.* 101, 13091–13095. doi: 10.1073/pnas.0405148101

Park, J., Carp, J., Hebrank, A., Park, D. C., and Polk, T. A. (2010). Neural specificity predicts fluid processing ability in older adults. *J. Neurosci.* 30, 9253–9259. doi: 10.1523/JNEUROSCI.0853-10.2010

Pinheiro, J. C., and Bates, D. M. (2000). *Mixed-Effects Models in s and s-Plus.* New York, NY: Springer.

Power, J. D., Cohen, A. L., Nelson, S. M., Wig, G. S., Barnes, K. A., Church, J. A., et al. (2011). Functional network organization of the human brain. *Neuron* 72, 665–678. doi: 10.1016/j.neuron.2011.09.006

Power, J. D., and Petersen, S. E. (2013). Control-related systems in the human brain. *Curr. Opin. Neurobiol.* 23, 223–228. doi: 10.1016/j.conb.2012.12.009

Reuter-Lorenz, P. A., and Cappell, K. A. (2008). Neurocognitive aging and the compensation hypothesis. *Curr. Dir. Psychol. Sci.* 17, 177–182. doi: 10.1111/j.1467-8721.2008.00570.x

Reuter-Lorenz, P. A., and Park, D. C. (2014). How does it STAC up? Revisiting the scaffolding theory of aging and cognition. *Neuropsychol. Rev.* 24, 355–370. doi: 10.1007/s11065-014-9270-9

Rhodes, R. E., and Katz, B. (2017). Working memory plasticity and aging. *Psychol. Aging* 32, 51–59. doi: 10.1037/pag0000135

Román, F. J., Iturria-Medina, Y., Martinez, K., Karama, S., Burgaleta, M., Evans, A. C., et al. (2017). Enhanced structural connectivity within a brain sub-network supporting working memory and engagement processes after cognitive training. *Neurobiol. Learn. Mem.* 141, 33–43. doi: 10.1016/j.nlm.2017.03.010

Rubinov, M., and Sporns, O. (2010). Complex network measures of brain connectivity: uses and interpretations. *Neuroimage* 52, 1059–1069. doi: 10.1016/j.neuroimage.2009.10.003

Sadaghiani, S., Poline, J.-B., Kleinschmidt, A., and D'Esposito, M. (2015). Ongoing dynamics in large-scale functional connectivity predict perception. *Proc. Natl. Acad. Sci. U.S.A.* 112, 8463–8468. doi: 10.1073/pnas.1420687112

Sala-Llonch, R., Bartrés-Faz, D., and Junqué, C. (2015). Reorganization of brain networks in aging: a review of functional connectivity studies. *Front. Psychol.* 6:663. doi: 10.3389/fpsyg.2015.00663

Salvador, R., Suckling, J., Schwarzbauer, C., and Bullmore, E. (2005). Undirected graphs of frequency-dependent functional connectivity in whole brain networks. *Philos. Trans. R. Soc. Lond. B Biol. Sci.* 360, 937–946. doi: 10.1098/rstb.2005.1645

Seeley, W. W., Menon, V., Schatzberg, A. F., Keller, J., Glover, G. H., Kenna, H., et al. (2007). Dissociable intrinsic connectivity networks for salience processing and executive control. *J. Neurosci.* 27, 2349–2356. doi: 10.1523/JNEUROSCI.5587-06.2007

Shrout, P. E., and Fleiss, J. L. (1979). Intraclass correlations: uses in assessing rater reliability. *Psychol. Bull.* 86, 420–428. doi: 10.1037/0033-2909.86.2.420

Song, J., Birn, R. M., Boly, M., Meier, T. B., Nair, V. A., Meyerand, M. E., et al. (2014). Age-related reorganizational changes in modularity and functional connectivity of human brain networks. *Brain Connect.* 4, 662–676. doi: 10.1089/brain.2014.0286

Sporns, O., and Betzel, R. F. (2015). Modular brain networks. *Annu. Rev. Psychol.* 67, 1–28. doi: 10.1146/annurev-psych-122414-033634

Sporns, O., Tononi, G., and Edelman, G. M. (2000). Theoretical neuroanatomy: relating anatomical and functional connectivity in graphs and cortical connection matrices. *Cereb. Cortex* 10, 127–141. doi: 10.1093/cercor/10.2.127

Stanley, M. L., Simpson, S. L., Dagenbach, D., Lyday, R. G., Burdette, J. H., and Laurienti, P. J. (2015). Changes in brain network efficiency and working memory performance in aging. *PLoS ONE* 10:e0123950. doi: 10.1371/journal.pone.0123950

Stepankova, H., Lukavsky, J., Buschkuehl, M., Kopecek, M., Ripova, D., and Jaeggi, S. M. (2014). The malleability of working memory and visuospatial skills: a randomized controlled study in older adults. *Dev. Psychol.* 50, 1049–1059. doi: 10.1037/a0034913

Sternberg, S. (1966). High-speed scanning in human memory. *Science* 153, 652–654. doi: 10.1126/science.153.3736.652

Stevens, A. A., Tappon, S. C., Garg, A., and Fair, D. A. (2012). Functional brain network modularity captures inter- and intra-individual variation in working memory capacity. *PLoS ONE* 7:e30468. doi: 10.1371/journal.pone.0030468

Sun, Y., Danila, B., Josić, K., and Bassler, K. E. (2009). Improved community structure detection using a modified fine-tuning strategy. *Europhys. Lett.* 86:28004. doi: 10.1209/0295-5075/86/28004

Sutton, B. P., Noll, D. C., and Fessler, J. A. (2003). Fast, iterative image reconstruction for MRI in the presence of field inhomogeneities. *IEEE Trans. Med. Imaging* 22, 178–188. doi: 10.1109/TMI.2002.808360

Telesford, Q. K., Morgan, A. R., Hayasaka, S., Simpson, S. L., Barret, W., Kraft, R. A., et al. (2010). Reproducibility of graph metrics in fMRI networks. *Front. Neuroinformatics* 4:117. doi: 10.3389/fninf.2010.00117

Tsvetanov, K. A., Henson, R. N. A., Tyler, L. K., Razi, A., Geerligs, L., Ham, T. E., et al. (2016). Extrinsic and intrinsic brain network connectivity maintains cognition across the lifespan despite accelerated decay of regional brain activation. *J. Neurosci.* 36, 3115–3126. doi: 10.1523/JNEUROSCI.2733-15.2016

Turner, G. R., and Spreng, R. N. (2015). Prefrontal engagement and reduced default network suppression co-occur and are dynamically coupled in older adults: the default–executive coupling hypothesis of aging. *J. Cogn. Neurosci.* 27, 2462–2476. doi: 10.1162/jocn_a_00869

van den Heuvel, M. P., de Lange, S. C., Zalesky, A., Seguin, C., Yeo, B. T. T., and Schmidt, R. (2017). Proportional thresholding in resting-state fMRI functional connectivity networks and consequences for patient-control connectome studies: issues and recommendations. *Neuroimage* 152, 437–449. doi: 10.1016/j.neuroimage.2017.02.005

van Wijk, B. C. M., Stam, C. J., and Daffertshofer, A. (2010). Comparing brain networks of different size and connectivity density using graph theory. *PLoS ONE* 5:e13701. doi: 10.1371/journal.pone.0013701

Vas, A. K., Chapman, S. B., Cook, L. G., Elliott, A. C., and Keebler, M. (2011). Higher-order reasoning training years after traumatic brain injury in adults. *J. Head Trauma Rehabil.* 26, 224–239. doi: 10.1097/HTR.0b013e318 218dd3d

Wang, J., Zuo, X., and He, Y. (2010). Graph-based network analysis of resting-state functional MRI. *Front. Syst. Neurosci.* 4:16. doi: 10.3389/fnsys.2010.00016

Wang, J.-H., Zuo, X.-N., Gohel, S., Milham, M. P., Biswal, B. B., and He, Y. (2011). Graph theoretical analysis of functional brain networks: test-retest evaluation on short- and long-term resting-state functional MRI data. *PLoS ONE* 6:e21976. doi: 10.1371/journal.pone.0021976

Welton, T., Kent, D. A., Auer, D. P., and Dineen, R. A. (2015). Reproducibility of graph-theoretic brain network metrics: a systematic review. *Brain Connect.* 5, 193–202. doi: 10.1089/brain.2014.0313

Whitfield-Gabrieli, S., and Nieto-Castanon, A. (2012). Conn: a functional connectivity toolbox for correlated and anticorrelated brain networks. *Brain Connect.* 2, 125–141. doi: 10.1089/brain.2012.0073

Yeo, B. T. T., Krienen, F. M., Sepulcre, J., Sabuncu, M. R., Lashkari, D., Hollinshead, M., et al. (2011). The organization of the human cerebral cortex estimated by intrinsic functional connectivity. *J. Neurophysiol.* 106, 1125–1165. doi: 10.1152/jn.00338.2011

Zalesky, A., Fornito, A., and Bullmore, E. (2012). On the use of correlation as a measure of network connectivity. *Neuroimage* 60, 2096–2106. doi: 10.1016/j.neuroimage.2012.02.001

Zalesky, A., Fornito, A., Cocchi, L., Gollo, L. L., van den Heuvel, M. P., and Breakspear, M. (2016). Connectome sensitivity or specificity: which is more important? *Neuroimage* 142, 407–420. doi: 10.1016/j.neuroimage.2016. 06.035

16

Resting State fMRI Reveals Increased Subthalamic Nucleus and Sensorimotor Cortex Connectivity in Patients with Parkinson's Disease under Medication

Bo Shen[1], Yang Gao[2], Wenbin Zhang[3], Liyu Lu[1], Jun Zhu[1], Yang Pan[1], Wenya Lan[1], Chaoyong Xiao[4] and Li Zhang[1]*

[1] Department of Geriatrics, Affiliated Brain Hospital of Nanjing Medical University, Nanjing, China, [2] Department of Computer Science and Technology, Nanjing University, Nanjing, China, [3] Department of Neurosurgery, Affiliated Brain Hospital of Nanjing Medical University, Nanjing, China, [4] Department of Radiology, Affiliated Brain Hospital of Nanjing Medical University, Nanjing, China

*Correspondence:
Li Zhang
neuro_zhangli@163.com

Functional connectivity (FC) between the subthalamic nucleus (STN) and the sensorimotor cortex is increased in off-medication patients with Parkinson's disease (PD). However, the status of FC between STN and sensorimotor cortex in on-medication PD patients remains unclear. In this study, resting state functional magnetic resonance imaging was employed on 31 patients with PD under medication and 31 healthy controls. Two-sample t-test was used to study the change in FC pattern of the STN, the FC strength of the bilateral STN was correlated with overall motor symptoms, while unilateral STN was correlated with offside motor symptoms. Both bilateral and right STN showed increased FC with the right sensorimotor cortex, whereas only right STN FC was correlated with left-body rigidity scores in all PD patients. An additional subgroup analysis was performed according to the ratio of mean tremor scores and mean postural instability and gait difficulty (PIGD) scores, only the PIGD subgroup showed the increased FC between right STN and sensorimotor cortex under medication. Increased FC between the STN and the sensorimotor cortex was found, which was related to motor symptom severity in on-medication PD patients. Anti-PD drugs may influence the hyperdirect pathway to alleviate motor symptoms with the more effect on the tremor subtype.

Keywords: Parkinson's disease, subthalamic nucleus, sensorimotor cortex, functional connectivity, hyperdirect pathway, on-medication

INTRODUCTION

Parkinson's disease (PD) is the second most common progressive neurological degenerative disorder caused by dopamine deficits in the substantia nigra pars compacta (Lees et al., 2009). Impairment of the respective functions of parallel cortico-basal ganglia-thalamo-cortical circuits causes various symptoms (DeLong, 1990; Helmich et al., 2010). The subthalamic nucleus (STN) is one of the preferred targets in deep brain stimulation (DBS) treatment of PD patients, with greater clinical benefits in motor symptom improvement than those obtained by stimulating other sites (Volkmann et al., 2004; Odekerken et al., 2013). However, the exact mechanism of this stimulation remains unknown. Therefore, STN may play a role in the motor control in PD patients (Chiken and Nambu, 2014).

In a healthy brain, the STN stimulates the internal segment of the globus pallidus, leading to increased inhibition of the ventrolateral thalamus. Consequently, the motor activity is increased within the primary somatosensory cortex (S1), primary motor cortex (M1), and premotor cortical area (Weintraub and Zaghloul, 2013). This phenomenon is an indirect pathway that is depressed by dopamine. The indirect pathway is overactive in PD patients, leading to hyperactivity of the STN (Alexander and Crutcher, 1990). Furthermore, the fast hyperdirect feedback loop from supplementary motor area and M1 cortical projections to the STN via glutamatergic neurons needs further investigation (Tewari et al., 2016).

Resting state functional MRI (rs-fMRI) is a relatively novel technique which is easily carried out in large populations. However, the biological origin and relevance of these slow neuronal activity components are still poorly understood, the latter observation that spontaneous BOLD activity is specifically organized in the resting human brain, which has generated a new avenue of neuroimaging research (Deco et al., 2011). Subsequently, rs-fMRI is also a well-accepted tool in the non-invasive study of neurological and psychiatric disorders at a network level in vivo (Zhang and Raichle, 2010). In off-medication PD patients, an increased functional connectivity (FC) between the STN and hand M1S1 areas was found in the non-tremor subgroup with the FC strength correlating with rigor scores (Baudrexel et al., 2011), while increased FC between these two areas was also discovered in early drug-naïve PD patients (Kurani et al., 2015). Primary data in the α- and β-frequency EEG bands showed a burst oscillatory local field activity in the STN and an increased FC between STN and motor cortical in PD patients (Hammond et al., 2007; Lalo et al., 2008). Therefore, increased oscillations in the STN may be a factual reason for the abnormal activity of the M1S1 cortex. A consistent conclusion was the increased FC of STN at different stages in off-medication PD patients.

Only two articles reported the FC of STN and motor area in normal PD patients while in the on-medication. Fernández-Seara et al. (2015) showed an increased FC between the STN and the motor cortex just like in off-medication PD patients using arterial spinlabeled (ASL) perfusion fMRI, whereas Mathys et al. (2016) did not find a change in the FC between the two areas. Aside from the different methods in these two articles, we speculate that choosing patients from a broad severity range may benefit FC change analysis, as previous research shows that a broad range of severity is needed when combining the de novo and moderate PD groups into the correlation analysis (Kurani et al., 2015), while Fernández-Seara et al. (2015) preferred early-state PD patients (mean HY = 1.83) and Mathys selected patients with a mean duration of 6 years. Litvak et al. (2011) found that dopaminergic medication modulated the resting beta network by combining magnetoencephalographic and subthalamic local field potential recordings. However, the

correlation between decreased FC strength and decreased motor symptoms in on-medication PD patients using fMRI technology was still unknown.

Hence, in this work, we selected PD patients with different severities (HY from 1 to 4 on-medication based, duration from 1 to 18 years) to assess the change in FC of STN. We tested whether changes in FC between STN and whole brain may exist, as well as the correlation with the motor symptom, because motor symptoms exist after drug administration.

MATERIALS AND METHODS

Participants
We conducted a prospective case – control study of 36 PD patients and 31 healthy controls in the Department of Geriatrics, Nanjing Brain Hospital between July 2015 and March 2016. Patients were included in the study if they were aged 18 years or older, satisfied the standard UK Brain Bank criteria for PD (Hughes et al., 1992), and experienced at least one of the following symptoms: severe response fluctuations, dyskinesias, painful dystonias, or bradykinesia. Exclusion criteria included history of other neurological or psychiatric diseases, and cognitive impairment based on the PDD criterion in 2007 (Dubois et al., 2007). We defined anti-Parkinsonian medication to include any drug designed to alter symptoms of PD or any drug that slows the progression of PD, levodopa equivalent daily dose (LEDD) was calculated with previous research (Tomlinson et al., 2010). All PD patients were scanned twice in off-medication and in 60–90 min after taking anti-Parkinsonian medication. Only the on-medication measurements were analyzed. All participants had written informed consent and the study was approved by the Medical Research Ethical Committee of Nanjing Brain Hospital, Nanjing, China.

Assessment of PD Motor and Cognition Symptoms
Motor impairment in patients with PD was assessed by items of Part III (motor part) of the Unified Parkinson's disease Rating Scale (UPDRS) and H&Y staging scale for both the "on" and "off" states. Unilateral limb tremor scores are the sum of hand tremor scores and lower limb scores from UPDRSIII. The mean tremor score was derived from the sum of items 16 and 20–26 on the UPDRS, while a mean score was derived from five postural instability and gait difficulty (PIGD) items (Stebbins et al., 2013). Patients were classified as having tremor-domain Parkinson's disease (TD-PD) when the ratio of the mean tremor score to the mean PIGD score was ≥ 1.5 and as having PIGD-PD when this ratio was ≤ 1, others were included as having mixed subtype PD. Overall cognition condition was assessed using the Mini-Mental State Examination (MMSE) and Montreal Cognitive Assessment (MoCA) (Chen et al., 2016).

MRI Data Acquisition Protocol
MR-imaging was carried out on a 3.0-T MR scanner system (Siemens, Verio, Germany) with an 8-channel phased-array head

coil for signal reception and a whole body coil for radio frequency transmission. Subjects were instructed to lie still, relax, and not think of anything in particular, while being required to keep their eyes open to avoid falling asleep. No subject reported to have fallen asleep when routinely asked immediately after examination.

Image Acquisition

Functional scans of the brain were acquired using a gradient echo EPI sequence with the following parameters: repetition time (TR) = 2000 ms, echo time (TE) = 25 ms, matrix size = 64 × 64, field of view (FoV) = 240 mm × 240 mm, 33 slices with 4 mm slice thickness and 0 mm inter-slice gap, and scan duration of 8 min and 6 s. Axial anatomical images were acquired using a 3D-MPRAGE sequence (TR = 1900 ms; TE = 2.48 ms; flip angle [FA] = 9°; matrix = 256 × 256; FoV = 250 mm × 250 mm; slice thickness = 1 mm; and gap = 0 mm; slices covered the whole brain, with registration and functional localization). Patients were scanned during on-state medication, resulting in a 4D data set consisting of 240 volumes of functional data for subsequent FC analysis.

Data Preprocessing

Preprocessing was carried out using Data Processing Assistant for Resting-State fMRI (DPARSF; Chao-Gan and Yu-Feng, 2010[1]) which is based on Statistical Parametric Mapping (SPM8)[2].

The first 10 volumes of the BOLD data for each subject were discarded, while the remaining images were corrected by realignment, accounting for head motion. Three patients with head motions exceeding 3 mm of translation, or a rotation of 3°, throughout the course of the scan were excluded from the study. The remaining functional images were coregistered to the individual T1-weighted images and were then segmented into gray matter (GM), white matter (WM), and cerebrospinal fluid (CSF) tissue maps using a unified segmentation algorithm followed by non-linear normalization into the Montreal Neurological Institute space. Resultant functional images were re-sampled to 3-mm isotropic voxels, and spatially smoothed with a Gaussian kernel full width at half maximum = 4 mm × 4 mm × 4 mm. The resulting fMRI data were band-pass filtered (0.01 < f < 0.08 Hz) to reduce low-frequency drift and high-frequency physiological, respiratory, and cardiac noise. Any linear trend was then removed. Subsequently, six head motion parameters and the mean time series of global activities, WM, and CSF signals were introduced as covariates into a random effects model to remove possible effects of head motion, global activities, WM, and CSF signals on the results. For each patient, the global signal is obtained by averaging the time series of voxels in all brain tissues, everyone has an unique global signal, global signals was thought as including the breath, heart rate, and other noise. So in the data preprocessing step, global signals are regressed out at the single-subject level.

---

[1]http://rfmri.org/DPARSF

[2]http://www.fil.ion.ucl.ac.uk/spm

Seed Region and FC Analysis

The bilateral STNs were defined as regions of interest from the WFU_pickatla (Talairach brain atlas theory), which automatically generated segmented atlas region of interest templates in the MNI space (Sakurai et al., 2017). Each STN was about 81 mm³, the centers of the left and right STN were [−9, −12, −8] and [9, −14, −8], the location and extent of STN are displayed in **Figure 1**. The mean time series of bilateral STN were extracted. Furthermore, a voxel-wise FC analysis was performed by computing the temporal correlation between the mean time series of the combined left and right STN and the time series of each voxel within the whole brain. The correlation coefficients of each voxel were normalized to z-scores with Fisher's r-to-z transformation. Therefore, a z-score map for the entire brain was created for the STN of each subject. Finally, the region where the significant difference between PD and HC, was used as the mask to extract the mean Z value for each PD patient. The correlation of Z-values and motor symptoms was measured with SPSS20, and motor symptoms included UPDRSIII, TD scores, PIGD scores, duration, bilateral tremor and rigidly scores, as the tremor and rigidly are the common symptoms of PD. The TD score was derived from the sum of items 16 and 20–26 on the UPDRS, while PIGD score was derived from five PIGD items.

Statistical Analysis

One-sample t-tests were conducted on the z-score maps of the two groups. Then, between-group two-sample t-tests were performed within the whole brain mask, with age, gender, education, and GM volumes as covariates, to detect significant differences between the two groups, GM volumes were calculated by the SPM in the latter voxel based morphometry step. With in-group multiple comparisons, all T maps had a threshold of $p < 0.005$, while the cluster extent was calculated according to alphasim correction based on REST software (voxel-level p value < 0.005; cluster size: >69 voxels; determined by a Monte-Carlo simulation resulted in a cluster-level significance threshold of $P < 0.005$). Correlation between the FC strength of the bilateral STN and overall motor symptoms have been evaluated, while unilateral STN FC was correlated with contralateral motor symptoms, and motor symptoms included UPDRSIII, TD scores,

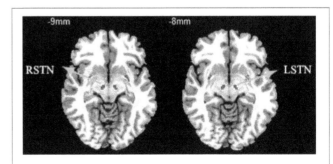

FIGURE 1 | ROI presentation of subthalamic nucleus (STN). ROI definition of the STN, bilateral STNs were defined as regions of interest from the WFU_pickatla, the centers of the left and right STN were [−9, −12, −8] and [9, −14, −8].

PIGD scores, duration, bilateral tremor and rigidly scores, as the tremor and rigidly are the common symptoms of PD. All correlation analyses were performed using the SPSS20.0 software package.

Voxel Based Morphometry (VBM)

To test whether the change in FC pattern was associated with the structural atrophy, gray and white matter volumes were measured based on the SPM8. VBM procedure involved the segmentation of the original structural MRI images in native space into GM, WM, and CSF tissues, then GM and WM images were normalized to templates in stereotactic space to acquire optimized normalization parameters, which were applied to the raw images. GM images were smoothed using an 8-mm full width at half maximum isotropic Gaussian kernel. The last, we employed a general linear model, using age and sex as covariates. Comparison between PD patients and healthy controls was again carried out with the two-sample t-test option provided in the SPSS software, with significant difference set at $p < 0.05$.

RESULTS

Clinical and Neuropsychological Evaluations

A total of 31 PD patients were included in our study (excluding three patients whose head motions exceeded 3 mm of translation and another two patients who could not bear the noise of the MRI). The 31 PD patients contained varying motor symptom severity and durations, with 18 of the 31 patients being more affected at the left side of the body in terms of UPDRS III. For subsequent analyses, due to the smaller size of TD patients, patients with tremor-dominant ($n = 5$) and mixed type ($n = 9$) were pooled and referred to as the tremor subgroup ($n = 14$)

similar to the previous study (Baudrexel et al., 2011). No significant differences in age, sex, education, MMSE, and MOCA were found for the three groups. **Table 1** summarizes the detailed demographic and clinical characteristics of the three groups (patients with PD and healthy controls).

STN FC in Healthy Controls

Mean resting state FC z-score maps of STN in healthy controls are displayed in **Figure 2**. The correlation of left and right STN with whole brain was measured with DPARSF and REST software, as a result, the left and right STN FC pattern were compared with the two-sample t-test to seek the differences, and there is no difference. The result showed that most of the positive z-score values were found bilaterally in the brainstem, caudate nucleus, putamen, thalamus, and the cerebellum. Moreover, relatively small positive z-score values were found in the Frontal Lobe, which included middle frontal gyrus, superior frontal gyrus, frontal eyes field, pre-motor, and supplementary motor cortex in the right cerebrum. In contrast, negative z-score values were found in bilateral precuneus, which is the core area of the DMN, cuneus, lingual gyrus, middle occipital gyrus, left superior occipital gyrus, right middle temporal gyrus, left primary visual cortex, and calcarine.

Between-Group Differences of STN FC

Compared with healthy controls, the PD patients exhibited increased right STN FC with the right M1S1, which contains the precentral and postcentral gyrus ($p < 0.005$, cluster size: >69 voxels, multiple-comparison correction using AlphaSim in REST), while no decreased areas were found as shown in **Figure 3** and **Table 2**. Increased FC patterns of bilateral STN with the right M1S1 were also found as shown in **Figure 3** and **Table 2**. The left STN FC pattern had no change in area, while all T maps showed no decrease in area. The PIGD showed the increased FC between

TABLE 1 | Demographic and neuropsychological characteristics of all subjects (on-medication).

Groups	PD ($n = 31$)	TD ($n = 14$)	PIGD ($n = 17$)	HC ($n = 31$)	P-value
Sex (male/female)	16/15	8/6	8/9	16/15	0.958[a]
Age, years	60.29 ± 9.03	61.07 ± 9.18	59.64 ± 9.14	59.71 ± 4.79	0.943
Education, years	11.71 ± 3.53	11.79 ± 3.85	11.64 ± 3.71	12.00 ± 2.42	0.642
MOCA	26.32 ± 2.65	26.00 ± 2.66	26.59 ± 2.69	27.03 ± 1.33	0.146
MMSE	27.71 ± 1.53	27.79 ± 1.63	27.65 ± 1.50	28.03 ± 1.49	0.405
Duration, years	6.64 ± 4.20	5.79 ± 2.33	7.35 ± 5.24	NA	0.588
H&Y stage	2.55 ± 0.97	2.43 ± 0.92	2.65 ± 1.03	NA	0.825
UPDRS	36.68 ± 14.45	32.43 ± 14.34	40.18 ± 14.00	NA	0.331
UPDRSIII	18.58 ± 9.03	16.86 ± 8.97	20.00 ± 9.11	NA	0.631
Termor scores	3.55 ± 3.64	4.86 ± 3.72	2.47 ± 2.70	NA	0.140
PIGD scores	3.84 ± 2.21	2.79 ± 1.81	4.71 ± 2.17	NA	0.050
Left lumbar tremor scores	0.81 ± 1.47	1.14 ± 1.40	0.53 ± 1.50	NA	0.514
Right lumber tremor scores	0.74 ± 1.18	1.21 ± 1.53	0.35 ± 0.61	NA	0.126
Left lumbar rigidly scores	1.84 ± 1.66	1.791.81	1.881.58	NA	0.987
Right lumbar rigidly scores	1.45 ± 1.35	1.43 ± 1.50	1.47 ± 1.28	NA	0.996
LEDD, mg/day	614.38 ± 269.62	619.46 ± 242.04	610.21 ± 297.75	NA	0.996

MMSE, Mini-Mental State Examination; TD, tremor-dominant; PIGD, postural instability and gait difficulty; UPDRS, unified Parkinson's disease rating scale; LEDD, levodopa equivalent daily dose; p[a]-value for the gender difference was obtained by chi-square test, others were obtained using one-way analyses of variance.

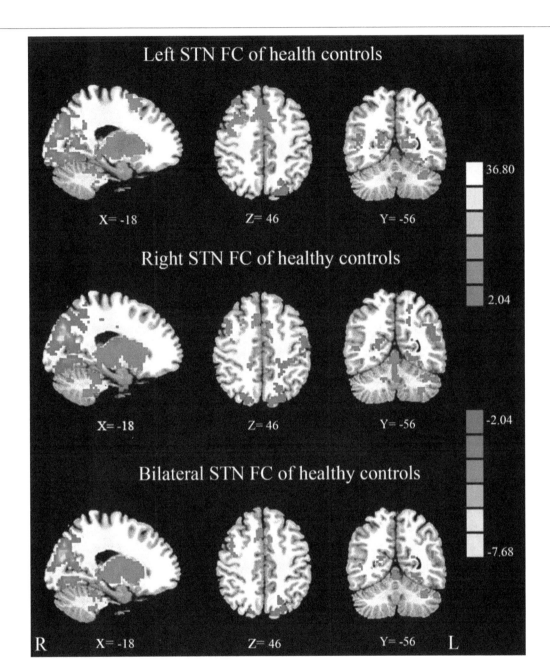

FIGURE 2 | Mean resting state functional connectivity (FC) z-score maps of the STN in healthy controls. STN FC map of healthy controls, results are in MNI space, red color represents the positive correlation while the blue color represents the negative correlation.

the right STN and bilateral M1S1 compared with the HC with on changed pattern in TD subgroup as shown in **Figure 4** and **Table 3**. Z-values of right STN and right M1S1 in the different groups as shown in **Figure 5**.

STN–M1S1 FC and Motor Symptom Correlation Analysis

Finally, the region where the significant M1S1 clustered, as a result of the between-group analysis, was used as the mask to extract the mean Z value for each PD patient. The Z-values of

right STN showed no correlation with tremor and PIGD scores. By contrast, the Z-values of right STN and right M1S1 showed a correlation with left lumbar rigidity scores from UPDRS ($r = 0.414$, $p = 0.021$) and LEDD (r = 0.435, $p = 0.014$) in 31 PD patients (**Figure 6**). What's more, there were no correlation of Z-values and motor symptoms in the PD subgroup.

ROI Analysis of Right STN–Right M1S1 FC

A special ROI centered at the t maximum from the previous experiments was used as functional representation of right M1S1 for further research. This special ROI was defined by the changed

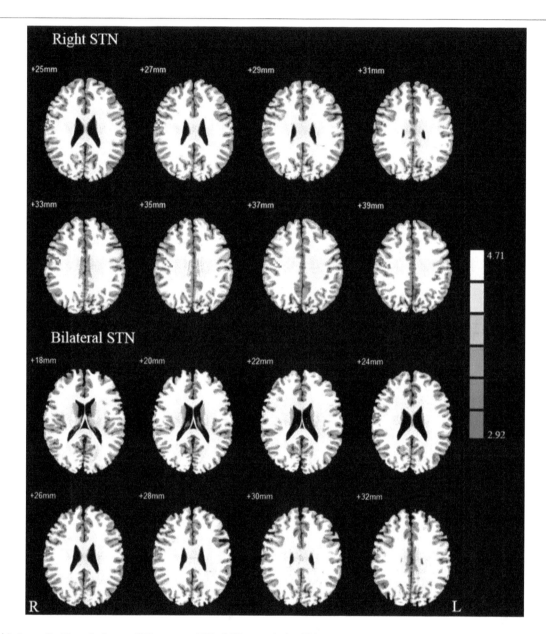

FIGURE 3 | Between Parkinson's disease (PD) group and HC of difference in the STN resting state FC. Between-group differences in the STN – sensorimotor cortex FC, results are in MNI space, red color represents the increased correlation while the blue color represents the decreased correlation.

area of STN FC pattern between PD and HC. It was in the right hemisphere and it's peak coordinate was (45, −11, 36), the detailed information of M1S1 were seen in **Table 2**. Compared with the HC, both the PD subgroup showed the increased FC (TD: $p = 0.002$, PIGD: $p < 0.001$), A direct statistical comparison of the two PD subgroups under medication again yielded no significant results similar to the previous study (Baudrexel et al., 2011) (**Figure 5**).

VBM

Voxel Based Morphometry did not reveal significant differences between patients and healthy controls for gray matter volume and WMV, with detailed information in **Table 4**.

DISCUSSION

The STN is the preferred target in DBS surgery to normalize aberrant patterns of STN and to improve cardinal motor symptoms. However, the mechanism is still unclear. The current study found that the combined bilateral STN and right STN showed increased FC with M1S1 in PD patients under medication. These findings provide new evidence of increased FC between STN–M1S1. Furthermore, severe motor symptoms related to the changes in STN–M1S1 FC may also exist in PD patients despite the effects of medication.

Resting state fMRI provided a new way of viewing the hyperdirect pathway, although its mechanism remains unknown.

TABLE 2 | REST group comparison results indicating increased STN FC in PD patients as compared to healthy controls.

	Voxels sizes (mm³)	T-value	Coordinates MNI		
			x	y	z
(A) Bilateral STN					
Cluster size 1404 (p < 0.05, corrected)					
Postcentral_R	1296	4.20	60	−6	36
Precentral_R	84	3.22	59	−2	42
(B) Right STN					
Cluster size 3294 (p < 0.005, corrected)					
Postcentral_R	2187	4.62	45	−9	33
Precentral_R	972	3.47	58	−2	42

Localization, voxels sizes, T-values, and MNI coordinates of bilateral (A) and right (B) STN FC pattern as compared with healthy controls. Spatial distribution of significant voxels with respect to their locations according to the automated anatomical labeling AAL template.

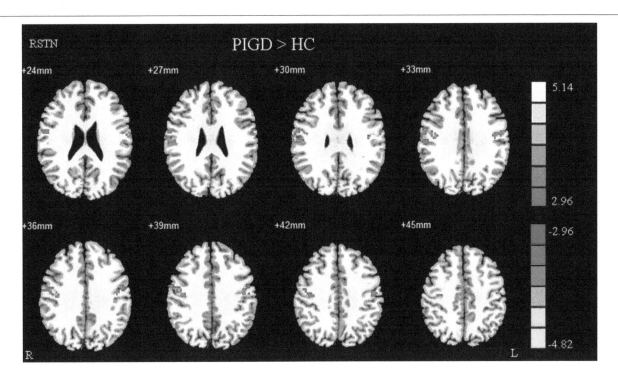

FIGURE 4 | Between postural instability and gait difficulty (PIGD) subgroup and HC of difference in the right STN resting state FC. Between PIGD subgroup and HC of difference in the STN resting state FC, results are in MNI space, red color represents the increased correlation while the blue color represents the decreased correlation.

TABLE 3 | REST group comparison results of right STN in PIGD patients.

	Voxels sizes (mm³)	T-value	Coordinates MNI		
Cluster 1 (Sizes 3699, p < 0.005, corrected)					
Postcentral_R	2097	5.14	45	−11	36
Precentral_R	999	3.15	47	−7	37
Cluster 2 (Sizes 1809, p < 0.01, corrected)					
Postcentral_L	1674	5.04	−62	−5	28
Precentral_L	54	3.57	−54	−5	32

Localization, voxels sizes, T-values, and MNI coordinates of right STN FC pattern as compared with healthy controls. Spatial distribution of significant voxels with respect to their locations according to the AAL template. PIGD, postural instability gait difficulty.

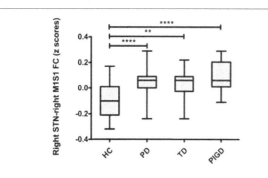

FIGURE 5 | Difference of right STN–right M1S1 FC values in PD subgroups and healthy controls. Box plots of right STN–right M1S1 FC values in PD subgroups and healthy controls. Significant differences between healthy controls and the respective PD subgroups are indicated with (*), **$p = 0.002$, ****$p < 0.0001$.

Moreover, the overactivity of the hyperdirect pathway was proven in the off-medication PD patients and animal PD models (Dejean et al., 2008). Kahan et al. (2014) found a decrease in the effective FC of the hyperdirect pathway with STN stimulation, with the relationship between decreased hyperdirect coupling strength and improved clinical severity being particularly interesting. Local field potential recordings from the STN of patients

undergoing surgery for DBS revealed strong oscillatory activity, particularly in the beta band (13–35 Hz) (Kuhn et al., 2004). STN beta oscillations were reduced by the application of levodopa and DBS (Priori et al., 2004; Kuhn et al., 2008). Furthermore, STN beta power reduction correlated with clinical improvement (Kuhn et al., 2008). The STN has also been involved in reactive global inhibition through the hyperdirect path (Vink et al., 2005; Zandbelt et al., 2013), with the increased 2.5–5 Hz phase activity of STN leading to increased response thresholds and slower responses (Tewari et al., 2016). Previous studies showed increased FC of STN with M1S1 in off- and on-medication patients. Adding our conclusions, the overactivity of the so-called hyperdirect loop and the occurrence of motor symptoms could be simultaneously depressed with the effects of medication.

Compared with the ASL research, the same conclusions regarding the increased correlation of bilateral STN and M1S1 and the similar correlation between FC and LEDD were seen, which may show the modulation of medication on brain activity (Litvak et al., 2011). Multi-model research correlating ASL, fMRI, and EEG research outputs would help us know more about the mechanism of this disease. The difference in the FC pattern was that changed areas in our research were all in right hemisphere, whereas they found the left part to be mainly

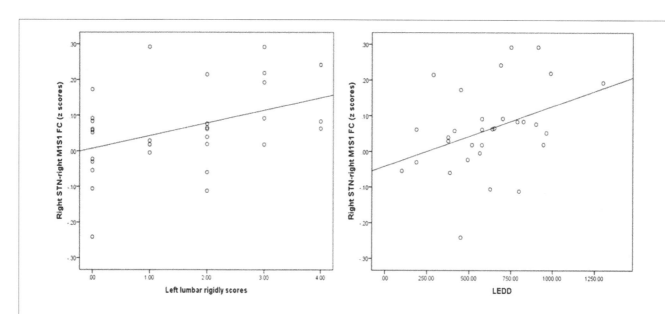

FIGURE 6 | Results of the correlation of FC values with levodopa equivalent daily dose (LEDD) and motor symptom. Left graph showed the correlation diagram of right STN–M1S1 area FC values with corresponding UPDRS III right lumbar rigor scores (hand scores plus leg scores) in patients, right graph showed the correlation diagram of same FC values with LEDD.

TABLE 4 | Results of VBM analysis between PD, PD subgroup, and HC groups.

	PD	TD	PIGD	HC	*F*-value	*P*
GMV (cm³)	543.50 ± 61.45	536.50 ± 60.40	549.26 ± 63.54	573.77 ± 59.25	1.811	0.151
WMV (cm³)	585.02 ± 65.62	593.80 ± 71.82	577.80 ± 61.30	577.92 ± 72.02	0.217	0.884

GMV, Gray matter volume; WMV, white matter volume; volumes are represented as the mean ± standard deviation. For comparisons of demographics, P-values were obtained using one-way analyses of variance. TD, tremor-dominant; PIGD, postural instability gait difficulty.

altered. This may be because our patients were more onset in the left side of body since the change in FC was only based on the seed of the right STN, while no significant difference was found in the seed of the left STN. Furthermore, previous research performed right-sided surgery faster but with higher errors (Obeso et al., 2013), which means that the right STN is more likely to be involved in action inhibition (Tewari et al., 2016). This abnormal FC in the unilateral cerebral hemisphere is consistent with previous studies wherein the unilateral hemispheric basal ganglia-thalamo-cortical circuit modulated the contralateral movement (Kahan et al., 2014).

We selected unilateral STN as the seed to find its relationship to the offside motor symptom because of the unsymmetrical severity of motor symptoms. Our findings were similar to that of Baudrexel's research wherein FC strength with right STN and right M1S1 were correlated with left-leg rigor scores. Previous studies showed an association between rigor strength and increased oscillatory activity within the STN (Kuhn et al., 2009). We found that the relationship between FC strength and rigidity scores may be because of the stability and objectivity of the rigidity symptoms, whereas tremors were always affected by mood. A little difference between our research with previous off-medication study is that the PIGD showed the most significant enhanced FC pattern. In our study, some people presented serious tremors in the off-state, which disappeared after taking anti-PD drugs. This finding is consistent with previous studies showing that tremors are more affected by drugs (Connolly and Lang, 2014), along with increased FC strength. Katz et al. (2015) found TD patients had greater mean overall motor improvement than PIGD patients after STN DBS, measured by UPDRS-III. Anti-PD drugs or DBS may have a more effect on the hyperdirect pathway of TD patients to resolve the abnormal activity of

STN. Therefore, in studies involving on-state PD patients, the burst FC pattern is also related with the motor symptoms and PD subgroup showed the different hyperdirect pathway under medication.

CONCLUSION

We are the first to prove the increased FC patterns and the correlations between rigidity symptoms of varying severity in PD patients under medication. Our findings further suggest that PIGD and tremor symptoms might be linked to an different coupling of these areas in on-medication PD patients. Moreover, anti-PD drugs may changed the hyperdirect pathway, thereby altering the motor symptoms.

AUTHOR CONTRIBUTIONS

LZ designed the study and revised it critically for important intellectual content. BS performed the research and drafted the manuscript, YG and YP helped in data analyses, WZ, CX, LL, and JZ help in clinical data collection and analyses, and made patient follow-ups, and WL edited the paper.

FUNDING

This study was supported by the Nanjing Science and Technology Development Program (201503039) and special funds of the Jiangsu Provincial Key Research and Development Projects (BE2016614).

REFERENCES

Alexander, G. E., and Crutcher, M. D. (1990). Functional architecture of basal ganglia circuits: neural substrates of parallel processing. Trends Neurosci. 13, 266–271. doi: 10.1016/0166-2236(90)90107-L

Baudrexel, S., Witte, T., Seifried, C., von Wegner, F., Beissner, F., Klein, J. C., et al. (2011). Resting state fMRI reveals increased subthalamic nucleus–motor cortex connectivity in Parkinson's disease. Neuroimage 55, 1728–1738. doi: 10.1016/j.neuroimage.2011.01.017

Chao-Gan, Y., and Yu-Feng, Z. (2010). DPARSF: a MATLAB toolbox for "Pipeline" data analysis of resting-state fMRI. Front. Syst. Neurosci. 4:13. doi: 10.3389/fnsys.2010.00013

Chen, L., Yu, C., Zhang, N., Liu, J., and Liu, W. (2016). Cognitive impairment in patients with Parkinson's disease: a 30-month follow-up study. Clin. Neurol. Neurosurg. 151, 65–69. doi: 10.1016/j.clineuro.2016.09.021

Chiken, S., and Nambu, A. (2014). Disrupting neuronal transmission: mechanism of DBS? Front. Syst. Neurosci. 8:33. doi: 10.3389/fnsys.2014.00033

Connolly, B. S., and Lang, A. E. (2014). Pharmacological treatment of Parkinson disease. JAMA 311, 1670–1683. doi: 10.1001/jama.2014.3654

Deco, G., Jirsa, V. K., and McIntosh, A. R. (2011). Emerging concepts for the dynamical organization of resting-state activity in the brain. Nat. Rev. Neurosci. 12, 43–56. doi: 10.1038/nrn2961

Dejean, C., Gross, C. E., Bioulac, B., and Boraud, T. (2008). Dynamic changes in the cortex-basal ganglia network after dopamine depletion in the rat. J. Neurophysiol. 100, 385–396. doi: 10.1152/jn.90466.2008

DeLong, M. R. (1990). Primate models of movement disorders of basal ganglia origin. Trends Neurosci. 13, 281–285. doi: 10.1016/0166-2236(90)90110-V

Dubois, B., Burn, D., Goetz, C., Aarsland, D., Brown, R. G., Broe, G. A., et al. (2007). Diagnostic procedures for Parkinson's disease dementia: recommendations from the movement disorder society task force. Mov. Disord. 22, 2314–2324. doi: 10.1002/mds.21844

Fernández-Seara, M. A., Mengual, E., Vidorreta, M., Castellanos, G., Irigoyen, J., Erro, E., et al. (2015). Resting state functional connectivity of the subthalamic nucleus in Parkinson's disease assessed using arterial spin-labeled perfusion fMRI. Hum. Brain Mapp. 36, 1937–1950. doi: 10.1002/hbm.22747

Hammond, C., Bergman, H., and Brown, P. (2007). Pathological synchronization in Parkinson's disease: networks, models and treatments. Trends Neurosci. 30, 357–364. doi: 10.1016/j.tins.2007.05.004

Helmich, R. C., Derikx, L. C., Bakker, M., Scheeringa, R., Bloem, B. R., and Toni, I. (2010). Spatial remapping of cortico-striatal connectivity in Parkinson's disease. Cereb. Cortex 20, 1175–1186. doi: 10.1093/cercor/bhp178

Hughes, A. J., Daniel, S. E., Kilford, L., and Lees, A. J. (1992). Accuracy of clinical diagnosis of idiopathic Parkinson's disease: a clinico-pathological study of 100 cases. J. Neurol. Neurosurg. Psychiatry 55, 181–184. doi: 10.1136/jnnp.55.3.181

Kahan, J., Urner, M., Moran, R., Flandin, G., Marreiros, A., Mancini, L., et al. (2014). Resting state functional MRI in Parkinson's disease: the impact of deep brain stimulation on 'effective' connectivity. Brain 137, 1130–1144. doi: 10.1093/brain/awu027

Katz, M., Luciano, M. S., Carlson, K., Luo, P., Marks, W. J., Larson, P. S., et al. (2015). Differential effects of deep brain stimulation target on motor subtypes in Parkinson's disease. Ann. Neurol. 77, 710–719. doi: 10.1002/ana.24374

Kuhn, A. A., Kempf, F., Brucke, C., Gaynor, D. L., Martinez-Torres, I., Pogosyan, A., et al. (2008). High-frequency stimulation of the subthalamic nucleus suppresses oscillatory beta activity in patients with Parkinson's disease in parallel with improvement in motor performance. *J. Neurosci.* 28, 6165–6173. doi: 10.1523/JNEUROSCI.0282-08.2008

Kuhn, A. A., Tsui, A., Aziz, T., Ray, N., Brucke, C., Kupsch, A., et al. (2009). Pathological synchronisation in the subthalamic nucleus of patients with Parkinson's disease relates to both bradykinesia and rigidity. *Exp. Neurol.* 215, 380–387. doi: 10.1016/j.expneurol.2008.11.008

Kuhn, A. A., Williams, D., Kupsch, A., Limousin, P., Hariz, M., Schneider, G. H., et al. (2004). Event-related beta desynchronization in human subthalamic nucleus correlates with motor performance. *Brain* 127, 735–746. doi: 10.1093/brain/awh106

Kurani, A. S., Seidler, R. D., Burciu, R. G., Comella, C. L., Corcos, D. M., Okun, M. S., et al. (2015). Subthalamic nucleus—sensorimotor cortex functional connectivity in de novo and moderate Parkinson's disease. *Neurobiol. Aging* 36, 462–469. doi: 10.1016/j.neurobiolaging.2014.07.004

Lalo, E., Thobois, S., Sharott, A., Polo, G., Mertens, P., Pogosyan, A., et al. (2008). Patterns of bidirectional communication between cortex and basal ganglia during movement in patients with Parkinson disease. *J. Neurosci.* 28, 3008–3016. doi: 10.1523/JNEUROSCI.5295-07.2008

Lees, A. J., Hardy, J., and Revesz, T. (2009). Parkinson's disease. *Lancet* 373, 2055–2066. doi: 10.1016/S0140-6736(09)60492-X

Litvak, V., Jha, A., Eusebio, A., Oostenveld, R., Foltynie, T., Limousin, P., et al. (2011). Resting oscillatory cortico-subthalamic connectivity in patients with Parkinson's disease. *Brain* 134, 359–374. doi: 10.1093/brain/awq332

Mathys, C., Caspers, J., Langner, R., Südmeyer, M., Grefkes, C., Reetz, K., et al. (2016). Functional connectivity differences of the subthalamic nucleus related to Parkinson's disease. *Hum. Brain Mapp.* 37, 1235–1253. doi: 10.1002/hbm.23099

Obeso, I., Wilkinson, L., Rodriguez-Oroz, M. C., Obeso, J. A., and Jahanshahi, M. (2013). Bilateral stimulation of the subthalamic nucleus has differential effects on reactive and proactive inhibition and conflict-induced slowing in Parkinson's disease. *Exp. Brain Res.* 226, 451–462. doi: 10.1007/s00221-013-3457-9

Odekerken, V. J., van Laar, T., Staal, M. J., Mosch, A., Hoffmann, C. F., Nijssen, P. C., et al. (2013). Subthalamic nucleus versus globus pallidus bilateral deep brain stimulation for advanced Parkinson's disease (NSTAPS study): a randomised controlled trial. *Lancet Neurol.* 12, 37–44. doi: 10.1016/S1474-4422(12)70264-8

Priori, A., Foffani, G., Pesenti, A., Tamma, F., Bianchi, A. M., Pellegrini, M., et al. (2004). Rhythm-specific pharmacological modulation of subthalamic activity in Parkinson's disease. *Exp. Neurol.* 189, 369–379. doi: 10.1016/j.expneurol.2004.06.001

Sakurai, K., Imabayashi, E., Tokumaru, A. M., Ito, K., Shimoji, K., Nakagawa, M., et al. (2017). Volume of interest analysis of spatially normalized PRESTO imaging to differentiate between Parkinson disease and atypical parkinsonian syndrome. *Magn. Reson. Med. Sci.* 16, 16–22. doi: 10.2463/mrms.mp.2015-0132

Stebbins, G. T., Goetz, C. G., Burn, D. J., Jankovic, J., Khoo, T. K., and Tilley, B. C. (2013). How to identify tremor dominant and postural instability/gait difficulty groups with the movement disorder society unified Parkinson's disease rating scale: comparison with the unified Parkinson's disease rating scale. *Mov. Disord.* 28, 668–670. doi: 10.1002/mds.25383

Tewari, A., Jog, R., and Jog, M. S. (2016). The striatum and subthalamic nucleus as independent and collaborative structures in motor control. *Front. Syst. Neurosci.* 10:17. doi: 10.3389/fnsys.2016.00017

Tomlinson, C. L., Stowe, R., Patel, S., Rick, C., Gray, R., and Clarke, C. E. (2010). Systematic review of levodopa dose equivalency reporting in Parkinson's disease. *Mov. Disord.* 25, 2649–2653. doi: 10.1002/mds.23429

Vink, M., Kahn, R. S., Raemaekers, M., van den Heuvel, M., Boersma, M., and Ramsey, N. F. (2005). Function of striatum beyond inhibition and execution of motor responses. *Hum. Brain Mapp.* 25, 336–344. doi: 10.1002/hbm.20111

Volkmann, J., Allert, N., Voges, J., Sturm, V., Schnitzler, A., and Freund, H. J. (2004). Long-term results of bilateral pallidal stimulation in Parkinson's disease. *Ann. Neurol.* 55, 871–875. doi: 10.1002/ana.20091

Weintraub, D. B., and Zaghloul, K. A. (2013). The role of the subthalamic nucleus in cognition. *Rev. Neurosci.* 24, 125–138. doi: 10.1515/revneuro-2012-0075

Zandbelt, B. B., Bloemendaal, M., Neggers, S. F., Kahn, R. S., and Vink, M. (2013). Expectations and violations: delineating the neural network of proactive inhibitory control. *Hum. Brain Mapp.* 34, 2015–2024. doi: 10.1002/hbm.22047

Zhang, D., and Raichle, M. E. (2010). Disease and the brain's dark energy. *Nat. Rev. Neurol.* 6, 15–28. doi: 10.1038/nrneurol.2009.198

17

Altered Functional and Causal Connectivity of Cerebello-Cortical Circuits between Multiple System Atrophy (Parkinsonian Type) and Parkinson's Disease

Qun Yao[1], Donglin Zhu[1], Feng Li[1], Chaoyong Xiao[2], Xingjian Lin[1], Qingling Huang[2] and Jingping Shi[1]*

[1] Department of Neurology, Affiliated Brain Hospital of Nanjing Medical University, Nanjing, China, [2] Department of Radiology, Affiliated Brain Hospital of Nanjing Medical University, Nanjing, China

Correspondence:
Jingping Shi
profshijp@163.com

Lesions of the cerebellum lead to motor and non-motor deficits by influencing cerebral cortex activity via cerebello-cortical circuits. It remains unknown whether the cerebello-cortical "disconnection" underlies motor and non-motor impairments both in the parkinsonian variant of multiple system atrophy (MSA-P) and Parkinson's disease (PD). In this study, we investigated both the functional and effective connectivity of the cerebello-cortical circuits from resting-state functional magnetic resonance imaging (rs-fMRI) data of three groups (26 MSA-P patients, 31 PD patients, and 30 controls). Correlation analysis was performed between the causal connectivity and clinical scores. PD patients showed a weakened cerebellar dentate nucleus (DN) functional coupling in the posterior cingulate cortex (PCC) and inferior parietal lobe compared with MSA-P or controls. MSA-P patients exhibited significantly enhanced effective connectivity from the DN to PCC compared with PD patients or controls, as well as declined causal connectivity from the left precentral gyrus to right DN compared with the controls, and this value is significantly correlated with the motor symptom scores. Our findings demonstrated a crucial role for the cerebello-cortical networks in both MSA-P and PD patients in addition to striatal-thalamo-cortical (STC) networks and indicated that different patterns of cerebello-cortical loop degeneration are involved in the development of the diseases.

Keywords: functional connectivity, granger causality analysis, multiple system atrophy, Parkinson's disease, resting-state fMRI

INTRODUCTION

The parkinsonian variant of multiple system atrophy (MSA-P) is a neurodegenerative disorder that is clinically difficult to differentiate from idiopathic Parkinson's disease (PD), especially in the early stages of the diseases (Wenning et al., 2000; Kim et al., 2016). Inchoate differentiation between MSA-P and PD has significant therapeutic and rehabilitative implications. At the neuronal level, these diseases are all characterized by extensive cell loss in the substantia nigra pars compacta

(Dickson, 2012). In the past, functional brain imaging had been proved to be of some value for the differential diagnosis of parkinsonism. Positron emission tomography, for instance, disclosed decreased striatal presynaptic uptake, binding, glucose metabolism, and post-synaptic binding in both MSA-P and PD (Ghaemi et al., 2002; Bohnen et al., 2006), especially the reduced post-synaptic binding in MSA-P. Liu et al. (2013) described that the dopamine deficits in striatal subregions impair the function of striatal-thalamo-cortical (STC) networks involved in motor, cognitive and emotional processing (Braak and Braak, 2000).

Considering the demonstrated alteration of pathology was found in the basal ganglia of PD and MSA-P (Galvan et al., 2015). The cerebellum is also an important component in motor control, higher cognitive, and emotional processing (Allen et al., 2005; Schutter and van Honk, 2005; Habas, 2010). It is known to affect cerebral cortical activity by cerebello-thalamo-cortical (CTC) circuits (Middleton and Strick, 2000). Previous studies have demonstrated the cerebellum to be involved in these diseases. For example, in MSA-P patients, morphological and microstructural alterations of cerebellum have been reported (Nicoletti et al., 2006a,b). The cerebellar functional activation was increased in MSA-P after repetitive transcranial magnetic stimulation (rTMS) treatment (Wang H. et al., 2016). Moreover, the cerebellum is anatomically and functionally connected with the basal ganglia and its connectivity changes in PD have been discovered (Wu and Hallett, 2013). Wu et al. (2009) found increased cerebellar activity in PD by a regional homogeneity method. Another causal connectivity study has shown that the connectivity of cortico-cerebellar motor regions is strengthened in PD during the performance of self-initiated movement (Wu et al., 2011). A PET research has also revealed that the cerebellum is a crucial node in the abnormal metabolic patterns of both MSA-P and PD (Poston et al., 2012), with decreased cerebellar 18F-fluorodeoxyglucose metabolism in MSA-P and increased in PD. It has been presumed that compensatory activity in CTC circuits in PD patients may act as a compensatory mechanism to overcome the deficits in the STC circuits (Cerasa et al., 2006; Palmer et al., 2010). However, the exact role of the cerebellum in Parkinsonism, especially the MSA-P, remains unclear.

The cerebellar outputs polymerize to the dentate nucleus (DN), which successively sends neural fibers to the thalamus and cerebral cortex via the superior cerebellar peduncles, thus completing the cerebello-cortical circuits (Middleton and Strick, 2000). Histological studies have demonstrated anatomically segregated cerebello-cortical circuits including motor and non-motor loops (Clower et al., 2001; Middleton and Strick, 2001). Available evidence regarding the cerebello-cortical circuits connecting the lateral cerebellum to motor and non-motor cortical areas is limited in humans, due to technical challenges in assessing the long polysynaptic connections between the cerebellum and the cerebral cortex *in vivo*. Although the established cerebellar involvement in Parkinsonism, subtle studies on cerebellum for the differential diagnosis of parkinsonian syndromes are still penurious to date. Recently, resting-state fMRI (rs-fMRI) has been widely used to discover abnormalities in spontaneous neuronal activity by measuring the functional connectivity between spatially distinct

brain regions (Biswal et al., 1995). Functional connectivity (FC) is defined as statistical dependencies among remote neurophysiological events. However, granger causality analysis (GCA) is another widely used method for identifying directed functional ('causal') connectivity in neural time series data (Roebroeck et al., 2005). GCA has been applied to human EEG data (Hesse et al., 2003). Moreover, GCA has recently also been applied to human fMRI data based on temporal order (Friston, 2009; Seth et al., 2013). It has been widely used in exploring cognitive functions such as working memory (Protopapa et al., 2014, 2016), as well as other neurological disorders (Brovelli et al., 2004; Jiao et al., 2011). The DN is the largest single structure linking the cerebellum to the rest of the brain. Accordingly, we selected the bilateral DN as regions of interest (ROIs) to explore the different roles of the cerebellum in PD and MSA-P.

Only a few studies have investigated DN connectivity changes in the resting state in PD (Liu et al., 2013; Ma et al., 2015). However, there has been no reported data about MSA-P. In this study, we focused on potential connectivity changes between the DN and cerebral cortices. We hypothesized that the connectivity between the DN and cortical or subcortical regions may be altered and implicate motor symptoms difference between PD and MSA-P. To test this hypothesis, the functional connectivity (FC) and multivariate granger causality analysis (mGCA) methods were combined to explore the connectivity differences within the cerebello-cortical circuits during resting state.

MATERIALS AND METHODS

Participants

All subjects were recruited from Nanjing Brain Hospital from June 2013 to December 2015. Twenty-six MSA-P patients, 31 PD patients and 30 normal subjects were recruited into this study. The patients were diagnosed by a movement disorders specialist using established criteria: PD based on United Kingdom PD Society Brain Bank criteria (Hughes et al., 1992) and probable MSA-P based on the American Academy of Neurology and American Autonomic Society criteria (Gilman et al., 2008). Five subjects (2 MSA-P, 2 PD, and 1 control) were excluded due to excessive head motion during the fMRI procedure or incomplete scanning data, yielding a total of 24 MSA-P patients, 29 PD patients and 29 controls for the final analysis. All subjects underwent comprehensive neuropsychological assessments. Overall cognitive condition was assessed by the Mini-Mental State Examination (MMSE), Montreal Cognitive Assessment (MoCA) and Frontal Assessment Battery (FAB). The severity of motor symptoms for all patients was assessed using the motor part of Unified Parkinson's Disease Rating Scale (UPDRS-III) and the Hoehn-Yahr (H-Y) scale. In this study, we used the sum of all left hemibody Part III items 20–26 (UPDRS-III L), the sum of all right hemibody Part III items 20–26 (UPDRS-III R) and the sum of all Part III items (UPDRS-III total). In addition, MSA-P patients were evaluated by the Unified Multiple System Atrophy Rating Scale (UMSARS), which was conducive to classification. Assessments were performed on the day before fMRI scanning in all subjects.

Patients who had hemorrhage, infarction, tumors, trauma, or severe white matter hyperintensity were excluded from the study. All participants had written informed consent and the study was approved by the Medical Research Ethical Committee of Nanjing Brain Hospital, Nanjing, China.

Image Acquisition

All scans were acquired using a Siemens 3.0 T singer scanner (Siemens, Verio, Germany) with an 8-channel radio frequency coil. All subjects lay supine with their head cozily fixed by sponge earplugs to minimize head movement. Participants were instructed to remain as still as possible, close their eyes, remain awake and not think of anything. Three-dimensional T1 weighted images were acquired in a sagittal orientation employing a 3D-SPGR sequence with the following parameters: TE = 3.34 ms; TR = 2530 ms; flip angle = 7°; 128 sagittal slices; 1.33 mm slice thickness; matrix = 256 × 256. Functional images were collected using a gradient-recalled echo-planar imaging pulse sequence: 140 time points (that were sufficient to assess resting state connectivity); TE = 30 ms; TR = 2000 ms; FOV = 240 mm × 240 mm; matrix = 64 × 64; flip angle = 90°; 30 axial slices; 3.0 mm thickness; section gap = 0 mm.

Definition of Regions of Interest (ROIs)

Regions of interest of the left and right DN were defined by WFU PickAtlas[1] and were resliced into Montreal Neurological Institute (MNI) space. The blood oxygen level dependent (BOLD) time series of the voxels within the ROI were extracted to generate the reference time series for each ROI.

Data Preprocessing

The fMRI data were preprocessed using Data Processing Assistant for Resting-State fMRI toolkit (DPARSF[2]), which is based on the Statistical Parametric Mapping software SPM8[3]. The first 10 volumes of the rest session were discarded for each subject. The remaining images were corrected for slice timing and motion correction. According to the record of head motion, all participants had less than 2.0 mm maximum displacement in the x, y, or z plane and less than 2° of angular rotation about each axis. After spatial normalization to T1 space, all images were resampled into 3 mm × 3 mm × 3 mm voxels and spatially smoothed with a Gaussian filter of 4 mm full-width at half-maximum (FWHM). The fMRI data were then temporally band-pass-filtered (0.01–0.08 Hz) to remove low-frequency drifts and physiological high-frequency noise. To further reduce the effects of confounding factors, linear drift, six motion parameters and the mean time series of all voxels within the entire brain, white matter and cerebrospinal fluid signals were removed from the data by linear regression.

In the fMRI data, global signal can be defined as the time series of signal intensity averaged across all brain voxels, which includes both the signal of the neural activity and the noise of the non-neural activity. Global signal regression (GSR) uses linear regression to remove variance between the global signal and the time course of each individual voxel. It can improve the specificity of positive correlations and improve the correspondence to anatomical connectivity. It helps remove non-neuronal sources of global variance such as respiration and movement. With the growing use of GSR, some problems it brings have led to some controversy. Different processing techniques likely produce different complementary insights into the brain's functional organization. Whether GSR should be useful or not depend on the scientific question and how we use it. If applied and interpreted correctly, they provide complementary information (Murphy and Fox, 2016). In this study, we are concerned with the neural activity of a particular brain area, and are not interested in the noise of those non-neural activities, so we applied GSR to remove global signal variance from all voxel time series.

The voxel based morphometry (VBM) was processed and examined using SPM8 software. The 3D-T1 weighted images were segmented into gray matter, white matter and cerebrospinal fluid. The gray matter and white matter images were then normalized and resampled to MNI space in 1.5 mm cubic resolution with modulation to preserve the local tissue volumes. The resulting images were smoothed using an 8 mm FWHM Gaussian kernel.

Statistical Analysis

To compare certain demographic information and clinical characteristics (age, education, MMSE, MoCA, FAB), one-way analysis of variance (ANOVA) was used. Disease duration, UPDRS-III, H-Y, and levodopa equivalent daily dose (LEDD) were compared using the two-sample t-test. A chi-squared test was used to compare sex distribution among the groups. VBM analysis among MSA-P, PD, and control groups was carried out with the ANOVA, followed by Bonferroni test for *post hoc* comparisons. All data were statistically analyzed using SPSS19.0 (SPSS, Inc., Chicago, IL, United States). Two-sided values of $p < 0.05$ were considered statistically significant.

Functional Connectivity Analysis

Functional connectivity analysis was performed between each seed reference and the entire brain in a voxel-wise manner using the REST Toolkit[2]. Correlation coefficients were transformed to z-values using the Fisher r-to-z transformation to enhance normality. Statistical analysis across the three groups was conducted using one-way analysis of covariance (ANCOVA), with age, gender, disease duration, and gray matter volume as covariates. Then, *post hoc* two-sample t-tests were followed. The multiple comparisons of ANCOVA result was AlphaSim corrected with a cluster-level significance threshold of $p < 0.01$ (cluster size > 32 voxels and voxel-level $p < 0.01$; determined by a Monte-Carlo simulation). The *post hoc* two-sample t-tests were performed within a mask showing conspicuous differences acquired from the ANCOVA results, with a significance threshold of $p < 0.01$ with AlphaSim correction (cluster size > 14 voxels; voxel-level $p < 0.01$; determined by a Monte-Carlo simulation). The ANOVA was also performed with the similar results of ANCOVA after correction.

---

[1] http://www.ansir.wfubmc.edu
[2] http://www.rest.restfmri.net
[3] http://www.fil.ion.ucl.ac.uk/spm/software/spm8

Granger Causality Analysis

Causal connectivity refers to the influence that one neural system exerts over another. The distinction between functional and causal connectivity is that functional connectivity is ambiguous with respect to underlying directed interactions that generated the observed correlations. While causal connectivity corresponds to the intuitive notion of coupling or directed causal influence (Friston, 2011). GCA is a feasible technique for analyzing fMRI data (Wen et al., 2013). It is based on the idea that, given two time series x and y, if knowing the past of y is useful for predicting the future of x, then y must have a causal influence on x. GC method shows distinct and complementary functions in relation to the detection of causality and does not need predefined model. To identify the informational influence on the functional interactions and infer their causal relationship within the cerebello-cortical circuits, the mGCA method was applied (Blinowska et al., 2004; Chen et al., 2014). This approach is based on the MATLAB toolbox (The MathWorks, Inc., Natick, MA, United States). Briefly, to determine the structure of the cerebello-cortical circuits, nine ROIs were selected according to the abnormal functional connectivity patterns identified in the group comparisons in this study (for details refer to **Table 1**). Each seed region was represented by a radius of 6 mm around the central coordinates. The average time series for each ROI was extracted and may be expressed in Eq. 1.

$$X(t) = (x_1(t), x_2(t), ..., x_m(t)) \qquad (1)$$

where m represented the number of ROIs. The values of causal connectivity strengths from all other regions to region j were measured by multivariate auto regression (MVAR) model (Eq. 2).

$$x_j(t) = \sum_{i=1}^{p} A_j(i)X(t-i) + E_j(t) \qquad (2)$$

The parameter p is the model order or the lag parameter. $A_j(i)$ is the regression coefficient matrix, X is the time series matrix of different regions, E is the residual error

matrix. The optimal lag parameter p is usually determined by minimizing Akaike Information Criterion (AIC) (Akaike, 1998). For each subject, random-effect Granger causality maps were calculated. Statistical thresholds for these maps was performed in the context of the bootstrap technique with corrections for multiple comparisons based on a permutation test ($p < 0.05$) (Chen et al., 2014). For each group, an average Granger causality map was created to illustrate the effective connectivity influence on the paired regions. Then, group comparisons were also conducted to identify the significantly altered causal influence between paired brain areas using the Kruskal–Wallis, followed by the Dunn–Bonferroni test for *post hoc* comparisons.

Connectivity-Behavior Correlation

To explore whether the alterations of causal connectivity are covariant with disease progression, a correlation analysis between altered causal connectivity and neuropsychological performance metrics, disease duration and LEDD was performed separately for MSA-P and PD patients. First, causal connectivity values for the significant group differences were extracted. Then, Pearson's correlative analysis was conducted to examine the relationships between causal connectivity and neuropsychological scores [including MMSE, MoCA, FAB, UPDRS-III (total, L, R) and H-Y staging scale] and LEDD.

RESULTS

Demographic and Clinical Characteristics

The demographic and clinical characteristics of the participants are presented in **Table 2**. There were no significant differences in age, gender, education level, MMSE, and MoCA scores among the three groups. No significant differences were found in UPDRS-III (total, L, R) and H-Y staging scores between MSA-P and PD groups. Difference in disease duration was significant between MSA-P and PD ($p < 0.001$). The FAB scores were significantly different between MSA-P versus control ($p = 0.001$) and PD versus control ($p = 0.037$).

Voxel Based Morphometry

Voxel based morphometry did not reveal significant differences between patients and controls for gray matter volume and white matter volume (for details refer to **Table 2**).

Functional Connectivity

The ANCOVA results revealed that the left DN had significantly different FC values in the frontal, parietal or cingulate cortices among MSA-P, PD, and controls (**Table 2** and **Figure 1**). A further detailed investigation of these alterations in the three groups showed that the FC values of both MSA-P and PD patients were significantly decreased in the left dorsolateral prefrontal cortex (DLPFC) compared with the controls. PD patients exhibited lower FC values in the bilateral inferior parietal lobe compared to MSA-P or the controls. Reduced FC values in the posterior

TABLE 1 | Brain regions for granger causality analysis across all subjects.

ROIs	Brain regions	Sides (L/R)	X	Y	Z
ROI 1	Posterior cingulate cortex	–	−3	−36	33
ROI 2	Medial prefrontal cortex	–	3	42	39
ROI 3	Dorsal lateral prefrontal cortex	L	−33	49	9
ROI 4	Dorsal lateral prefrontal cortex	R	48	27	27
ROI 5	Precentral gyrus	L	−51	9	39
ROI 6	Inferior parietal cortex	L	−34	−62	46
ROI 7	Inferior parietal cortex	R	39	−66	45
ROI 8	Cerebellar dentate nucleus	L	−16	−54	−32
ROI 9	Cerebellar dentate nucleus	R	15	−56	−30

Brain regions obtained from differential functional connectivity of cerebello-cortical network among MSA-P, PD, and controls; MNI, Montreal Neurological Institute; L, left; R, right.

TABLE 2 | Demographic and clinical characteristics of the participants.

Groups	MSA-P (n = 24)	PD (n = 29)	Control (n = 29)	p-Value
Age, years	63.00 ± 6.99	66.52 ± 6.98	63.21 ± 8.01	0.141
Gender, male/female	13/11	18/11	12/17	0.282
Education, years	8.45 ± 1.18	8.52 ± 1.09	8.41 ± 1.21	0.944
Disease duration years	2.37 ± 0.92	4.62 ± 1.26	NA	<0.001[a]
GMV, ml	489.01 ± 49.59	511.77 ± 54.47	521.38 ± 41.75	0.064
WMV, ml	515.92 ± 62.10	528.05 ± 53.29	541.06 ± 68.25	0.337
MMSE	27.71 ± 0.86	27.59 ± 1.40	27.93 ± 0.88	0.373
MoCA	25.17 ± 1.43	24.79 ± 1.40	25.58 ± 1.21	0.087
FAB	14.63 ± 1.10	15.00 ± 1.22	15.72 ± 0.88	0.001[bc]
UPDRS-III, total	28.42 ± 7.22	24.45 ± 9.01	NA	0.087
UPDRS-III, right	8.08 ± 5.05	7.45 ± 3.33	NA	0.586
UPDRS-III, left	7.58 ± 3.94	6.51 ± 2.63	NA	0.245
H-Y	2.79 ± 0.76	2.43 ± 0.80	NA	0.102
LEDD, mg/day	543.23 ± 100.8	504.31 ± 85.65	NA	0.135

GMV, gray matter volume; WMV, white matter volume; MMSE, Mini-Mental State Examination; MoCA, Montreal Cognitive Assessment; FAB, Frontal Assessment Battery; UPDRS-III, Unified Parkinson's Disease Rating Scale-motor part III; H-Y, Hoehn-Yahr staging scale; LEDD, levodopa equivalent daily dose; NA, not applicable; p < 0.05 was considered significant. [a]Means significant difference between the two groups (MSA-P versus PD). [bc]Means significant group differences between (MSA-P versus control), (PD versus control) by post hoc comparisons.

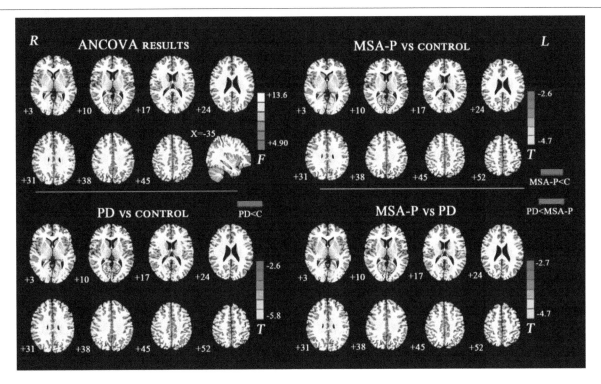

FIGURE 1 | Statistical maps showing FC differences of left DN in different brain regions among the MSA-P, PD, and control groups. The threshold for display was set to p < 0.01 corrected by AlphaSim; Results are in MNI space; Red color represents the increased correlation while the blue color represents the decreased correlation; R, right; L, left; C, controls.

cingulate cortex (PCC) were also observed in the PD patients relative to the controls. Moreover, abnormal FC values of the right DN were observed throughout the frontal, parietal, and cingulate cortices by ANCOVA analysis (**Table 3** and **Figure 2**). Decreased FC values in the left precentral gyrus (M1) and right DLPFC were shown in MSA-P patients compared with the controls. PD patients produced attenuated connectivity in the PCC, medial PFC and bilateral DLPFC compared to the controls, as well as decreased FC values of the PCC compared to MSA-P.

Causal Connectivity

We further attested that the DN, as core regions of the neural circuitry, is causally influenced in the cerebello-cortical circuits. As shown in **Figure 3**, MSA-P and PD patients presented with different patterns of the connectivity strength of causal flow between the previously defined paired regions compared to controls. MSA-P patients showed significantly enhanced causal information from the left DN to the PCC compared to PD or controls, as well as lower information flow from the left M1 to the right DN relative to the controls. In the PD group, the right DLPFC exhibited obvious causal interaction disruption with the left DN compared to the controls, as shown in **Figure 3B**.

Correlation Analysis with Clinical Behavior Scores

As shown in **Figure 3D**, the connectivity of the causal path from the left M1 to the right DN was significantly decreased in the MSA-P group, which was negatively correlated with UPDRS-III R scores.

TABLE 3 | Regions showing significant differences in DN FC among MSA-P, PD, and control group.

Brain region	Cluster size	MNI coordinates			T-value
		X	Y	Z	
Left dentate nucleus					
MSA-P < Controls					
Left dorsolateral prefrontal cortex	44	−33	48	3	−5.14
PD < Controls					
Left dorsolateral prefrontal cortex	70	−33	49	9	−4.57
Posterior cingulate cortex	33	−3	−32	38	−3.94
Left inferior parietal lobe	39	−34	−62	46	−4.59
Right inferior parietal lobe	34	39	−66	45	−3.88
PD < MSA-P					
Left inferior parietal lobe	38	−29	−68	45	−4.61
Right inferior parietal lobe	30	37	−70	45	−3.37
Right dentate nucleus					
MSA-P < Controls					
Left precentral gyrus	20	−51	9	39	−4.08
Right dorsolateral prefrontal cortex	26	48	30	24	−3.95
PD < Controls					
Medial prefrontal cortex	27	3	42	39	−4.44
Left dorsolateral prefrontal cortex	28	−42	27	42	−3.89
Right dorsolateral prefrontal cortex	41	48	27	27	−4.04
Posterior cingulate cortex	180	−3	−36	33	−5.63
PD < MSA-P					
Posterior cingulate cortex	30	−9	−39	36	−3.82

MNI, Montreal Neurological Institute; Significance set at p < 0.01 corrected by AlphaSim; Cluster size is in mm³; Results are given in MNI space.

DISCUSSION

Recently, many efforts have been made to detect early differences between MSA-P and PD patients (Wang et al., 2012; Ji et al., 2015). The novelty of this study lies in the fact that we have used unidirectional and directional connectivity methods to explore the unique association between altered cerebello-cortical connectivity and motor and non-motor defects in both MSA-P and PD patients. Our research yielded several major findings. First, MSA-P an PD patients exhibited both functional and causal connectivity differences within cerebello-cortical networks compared with controls. Second, the comparison of MSA-P patients with PD patients by BOLD signal mainly revealed differences in the DN-PCC connectivity. Third, in the MSA-P group, a significant correlation was found between the UPDRS-III R scores and the causal connectivity from the left M1 to right DN.

Relative to the controls, MSA-P patients displayed disrupted functional and causal coupling between the left M1 and right DN. The classical view of M1, which was based principally on direct cortical stimulation and attributed to select the muscles and force for executing an intended movement. A recent diffusion tensor imaging study has reported stronger connections between the cerebellum and the precentral gyrus as well as the superior frontal gyrus (Doron et al., 2010), which indicated that the cerebellum involved in the processing of motor, oculomotor, and spatial working memory by cerebello-cortical circuits (du Boisgueheneuc et al., 2006). Rs-fMRI in MSA has shown reduced regional homogeneity of the spontaneous BOLD fluctuations in left M1 compared with controls (You et al., 2011). Wang H. et al. (2016) also found that the induced motor improvement in MSA-P patients by rTMS over left M1 may be associated with increased activation in the cerebellum. The cerebellum receives input from the M1 and then projects to thalamus, M1 (Kelly and Strick, 2003). In this study, the causal influence from M1 to the cerebellum in MSA-P patients was attenuated. This result could imply that the cerebellum exerts its influence on cortical inhibitory activity (Picazio and Koch, 2015). It may be one explanation for the underlying pathophysiology of motor deficits. Noticeably, the decreased causal connectivity from left M1 to right DN is significantly correlated with the contralateral motor symptom scores for the MSA-P group, which emphasized that the motor impairments in MSA-P patients could be influenced by cerebello-cortical loop degeneration in addition to striatal pathology.

In this study, the cerebellar functional connectivity was disrupted in several default mode network (DMN) regions (the PCC, medial PFC, and inferior parietal lobe) in PD patients compared with MSA-P patients or controls. In the baseline state, the PCC appears a high metabolic rate (Raichle et al., 2001) and plays a crucial role in modulating the balance between internal and external information for maintaining normal brain functions (Leech and Sharp, 2014). Lin et al. (2016) found that the PCC is a core node of the DMN and it is closely related with cognitive task performance, by aggregating information to allow functional cooperation within the DMN. A previous study reported that cognitively unimpaired patients with PD

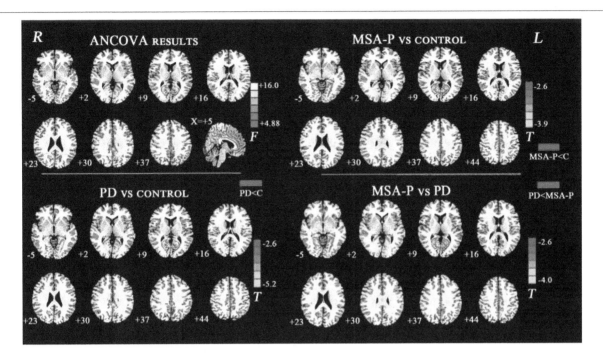

FIGURE 2 | Statistical maps showing FC differences of right DN in different brain regions among the MSA-P, PD, and control groups. The threshold for display was set to $p < 0.01$ corrected by AlphaSim; Results are in MNI space; Red color represents the increased correlation while the blue color represents the decreased correlation; R, right; L, left; C, controls.

tend to show attenuated DMN activity compared to controls (Tessitore et al., 2012). The study associated DMN deficits with cognitive decline, because cognitive function was correlated with DMN connectivity. It suggested that there is an early functional disruption of the DMN in PD prior to clinical evidence of cognitive impairment. The DMN sub-regions play important roles in remembering, self-reflection, mental imagery, and stream-of-consciousness processing (Greicius et al., 2004; Buckner and Carroll, 2007). The consolidation and maintenance of brain function might be facilitated through the DMN plasticity. However, the mechanisms underlying modulations of the DMN are not yet clear. We hypothesized that the DN dysfunction contributed to abnormal recruitment of the PCC node of the DMN. The DN, which represents the capital cerebellar output channel, is considered to be implicated with salience and sensorimotor networks (Habas et al., 2009). The DMN deactivates during externally goal-directed activity (Gusnard et al., 2001) and is causally influenced by the salience network (Chiong et al., 2013). In a recent report, a whole-brain functional connectivity analysis method was used to uncover connectivity changes following rTMS intervention over M1 for MSA-P patients. This result indicated that the rTMS-related functional links were mainly connected to the cerebellar and limbic networks from the DMN (Chou et al., 2015). It seems plausible that DMN plasticity might be sensitive to the cerebellar network effects. Only one study has described reduced DMN activity in MSA-P (with a average disease duration of 3.9 years) (Franciotti et al., 2015). In this study, MSA-P patients showed significant strengthened causal connectivity from the left DN

to the PCC compared with both PD patients and controls. The DN exerted a causal influence on the PCC, perhaps as a compensatory mechanism for DMN functions in the early stages. In previous study, the DMN activity was enhanced in dementia with lewy bodies (DLB), the explanatory hypothesis was that the preserved DMN activity could depend on compensatory mechanisms attempting to maintain DMN functions, in the face of developing pathology (Kenny et al., 2012). The consolidated DMN connectivity was similar to the enhancement observed in DLB, as we found no cellular loss, and this finding supports that functional modulatory mechanisms are relevant rather than structural differences.

The inferior parietal lobe within the executive network is involved with sustained attention and working memory information for action preparation (Seeley et al., 2007). In patients with PD, the functional parieto-motor impairment could be related to bradykinesia (Palomar et al., 2013). The cerebellar damage may impair the competence to convert a programmed motion sequence into action before the launch of movement (Bhanpuri et al., 2014; Brunamonti et al., 2014). The interruption of the dynamic equilibrium between the cerebellar and executive network may weaken the ability of the motor system to prepare for future task execution. Evidence from previous studies has demonstrated the existed functional connectivity between the cerebellum and parietal cortex (Macher et al., 2014). The decline in functional connectivity between the DN and the inferior parietal lobe may contribute to the impaired function of PD patients in linking simple movements together into complicated and sequential movements (Liu et al., 2013).

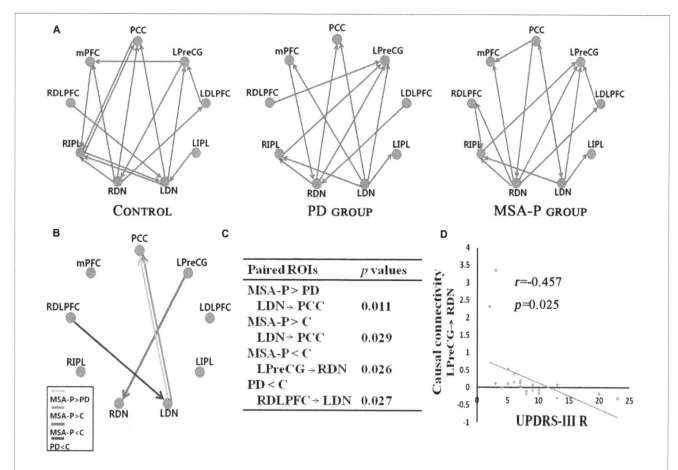

FIGURE 3 | Granger causality (GC) analysis of alterations within the cerebello-cerebral circuits among the MSA-P, PD, and control groups. **(A)** Significant GC patterns within the controls, PD group and MSA-P group (p < 0.05). The red arrow indicates the direction of informational influence between paired regions; **(B)** significant differences in GC values between the groups: MSA-P versus controls, PD versus controls and MSA-P versus PD; **(C)** the p-value of each paired region is presented; **(D)** significant correlation between causal connectivity and UPDRS-III R scores in MSA-P group; PCC, posterior cingulate cortex; mPFC, medial prefrontal cortex; LDLPFC, left dorsolateral prefrontal cortex; RDLPFC, right dorsolateral prefrontal cortex; LPreCG, left precentral gyrus; LIPL, left inferior parietal lobe; RIPL, right inferior parietal lobe; LDN, left dentate nucleus; RDN, right dentate nucleus.

However, such correlations between clinical observations and neural connectivity patterns need further explorations.

Both MSA-P and PD patients showed decreased connectivity between the DN and the DLPFC compared with the controls. Reduced causal information flows from the DLPFC to the DN were also found in the PD group compared to the controls. The DLPFC, a crucial node in the cognition control network (Wang Y.L. et al., 2016), is involved in attention, working memory and executive control (Pope et al., 2015). MSA patients presented with a distinctive pattern of cognitive deficits in frontal executive dysfunction (Siri et al., 2013). A PET study suggested that MSA patients with memory and frontal executive dysfunction tended to show hypometabolism in the anterior cerebellum and frontal cortex in the early stage of the disease (Lyoo et al., 2008). In addition, the hypoactivity of the DLPFC in PD patients with depression has also been identified in previous studies (Zhu et al., 2016). The impaired striatal cells in parkinsonism could lead to secondary frontal lobe dysfunction, including disruption of the cognitive loop linking the striatum with the DLPFC (Jokinen et al., 2013). Recently, the possibility of cerebellar influence on

cognitive function in parkinsonism has also been raised (Hirata et al., 2006; Wu and Hallett, 2013; Kim et al., 2015). Abundant structural and functional investigations in both human and non-human primates revealed that the cerebellum is involved in higher-order cognitive and emotional processes by sending fibers from the DN to PFC via the thalamus (Allen et al., 2005; Ramnani, 2006). The decreased DLPFC connectivity may be significantly associated with executive control and emotional processes in both MSA-P and PD patients, although no significant correlations were obtained in this study. These results illustrated that the connectivity of the cerebellum with the motor and non-motor cortical domains is significantly involved in the PD and MSA-P disease process.

This analysis demonstrated the cerebellum to be a causal flow hub of the cerebello-cortical network, with the high number of causal flow connections. A possible correspondence of tractography between cortices with similar functional roles, as reported here, suggests that the cerebellum contributes to parallel associative cerebello-cortical networks involved in various aspects of motor and cognition. The converging results strongly indicated that the causal topology of the cerebello-cortical circuits may be disrupted in both MSA-P and PD patients, adding an additional hint for comprehending the neurobiology underlying patients with MSA-P and PD.

CONCLUSION

This rs-fMRI study provides evidence that the dysfunction reported within the cerebello-cortical networks, typically related to motor and cognitive defects in MSA-P and PD. It may be associated with impaired interactions between the cerebellum and key cerebral cortical regions. In conclusion, our findings indicate a crucial role for the cerebello-cortical network in both MSA-P and PD patients in addition to STC network and revealed that different patterns of cerebello-cortical loop degeneration are involved in the development of the diseases. Furthermore, the alterations of the functional link within the cerebello-cortical circuits, especially the DN-PCC connectivity, may facilitate early differential diagnosis and the monitoring of disease progression.

AUTHOR CONTRIBUTIONS

JS designed the study and revised it critically for important intellectual content. QY performed the research and drafted the manuscript, DZ and FL helped in data analyses, XL, CX, and QH help in clinical data collection, analyses and made patients follow-ups.

FUNDING

This work was supported by the Nanjing Bureau of Science and Technology (No. 201605040).

REFERENCES

Akaike, H. (1998). "A new look at the statistical model identification," in *Selected Papers of Hirotugu Akaike*, eds E. Parzen, K. Tanabe, and G. Kitagawa (New York, NY: Springer), 215–222.

Allen, G., McColl, R., Barnard, H., Ringe, W. K., Fleckenstein, J., and Cullum, C. M. (2005). Magnetic resonance imaging of cerebellar-prefrontal and cerebellar-parietal functional connectivity. *Neuroimage* 28, 39–48. doi: 10.1016/j.neuroimage.2005.06.013

Bhanpuri, N. H., Okamura, A. M., and Bastian, A. J. (2014). Predicting and correcting ataxia using a model of cerebellar function. *Brain* 137(Pt 7), 1931–1944. doi: 10.1093/brain/awu115

Biswal, B., Yetkin, F. Z., Haughton, V. M., and Hyde, J. S. (1995). Functional connectivity in the motor cortex of resting human brain using echo-planar MRI. *Magn. Reson. Med.* 34, 537–541.

Blinowska, K. J., Kus, R., and Kaminski, M. (2004). Granger causality and information flow in multivariate processes. *Phys. Rev. E Stat. Nonlin. Soft Matter Phys.* 70:050902. doi: 10.1103/PhysRevE.70.050902

Bohnen, N. I., Albin, R. L., Koeppe, R. A., Wernette, K. A., Kilbourn, M. R., Minoshima, S., et al. (2006). Positron emission tomography of monoaminergic vesicular binding in aging and Parkinson disease. *J. Cereb. Blood Flow Metab.* 26, 1198–1212. doi: 10.1038/sj.jcbfm.9600276

Braak, H., and Braak, E. (2000). Pathoanatomy of Parkinson's disease. *J. Neurol.* 247(Suppl. 2), II3–II10. doi: 10.1007/pl00007758

Brovelli, A., Ding, M., Ledberg, A., Chen, Y., Nakamura, R., and Bressler, S. L. (2004). Beta oscillations in a large-scale sensorimotor cortical network: directional influences revealed by Granger causality. *Proc. Natl. Acad. Sci. U.S.A.* 101, 9849–9854. doi: 10.1073/pnas.0308538101

Brunamonti, E., Chiricozzi, F. R., Clausi, S., Olivito, G., Giusti, M. A., Molinari, M., et al. (2014). Cerebellar damage impairs executive control and monitoring of movement generation. *PLoS ONE* 9:e85997. doi: 10.1371/journal.pone.0085997

Buckner, R. L., and Carroll, D. C. (2007). Self-projection and the brain. *Trends Cogn. Sci.* 11, 49–57. doi: 10.1016/j.tics.2006.11.004

Cerasa, A., Hagberg, G. E., Peppe, A., Bianciardi, M., Gioia, M. C., Costa, A., et al. (2006). Functional changes in the activity of cerebellum and frontostriatal regions during externally and internally timed movement in Parkinson's disease. *Brain Res. Bull.* 71, 259–269. doi: 10.1016/j.brainresbull.2006.09.014

Chen, G., Ward, B. D., Chen, G., and Li, S. J. (2014). Decreased effective connectivity from cortices to the right parahippocampal gyrus in Alzheimer's disease subjects. *Brain Connect.* 4, 702–708. doi: 10.1089/brain.2014.0295

Chiong, W., Wilson, S. M., D'Esposito, M., Kayser, A. S., Grossman, S. N., Poorzand, P., et al. (2013). The salience network causally influences default mode network activity during moral reasoning. *Brain* 136(Pt 6), 1929–1941. doi: 10.1093/brain/awt066

Chou, Y. H., You, H., Wang, H., Zhao, Y. P., Hou, B., Chen, N. K., et al. (2015). Effect of repetitive transcranial magnetic stimulation on fMRI resting-state connectivity in multiple system atrophy. *Brain Connect.* 5, 451–459. doi: 10.1089/brain.2014.0325

Clower, D. M., West, R. A., Lynch, J. C., and Strick, P. L. (2001). The inferior parietal lobule is the target of output from the superior colliculus, hippocampus, and cerebellum. *J. Neurosci.* 21, 6283–6291.

Dickson, D. W. (2012). Parkinson's disease and parkinsonism: neuropathology. *Cold Spring Harb. Perspect. Med.* 2:a009258. doi: 10.1101/cshperspect.a009258

Doron, K. W., Funk, C. M., and Glickstein, M. (2010). Fronto-cerebellar circuits and eye movement control: a diffusion imaging tractography study of human cortico-pontine projections. *Brain Res.* 1307, 63–71. doi: 10.1016/j.brainres.2009.10.029

du Boisgueheneuc, F., Levy, R., Volle, E., Seassau, M., Duffau, H., Kinkingnehun, S., et al. (2006). Functions of the left superior frontal gyrus in humans: a lesion study. *Brain* 129, 3315–3328. doi: 10.1093/brain/awl244

Franciotti, R., Delli Pizzi, S., Perfetti, B., Tartaro, A., Bonanni, L., Thomas, A., et al. (2015). Default mode network links to visual hallucinations: a comparison between Parkinson's disease and multiple system atrophy. *Mov. Disord.* 30, 1237–1247. doi: 10.1002/mds.26285

Friston, K. (2009). Causal modelling and brain connectivity in functional magnetic resonance imaging. *PLoS Biol.* 7:e33. doi: 10.1371/journal.pbio.1000033

Friston, K. J. (2011). Functional and effective connectivity: a review. *Brain Connect.* 1, 13–36. doi: 10.1089/brain.2011.0008

Galvan, A., Devergnas, A., and Wichmann, T. (2015). Alterations in neuronal activity in basal ganglia-thalamocortical circuits in the parkinsonian state. *Front. Neuroanat.* 9:5. doi: 10.3389/fnana.2015.00005

Ghaemi, M., Hilker, R., Rudolf, J., Sobesky, J., and Heiss, W. D. (2002). Differentiating multiple system atrophy from Parkinson's disease: contribution of striatal and midbrain MRI volumetry and multi-tracer PET imaging. *J. Neurol. Neurosurg. Psychiatry* 73, 517–523.

Gilman, S., Wenning, G. K., Low, P. A., Brooks, D. J., Mathias, C. J., Trojanowski, J. Q., et al. (2008). Second consensus statement on the diagnosis of multiple system atrophy. *Neurology* 71, 670–676. doi: 10.1212/01.wnl.0000324625.00404.15

Greicius, M. D., Srivastava, G., Reiss, A. L., and Menon, V. (2004). Default-mode network activity distinguishes Alzheimer's disease from healthy aging: evidence from functional MRI. *Proc. Natl. Acad. Sci. U.S.A.* 101, 4637–4642. doi: 10.1073/pnas.0308627101

Gusnard, D. A., Raichle, M. E., and Raichle, M. E. (2001). Searching for a baseline: functional imaging and the resting human brain. *Nat. Rev. Neurosci.* 2, 685–694. doi: 10.1038/35094500

Habas, C. (2010). Functional imaging of the deep cerebellar nuclei: a review. *Cerebellum* 9, 22–28. doi: 10.1007/s12311-009-0119-3

Habas, C., Kamdar, N., Nguyen, D., Prater, K., Beckmann, C. F., Menon, V., et al. (2009). Distinct cerebellar contributions to intrinsic connectivity networks. *J. Neurosci.* 29, 8586–8594. doi: 10.1523/jneurosci.1868-09.2009

Hesse, W., Moller, E., Arnold, M., and Schack, B. (2003). The use of time-variant EEG Granger causality for inspecting directed interdependencies of neural assemblies. *J. Neurosci. Methods* 124, 27–44.

Hirata, K., Tanaka, H., Zeng, X. H., Hozumi, A., and Arai, M. (2006). The role of the basal ganglia and cerebellum in cognitive impairment: a study using event-related potentials. *Suppl. Clin. Neurophysiol.* 59, 49–55.

Hughes, A. J., Daniel, S. E., Kilford, L., and Lees, A. J. (1992). Accuracy of clinical diagnosis of idiopathic Parkinson's disease: a clinico-pathological study of 100 cases. *J. Neurol. Neurosurg. Psychiatry* 55, 181–184.

Ji, L., Wang, Y., Zhu, D., Liu, W., and Shi, J. (2015). White matter differences between multiple system atrophy (parkinsonian type) and Parkinson's disease: a diffusion tensor image study. *Neuroscience* 305, 109–116. doi: 10.1016/j.neuroscience.2015.07.060

Jiao, Q., Lu, G., Zhang, Z., Zhong, Y., Wang, Z., Guo, Y., et al. (2011). Granger causal influence predicts BOLD activity levels in the default mode network. *Hum. Brain Mapp.* 32, 154–161. doi: 10.1002/hbm.21065

Jokinen, P., Karrasch, M., Bruck, A., Johansson, J., Bergman, J., and Rinne, J. O. (2013). Cognitive slowing in Parkinson's disease is related to frontostriatal dopaminergic dysfunction. *J. Neurol. Sci.* 329, 23–28. doi: 10.1016/j.jns.2013.03.006

Kelly, R. M., and Strick, P. L. (2003). Cerebellar loops with motor cortex and prefrontal cortex of a nonhuman primate. *J. Neurosci.* 23, 8432–8444.

Kenny, E. R., Blamire, A. M., Firbank, M. J., and O'Brien, J. T. (2012). Functional connectivity in cortical regions in dementia with Lewy bodies and Alzheimer's disease. *Brain* 135, 569–581. doi: 10.1093/brain/awr327

Kim, H. J., Stamelou, M., and Jeon, B. (2016). Multiple system atrophy-mimicking conditions: diagnostic challenges. *Parkinsonism Relat. Disord.* 22(Suppl. 1), S12–S15. doi: 10.1016/j.parkreldis.2015.09.003

Kim, J. S., Yang, J. J., Lee, D. K., Lee, J. M., Youn, J., and Cho, J. W. (2015). Cognitive impairment and its structural correlates in the parkinsonian subtype of multiple system atrophy. *Neurodegener. Dis.* 15, 294–300. doi: 10.1159/000430953

Leech, R., and Sharp, D. J. (2014). The role of the posterior cingulate cortex in cognition and disease. *Brain* 137, 12–32. doi: 10.1093/brain/awt162

Lin, P., Yang, Y., Jovicich, J., De Pisapia, N., Wang, X., Zuo, C. S., et al. (2016). Static and dynamic posterior cingulate cortex nodal topology of default mode network predicts attention task performance. *Brain Imaging Behav.* 10, 212–225. doi: 10.1007/s11682-015-9384-6

Liu, H., Edmiston, E. K., Fan, G., Xu, K., Zhao, B., Shang, X., et al. (2013). Altered resting-state functional connectivity of the dentate nucleus in Parkinson's disease. *Psychiatry Res.* 211, 64–71. doi: 10.1016/j.pscychresns.2012.10.007

Lyoo, C. H., Jeong, Y., Ryu, Y. H., Lee, S. Y., Song, T. J., Lee, J. H., et al. (2008). Effects of disease duration on the clinical features and brain glucose metabolism in patients with mixed type multiple system atrophy. *Brain* 131, 438–446. doi: 10.1093/brain/awm328

Ma, H., Chen, H., Fang, J., Gao, L., Ma, L., Wu, T., et al. (2015). Resting-state functional connectivity of dentate nucleus is associated with tremor in Parkinson's disease. *J. Neurol.* 262, 2247–2256. doi: 10.1007/s00415-015-7835-z

Macher, K., Bohringer, A., Villringer, A., and Pleger, B. (2014). Cerebellar-parietal connections underpin phonological storage. *J. Neurosci.* 34, 5029–5037. doi: 10.1523/jneurosci.0106-14.2014

Middleton, F. A., and Strick, P. L. (2000). Basal ganglia and cerebellar loops: motor and cognitive circuits. *Brain Res. Brain Res. Rev.* 31, 236–250.

Middleton, F. A., and Strick, P. L. (2001). Cerebellar projections to the prefrontal cortex of the primate. *J. Neurosci.* 21, 700–712.

Murphy, K., and Fox, M. D. (2016). Towards a consensus regarding global signal regression for resting state functional connectivity MRI. *Neuroimage* 154, 169–173. doi: 10.1016/j.neuroimage.2016.11.052

Nicoletti, G., Fera, F., Condino, F., Auteri, W., Gallo, O., Pugliese, P., et al. (2006a). MR imaging of middle cerebellar peduncle width: differentiation of multiple system atrophy from Parkinson disease. *Radiology* 239, 825–830. doi: 10.1148/radiol.2393050459

Nicoletti, G., Lodi, R., Condino, F., Tonon, C., Fera, F., Malucelli, E., et al. (2006b). Apparent diffusion coefficient measurements of the middle cerebellar peduncle differentiate the Parkinson variant of MSA from Parkinson's disease

and progressive supranuclear palsy. *Brain* 129, 2679–2687. doi: 10.1093/brain/awl166

Palmer, S. J., Li, J., Wang, Z. J., and McKeown, M. J. (2010). Joint amplitude and connectivity compensatory mechanisms in Parkinson's disease. *Neuroscience* 166, 1110–1118. doi: 10.1016/j.neuroscience.2010.01.012

Palomar, F. J., Conde, V., Carrillo, F., Fernandez-del-Olmo, M., Koch, G., and Mir, P. (2013). Parieto-motor functional connectivity is impaired in Parkinson's disease. *Brain Stimul.* 6, 147–154. doi: 10.1016/j.brs.2012.03.017

Picazio, S., and Koch, G. (2015). Is motor inhibition mediated by cerebello-cortical interactions? *Cerebellum* 14, 47–49. doi: 10.1007/s12311-014-0609-9

Pope, P. A., Brenton, J. W., and Miall, R. C. (2015). Task-specific facilitation of cognition by anodal transcranial direct current stimulation of the prefrontal cortex. *Cereb. Cortex* 25, 4551–4558. doi: 10.1093/cercor/bhv094

Poston, K. L., Tang, C. C., Eckert, T., Dhawan, V., Frucht, S., Vonsattel, J. P., et al. (2012). Network correlates of disease severity in multiple system atrophy. *Neurology* 78, 1237–1244. doi: 10.1212/WNL.0b013e318250d7fd

Protopapa, F., Siettos, C. I., Evdokimidis, I., and Smyrnis, N. (2014). Granger causality analysis reveals distinct spatio-temporal connectivity patterns in motor and perceptual visuo-spatial working memory. *Front. Comput. Neurosci.* 8:146. doi: 10.3389/fncom.2014.00146

Protopapa, F., Siettos, C. I., Myatchin, I., and Lagae, L. (2016). Children with well controlled epilepsy possess different spatio-temporal patterns of causal network connectivity during a visual working memory task. *Cogn. Neurodyn.* 10, 99–111. doi: 10.1007/s11571-015-9373-x

Raichle, M. E., MacLeod, A. M., Snyder, A. Z., Powers, W. J., Gusnard, D. A., and Shulman, G. L. (2001). A default mode of brain function. *Proc. Natl. Acad. Sci. U.S.A.* 98, 676–682. doi: 10.1073/pnas.98.2.676

Ramnani, N. (2006). The primate cortico-cerebellar system: anatomy and function. *Nat. Rev. Neurosci.* 7, 511–522. doi: 10.1038/nrn1953

Roebroeck, A., Formisano, E., and Goebel, R. (2005). Mapping directed influence over the brain using Granger causality and fMRI. *Neuroimage* 25, 230–242. doi: 10.1016/j.neuroimage.2004.11.017

Schutter, D. J., and van Honk, J. (2005). The cerebellum on the rise in human emotion. *Cerebellum* 4, 290–294. doi: 10.1080/14734220500348584

Seeley, W. W., Menon, V., Schatzberg, A. F., Keller, J., Glover, G. H., Kenna, H., et al. (2007). Dissociable intrinsic connectivity networks for salience processing and executive control. *J. Neurosci.* 27, 2349–2356. doi: 10.1523/JNEUROSCI.5587-06.2007

Seth, A. K., Chorley, P., and Barnett, L. C. (2013). Granger causality analysis of fMRI BOLD signals is invariant to hemodynamic convolution but not downsampling. *Neuroimage* 65, 540–555. doi: 10.1016/j.neuroimage.2012.09.049

Siri, C., Duerr, S., Canesi, M., Delazer, M., Esselink, R., Bloem, B. R., et al. (2013). A cross-sectional multicenter study of cognitive and behavioural features in multiple system atrophy patients of the parkinsonian and cerebellar type. *J. Neural Transm.* 120, 613–618. doi: 10.1007/s00702-013-0997-x

Tessitore, A., Esposito, F., Vitale, C., Santangelo, G., Amboni, M., Russo, A., et al. (2012). Default-mode network connectivity in cognitively unimpaired patients with Parkinson disease. *Neurology* 79, 2226–2232. doi: 10.1212/WNL.0b013e31827689d6

Wang, H., Li, L., Wu, T., Hou, B., Wu, S., Qiu, Y., et al. (2016). Increased cerebellar activation after repetitive transcranial magnetic stimulation over the primary motor cortex in patients with multiple system atrophy. *Ann. Transl. Med.* 4, 103. doi: 10.21037/atm.2016.03.24

Wang, Y. L., Yang, S. Z., Sun, W. L., Shi, Y. Z., and Duan, H. F. (2016). Altered functional interaction hub between affective network and cognitive control network in patients with major depressive disorder. *Behav. Brain Res.* 298, 301–309. doi: 10.1016/j.bbr.2015.10.040

Wang, Y., Butros, S. R., Shuai, X., Dai, Y., Chen, C., Liu, M., et al. (2012). Different iron-deposition patterns of multiple system atrophy with predominant parkinsonism and idiopathetic Parkinson diseases demonstrated by phase-corrected susceptibility-weighted imaging. *AJNR Am. J. Neuroradiol.* 33, 266–273. doi: 10.3174/ajnr.A2765

Wen, X., Rangarajan, G., and Ding, M. (2013). Is Granger causality a viable technique for analyzing fMRI data? *PLoS ONE* 8:e67428. doi: 10.1371/journal.pone.0067428

Wenning, G. K., Ben-Shlomo, Y., Hughes, A., Daniel, S. E., Lees, A., and Quinn, N. P. (2000). What clinical features are most useful to distinguish definite multiple system atrophy from Parkinson's disease? *J. Neurol. Neurosurg. psychiatry* 68, 434–440.

Wu, T., and Hallett, M. (2013). The cerebellum in Parkinson's disease. *Brain* 136, 696–709. doi: 10.1093/brain/aws360

Wu, T., Long, X., Zang, Y., Wang, L., Hallett, M., Li, K., et al. (2009). Regional homogeneity changes in patients with Parkinson's disease. *Hum. Brain Mapp.* 30, 1502–1510. doi: 10.1002/hbm.20622

Wu, T., Wang, L., Hallett, M., Chen, Y., Li, K., and Chan, P. (2011). Effective connectivity of brain networks during self-initiated movement in Parkinson's

disease. *Neuroimage* 55, 204–215. doi: 10.1016/j.neuroimage.2010.11.074

You, H., Wang, J., Wang, H., Zang, Y. F., Zheng, F. L., Meng, C. L., et al. (2011). Altered regional homogeneity in motor cortices in patients with multiple system atrophy. *Neurosci. Lett.* 502, 18–23. doi: 10.1016/j.neulet.2011.07.015

Zhu, Y., Song, X., Xu, M., Hu, X., Li, E., Liu, J., et al. (2016). Impaired interhemispheric synchrony in Parkinson's disease with depression. *Sci. Rep.* 6:27477. doi: 10.1038/srep27477

18

Cognitive Training Enhances Auditory Attention Efficiency in Older Adults

Jennifer L. O'Brien[1]*, Jennifer J. Lister[2], Bernadette A. Fausto[3], Gregory K. Clifton[2] and Jerri D. Edwards[4]

[1] *Department of Psychology, University of South Florida St. Petersburg, St. Petersburg, FL, United States,* [2] *Department of Communication Sciences and Disorders, University of South Florida, Tampa, FL, United States,* [3] *School of Aging Studies, University of South Florida, Tampa, FL, United States,* [4] *Department of Psychiatry and Behavioral Neurosciences, College of Medicine, University of South Florida, Tampa, FL, United States*

*Correspondence:
Jennifer L. O'Brien
jenobrien@usf.edu

Auditory cognitive training (ACT) improves attention in older adults; however, the underlying neurophysiological mechanisms are still unknown. The present study examined the effects of ACT on the P3b event-related potential reflecting attention allocation (amplitude) and speed of processing (latency) during stimulus categorization and the P1-N1-P2 complex reflecting perceptual processing (amplitude and latency). Participants completed an auditory oddball task before and after 10 weeks of ACT ($n = 9$) or a no contact control period ($n = 15$). Parietal P3b amplitudes to oddball stimuli decreased at post-test in the trained group as compared to those in the control group, and frontal P3b amplitudes show a similar trend, potentially reflecting more efficient attentional allocation after ACT. No advantages for the ACT group were evident for auditory perceptual processing or speed of processing in this small sample. Our results provide preliminary evidence that ACT may enhance the efficiency of attention allocation, which may account for the positive impact of ACT on the everyday functioning of older adults.

Keywords: aging, cognitive training, auditory cognition, attention, event-related potentials

INTRODUCTION

Hearing loss is a distressing impairment that becomes increasingly prevalent with age, affecting 30% of adults aged 65 to 74 and almost 50% of older adults over the age of 75 (National Institute on Deafness and Other Communication Disorders [NIDCD], 2010). Hearing loss causes speech perception difficulties (Humes et al., 2012) and has been linked to subsequent cognitive impairment (Lin, 2011; Lin et al., 2011a,b,c, 2013; Harrison Bush et al., 2015) as well as increased social isolation (Mick et al., 2014), reduced quality of life (Ciorba et al., 2012), increased risk for depression (Li et al., 2014), and reduced engagement in independent activities of daily living (Dalton et al., 2003). Because hearing loss results in effortful auditory processing in normal aging (Pichora-Fuller et al., 2016), remediation of auditory processing may improve cognition and enhance quality of life in older adults. The current study investigates the efficacy of auditory cognitive training (ACT) to improve underlying neurophysiological mechanisms of auditory perception and cognition.

Incipient, age-related hearing loss has been conventionally corrected with hearing aids. Despite improved audibility provided by current hearing aid technology, hearing aids alone often do not compensate for decreased ability to comprehend meaningful auditory stimuli among background noise. Speech perception, for instance, depends not only on intact auditory function but also intact cognitive function including the ability to attend to relevant stimuli, to process incoming stimuli, and to maintain new information all while actively manipulating temporarily stored stimuli. These cognitive functions all appear to decline in normal aging (for reviews, see Akeroyd, 2008; Arlinger et al., 2009). Thus, while hearing aids can enhance audibility, concomitant and subsequent age-related cognitive decline may persist, impairing older adults' ability to process meaningful sound in challenging listening situations.

There is growing evidence that cognitive training programs can ameliorate or minimize age-related sensory and cognitive decline through neuroplastic change (Smith et al., 2009). However, the neural mechanisms underlying these changes are still relatively unknown (although see O'Brien et al., 2013, 2015). The purpose of the current study is to investigate the neural mechanisms underlying cognitive gains following auditory-based cognitive training.

The current study employs computerized ACT in an attempt to improve auditory perception and cognition (attention, speed of processing) in older adults. ACT is a process-based training targeting certain neural circuits via perceptual information processing. Process-based training is hypothesized to lead to transfer to other tasks that engage the same or overlapping neural circuit(s) regardless of whether the other tasks were specifically trained (Jonides, 2004). ACT has a positive effect on behavior reflecting auditory perception, memory, attention, and speed of processing (Mahncke et al., 2006; Smith et al., 2009; Anderson et al., 2013) and there is some evidence for far transfer (Strenziok et al., 2014). However, the underlying mechanisms of these gains remain relatively unexplored. Most of the extant literature has measured efficacy of cognitive training behaviorally through neuropsychological and psychometric tests. Behavioral measures reflect combined effort stemming from several stages of processing (i.e., sensory, cognitive, and motor) and performance is influenced by outside factors such as motivation and physical function, making it difficult to draw conclusions about the neurophysiological processes underlying behavioral changes.

An alternate approach used in the current study is measuring event-related potentials (ERPs), which are averaged signals from electroencephalogram (EEG) time-locked to a perceptual and/or cognitive event. ERPs are reflective of ongoing brain activity and are particularly sensitive to the timing of mental processes (on the order of ms), such that early perceptual activity can be distinguished from post-perceptual cognitive processes (Luck and Kappenman, 2012). Of particular interest in the current study is the P1-N1-P2 complex and the P3b component. The P1-N1-P2 complex is a fronto-centrally occurring series of ERP components measuring the physiological response of the auditory cortex to a stimulus, reflective of the neural detection of sound (for a review, see Key et al., 2005). The effect of age on these components is unclear. Data from numerous studies show both increases and decreases to amplitudes and latencies with age depending on methodological differences such as the attentional demands of the task (for a review, see Čeponienė et al., 2008).

The P3b component is a posterior-parietal component thought to reflect the attentional resources allocated for categorization of a target (Donchin, 1981; Pfefferbaum et al., 1984; Kok, 2001). It is sensitive to target probability, with unexpected or deviant stimuli eliciting a larger P3b than stimuli occurring with a high probability. Effects of aging on the P3b show a more frontally distributed, attenuated P3b amplitude and longer P3b latency (Anderer et al., 1996; Polich, 1997). This is consistent with recent theories of cognitive aging (Davis et al., 2008; Park and Reuter-Lorenz, 2009) indicating that prefrontal cortex (PFC) processing is recruited to counteract sensory, cognitive, and physical brain changes associated with normal aging. O'Brien et al. (2013) demonstrated an increase in older adults' parietal P3b amplitude following process-based training in the visual modality compared to no-contact controls. Supporting evidence shows that P3b latency decreases after visual training are associated with better Useful Field of View performance (O'Brien et al., 2015).

In the present study, we predicted that ACT would result in improved attention consistent with previous evidence (Smith et al., 2009) and reflected cortically by a change in parietal P3b amplitude. Speed of processing improvements would be reflected in changes to parietal P3b latency. We also predicted that a frontal P3b would be present for all participants at baseline and would change following training. Also, if ACT impacts early cortical perception of auditory stimuli, we predicted a change to one or more components in the P1-N1-P2 complex in the form of amplitude or latency shifts, or a combination of both. Behavioral measures of cognition (Cognitive Self-Report Questionnaire, CSRQ) and speed of processing (Time-compressed speech, TCS) were included as corresponding evidence of neurophysiological changes. Changes in neurophysiological measures were predicted to correspond with changes in behavioral measures as a result of training.

MATERIALS AND METHODS

Participants

Twenty-four experimentally naïve healthy older adult subjects (17 female, mean age = 70.88 years, mean years of education = 15.29) participated in exchange for cognitive training (see **Table 1** for demographic information). Participants were recruited from a list compiled of older adults who contacted the lab in response to a newspaper article or an ad placed in

TABLE 1 | Summary statistics for participants by group.

Measure	Trained (n = 9)		Control (n = 15)	
	M %	**SD**	**M %**	**SD**
Age (years)	69.69	7.66	71.60	8.29
Sex (female)	[7]		[10]	
Race (Caucasian)	[9]		[13]	
Education (years)	15.00	2.06	15.47	2.72
PTA of right ear	11.85	10.75	26.22	14.27
PTA of left ear	16.67	6.92	29.44	14.70

PTA, pure tone average. Count in brackets.

local media. This study was carried out in accordance with the recommendations of the University of South Florida institutional review board with written informed consent from all subjects in accordance with the Declaration of Helsinki. The protocol was approved by the University of South Florida institutional review board.

Inclusion and Exclusion Criteria

Participants were required to: have a Mini-Mental State Examination (Folstein et al., 1975) score of 24 or greater (no severe cognitive impairment or dementia), have no self-reported neurological disorders, major strokes, or head injuries, have sufficient hearing (pure tone hearing thresholds <70 dB HL at 1000 and 2000 Hz in both ears), be a native English speaker, be available and willing to commit to the time and travel requirements of the study (maximum 22 visits), not be concurrently enrolled in another cognitive or training-related study, and not have previously completed a cognitive training program before participating.

Group Assignment

Training-eligible participants were randomly assigned to computer-based ACT using Brain Fitness© ($n = 9$) or a no-contact control group ($n = 15$). During recruitment, participants were informed that they would be receiving cognitive training either immediately after baseline testing or subsequent to a second testing session 10 weeks after their baseline session. Chi-square analysis showed no significant differences between groups based on sex, $p = 0.668$. Independent samples t-tests revealed no significant differences between the groups in age or education, $ts < 1$.

Measures
Audiometric Testing

A standard comprehensive audiometric evaluation was completed (American Speech-Language-Hearing Association, 2005) for both ears at octave frequencies between 250 and 8000 Hz to determine sufficient hearing to discern testing and training stimuli (pure tone hearing thresholds < 70 dB HL at 1000 and 2000 Hz in both ears). Testing was completed in a single-walled sound-treated booth suitable for audiometric testing. A three-frequency pure tone average (PTA) was calculated for each ear for using thresholds measured at 500, 1000, and 2000 Hz. PTAs lower than 25 dB are considered within normal hearing limits, 26–40 dB constitutes mild hearing loss, and moderate hearing loss at 41–55 dB. Participants in the trained group had PTAs ranging from 0 to 27 dB, significantly lower than those in the control group, $ps < 0.025$, which ranged from 5 to 55 dB (see **Table 1** for more descriptives).

Auditory Oddball Task

Frequent pure tone stimuli were presented (80% of the time) at 1000 Hz; oddball pure tone stimuli were presented (20% of the time) at 1500 Hz. Participants indicated the presence of an oddball stimulus by pressing a key on a computer keyboard. The task contained 8 blocks of 60 trials each (12 oddballs made up

20% and 48 frequents made up the remaining 80% of the stimuli presented) for a total of 480 stimuli (96 oddballs, 384 frequents) for each stimulus condition. The stimuli were 60 ms in duration and were presented at 80 dB SPL and the same wav file was used on each presentation. The task took approximately 15 min to complete.

Cognitive Self-Report Questionnaire (CSRQ)

The CSRQ is a 25-item self-report questionnaire comprising statements about an individual's self-reported perceptions of hearing, cognition, and mood (Spina et al., 2006). Participants are asked to rate each statement (e.g., "I have had trouble hearing conversations on the telephone"; "I have felt I have a good memory"; "I have been in a bad mood" on a 5-point Likert scale from 1 "Almost Always" to "Hardly Ever." The sum of all 25 items is calculated for a total score, with higher scores indicating more cognitive difficulties. The CSRQ has been reported to have excellent internal consistency ($\alpha = 0.91$) and good 2-month test–retest reliability ($r = 0.85$) and has been used as a pre-and-post cognitive training tool to examine cognitive training effects on hearing, cognition, and mood in older adults (Spina et al., 2006).

Time-Compressed Speech (TCS)

The TCS is a low redundancy measure of auditory processing speed in which speech is digitally accelerated (compressed) to resemble fast speech (Beasley et al., 1980). For the current study, the TCS stimuli comprised the Northwestern University Number 6 words. Fifty words spoken by a female were presented binaurally at a 65% compression rate. Immediately after each word presentation, the participant was asked to repeat the word, even if he or she was unsure of the answer. TCS performance was defined as the percent of words correctly recognized with higher scores indicating better performance. Performance typically decreases with age (Sticht and Gray, 1969; Gordon and Fitzgibbons, 2001). The TCS is a routinely used clinical measure for auditory processing deficits and has been previously validated in older adults (Letowski and Poch, 1996).

Procedure

Participants completed a screening visit to determine eligibility for the study and a baseline assessment of behavioral tasks (detailed above). EEG was recorded at baseline during performance of an auditory oddball task (detailed above). After baseline assessment, participants in the cognitive training group worked on computerized training exercises with the goal of completing a minimum of 16 training hours. Participants completed the auditory training program Brain Fitness (Posit Science). The program consists of six adaptive auditory exercises that are aimed at enhancing speed and accuracy of auditory processing. **Table 2** describes each exercise. The exercises are designed to simulate realistic listening contexts in a progressive fashion, moving from simple to complex auditory stimuli across exercises. Within each exercise, the stimuli become less discriminable and duration of stimulus presentation decreases as performance improves.

TABLE 2 | Brain fitness exercises.

Exercise	Description
Frequency sweeps	Identify order of tone sweeps; shorter & faster sweeps
Tell us apart	Discriminate speech syllables; decreasing differences between syllables and increasing speed
Match it	Identify and remember speech syllables; increasing number of items and speed
Sound replay	Remember and identify order of words; increasing number of words and speed
Listen and do	Remember and follow instructions; increasing complexity of instructions and speed
Story teller	Comprehend story and answer questions; increasing story length and speed

Training sessions were 60 min in duration, 2 days per week, for up to 10 weeks, based on prior study protocols of cognitive training (e.g., Edwards et al., 2002, 2005; Ball et al., 2007). On average, participants completed training in 62 days (Min = 56, Max = 70, SD = 6.01), missing at most 1 week between sessions. During each training session, individuals were required to take at least one 5-min break, and were allowed to take additional breaks as necessary. Based on prior findings that the interval between sessions could vary without affecting efficacy (Vance et al., 2007), participants could skip training days if necessary, although frequent or extended missing of sessions was discouraged. Participants were supervised by a trainer in a group computer lab setting. The trainer was present to ensure on-task participation for the full session, as well as to clarify task instructions and handle any technical difficulties if necessary. On average, participants completed 18.78 h of training (Min = 14, Max = 20, SD = 1.99). Following training, participants repeated the same behavioral and auditory oddball tasks as completed at baseline.

Participants in the no-contact control group completed a second testing session 10 weeks following their baseline assessment, during which they repeated the same behavioral and auditory oddball tasks as completed at baseline. They were then invited to complete 10 weeks of training. We chose a no-contact control because previous research of cognitive training has revealed no differences between no-contact and social- and computer-activity control conditions (Wadley et al., 2006) on behavioral outcome measures.

EEG Recording

Continuous EEG activity was recorded from 64 Ag/AgCl electrodes at standard 10/20 locations using Neuroscan™ (SCAN version 4.3.1) with a SynAmps2 amplifier, with a vertex midline electrode position halfway between Cz and CPz as reference. For five trained and five control participants, continuous EEG activity was recorded using the NuAmps (NuAmp, Neuroscan, Inc., El Paso, TX, United States) single-ended, 40-channel amplifier according to the NuAmps International 10–20 electrode system using a Quikcap with sintered Ag/AgCl electrodes, and a continuous acquisition system (Scan 4.3 Acquisition Software, Neuroscan, Inc.). A right mastoid electrode was used as a reference. For all participants, four additional electrodes were placed on the outer canthus of each eye and on the supra and infraorbital ridges of the left eye to monitor eye movement and blink activity. Data was sampled at 1000 Hz with a 100 Hz low pass filter (time constant: DC). Electrode impedances were kept below 5 kΩ for most electrodes.

The experiment took place in a dimly lit, sound-attenuating booth. A Pentium 4 PC running E-Prime 1.1 (Schneider et al., 2002) recorded behavioral data and presented auditory stimuli. Responses were registered using a keyboard.

Data Analysis and Predictions

Continuous EEG was high-pass filtered at a corner frequency of.1 Hz and low-pass filtered at a corner frequency of 30 Hz with a squared Butterworth zero-phase filter (12 dB/octave roll-off). Ocular artifact from eye movement and blinks were corrected for each subject by extracting the electroocular signals from the EEG. EEG for frequent and oddball trials was separated into epochs of 1000 ms (−200 ms before trial onset to 1200 ms after) and baseline corrected (−100 to 0 ms). Epochs in which EEG amplitude exceeded criteria of ±100 μV were rejected prior to averaging ($M = 6\%$, $MAX = 17\%$). Data were then averaged separately for each stimulus type (frequent, oddball). Data for the P3b component were re-referenced to averaged mastoids. Mean amplitudes and peak latencies were measured at parietal electrode site Pz and frontal electrode FCz for frequent and oddball stimuli in a 250 – 750 ms post-stimulus time window. Data for the P1-N1-P2 complex were re-referenced to a global reference. Mean amplitudes and peak latencies were measured at FCz for frequent stimuli in a 45 – 95 ms post-stimulus time window for P1, 105 – 155 ms post-stimulus time window for N1, and 225 – 275 ms post-stimulus time window for P2.

For each component, an Analysis of Variance (ANOVA) (or independent t-test where applicable) was first used to compare the two conditions at baseline, and repeated-measures ANOVA was used to examine training effects. All tests were two-sided and had an alpha level of.05. P3b analyses at Pz included within-participant factors of Testing Session and Stimulus Type, and the between-participants factor of Group. Effect sizes were calculated using omega squared (ω^2). A significant Testing Session × Stimulus Type × Group interaction for P3b amplitude was expected to support the hypothesis that attentional allocation is enhanced post-training and the same interaction for P3b latency was expected to support the hypothesis that speed of processing is enhanced post-training. Frontal P3b analyses at FCz were conducted in the same manner with the same expected results. P1-N1-P2 analyses for frequent stimuli included the within-participant factors of Testing Session and the between-participants factor of Group. For all the above analyses, follow-up ANOVAs and t-tests were conducted to examine any significant effects within each subgroup.

Behavioral data from the oddball task were analyzed with repeated measures ANOVAs including within-participant factors of Testing Session and the between-participants factor of Group. The auditory oddball task was designed to be very easy to ensure high accuracy rates to preserve as many trials as possible for the electrophysiological analyses. Therefore, behavior from the oddball task was not predicted to change following training.

TABLE 3 | Mean amplitudes and peak latencies for P3b and P1-N1-P2 at baseline and post-test per group.

| | Trained (n = 9) | | | | Control (n = 15) | | | |
| | Amplitude (μV) | | Latency (ms) | | Amplitude (μV) | | Latency (ms) | |
	Baseline	Post-test	Baseline	Post-test	Baseline	Post-test	Baseline	Post-test
P3b[a†]	5.14 (3.96)	3.12 (3.64)	473.78 (133.80)	397.89 (93.71)	3.12 (3.26)	3.21 (3.86)	509.07 (169.58)	445.07 (141.94)
P3b[a‡]	−0.17 (1.52)	−0.48 (1.03)	412.33 (204.69)	357.67 (143.44)	0.12 (1.04)	0.33 (0.81)	392.40 (177.92)	398.33 (168.62)
P3b[b†]	1.42 (4.93)	−0.84 (4.95)	531.33 (207.67)	505.89 (180.59)	2.75 (4.57)	2.41 (5.44)	414.07 (163.42)	475.27 (183.15)
P3b[b‡]	0.43 (1.08)	0.42 (1.10)	310.56 (162.90)	331.44 (154.46)	0.96 (1.09)	1.28 (1.54)	288.20 (72.31)	354.47 (187.56)
P1[b‡]	0.17 (0.53)	−0.16 (0.67)	61.67 (16.55)	66.89 (20.03)	0.14 (0.75)	0.23 (0.74)	68.40 (14.51)	66.93 (13.18)
N1[b‡]	−1.21 (1.11)	−1.67 (1.55)	122.89 (15.31)	124.67 (16.29)	−1.69 (1.55)	−1.85 (1.44)	128.07 (16.03)	124.47 (11.67)
P2[b‡]	2.50 (1.24)	2.21 (1.24)	243.22 (18.88)	249.89 (20.52)	1.73 (1.41)	1.89 (1.56)	245.20 (16.31)	247.73 (19.21)

a, electrode site Pz; b, electrode site FCz. Standard deviations in parentheses; †Oddball stimuli; ‡Frequent stimuli.

Due to the small sample size, the sample was underpowered to be able to detect behavioral changes in the two auditory behavioral measures (CSRQ and TCS). However, prior research (Smith et al., 2009) has documented the positive effect of ACT on the CSRQ.

Finally, Pearson correlations were conducted to determine the relationship between any significant neurophysiological training gains and changes in auditory behavior measures. Alpha was set to 0.05. Mean amplitudes and peak latencies for all components are reported in **Table 3**. Behavioral scores for the CSRQ and TCS are reported in **Table 4**. Effects relevant to the proposed hypotheses are summarized below and all main effects and interactions are reported in **Tables 5–9**.

RESULTS

Auditory Oddball Task Accuracy
Behavioral performance, accuracy for detecting the occurrence of oddballs, was above 99% (SDs below 2%) for both groups at both time points. ANOVA of behavioral accuracy revealed that performance did not significantly differ by group or by time, $Fs < 1$. Reaction times to oddball stimuli also did not significantly vary by group or time point, $ps > 0.200$.

Parietal P3b Amplitude
Figure 1 illustrates the grand average ERP waveforms of the oddball and frequent stimuli for the trained and control groups at both testing points at electrode Pz. ANOVA of initial P3b

TABLE 4 | Mean behavioral scores for Cognitive Self-Report Questionnaire and time-compressed speech at baseline and post-test per group.

| | Trained (n = 9) | | Control (n = 15) | |
	Baseline	Post-test	Baseline	Post-test
CSRQ*	61.25 (15.39)	56.50 (15.20)	56.87 (10.64)	58.33 (10.70)
TCS	68.22 (8.63)	66.22 (11.81)	48.00 (12.67)	54.13 (20.11)

*CSRQ, Cognitive Self-Report Questionnaire; TCS, time-compressed speech at 65% compression; *Score for one training group participant is missing (n = 8). Standard deviations in parentheses.*

amplitudes at baseline revealed that they did not significantly differ between groups, $F(1,22) = 1.17$, $p = 0.292$, $\omega^2 = 0.007$. When comparing P3b amplitudes across time, the hypothesized interaction between Stimulus Type, Testing Session, and Group was marginally significant, $F(1,22) = 4.01$, $p = 0.058$, $\omega^2 = 0.007$; there was also a significant interaction of Testing Session and Group $F(1,22) = 14.58$, $p < 0.001$, $\omega^2 = 0.025$. Follow-up analysis of the trained group showed a significant interaction of Stimulus Type and Testing Session, $F(1,8) = 11.03$, $p = 0.011$, $\omega^2 = 0.036$, reflecting a significant decrease in P3b amplitude to the oddball stimulus from baseline ($M = 5.14$, $SD = 3.96$) to post-test ($M = 3.12$, $SD = 3.64$), $t(8) = 5.60$, $p = 0.001$. There were no significant changes in amplitude across testing sessions after 10 weeks of no contact for the control group, $F < 1$.

Given the difference between the trained and control groups' hearing PTAs at baseline, it is possible that the pattern of results were associated with this difference. To test this, we removed six participants from the control group who had average PTAs greater than 2.5 SDs from that of the trained group to conduct sensitivity analyses. Initial P3b amplitudes at baseline did not significantly differ between groups, $F(1,16) = 1.32$, $p = 0.268$, $\omega^2 = 0.017$. When comparing P3b amplitudes across time, the hypothesized interaction between Stimulus Type, Testing Session, and Group was now not significant, $F(1,16) = 2.68$, $p = 0.121$, $\omega^2 = 0.005$; however, there was still a significant interaction of Testing Session and Group $F(1,22) = 13.20$, $p = 0.002$, $\omega^2 = 0.030$. Critically, there remained no significant changes in amplitude across testing sessions for the control group, $F < 1$.

Frontal P3b Amplitude
Figure 2 illustrates the grand average ERP waveforms of the oddball and frequent stimuli for the trained and control groups at both testing points at electrode FCz. ANOVA of initial P3b amplitudes at baseline revealed that they did not significantly differ between groups, $F < 1$. When comparing P3b amplitudes across time, the hypothesized interaction between Stimulus Type, Testing Session, and Group was not significant, $F(1,22) = 1.60$, $p = 0.220$, $\omega^2 = 0.002$. However, there was a significant interaction of Testing Session and Stimulus, $F(1,22) = 5.46$,

TABLE 5 | Results of P3b amplitude at Pz repeated measures ANOVA.

Variable	Overall			Trained			Control		
	F	p	ω^2	F	p	ω^2	F	p	ω^2
Group	0.07	0.797	−0.040	−	−	−	−	−	−
Testing session	8.66	0.008	0.014	30.12	0.001	0.070	0.42	0.529	−0.002
Stimulus type	23.70	<0.001	0.317	12.57	0.008	0.369	10.55	0.006	0.235
Group × testing session	14.58	0.001	0.025	−	−	−	−	−	−
Group × stimulus type	1.00	0.328	0.000	−	−	−	−	−	−
Testing session × stimulus type	5.37	0.030	0.011	11.03	0.011	0.036	0.06	0.817	−0.067
Group × testing session × stimulus type	4.01	0.058	0.007	−	−	−	−	−	−

TABLE 6 | Results of P3b amplitude at FCz repeated measures ANOVA.

Variable	Overall			Trained			Control		
	F	p	ω^2	F	p	ω^2	F	p	ω^2
Group	2.06	0.166	0.042	−	−	−	−	−	−
Testing session	3.50	0.075	0.009	11.82	0.009	0.044	0.00	0.988	−0.007
Stimulus type	0.40	0.532	−0.013	0.01	0.935	−0.057	1.29	0.274	0.010
Group × testing session	3.42	0.078	0.008	−	−	−	−	−	−
Group × stimulus type	0.59	0.452	−0.009	−	−	−	−	−	−
Testing session × stimulus type	5.46	0.029	0.016	7.38	0.026	0.040	0.66	0.432	−0.023
Group × testing session × stimulus type	1.60	0.220	0.002	−	−	−	−	−	−

TABLE 7 | Results of P3b latency at Pz and FCz repeated measures ANOVA.

Variable	Pz			FCz		
	F	p	ω^2	F	p	ω^2
Group	0.26	0.615	−0.032	0.46	0.503	−0.023
Testing session	5.63	0.027	0.026	1.81	0.192	0.005
Stimulus type	4.38	0.048	0.040	25.41	<0.001	0.215
Group × testing session	0.83	0.372	−0.001	2.09	0.162	0.007
Group × stimulus type	0.24	0.631	−0.009	1.36	0.256	0.004
Testing session × stimulus type	0.92	0.347	−0.001	0.38	0.542	−0.003
Group × testing session × stimulus type	0.26	0.613	−0.006	0.25	0.624	−0.004

TABLE 8 | Results of P1-N1-P2 Amplitudes at FCz Repeated Measures ANOVA.

Variable	P1			N1			P2		
	F	p	ω^2	F	p	ω^2	F	p	ω^2
Group	0.63	0.435	−0.015	0.39	0.539	−0.026	1.01	0.327	0.000
Testing session	0.13	0.723	−0.017	0.86	0.364	−0.002	0.00	0.965	−0.006
Group × testing session	1.22	0.282	0.004	0.24	0.630	−0.008	1.03	0.321	0.000

TABLE 9 | Results of P1-N1-P2 latencies at FCz repeated measures ANOVA.

Variable	P1			N1			P2		
	F	p	ω^2	F	p	ω^2	F	p	ω^2
Group	0.33	0.574	−0.029	0.22	0.643	−0.034	0.00	0.990	−0.043
Testing session	0.14	0.712	−0.007	0.26	0.617	−0.009	1.23	0.280	0.002
Group × testing session	1.35	0.257	0.003	0.70	0.413	−0.004	0.30	0.592	−0.007

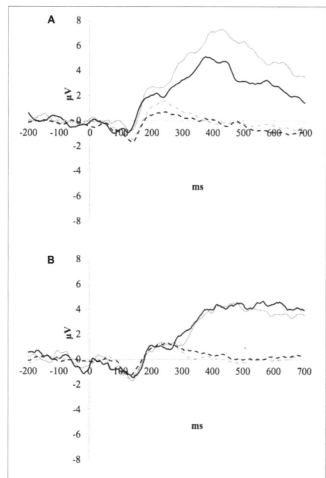

FIGURE 1 | (A) Grand average ERP waveforms of the oddball (solid line) and frequent (dotted line) stimuli for the trained group at baseline (gray line) and post-test (black line) at electrode Pz. **(B)** Grand average ERP waveforms of the oddball (solid line) and frequent (dotted line) stimuli for the control group at baseline (gray line) and post-test (black line) at electrode Pz.

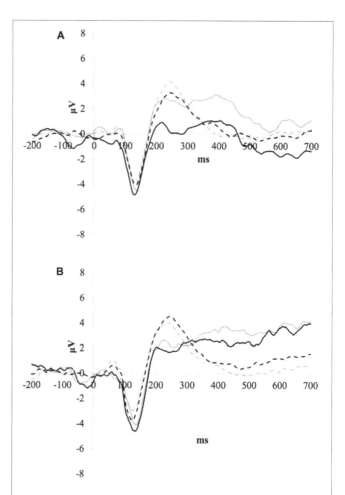

FIGURE 2 | (A) Grand average ERP waveforms of the oddball (solid line) and frequent (dotted line) stimuli for the trained group at baseline (gray line) and post-test (black line) at electrode FCz. **(B)** Grand average ERP waveforms of the oddball (solid line) and frequent (dotted line) stimuli for the control group at baseline (gray line) and post-test (black line) at electrode Pz.

$p = 0.029$, $\omega^2 = 0.016$ and a marginally significant interaction of Testing Session and Group, $F(1,22) = 3.42$, $p = 0.078$, $\omega^2 = 0.008$.

Given these effects and the *a priori* hypothesis of frontal shifts of P3b with aging, we conducted follow-up analyses to determine if significant P3b amplitude decreases occurred frontally as well for trained participants. Follow-up analysis of the trained group showed a significant interaction of Stimulus Type and Testing Session, $F(1,8) = 7.38$, $p = 0.026$, $\omega^2 = 0.040$, indeed reflecting a decrease in P3b amplitude to the oddball stimulus from baseline ($M = 1.42$, $SD = 4.93$) to post-test ($M = -0.84$ $SD = 4.95$), $t(8) = 3.28$, $p = 0.011$. There were no significant changes in amplitude across testing sessions after 10 weeks of no contact for the control group, $F < 1$.

P3b and Frontal P3b Latencies

ANOVA of initial P3b latencies at baseline revealed that they did not significantly differ between groups, $F < 1$. When comparing P3b latencies across time, there was a significant main effect of

Testing Session, $F(1,22) = 5.63$, $p = 0.027$, $\omega^2 = 0.026$. P3b latencies decreased from baseline ($M = 447.85$, $SD = 132.63$) to post-testing ($M = 405.23$, $SD = 121.31$), with no significant interaction of Group or Stimulus Type, $Fs < 1$. There were no noteworthy significant latency effects at the frontal P3b.

P1-N1-P2 Amplitude and Latencies

Figure 3 illustrates the grand average ERP waveforms of the frequent stimuli for the trained and control groups at both testing points. Comparison of initial P1-N1-P2 amplitudes and latencies at baseline revealed that neither significantly differed between groups, $ps > 0.187$. When comparing P1-N1-P2 amplitudes across time, there were no significant effects of time, group, or interactions for any of the three components, $ps > 0.281$. This was also the case for P1-N1-P2 latencies, $ps > 0.256$.

ERP Correlations with Behavioral Data

To determine whether significant training effects on the P3b component corresponded with positive auditory behavioral

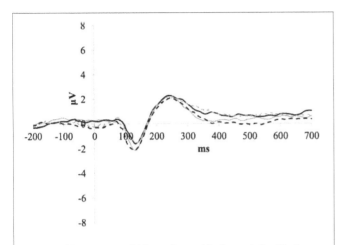

FIGURE 3 | Grand average ERP waveforms of the frequent stimuli for the trained (solid line) and control (dotted line) groups at baseline (gray) and post-test (black) at electrode FCz.

gains, we first conducted a Pearson correlation between posterior P3b amplitude differences and differences self-reported perceptions of cognition (CSRQ) from baseline to post-test. A significant positive correlation was found between scores on the CSRQ and P3b amplitudes, with larger P3b amplitudes for the individuals with more self-reported auditory cognitive difficulties, $r = 0.53$, $p = 0.010$. We also conducted a Person correlation between posterior P3b latency differences and differences in our behavioral measure of auditory processing speed (TCS) from baseline to post-test, which was not significant, $p = 0.501$.

DISCUSSION

The goal of the current study was to elucidate the role of ACT on attentional and perceptual processing as measured by ERPs to help determine the underlying mechanisms of training gains and transfer. We provide electrophysiological evidence showing that engaging in process-based ACT can enhance attentional mechanisms in older adults.

Training-Related Effect on P3b Amplitude

P3b amplitude is considered to reflect the attentional resources involved in comparing a significant or relevant event with an internal representation to categorize as a match or mismatch (Kok, 2001). Rare events, as a mismatch to internal representations, typically capture more attentional resources and result in larger P3b amplitudes than expected frequent events. Consistent with this, oddball stimuli (rare events) did elicit a larger P3b than frequent stimuli for both groups at both testing time points in the current study. However, oddball stimuli elicited a P3b following ACT that was smaller compared to pre-training amplitudes, while oddball amplitudes showed no change for controls across time. There was no significant difference between groups in baseline P3b amplitudes for oddball stimuli, but visual

inspection shows a descriptively larger baseline amplitude for the trained group compared to the control group (see **Table 3**, **Figure 1**). Further study is needed to determine how baseline differences in cognitive abilities such as attention may impact neurophysiological measures after training.

While decreases in P3b amplitude are usually interpreted as diminished attentional resources, it is also possible that decreased P3b amplitude reflects diminished allocation due to the need for fewer attentional resources to categorize a stimulus. This interpretation suggests that ACT leads to an efficiency of attentional resource allocation and/or interaction with working memory updating. There is some prior evidence to support this hypothesis. Using meditation training, which promotes a broader attentional state, Slagter et al. (2007, 2009) showed decreased P3b amplitude to the first target in an attentional blink task following training compared to untrained controls. The attentional blink task requires attention to a rapid stream of stimuli and the subsequent report of two embedded target stimuli. Ability to report the second target in the stream is typically reduced if it appears within 500 ms after the first target ("attentional blink," Raymond et al., 1992). A reduction in P3b amplitude to the first target suggests that training improved efficiency of attentional engagement such that resources were not solely devoted to the first target and were instead balanced between the two. In support of this, behavioral results showed a parallel reduction in the attentional blink following training. Mindfulness training has also been shown to reduce the P3b amplitude to incongruent words in a Stroop task possibly reflecting more efficient allocation of attentional resources during stimulus processing (Moore et al., 2012).

In a sample of young adults, Ben-David et al. (2010) showed a reduction in the late positive complex (LPC), a parietal response of which P3b is considered to be a subcomponent (Rushby et al., 2005), following an hour of auditory perceptual training of speech sounds. This was interpreted to reflect improvement in stimulus categorization and perceptual processes and possibly improvement in memory updating. Interestingly, Ben-David et al. (2010) showed the opposite effect of speech sound practice on the LPC, an increased LPC amplitude following training. They cite differences in experimental design between the two studies as a possible cause of amplitude reversal. Similar to this, O'Brien et al. (2015) reported larger P3b amplitudes following visual cognitive training compared to controls. In addition to being in a different modality, the oddball task used in their study was significantly more complex involving locating a perceptually different (tilted) target among an array of identical (horizontal) distractors. The possibility that visual and auditory process-based training impacts P3b amplitude differently needs to be further explored.

P3b amplitude was also significantly correlated with participants' self-reported perceptions of their own auditory cognition (CSRQ). Participants who reported more cognitive difficulties had larger P3b amplitudes compared to those with fewer cognitive difficulties. ACT has previously been shown to result in CSRQ self-reported improvements by participants (Smith et al., 2009), suggesting that the neurophysiological changes occurring due to training may be behaviorally significant. Taken together, these findings show that a reduction in P3b amplitude can reflect efficiency in attentional resource allocation, such as flexibility in engaging and disengaging from relevant target stimuli. Attentional resource allocation following ACT is likely more efficient, resulting in fewer resources needed to categorize an oddball stimulus.

Training-Related Effect on Frontal P3b Amplitude

Auditory cognitive training also resulted in a marginally significant decrease in frontal P3b amplitude compared to untrained controls. P3b activity shifts to a more frontal distribution with age and this shift has been interpreted as reflecting frontal lobe activity (for meta-analysis studies supporting this, see Friedman et al., 1997). Friedman and colleagues (Friedman et al., 1993; Friedman and Simpson, 1994; Fabiani and Friedman, 1995) report that older adults have two scalp distributions in response to auditory oddball stimuli – one frontal and the other parietal – suggesting that older adults activate frontal lobe processes to help encode these stimuli. Frontal areas are often activated in target detection tasks, corresponding with P3b generation (for reviews, see Polich, 2003; Fjell et al., 2007). As previously described, current theories of cognitive aging propose that PFC processing is recruited for cognitive tasks to compensate for parietal network functions that decline with age. Reduction in amplitude of the frontal P3b following training suggests that ACT potentially reduces the demand for PFC recruitment during attention processing.

P3b Latency Changes

P3b latency did not show any change based on training as hypothesized but instead showed an effect of testing. Participants showed faster processing for both stimuli types during their post-test regardless of whether they were in the training or the control group. This is consistent with evidence that P3b latency reliability in an auditory oddball task is low in older adults both within a session ($r = 0.07–0.24$) and from 1 year to the next ($r = 0.14–0.40$) (Walhovd and Fjell, 2002). In addition, the correlation between P3b latency and behavioral auditory processing speed (TCS) was not significant.

Auditory cognitive training is designed to target speed of processing and has previously been shown to improve auditory processing speed in a sample of healthy older adults (Anderson et al., 2013) as well as in a sample of older adults with heart failure (Athilingam et al., 2015). It is possible that P3b latency as a measure of processing speed in the current study did not have enough power to detect an effect given the inconsistencies likely occurring within subjects. However, it is also possible that ACT primarily enhances allocation of attention rather than speed of processing.

No P1-N1-P2 Changes

Auditory cognitive training did not impact auditory perceptual processing in the current study, as measured by P1-N1-P2 amplitude and latency. Enhancements in subcortical neural timing and speech perception following ACT have previously

been observed using evoked potentials representing auditory brainstem responses to a speech syllable in noise (Anderson et al., 2013). It is possible that changes to early auditory perception following ACT are only measurable subcortically and that our later ERP measure was insensitive to these changes. The stimuli used in the current study – pure tones in quiet – were likely much easier to perceive than the speech in noise condition used in Anderson et al. (2013) study and it is therefore plausible that the insensitivity of our measure is due to a ceiling effect.

Limitations

A significant limitation to this study is the small sample size. Randomized controlled studies involving cognitive training with older adults across a significant period of time are resource-intensive and prone to high levels of attrition for multiple reasons (e.g., voluntary withdrawal of consent, no longer meeting inclusion/exclusion criteria during course of study, poor adherence to training regimen). A large-scale, multi-site trial investigating the cognitive impact of ACT in older adults has been conducted (Smith et al., 2009), but this did not include any ERP measures to determine underlying mechanisms of training gains. To further investigate these underlying mechanisms, a study using neurophysiological measures similar in scope to Smith et al. (2009), utilizing intent-to-treat analysis modeling for attrition needs to be conducted.

Study demographics (primarily female, Caucasian, and well educated) also limit the interpretation of the current findings. Given the proposal that ACT targets speed of processing, and the current finding that ACT benefits attention and not speed of processing, multiple converging measures of these two functions should be included in future studies to clarify their role in training gains. Finally, the impact of ACT on functional outcomes as well as the long-term maintenance of training gains need to be investigated.

CONCLUSION

The present finding of decreased P3b amplitudes following ACT reinforces the hypothesis that there is plasticity in the attentional control systems of older adults. Control over attentional resource allocation is vulnerable to age-related decline, but is shown here to be ameliorated by ACT. In light of previous findings demonstrating that portions of this training program result in improved cognition and transfer of gains to functional tasks (e.g., Smith et al., 2009; Anderson et al., 2013; Strenziok et al., 2014), our study is the first to provide preliminary neurophysiological evidence that ACT may particularly be enhancing the efficiency of attention allocation, which may account for the positive impact of ACT on the everyday functioning of older adults.

AUTHOR CONTRIBUTIONS

JO, JL, GC, and JE contributed to the conception and design of the work; JO and GC contributed to the acquisition of the data, JO, JL, BF, GC, and JE contributed to the analysis and interpretation of the data, drafted the work, JO, JL, BF, and JE revised the work critically for important intellectual content, JO, JL, BF, GC, and JE gave final approval of the version to be published and agree to be accountable for all aspects of the work.

ACKNOWLEDGMENTS

Special thanks to Courtney Matthews and Amanda Brandino for assistance in data collection.

REFERENCES

Akeroyd, M. A. (2008). Are individual differences in speech reception related to individual differences in cognitive ability? A survey of 20 experimental studies with normal and hearing-impaired adults. *Int. J. Audiol.* 47, S53–S71. doi: 10.1080/14992020802301142

American Speech-Language-Hearing Association (2005). Guidelines for manual pure-tone threshold audiometry. *ASHA* 20, 297–301.

Anderer, P., Semlitsch, H. V., and Saletu, B. (1996). Multichannel auditory event-related brain potentials: effects of normal aging on the scalp distribution of N1, P2, N2 and P300 latencies and amplitudes. *Electroencephalogr. Clin. Neurophysiol.* 99, 458–472. doi: 10.1016/S0013-4694(96)96518-9

Anderson, S., White-Schwoch, T., Parbery-Clarka, A., and Kraus, N. (2013). Reversal of age-related neural timing delays with training. *Proc. Natl. Acad. Sci. U.S.A.* 110, 4357–4362. doi: 10.1073/pnas.1213555110

Arlinger, S., Lunner, T., Lyxell, B., and Pichora-Fuller, M. K. (2009). The emergence of cognitive hearing science. *Scand. J. Psychol.* 50, 371–384. doi: 10.1111/j.1467-9450.2009.00753.x

Athilingam, P., Edwards, J. D., Valdes, E. G., Ji, M., and Guglin, M. (2015). Computerized auditory cognitive training to improve cognition and functional outcomes in patients with heart failure: results of a pilot study. *Heart Lung* 44, 120–128. doi: 10.1016/j.hrtlng.2014.12.004

Ball, K., Edwards, J. D., and Ross, L. A. (2007). The impact of speed of processing training on cognitive and everyday functions. *J. Gerontol. B Psychol. Sci. Soc. Sci.* 62, 19–31. doi: 10.1093/geronb/62.special_issue_1.19

Beasley, D. S., Bratt, G. W., and Rintelmann, W. F. (1980). Intelligibility of time-compressed sentential stimuli. *J. Speech Lang. Hear. Res.* 23, 722–731. doi: 10.1044/jshr.2304.722

Ben-David, B. M., Campeanu, S., Tremblay, K. L., and Alain, C. (2010). Auditory evoked potentials dissociate rapid perceptual learning from task repetition without learning. *Psychophysiology* 48, 797–807. doi: 10.1111/j.1469-8986.2010.01139.x

Čeponienė, R., Westerfield, M., Torki, M., and Townsend, J. (2008). Modality-specificity of sensory aging in vision and audition: evidence from event-related potentials. *Brain Res.* 1215, 53–68. doi: 10.1016/j.brainres.2008.02.010

Ciorba, A., Bianchini, C., Pelucchi, S., and Pastore, A. (2012). The impact of hearing loss on the quality of life of elderly adults. *Clin. Interv. Aging* 7, 159–163. doi: 10.2147/CIA.S26059

Dalton, D. S., Cruickshanks, K. J., Klein, B. E., Klein, R., Wiley, T. L., and Nondahl, D. M. (2003). The impact of hearing loss on quality of life in older adults. *Gerontologist* 43, 661–668. doi: 10.1093/geront/43.5.661

Davis, S. W., Dennis, N. A., Daselaar, S. M., Fleck, M. S., and Cabeza, R. (2008). Qué PASA? The posterior-anterior shift in aging. *Cereb. Cortex* 18, 1201–1209. doi: 10.1093/cercor/bhm155

Donchin, E. (1981). Surprise!... Surprise? *Psychophysiology* 18, 493–513. doi: 10.1111/j.1469-8986.1981.tb01815.x

Edwards, J. D., Wadley, V. G., Myers, R. S., Roenker, D. L., Cissell, G. M., and Ball, K. (2002). Transfer of a speed of processing intervention to near and far cognitive functions. *Gerontology* 48, 329–340. doi: 10.1159/000065259

Edwards, J. D., Wadley, V. G., Vance, D. E., Wooda, K., Roenker, D. L., and Ball, K. (2005). The impact of speed of processing training on cognitive and everyday performance. *Aging Ment. Health* 9, 262–271. doi: 10.1080/13607860412331336788

Fabiani, M., and Friedman, D. (1995). Changes in brain activity patterns in aging: the novelty oddball. *Psychophysiology* 32, 579–594. doi: 10.1111/j.1469-8986.1995.tb01234.x

Fjell, A. M., Walhovd, K. B., Fischl, B., and Reinvang, I. (2007). Cognitive function, P3a/P3b brain potentials, and cortical thickness in aging. *Hum. Brain Mapp.* 28, 1098–1116. doi: 10.1002/hbm.20335

Folstein, M. F., Folstein, S. E., and McHugh, P. R. (1975). "Mini-mental state". A practical method for grading the cognitive state of patients for the clinician. *J. Psychiatr. Res.* 12, 189–198. doi: 10.1016/0022-3956(75)90026-6

Friedman, D., Kazmerski, V., and Fabiani, M. (1997). An overview of age-related changes in the scalp distribution of P3b. *Electroencephalogr. Clin. Neurophysiol.* 104, 498–513. doi: 10.1016/S0168-5597(97)00036-1

Friedman, D., and Simpson, G. (1994). ERP amplitude and scalp distribution to target and novel events: effects of temporal order in young, middle-aged and older adults. *Cogn. Brain Res.* 2, 49–63. doi: 10.1016/0926-6410(94)90020-5

Friedman, D., Simpson, G., and Hamberger, M. (1993). Age-related changes in scalp topography to novel and target stimuli. *Psychophysiology* 30, 383–396. doi: 10.1111/j.1469-8986.1993.tb02060.x

Gordon, S., and Fitzgibbons, P. J. (2001). Sources of age-related recognition difficulty for time-compressed speech. *J. Speech Lang. Hear. Res.* 44, 709–719.

Harrison Bush, A. L., Lister, J. J., Edwards, J. D., Lin, F., and Betz, J. (2015). Peripheral hearing and cognition: evidence from the staying keen in later life (SKILL) study. *Ear Hear.* 36, 395–407. doi: 10.1097/AUD.0000000000000142

Humes, L., Dubno, J. R., Gordon-Salant, S., Lister, J. J., Cacace, A. T., Cruickshanks, K. J., et al. (2012). Central presbycusis: a review and evaluation of the evidence. *J. Am. Acad. Audiol.* 23, 635–666. doi: 10.3766/jaaa.23.8.5

Jonides, J. (2004). How does practice makes perfect? *Nat. Neurosci.* 7, 10–11. doi: 10.1038/nn0104-10

Key, A. P. F., Dove, G. O., and Maguire, M. J. (2005). Linking brainwaves to the brain: an ERP primer. *Dev. Neuropsychol.* 27, 183–215. doi: 10.1207/s15326942dn2702_1

Kok, A. (2001). On the utility of P3 amplitude as a measure of processing capacity. *Psychophysiology* 38, 557–577. doi: 10.1017/S0048577201990559

Letowski, T., and Poch, N. (1996). Comprehension of time-compressed speech: effects of age and speech complexity. *J. Am. Acad. Audiol.* 7, 447–457. doi: 10.1121/1.408759

Li, C., Zhang, X., Hoffman, H. J., Cotch, M. F., Themann, C. L., and Wilson, M. R. (2014). Hearing impairment associated with depression in us adults, national health and nutrition examination survey 2005-2010. *JAMA Otolaryngol. Head Neck Surg.* 140, 293–302. doi: 10.1001/jamaoto.2014.42

Lin, F. R. (2011). Hearing loss and cognition among older adults in the United States. *J. Gerontol. A Biol. Sci. Med. Sci.* 66, 1131–1136. doi: 10.1093/gerona/glr115

Lin, F. R., Ferrucci, L., Metter, E. J., An, Y., Zonderman, A. B., and Resnick, S. M. (2011a). Hearing loss and cognition in the Baltimore longitudinal study of aging. *Neuropsychology* 25, 763–770. doi: 10.1037/a0024238

Lin, F. R., Metter, E. J., O'Brien, R. J., Resnick, S. M., Zonderman, A. B., and Ferrucci, L. (2011b). Hearing loss and incident dementia. *Arch. Neurol.* 68, 214–220. doi: 10.1001/archneurol.2010.362

Lin, F. R., Thorpe, R., Gordon-Salant, S., and Ferrucci, L. (2011c). Hearing loss prevalence and risk factors among older adults in the United States. *J. Gerontol. A Biol. Sci. Med. Sci.* 66A, 582–590. doi: 10.1093/gerona/glr002

Lin, F. R., Yaffe, K., Xia, J., Xue, Q. L., Harris, T. B., Purchase-Helzner, E., et al. (2013). Hearing loss and cognitive decline in older adults. *J. Am. Med. Assoc.* 173, 293–299. doi: 10.1001/jamainternmed.2013.1868

Luck, S. J., and Kappenman, E. S. (2012). "ERP components and selective attention," in *The Oxford Handbook of Event-Related Potential Components*, ed. P. E. Nathan (New York, NY: Oxford University Press).

Mahncke, H. W., Connor, B. B., Appelman, J., Ahsanuddin, O. N., Hardy, J. L., Wood, R. A., et al. (2006). Memory enhancement in healthy older adults using a brain plasticity-based training program: a randomized, controlled study. *Proc. Natl. Acad. Sci. U.S.A.* 103, 12523–12528. doi: 10.1073/pnas.0605194103

Mick, P., Kawachi, I., and Lin, F. R. (2014). The association between hearing loss and social isolation in older adults. *Otolaryngol. Head Neck Surg.* 150, 378–384. doi: 10.1177/0194599813518021

Moore, A., Gruber, T., Derose, J., and Malinowski, P. (2012). Regular, brief mindfulness meditation practice improves electrophysiological markers of attentional control. *Front. Hum. Neurosci.* 6:18. doi: 10.3389/fnhum.2012.00018

National Institute on Deafness and Other Communication Disorders [NIDCD] (2010). *Quick Statistics.* Available at: http://www.nidcd.nih.gov/health/statistics/pages/quick.aspx [accessed August 15, 2014].

O'Brien, J. L., Edwards, J. D., Maxfield, N. D., Peronto, C. L., Williams, V. A., and Lister, J. J. (2013). Cognitive training and selective attention in the aging brain: an electrophysiological study. *Clin. Neurophysiol.* 124, 2198–2208. doi: 10.1016/j.clinph.2013.05.012

O'Brien, J. L., Lister, J. J., Peronto, C. L., and Edwards, J. D. (2015). Perceptual and cognitive neural correlates of the Useful Field of View test in older adults. *Brain Res.* 1624, 167–174. doi: 10.1016/j.brainres.2015.07.032

Park, D. C., and Reuter-Lorenz, P. (2009). The adaptive brain: aging and neurocognitive scaffolding. *Annu. Rev. Psychol.* 60, 173–196. doi: 10.1146/annurev.psych.59.103006.093656

Pfefferbaum, A., Ford, J. M., Wenegrat, B. G., Roth, W. T., and Kopell, B. S. (1984). Clinical application of the P3 component of event-related potentials. *Electroencephalogr. Clin. Neurophysiol.* 59, 85–103. doi: 10.1016/0168-5597(84)90026-1

Pichora-Fuller, M. K., Kramer, S. E., Eckert, M. A., Edwards, B., Hornsby, B. W. Y., Humes, L., et al. (2016). Hearing impairment and cognitive energy: the framework for understanding effortful listening (FUEL). *Ear Hear.* 37, 5S–27S.

Polich, J. (1997). EEG and ERP assessment of normal aging. *Electroencephalogr. Clin. Neurophysiol.* 104, 244–256. doi: 10.1016/S0168-5597(97)96139-6

Polich, J. (2003). "Theoretical overview of P3a and P3b," in *Detection of Change: Event-Related Potential and fMRI Findings*, ed. J. Polich (Boston, MA: Springer), 83–98.

Raymond, J. E., Shapiro, K. L., and Arnell, K. M. (1992). Temporary suppression of visual processing in an RSVP task: An attentional blink? *J. Exp. Psychol. Hum. Percept. Perform.* 18, 849–860. doi: 10.1037/0096-1523.18.3.849

Rushby, J. A., Barry, R. J., and Doherty, R. J. (2005). Separation of the components of the late positive complex in an ERP dishabituation paradigm. *Clin.*

Neurophysiol. 116, 2363–2380. doi: 10.1016/j.clinph.2005.06.008

Schneider, W., Eschman, A., and Zuccolotto, A. (2002). *E-Prime User's Guide.* Pittsburgh, PA: Psychology Software Tools, Inc.

Slagter, H. A., Lutz, A., Greischar, L. L., Francis, A. D., Nieuwenhuis, S., Davis, J. M., et al. (2007). Mental training affects distribution of limited brain resources. *PLOS Biol.* 5:e138. doi: 10.1371/journal.pbio.0050138

Slagter, H. A., Lutz, A., Greischar, L. L., Nieuwenhuis, S., and Davidson, R. J. (2009). Theta phase synchrony and conscious target perception: impact of intensive mental training. *J. Cogn. Neurosci.* 21, 1536–1549. doi: 10.1162/jocn.2009.21125

Smith, G. E., Housen, P., Yaffe, K., Ruff, R., Kennison, R. F., Mahncke, H. W., et al. (2009). A cognitive training program based on principles of brain plasticity: results from the improvement in memory with plasticity-based adaptive cognitive training (IMPACT) study. *J. Am. Geriatr. Soc.* 57, 594–603. doi: 10.1111/j.1532-5415.2008.02167.x

Spina, L. M. R., Ruff, R. M., and Mahncke, H. W. (2006). *Cognitive Self-Report Questionnaire (CSRQ) Manual.* San Francisco, CA: Posit Science Corporation.

Sticht, T. G., and Gray, B. B. (1969). The intelligibility of time compressed words as a function of age and hearing loss. *J. Speech Lang. Hear. Res.* 12, 443–448. doi: 10.1044/jshr.1202.443

Strenziok, M., Parasuraman, R., Clarke, E., Cisler, D. S., Thompson, J. C., and Greenwood, P. M. (2014). Neurocognitive enhancement in older adults: comparison of three cognitive training tasks to test a hypothesis of training transfer in brain connectivity. *Neuroimage* 85, 1027–1039. doi: 10.1016/j.neuroimage.2013.07.069

Vance, D., Dawson, J., Wadley, V., Edwards, J. D., Roenker, D., Rizzo, M., et al. (2007). The accelerate study: the longitudinal effect of speed of processing training on cognitive performance of older adults. *Rehabil. Psychol.* 52, 89–96. doi: 10.1037/0090-5550.52.1.89

Wadley, V. G., Benz, R. L., Ball, K., Roenker, D. L., Edwards, J. D., and Vance, D. E. (2006). Development and evaluation of home-based speed-of-processing training for older adults. *Arch. Phys. Med. Rehabil.* 87, 757–763. doi: 10.1016/j.apmr.2006.02.027

Walhovd, K. B., and Fjell, A. M. (2002). One-year test–retest reliability of auditory ERPs in young and old adults. *Int. J. Psychophysiol.* 46, 29–40. doi: 10.1016/S0167-8760(02)00039-9

19

Altered Neuronal Activity Topography Markers in the Elderly with Increased Atherosclerosis

Takashi Shibata[1]*, Toshimitu Musha[2], Yukio Kosugi[2], Michiya Kubo[1], Yukio Horie[1],
Naoya Kuwayama[3], Satoshi Kuroda[3], Karin Hayashi[4], Yohei Kobayashi[2], Mieko Tanaka[2],
Haruyasu Matsuzaki[2,5], Kiyotaka Nemoto[6] and Takashi Asada[7]

[1] Department of Neurosurgery, Stroke Center, Saiseikai Toyama Hospital, Toyama, Japan, [2] Brain Functions Laboratory Inc.,
Yokohama, Japan, [3] Department of Neurosurgery, Graduate School of Medicine and Pharmacological Science, University of
Toyama, Toyama, Japan, [4] Department of Neuropsychiatry, Toho University Medical Center Sakura Hospital, Chiba, Japan,
[5] Department of Medical Course, Teikyo Heisei University, Tokyo, Japan, [6] Department of Neuropsychiatry, Institute of Clinical
Medicine, University of Tsukuba, Tsukuba, Japan, [7] Department of Neuropsychiatry, University of Tokyo Medical and Dental
University, Tokyo, Japan

*Correspondence:
Takashi Shibata
sibata@dj8.so-net.ne.jp

Background: Previously, we reported on vascular cognitive impairment (VCI) templates, consisting of patients with VCI associated with carotid stenosis (>60%) using a quantitative electroencephalographic (EEG) technique called neuronal activity topography (NAT). Here using the VCI templates, we investigated the hypothesis that internal carotid artery–intima-media thickness (ICA–IMT) is associated with EEG spectrum intensity (sNAT) and spectrum steepness (vNAT).

Methods: A total of 221 community-dwelling elderly subjects were recruited. Four groups were classified according to quartiles of ICA–IMT as assessed by ultrasonography: control group A, normal ($\leq$0.9 mm); group B, mild atherosclerosis (1−1.1 mm); group C, moderate atherosclerosis (1.2−1.8 mm); and group D, severe atherosclerosis ($\geq$1.9 mm). EEG markers of power ratio index (PRI), and the binary likelihood of being in the VCI group vs. the that of being in control group A ($sL_{x:VCI-A}$, $vL_{x:VCI-A}$) were assessed, respectively. Differences in mean total scores for PRI, $sL_{x:VCI-A}$, $vL_{x:VCI-A}$, between control group A and the other groups were compared using Dunnett's test, respectively.

Results: The mean total scores of the PRI were 3.25, 3.00, 2.77, and 2.26 for groups A, B, C, and D, respectively. There was a significant decrease in the PRI in group D compared with group A ($P = 0.0066$). The mean total scores of the $sL_{x:VCI-A}$ were −0.14, −0.11, −0.1, and −0.03 for groups A, B, C, and D, respectively. The $sL_{x:VCI-A}$ in group D was significantly higher compared to that in group A ($P < 0.0001$). The mean total scores of the $vL_{x:VCI-A}$ were −0.04,−0.01, 0.01, and 0.06 for group A, B, C, and D, respectively. The $vL_{x:VCI-A}$ in group D and group C was significantly higher compared to that in group A, respectively ($P < 0.0001$, $P = 0.02$).

Conclusion: Community-dwelling elderly subjects in the increased carotid atherosclerosis of ICA–IMT ($\geq$1.9 mm) were at greatest risk of an EEG change as assessed by NAT.

Keywords: EEG, vascular cognitive impairment, neuronal activity topography, atherosclerosis, elderly

INTRODUCTION

The carotid bifurcation and the proximal part of the internal carotid artery (ICA) are predilection sites for atherosclerotic plaques. Changes in the ICA–intima-media thickness (IMT) in this area, as assessed by ultrasonography, are a first sign of subclinical atherosclerosis (Polak et al., 2010; Bauer et al., 2012). Ultrasonography is an easily accessible and noninvasive method to measure different stages of the carotid artery atherosclerotic process, and it is widely used in clinical assessments and for epidemiological and clinical research (Arntzen and Mathiesen, 2011).

Carotid disease is a known risk factor for stroke and vascular cognitive impairment (VCI), but the relationship between carotid artery stenosis and cognitive function in asymptomatic people is unclear. The role of subclinical atherosclerosis in cognitive function can be studied by ultrasound measurement of the carotid arteries and neuropsychological tests. Previous studies indicate that patients with carotid stenosis have markedly poorer scores on cognitive tests compared with control subjects (Rao, 2001; Johnston et al., 2004; Mathiesen et al., 2004; Arntzen and Mathiesen, 2011). One cross-sectional study found that subjects with carotid stenosis (>35%) had lower levels of performance on cognitive function tests than subjects without stenosis (Mathiesen et al., 2004). In a cohort from the Cardiovascular Health Study (Haan et al., 1999), cognitive decline was markedly increased in subjects with an ICA–IMT > 2.01 mm. Most patients with subclinical carotid atherosclerosis have only minor impairments of cognitive function, and standard tests (e.g., the Mini-Mental State Examination: MMSE) are not sufficiently sensitive to detect such impairments. However, early detection of VCI is of particular importance because pharmacological intervention to prevent or delay dementia will prove effective for most patients with subclinical carotid atherosclerosis.

Electroencephalographic (EEG) signals are generated by electrical activity in the brain and are rich in information regarding cerebral function. In 2013, Musha et al developed a neuroimaging tool called Neuronal Activity Topography (NAT), which gives direct information on neuronal activity using quantitative EEG analysis (Musha et al., 2013). This tool categorizes cerebral neuronal activity by EEG spectrum intensity (sNAT) and spectrum steepness (vNAT). NAT consists of 210 submarkers referring to 10 frequency components ranging from 4 to 20 Hz (more precisely, from 4.7 to 18.8 Hz). Each submarker has its own role in the characterization of cerebral neuronal activity, which is represented by the 210-dimensional NAT spaces. The NAT system has been used to detect Alzheimer's disease (AD) and to discriminate AD from other forms of dementia, VCI, dementia with lewy bodies, and is currently undergoing testing for its practical use in the clinical setting (Musha et al., 2002, 2004, 2013). Recently, we reported on VCI templates, consisting of patients with VCI associated with moderate carotid stenosis (>60%) and normal controls (NLc) (Shibata et al., 2014). In brief, the binary likelihood of being in the VCI group vs. that of being in NLc group ($sL_{x:VCI-NLc}$, $vL_{x:VCI-NLc}$) was assessed in each of the sNAT and vNAT spaces. Separation of the VCI group and NLc group was made with a

sensitivity of 92 and 88%, as well as a false-positive rate of 8 and 12% for $sL_{x:VCIc-NLc}$ and $vL_{x:VCI-NLc}$, respectively. Therefore, the VCI templates based on NAT might be applied to community-dwelling elderly people to detect an EEG change reflecting VCI.

If EEG markers of NAT combined with ICA–IMT measurement could detect cognitive decline in subclinical atherosclerosis, then a combination of EEG and ultrasonography could be used to detect cognitive decline during routine medical checkups, because both EEG and ultrasonography are inexpensive, reliable, and noninvasive. To the best of our knowledge, the relationship between EEG finding and ICA–IMT has not yet been explored in elderly subjects. In the present study, using the VCI templates previously obtained from Toyama city, we investigated the hypothesis that increased ICA–IMT are associated with altered EEG markers of NAT for community-dwelling elderly people in Tsukuba city.

SUBJECTS AND METHODS

Characteristics of Survey Subjects

The present investigation is part of the Tsukuba epidemiological investigation project for the prevalence of dementia among inhabitants older than 65 years of age in Tsukuba, Ibaraki, Japan. This study was approved by the ethical committees from the University of Tsukuba (Tsukuba, Japan). All subjects gave written informed consent in accordance with the Declaration of Helsinki. As part of this project, a three-phase survey was carried out in the Tsukuba area. The survey protocol has been described in detail in a previous report (Ikejima et al., 2012). Between February 2012 and October 2012, 221 community-dwelling elderly subjects were enrolled. The 221 subjects underwent ultrasonography, EEG recording, and magnetic resonance imaging (MRI; 1.5T ECHELON RX; Hitachi Medical Corporation, Tokyo, Japan). Deep and periventricular white matter hyperintensities (WMH) were coded from 0 to 3 according to the Fazekas scale (Fazekas et al., 1987). Each EEG finding was independently interpreted by two EEG specialists who were blind to other data about the patients except their age and sex. All subjects underwent the MMSE to screen for cognitive function (cut-off score for cognitive impairment = 26/27).

Characteristics of VCI Group (Shibata et al., 2014)

The selected 55 VCI inpatients previously admitted at our hospital in Toyama city included 47 men and 8 women aged 58–87 years [mean ± standard deviation (SD), 72.6 ± 7.1 years]. Patients were selected based on the following criteria: (i) evidence of unilateral carotid stenosis of >60% (symptomatic or asymptomatic) confirmed with conventional angiography or computed tomography (CT) angiography and a degree of carotid artery stenosis determined using the criteria of the North American Symptomatic Carotid Endarterectomy Trial and (ii) mild cognitive impairment, considered as a score of <90 (low average) on the Repeatable Battery for the Assessment of Neuropsychological Status (RBANS) (Takaiwa et al., 2006, 2009). Of the 55 VCI patients with proximal carotid stenosis, 23 had right-sided lesions (stenosis or occlusion), 19 had left-sided lesions, and 13 had bilateral lesions. The mean score ($\pm$ SD) on the MMSE and RBANS for the 55 VCI patients was 27.1 $\pm$ 1.5 and 74.5 $\pm$ 13.6, respectively. Exclusion criteria included (i) evidence of a previous major stroke and brain damage revealed through MRI; (ii) rapidly evolving symptoms with any hemiparesis, aphasia, and apraxia; and (iii) evidence of dementia, considered as MMSE score of <24, (iv) history of cerebral surgery, obvious psychiatric or neurological disorders, or (v) uncontrolled or malignant general complications. All VCI patients had good levels of daily living activities.

We showed a flow chart for understanding two groups: (1) elderly group: community-dwelling elderly subjects from Tsukuba city, $n = 221$, (2) VCI group: VCI patients from Toyama city, $n = 55$ (**Figure 1**).

EEG Recording and Preprocessing

Electroencephalographic (EEG) recordings (EEG-1200/9100; Nihon Kohden Corporation, Tokyo, Japan) were performed in an awake, resting state with eyes closed for 10 min. Scalp potentials were recorded with 21 electrodes arranged according to the international 10–20 System (Fp1, Fp2, F3, F4, F7, F8, Fpz, Fz, T3, T4, T5, T6, C3, C4, Cz, P3, P4, Pz, O1, O2, and Oz). The contact impedance between the electrode and the scalp was < 50 kΩ. The reference electrode was on the right earlobe, and then the average reference for NAT analysis is computed as a mean of all electrodes. The raw EEG data were recorded at 0.08~300 Hz with 1,000 Hz sampling rate, and then the converted EEG data for NAT analysis were sampled at 200 Hz per channel and bandpass filtered to pick up signals in a frequency range of 4–20 Hz, which minimizes the effect of artifacts contaminating the recorded signals. The recorded signal sequence was divided into 0.64-s segments. To make the EEG data as high quality as possible and exclude the artifacts, each EEG finding was independently interpreted by EEG specialist who was blind to other data about the subjects except their age and sex. We carefully avoided particular epochs containing ocular movements, baseline shifts, drowsiness signs, and muscle or cardiac contamination.

EEG Data Analysis

The average power ratio index (PRI) was calculated for the 221 subjects by dividing the total sum of low frequency (4–8 Hz) power spectrum by the total sum of high frequency (8–20 Hz) power spectrum at each electrode (Cz, C3, C4, Pz, P3, P4, Oz, O1, and O2), respectively, because of an efficient calculation of dominant parieto-occipital rhythm prior to *Normalized Power Spectrum (NPS)* analyses using the following formula:

$$PRI \equiv \Sigma PS_h / \Sigma PS_l \qquad (1)$$

The PS_l and PS_h represent power spectrum of low frequency (4–8 Hz) and that of high frequency (8–20 Hz), respectively.

The mathematical background of NAT (Brain Functions Laboratory, Inc., Yokohama, Japan) was previously described in detail (Musha et al., 2013).

1) Normalized Power Spectrum

We are going to derive dimensionless markers from the EEG signals which characterize stochastic nature of the cerebral neuronal activities generating these signals. The discrete power spectrum PS consists of the ten frequency components $\left\langle |X_{j,m}|^2 \right\rangle_{seg}$ for $m = 3$–12 on signal channel j. The subscript attached to the averaging symbol denotes, hereafter, that the averaging is performed on this variable. In the present case, the averaging is performed across all of the segments. Dependence of the EEG signal level on individual subject is eliminated by normalizing it to its mean level. The NPS consists of 10 ($m = 3$–12) such components NPS$_{j,m}$ defined as,

$$NPS_{j,m} = \left\langle |X_{j,m}|^2 \right\rangle_{seg} / \left\langle |X_{j,m'}|^2 \right\rangle_{seg,m'} . \qquad (2)$$

They make a set of 10 submarkers for each signal channel. This marker characterizes the fractional partition of the EEG power over the 10 frequency components.

Another role of the collective neuronal activities is the signal transmission through the neuronal networks. The biological signal is encoded as the modulation of the occurrence rate of neuronal activities. The organized modulation mode introduces coherence in the collective neuronal activities, and the coherence causes spiky variations of the power spectrum. The modulation is characterized by a ratio $p_{j,m}$ between the adjacent power components given as $p_{j,m} = \left\langle |x_{j,m+1}|^2 \right\rangle_{seg} / \left\langle |x_{j,m}|^2 \right\rangle_{seg}$. Such ratios derive the 10 ($m = 3$–13) dimensionless submarkers NPV$_{j,m}$ on the signal channel j,

$$NPV_{j,m} = \frac{4p_{j,m}}{(1 + p_{j,m})^2} . \qquad (3)$$

2) Zero-Level Resetting

Averages (NPS$_{j\,l,m}$)$_{seg,jl}$ and (NPV$_{j\,l,m}$)$_{seg,jl}$ across the signal channels are left with offset values. The offset values lower the quality of discrimination between different brain diseases, and new markers sNAT$_{j,m}$ and vNAT$_{j,m}$ are introduced after removing the offset as,

$$sNAT_{j,m} \equiv \left\langle NPS_{j,m} \right\rangle_{seg} - \left\langle NPS_{j',m} \right\rangle_{seg,j'} \qquad (4)$$

$$vNAT_{j,m} \equiv \left\langle NPV_{j,m} \right\rangle_{seg} - \left\langle NPV_{j',m} \right\rangle_{seg,j'} . \qquad (5)$$

3) Likelihood

Briefly, a template marker sNAT map is prepared from data for 55 previously diagnosed VCI patients using the mean and SD of a number of sNAT states. The sNAT state of a test subject was assigned to a point in the 210-dimensional sNAT space, whereas the template state of the VCI patients was assigned to another

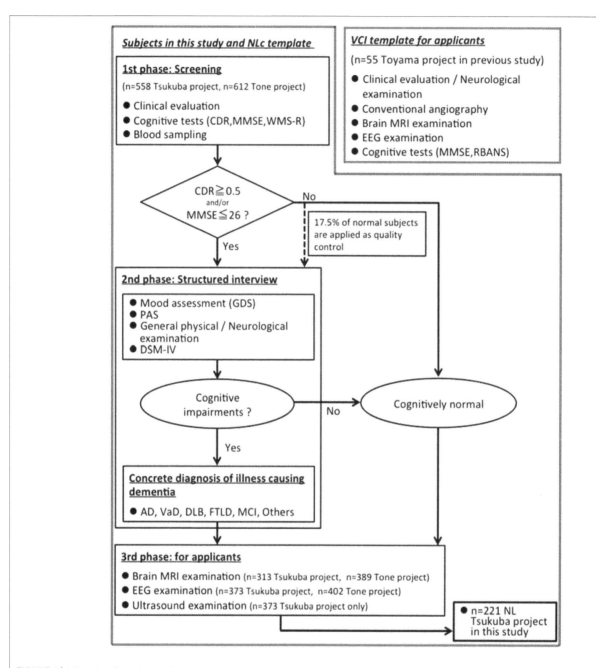

FIGURE 1 | A flow chart for understanding two groups: (1) elderly group: community-dwelling elderly subjects from Tsukuba city, $n = 221$, (2) VCI group: VCI patients from Toyama city (Shibata et al., 2014), $n = 55$. MMSE, Mini-Mental State Examination; CDR, Clinical Dementia Rating; WMS-R, "logical memory A" from the Wechsler Memory Scale-Revised; PAS, Psychogeriatric Assessment Scales; RBANS, Repeatable Battery for the Assessment of Neuropsychological Status; GDS, Geriatric Depression Scale-Short Form; DSM-IV, Diagnostic and Statistical Manual of Mental Disorders, 4th edition; AD, Alzheimer disease; VaD, Vascular dementia; DLB, Dementia with Lewy Bodies; FTLD, FrontoTemporal Lober Degeneration; MCI, Mild Cognitive Impairment.

point in this space. The states of patients with VCI are distributed within these spaces making clusters around their mean states, which are regarded as the template states $sNAT_{j,m}^{VCI}$ together with the standard deviations $s\sigma_{j,m}^{VCI}$ around them. $sNAT_{j,m}^{VCI}$ of VCI is defined as $sZ_{j,m}^{x:VCI}$ which is

$$sZ_{j,m}^{x:VCI} \equiv \left(sNAT_{j,m}^{x} - sNAT_{j,m}^{VCI} \right) / s\sigma_{j,m}^{VCI} \qquad (6)$$

The likelihood of the test subject x being in the VCI group, $sL_{x:VCI}$, was given as a function of the effective distance between the two points properly normalized in terms of the mean and SD related to the VCI template. The likelihood $sL_{x:VCI}$ of a test subject x to be in VCI is defined as,

$$sL_{x:VCI} \equiv \exp\left\langle -\left(sZ_{j,m}^{x:VCI} \right)^2 \right\rangle_{j,m} \qquad (7)$$

The differential (binary) likelihood of being in the VCI group vs. the control group A, $sL_{x:VCI-A}$ was defined as,

$$sL_{x:VCI-A} \equiv sL_{x:VCI} - sL_{x:A} \qquad (8)$$

Similarly, another differential likelihood in reference to vNAT was introduced as $vL_{x:VCI-A}$. The subject was more likely to be in the VCI group than in the control group A when this value was more positive and vice versa.

Ultrasonography Protocol

The same sonographer, who was blinded to the subjects' case status and risk factor levels, carried out all ultrasound examinations. High-resolution B-mode ultrasonography of the ICA was performed with an EUB-5500 ultrasound machine (Hitachi Medical Corporation, Tokyo, Japan). Subjects were examined in the supine position for about 15–20 min. Longitudinal images of the ICA were obtained by combined B-mode and color Doppler ultrasound examinations. With this technique, two parallel echogenic lines separated by an anechoic space can be visualized at the level of the artery wall. These lines are generated by the blood-intima and media-adventitia interfaces. The distance between the two lines gives a reliable index of the thickness of the intima-media complex. The posterior (far) wall IMT was measured with the electronic calipers of the ultrasound machines, as described by Pignoli et al. (1986). On a longitudinal, 2-dimensional ultrasound image of the ICA, images of the posterior wall are displayed as two bright white lines separated by a hypoechoic space. The distance between the leading edge of the first bright line and the leading edge of the second bright line indicates the IMT. We assessed the maximum IMT, which was defined as the single thickest part of the wall among the near and far right and left walls of the ICA.

Statistical Analysis

All data were analyzed using JMP® 12 (SAS Institute Inc., Japan). Mean ± SD values of age, total MMSE score, and years of education were used as descriptive measures of normally distributed variables. The results were compared among the 4 groups included VCI group by analysis of Dunnett's test as control group A. Tukey's HSD (honest significant difference) was used for quantitative variables (age, total MMSE score and years of education), and the χ^2 test was used for categorical variables (Fazekas score, EEG finding). Linear regression analysis among PRI, the binary likelihoods $sL_{x:VCI-A}$ and $vL_{x:VCI-A}$, and the ICA–IMT was performed. Differences with a P-value of <0.05 were considered statistically significant.

RESULTS

The clinical characteristics of the 221 study subjects grouped according to quartiles of ICA–IMT are shown in **Table 1**. The 221 subjects included 110 men and 111 women with a mean (± SD) age of 74.9 ± 6.5 years. The mean MMSE score (± SD) was 28.8 ± 1.2, and the mean education period (± SD) was 12.7 ± 3.1 years. The quartiles of ICA–IMT were defined based on the maximum ICA–IMT and were 1, 1.2, and 1.9

TABLE 1 | Clinical and radiological characteristics of the study population.

	Group A	Group B	Group C	Group D
Subjects	57	49	54	61
Sex (men/women)	18/39	27/22	30/24	35/26
Age	73.6 ± 6.2	74.4 ± 6.1	74.8 ± 6.2	76.6 ± 6.9
MMSE	28.9 ± 1.3	28.6 ± 1.1	28.9 ± 1.3	28.7 ± 1.2
Education	12.6 ± 2.8	13.1 ± 3.3	12.2 ± 3.2	12.8 ± 2.9
Max-IMT(Mean ± SD) mm	0.83 ± 0.13	1.07 ± 0.14	1.49 ± 0.31	2.79 ± 0.83
Max-IMT(Minimum − Max)	0.5–0.9	1–1.1	1.2–1.8	1.9–5.6
EEG				
Within Nomal Limits	47	34	41	42
No abnormality	2	7	2	2
Borderline	3	6	10	12
Sligtly slow abnormality	4	2	1	5
Moderately slow abnormality	1	0	0	0
FAZEKAS CLASS				
0	15	16	9	15
1	14	12	12	17
2	14	10	19	21
3	0	0	2	4

Mean values ± standard deviation of demographic characteristics (age, MMSE score, years of education, and ICA–IMT, EEG finding, Fazekas score on MRI). Age and education are expressed in years. Group A, normal (ICA–IMT ≤ 0.9 mm); Group B, mild atherosclerosis (1–1.1 mm); Group C, moderate atherosclerosis (1.2–1.8 mm); Group D, severe atherosclerosis (≥1.9 mm). MMSE, Mini-Mental State Examination; IMT, intima-media thickness; and SD, standard deviation.

mm. The groups were as follows: Group A, normal (ICA−IMT ≤0.9 mm); group B, mild atherosclerosis (1−1.1 mm); Group C, moderate atherosclerosis (1.2−1.8 mm); and Group D, severe atherosclerosis (≥1.9 mm). There were no significant differences in age, total MMSE score, years of education among the four groups. Although the cerebral white matter lesions on Fazekas class four and borderline on EEG findings were associated with an increased IMT, there were no significant differences in Fazekas score and EEG finding among the four groups (χ^2 test).

The characteristics distributions of sNAT in the elderly with increased IMT have appeared at a specific frequency range of 7.8 Hz, 10.9 Hz as follows. (1) At theta frequency of 7.8 Hz, there were statistically significant increased activities over occipital-temporal areas (O1, O2, T5, T6, F7, and F8) and decreased activities over bilateral frontal areas (F7, F8) in comparison with control group A (**Figure 2A**). Mean z-score sNAT map at 7.8 Hz frequency range was shown for group B, group C, group D, VCI group in comparison with control group A, respectively (**Figure 3**). (2) At alpha frequency range of 10.9 Hz, there were statistically significant decreased activities over occipital areas (O1, O2, and Oz) and increased activities over bilateral fronto-temporal areas (F7, F8, T3, and T4) in comparison with control group A (**Figure 2B**).

The characteristics distributions of vNAT in the elderly with increased IMT have appeared at a specific frequency range of 7.8 Hz, 9.4 Hz, respectively as follows. (1) At theta frequency range of 7.8 Hz, there were statistically significant increased activities over occipital areas and decreased activities over bilateral fronto-temporal areas in comparison with control group A (**Figure 4A**). (2) At alpha frequency range of 9.4 Hz, there were statistically significant decreased activities over occipital areas

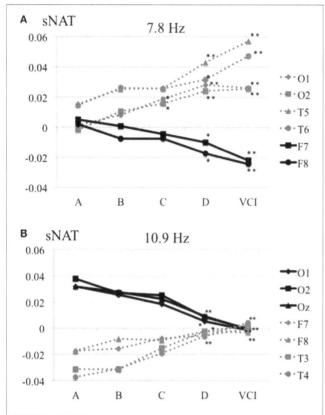

FIGURE 2 | (A) Mean sNAT plot at 7.8 Hz frequency range over occipital-temporal areas (O1, O2, T5, T6) and frontal areas (F7, F8) for group A, group B, group C, group D, VCI group, respectively. (B) Mean sNAT plot at 10.9 Hz frequency range over occipital areas (O1, O2, Oz) and fronto-temporal areas (F7, F8, T3, T4) for group A, group B, group C, group D, VCI group, respectively. *P <0.05, **P < 0.01 (Dunnett 's test as control group A).

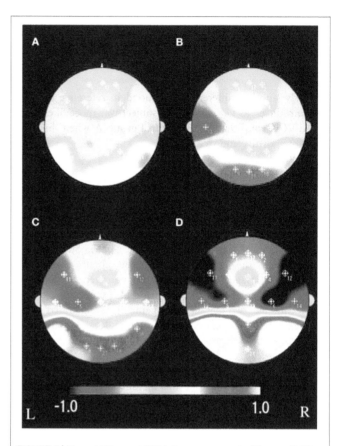

FIGURE 3 | Mean sNAT map at 7.8 Hz frequency range for (A) group B, (B) group C, (C) group D, (D) VCI group, respectively. The colorbar indicates the range of z-scores in comparison with control group A: Green indicates normal spectrum intensity. Red and blue indicate hyperspectrum intensity and hypospectrum intensity, respectively. L, left; R, right.

and increased activities over bilateral parieto-temporal areas in comparison with control group A (**Figure 4B**). Mean z-score vNAT map at 9.4 Hz frequency range was shown for group B, group C, group D, VCI group in comparison with control group A, respectively (**Figure 5**).

A comparison of the PRI among the normal group A and the subclinical atherosclerosis groups (B, C, D), VCI group is shown in **Figure 6A**. The mean total scores (± SD) for the PRI were 3.25 ± 1.64, 3.00 ± 1.87, 2.77 ± 1.8, 2.26 ± 1.17, and 1.41 ± 0.69 for group A, B, C, D, and VCI, respectively. In results of Dunnett's test as control group A, there was a significant decrease of the PRI in the group D and VCI compared with the normal group A, respectively ($P = 0.0018$, $P < 0.0001$).

Comparison of the binary likelihood $sL_{x:VCI-A}$ among the control group A and the subclinical atherosclerosis groups (B, C, D), VCI group is shown in **Figure 6B**. The mean total scores (± SD) for the binary likelihood $sL_{x:VCI-A}$ were −0.14 ± 0.1, −0.11 ± 0.13, −0.1 ± 0.12, −0.03 ± 0.13, and 0.09 ± 0.08 for group A, B, C, D, and VCI, respectively. In results of Dunnett's test as control group A, there was a significant increase in the binary likelihood $sL_{x:VCI-A}$ in the group D and VCI in comparison with control groups A, respectively ($P < 0.0001$, $P < 0.0001$).

Comparison of the binary likelihood $vL_{x:VCI-A}$ among the control group A and the subclinical atherosclerosis groups (B, C, D), VCI group is shown in **Figure 6C**. The mean total scores (± SD) for the binary likelihood $vL_{x:VCI-A}$ were −0.04 ± 0.09, −0.01 ± 0.09, 0.01 ± 0.1, 0.06 ± 0.1, and 0.1 ± 0.07 for groups A, B, C, D, and VCI, respectively. In results of Dunnett's test as control group A, there was a significant increase in the binary likelihood $vL_{x:VCI-A}$ in group C, D, and VCI in comparison with control group A, respectively ($P = 0.021$, $P < 0.0001$, $P < 0.0001$).

The correlation of the ICA–IMT and the PRI, the binary likelihood $sL_{x:VCI-A}$ and the binary likelihood $vL_{x:VCI-A}$ was examined, respectively (**Figure 7**). Linear regression analysis showed a weak negative correlation between the ICA–IMT and the PRI ($r = -0.25$, $P = 0.0002$), and a weak positive correlation between ICA–IMT and the binary likelihoods $sL_{x:VCI-NLc}$ ($r = 0.31$, $P < 0.0001$) and $vL_{x:VCI-NLc}$ ($r = 0.3$, $P < 0.0001$).

DISCUSSION

In the present study, a relationship between subclinical atherosclerosis and EEG markers of PRI, sNAT, vNAT in an elderly population was investigated, respectively. In results, we identified 2 important findings. First, it was confirmed that EEG

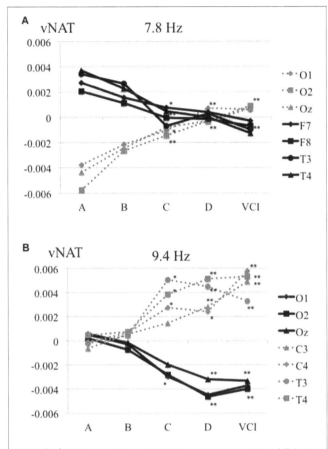

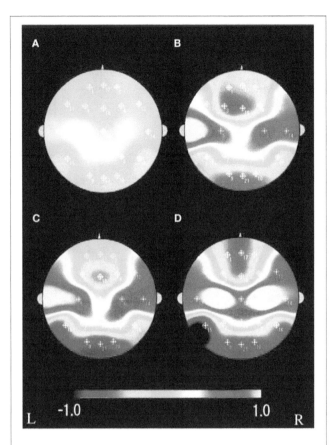

FIGURE 4 | (A) Mean vNAT plot at 7.8 Hz frequency range over occipital areas (O1, O2, Oz) and fronto-temporal areas (F7, F8, T3, T4) for group A, group B, group C, group D, VCI group, respectively. (B) Mean vNAT plot at 9.3 Hz frequency range over occipital areas (O1, O2, Oz) and centro-temporal areas (C3, C4, T3, T4) for group A, group B, group C, group D, VCI group, respectively. *$P < 0.05$, **$P < 0.01$ (Dunnett 's test as control group A).

FIGURE 5 | Mean vNAT map at 9.3 Hz frequency range for (A) group B, (B) group C, (C) group D, (D) VCI group, respectively. The colorbar indicates the range of z-scores in comparison with control group A: Green indicates normal spectrum steepness. Red and blue indicate spectrum blur and spectrum sharpness, respectively. L, left; R, right.

spectrum intensity (sNAT) and spectrum steepness (vNAT) are related to pathological changes indicative of subclinical carotid atherosclerosis. In particular, the binary likelihoods $sL_{x:VCI-A}$ and $vL_{x:VCI-A}$ in group D (ICA–IMT, ≥ 1.9 mm) suggests a risk of an EEG pathological change. Second, NAT might visually show topographic information about EEG alterations in the elderly with increased ICA–IMT. Although there was difficult to interpret an association between all the 210-dimensional NAT spaces and EEG alterations regarding subclinical atherosclerosis, the characteristics distributions of sNAT and vNAT in the elderly with increased ICA–IMT might have appeared at a specific frequency range (e.g., 7.8 Hz). As far as EEG alterations of a dominant parieto-occipital alpha rhythm goes, in sNAT, there were decreased activities over occipital areas at alpha frequency range of 10.9 Hz, and increased activities over occipital areas at theta frequency range of 7.8 Hz, suggesting the alterations of EEG spectrum intensity from alpha to upper theta ranges. Similarly, in vNAT, there were decreased activities over occipital areas at alpha frequency range of 9.4 Hz and increased activities over occipital areas at theta frequency range of 7.8 Hz, suggesting the alterations of EEG spectrum steepness, that is, more spectrum blur (i.e.,

undersynchrony) at upper theta frequency range and more spectrum sharpness (i.e., oversynchrony) at alpha frequency range.

There were many quantitative EEG markers of PRI, EEG global power, an asymmetry-based EEG marker, and NAT for detecting mild cognitive impairment (MCI). Previous findings in patients with MCI secondary to ischemic vascular damage, have demonstrated an increase in low frequency power and a decrease in high frequency power (Nagata, 1988; Nagata et al., 1989). Other studies of subjects with cognitive decline have identified an increase in theta relative power and a decrease in gamma relative power (Moretti et al., 2007a,b, 2009). Recently, Sheorajpanday et al reported about EEG global power in subcortical VCI, no dementia independently predicts vascular impairment, and brain symmetry index reflects severity of cognitive decline (Sheorajpanday et al., 2014). Although in this study, NAT was not compared with other markers of EEG global power or an asymmetry-based EEG marker, we have previously demonstrated a decrease of the PRI in VCI patients compared with normal controls, namely an increase in low frequency power and a decrease in high frequency power (Shibata et al., 2014). In the present study, we confirmed a decrease of the PRI in severe atherosclerosis group D compared

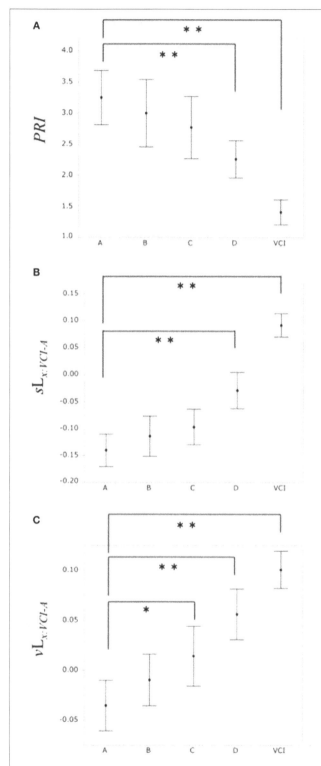

FIGURE 6 | (A) Comparison of PRI among the control group A and subclinical atherosclerosis groups (B, C, D), VCI group, respectively. **(B)** Comparison of the binary likelihood $sL_{x:VCI-A}$ among the control group (A) and subclinical atherosclerosis groups (B, C, D), VCI group, respectively. **(C)** Comparison of the binary likelihood $vL_{x:VCI-A}$ among the normal group (A) and subclinical atherosclerosis groups (B, C, D), VCI group, respectively. Each filled circle indicates the mean of the PRI, $sL_{x:VCI-A}$, $vL_{x:VCI-A}$, respectively, and each vertical line indicates 95% confidence intervals. $^*P < 0.05$, $^{**}P < 0.01$.

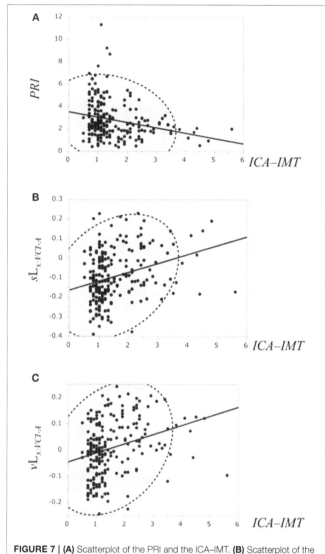

FIGURE 7 | (A) Scatterplot of the PRI and the ICA–IMT. **(B)** Scatterplot of the binary likelihood $sL_{x:VCI-A}$ and the ICA–IMT. **(C)** Scatterplot of the binary likelihood $vL_{x:VCI-A}$ and the ICA–IMT. Broken elliptical shape indicates a 95% confidence ellipse for normally distributed data.

with normal control group A. Further investigations are needed in order to widen the clinical applicability of EEG markers, that is, what is a best practical and cost-effective analysis for detecting MCI among many EEG markers of PRI, EEG global power, asymmetry-based EEG marker, NAT (sNAT, vNAT), and so on.

Carotid atherosclerosis might act as a marker of intracerebral and generalized atherosclerosis and small vessel disease, and has been associated with increased cognitive decline. Some studies have suggested that stenosis of the ICA may be an independent risk factor for cognitive impairment (Rao, 2001; Johnston et al., 2004; Mathiesen et al., 2004). High-grade stenosis of the ICA may be associated with MCI, even without evidence of infarction on MRI (Sztriha et al., 2009). In a large cohort study, high-grade stenosis was seen as an important predictor of cognitive decline (Johnston et al., 2004). Several population-based studies of elderly subjects (aged > 65 years) have found associations between carotid IMT and subsequent cognitive decline (Haan et al., 1999; Sander et al., 2010). However, the pathophysiology of VCI in carotid atherosclerosis without evidence of infarction on MRI is unclear (Mathiesen et al., 2004). In a previous study using magnetoencephalography (MEG), a theta rhythm (6–8 Hz) over parieto-temporal areas, which was separated from a occipital alpha rhythm, appeared in patients with internal carotid artery occlusive disease (Seki et al., 2005). Although conventional EEG in general may not be suitable to separate the upper theta rhythm of 6–8 Hz from the occipital alpha rhythm of 8–12 Hz, NAT might detect the increase of the upper theta frequency bands (more precisely, from 6.3 to 7.8 Hz) and the decrease of the alpha frequency bands over temporo-occipital areas in the elderly with increased atherosclerosis, which of regions might be in part corresponding to the characteristic findings of parieto-temporal upper theta activity (6–8 Hz) measured by MEG (Seki et al., 2005). Although another EEG study (Hsiao et al., 2016) pointed out that a carotid stenosis <50% did not alter theta (4–8 Hz) oscillations, the present study suggests that, at a specific frequency band from alpha to upper theta range, a subtle EEG alternation might appear in the elderly at an early stage of atherosclerosis (ICA–IMT $\geq$ 1.9 mm) before misery perfusion. Therefore, EEG markers included MEG might be more useful for detecting subtle cognitive decline, rather than MRI and conventional visual EEG analysis. To detect subtle cognitive decline with alternation of EEG, prospective studies are needed to investigate the precise association between EEG markers included MEG and several neuropsychological tests (e.g., Wechsler Adult Intelligence Scale -III, Raven's progressive matrices, Rey–Osterrieth complex figure test, and Montreal Cognitive Assessment) (Larner, 2012; Kirkpatrick et al., 2014; Sheorajpanday et al., 2014).

In general, EEG oscillations in the alpha and theta band reflect cognitive and memory performance (Klimesch, 1999). A recent study confirms the major role of the interplay of theta (5–7 Hz) and alpha (8–12 Hz) frequency in the cognitive impairment, that is, the local compensation in the baseline activity at a theta and alpha frequency range (Abuhassan et al., 2014). The structure of the model suggests that cortical oscillations respond differently to compensation mechanisms in the cognitive impairment. In the present study, changes of characteristics distributions regarding sNAT in the elderly with increased IMT have appeared at specific frequency ranges (anchor frequencies) of theta (7.8 Hz) and alpha (10.9 Hz), suggesting an insufficient interplay between a theta and alpha frequency band in the Default Mode Network (DMN). Similarly, changes of characteristics distributions regarding vNAT in the elderly with increased IMT have appeared at specific frequency ranges of theta (7.8 Hz) and alpha (9.3 Hz) (anchor frequencies), suggesting that disruptions of a balance in the DMN might be projected on the mapping of vNAT through a spectrum steepness on EEG.

Although NAT might detect abnormal cortical neuronal activity in VCI patients, our results should be interpreted with caution based on the following limitations. One limitation is that it seems to be very far away from understanding a concept and

getting a clinical merit of sNAT and vNAT markers. It is easier to understand a concept of sNAT than that of vNAT, because sNAT abnormality in the power partition over the spectrum of EEG signals (i.e., hyperspectrum intensity or hypospectrum intensity) is partially similar to PRI (see Supplementary Material). On the other hand, it is likely to confuse a concept of vNAT characterized by a ratio of power spectrum between the adjacent power component, with a well-known EEG coherence which indicating the spectral correlation between electrodes. Although, at this time, we have no obvious findings about the relation between vNAT and the well-known EEG coherence, Musha thought that the coherence causes spiky variations of the PS, suggesting a relationship between EEG coherence and spectrum steepness in vNAT. When vNAT is larger or smaller than that of the NLc, the collective neuronal activities are in the undersynchrony or oversynchrony, in other words, power spectrum blur or power spectrum sharpness, respectively. In case of flat variations or gentle gradient of PS (i.e., power spectrum blur), the collective randomly activated neurons have no modulation and no meaningful biological signals are transmitted, because the neuronal activities are generated at random. In case of spiky variations or steep gradient of PS at a specific frequency band (i.e., power spectrum sharpness), the collective neuronal activities are partly coherent and partly random, and some signal contents are transmitted through the collective neuronal activities. However, not to confuse vNAT with the well-known EEG coherence, we would like to change a mode of expression from the EEG coherence to EEG spectrum steepness regarding vNAT in this paper. Therefore, a precise relationship between vNAT marker and EEG coherence needs to be investigated. Second, EEG analysis is characterized by low spatial resolution (several centimeters) when compared to structural MRI. However, NAT includes 10 frequency bands ranging from 4.7 to 18.8 Hz, which might convey peculiar physiological information on cortical activity beyond MRI. Therefore, we would like to investigate the integration of brain structure based on MRI with brain function based on EEG at a specific frequency range (e.g., 7.8 Hz). Anatomical MRI and functional EEG might provide complementary information into the process of MCI in future.

The prevention of carotid atherosclerosis could protect against vascular cognitive decline, but properly designed intervention studies are needed to demonstrate whether treatment of carotid atherosclerosis could lower the risk of cognitive decline in people without prior cerebrovascular disease. In previous studies, the highest quintile of carotid IMT was associated with dementia risk (Van et al., 2007; Wendell et al., 2012). Although ICA–IMT must reach a criterion thickness to become predictive of dementia from large-scale epidemiologic investigations, the present study did not prove that the abnormality of NAT is an independent risk factor for cognitive decline in future. Therefore, longitudinal studies are needed to examine these associations between EEG markers and ICA–IMT, and neuropsychological tests in the elderly with subclinical carotid atherosclerosis. In a first checkup for cognitive decline in community-dwelling elderly people, a combination with neuropsychological test, ultrasonography, and EEG might be useful for screening subclinical cognitive impairment.

Electroencephalographic (EEG) analysis has practical advantages for neuronal activity assessment because it is inexpensive, portable, noninvasive, sensitive to MCI, and it provides direct, real-time physiological information regarding 4–8 Hz (theta), 8–13 Hz (alpha), 13–30 Hz (beta) frequency range. To widen the applicability of EEG for detecting MCI, reliable, standardized, and user-friendly methods should be needed and developed. NAT could provide information on pathophysiology at a specific frequency band, and asymmetrical visual information of cortical neuronal activity to assess cognitive decline. The present study suggests that physiological aging accompanied by EEG alpha (8–13 Hz) decreasing (Rossini et al., 2007) and MEG theta (6–8 Hz) increasing over the posterior parietal and occipital areas (Puligheddu et al., 2005) might be affected by a increased atherosclerosis to some extent. Bamidis have proposed the neuroscience of physical and cognitive interventions in aging (Bamidis et al., 2014). Further improvements in the NAT system are needed to detect prior cognitive decline in aging and support a monitor of physical and cognitive interventions to maintain a healthy brain.

CONCLUSION

Community-dwelling elderly subjects in the upper quintile for ICA–IMT (≥1.9 mm) were at greater risk of an EEG change reflecting VCI as assessed by NAT. Our study highlights the importance of early intervention for carotid atherosclerosis to minimize the risk of an EEG change that might be related to subsequent VCI.

AUTHOR CONTRIBUTIONS

The authors contributed to this manuscript in the following manner: study design (TS, TM, YK, HM, and TS), data acquisition and analysis (YK, MT, HM, and KN), interpretation of results (MK, YH, NK, and SK). All authors contributed to revise and approve the final version of the manuscript and agree to be accountable for this work.

FUNDING

Part of the present study was financially supported by SENTAN, JST (Japan Science and Technology Agency).

ACKNOWLEDGMENTS

We acknowledge collaboration of the members involved in the TONE epidemiological project and the Tsukuba project, in particular, Masanori Ishikawa. We thank Kazuo Ogino, chairman and CEO of Nihon Koden Corporation, and Kaoru Imajo, its deputy senior manager, for technical support.

SUPPLEMENTARY MATERIAL

Supplementary Figure1 | Two normalizations for understanding sNAT figuratively. Normalization of sNAT is often likened to a photograph processing. **(a)** PS, **(b)** NPS, **(c)** sNAT corresponds to **(d–f)**, respectively. **(d)** means a original subject (e.g., ship) in a frame, **(e)** means the adjustment of the size to frame the subject, and **(f)** means that the centroid of the subject is moved to the center of the frame.

REFERENCES

Abuhassan, K., Coyle, D., Belatreche, A., and Maguire, L. (2014). Compensating for synaptic loss in Alzheimer's disease. *J. Comput. Neurosci.* 36,19–37. doi: 10.1007/s10827-013-0462-8

Arntzen, K. A., and Mathiesen, E. B. (2011). Subclinical carotid atherosclerosis and cognitive function. *Acta Neurol. Scand. Suppl.* 191, 18–22. doi: 10.1111/j.1600-0404.2011.01538.x

Bamidis, P. D., Vivas, A. B., Styliadis, C., Frantzidis, C., Klados, M., Schlee, W., et al. (2014). A review of physical and cognitive interventions in aging. *Neurosci. Biobehav. Rev.* 44, 206–220. doi: 10.1016/j.neubiorev.2014.03.019

Bauer, M., Caviezel, S., Teynor, A., Erbel, R., Mahabadi, A. A., and Schmidt-Trucksäss, A. (2012). Carotid intima-media thickness as a biomarker of subclinical atherosclerosis. *Swiss Med. Wkly.* 25:142. doi: 10.4414/smw.2012.13705

Fazekas, F., Chawluk, J. B., Alavi, A., Hurtig, H. I., and Zimmerman, R. A. (1987). MR signal abnormalities at 1.5 T in Alzheimer's dementia and normal aging. *Am. J. Roentgenol.* 149, 351–356. doi: 10.2214/ajr.149.2.351

Haan, M. N., Shemanski, L., Jagust, W. J., Manolio, T. A., and Kuller, L. (1999). The role of APOE epsilon4 in modulating effects of other risk factors for cognitive decline in elderly persons. *JAMA* 282, 40–46. doi: 10.1001/jama.282.1.40

Hsiao, F. J., Hsieh, F. Y., Chen, W. T., Chu, D. C., and Lin, Y. Y. (2016). Altered resting-state cortical EEG oscillations in patients with severe asymptomatic carotid stenosis. *Clin. EEG Neurosci.* 47, 142–149. doi: 10.1177/1550059414560396

Ikejima, C., Hisanaga, A., Meguro, K., Yamada, T., Ouma, S., Kawamuro, Y., et al. (2012). Multicentre population-based dementia prevalence survey in Japan: a preliminary report. *Psychogeriatrics* 12, 120–123. doi: 10.1111/j.1479-8301.2012.00415.x

Johnston, S. C., O'Meara, E. S., Manolio, T. A., Lefkowitz, D., O'Leary, D. H., Goldstein, S., et al. (2004). Cognitive impairment and decline are associated with carotid artery disease in patients without clinically evident cerebrovascular disease. *Ann. Intern. Med.* 140, 237–247. doi: 10.7326/0003-4819-140-4-200402170-00005

Kirkpatrick, A. C., Vincent, A. S., Guthery, L., and Prodan, C. I. (2014). Cognitive impairment is associated with medication nonadherence in asymptomatic carotid stenosis. *Am. J. Med.* 127, 1243–1246. doi: 10.1016/j.amjmed.2014.08.010

Klimesch, W. (1999). EEG alpha and theta oscillations reflect cognitive and memory performance: a review and analysis. *Brain Res. Brain Res. Rev.* 29, 169–195. doi: 10.1016/S0165-0173(98)00056-3

Larner, A. J. (2012). Screening utility of the Montreal Cognitive Assessment (MoCA): in place of-or as well as-the MMSE ? *Int. Psychogeriatr.* 24, 391–396. doi: 10.1017/s1041610211001839

Mathiesen, E. B., Waterloo, K., Joakimsen, O., Bakke, S. J., Jacobsen, E. A., and Bønaa, K. H. (2004). Reduced neuropsychological test performance in asymptomatic carotid stenosis: the Tromsø study. *Neurology* 62, 695–701. doi: 10.1212/01.WNL.0000113759.80877.1F

Moretti, D. V., Miniussi, C., Frisoni, G. B., Geroldi, C., Zanetti, O., Binetti, G., et al. (2007a). Hippocampal atrophy and EEG markers in subjects with mild cognitive impairment. *Clin. Neurophysiol.* 118, 2716–2729. doi: 10.1016/j.clinph.2007.09.059

Moretti, D. V., Miniussi, C., Frisoni, G., Zanetti, O., Binetti, G., Geroldi, C., et al. (2007b). Vascular damage and EEG markers in subjects with mild cognitive impairment. *Clin. Neurophysiol.* 118, 1866–1876. doi: 10.1016/j.clinph.2007.05.009

Moretti, D. V., Pievani, M., Fracassi, C., Binetti, G., Rosini, S., Geroldi, C., et al. (2009). Increase of theta/gamma and alpha3/alpha2 ratio is associated with amygdalo-hippocampal complex atrophy. *J. Alzheimers Dis.* 17, 349–357. doi: 10.3233/JAD-2009-1059

Musha, T., Asada, T., Yamashita, F., Kinoshita, T., Chen, Z., Matsuda, H., et al. (2002). A new EEG method for estimating cortical neuronal impairment that is sensitive to early stage Alzheimers disease. *Clin. Neurophysiol.* 113:1052–1058. doi: 10.1016/S1388-2457(02)00128-1

Musha, T., Matsuzaki, H., Kobayashi, Y., Okamoto, Y., Tanaka, M., and Asada, T. (2013). EEG markers for characterizing anomalous activities of cerebral neurons in NAT (neuronal activity topography) method. *IEEE Trans. Biomed. Eng.* 60, 2332–2338. doi: 10.1109/TBME.2013. 2255101

Musha, T., Mochidukib, T., Kurachia, T., Matsuda, H., and Asada, T. (2004). Localization of impaired cortical neurons by EEG power fluctuation analysis. *Int. Congr. Ser.* 1270, 20–25. doi: 10.1016/j.ics.2004.04.051

Nagata, K. (1988). Topographic EEG in brain ischemia: correlation with blood flow and metabolism. *Brain Topogr.* 1, 97–106. doi: 10.1007/BF01129174

Nagata, K., Tagawa, K., Hiroi, S., Shishido, F., and Uemura, K. (1989). Electroencephalographic correlates of blood flow and oxygen metabolism provided by positron emission tomography in patients with cerebral infarction. *Electroencephalogr. Clin. Neurophysiol.* 72, 16–30. doi: 10.1016/0013-4694(89)90027-8

Pignoli, P., Tremoli, E., Poli, A., Oreste, P., and Paoletti, R. (1986). Intima plus media thickness of the arterial wall: a direct measurement with ultrasound imaging. *Circulation* 74, 1399–1406. doi: 10.1161/01.CIR.74.6.1399

Polak, J. F., Pencina, M. J., Meisner, A., Pencina, K. M., Brown, L. S., Wolf, P. A., et al. (2010). Associations of carotid artery intima-media thickness (IMT) with risk factors and prevalent cardiovascular disease: comparison of mean common carotid artery IMT with maximum internal carotid artery IMT. *J. Ultrasound Med.* 29, 1759–1768. doi: 10.7863/jum.2010.29.12.1759

Puligheddu, M., de Munck, J. C., Stam, C. J., Verbunt, J., de Jongh, A., van Dijk, B. W., et al. (2005). Age distribution of MEG spontaneous theta activity in healthy subjects. *Brain Topogr.* 17, 165–175. doi: 10.1007/s10548-005-4449-2

Rao, R. (2001). The role of carotid stenosis in vascular cognitive impairment. *Eur. Neurol.* 46, 63–69. doi: 10.1159/000050765

Rossini, P. M., Rossi, S., Babiloni, C., and Polich, J. (2007). Clinical neurophysiology of aging brain: from normal aging to neurodegeneration. *Progr. Neurobiol.* 83, 375–400. doi: 10.1016/j.pneurobio.2007.07.010

Sander, K., Bickel, H., Förstl, H., Etgen, T., Briesenick, C., Poppert, H., et al. (2010). Carotid-intima media thickness is independently associated with cognitive decline. The INVADE study. *Int. J. Geriatr. Psychiatry* 25, 389–394. doi: 10.1002/gps.2351

Seki, S., Nakasato, N., Ohtomo, S., Kanno, A., Shimizu, H., and Tominaga, T. (2005). Neuromagnetic measurement of unilateral temporo-parietal theta rhythm in patients with internal carotid artery occlusive disease. *Neuroimage* 25, 502–510. doi: 10.1016/j.neuroimage.2004.11.025

Sheorajpanday, R. V., Mariën, P., Nagels, G., Weeren, A. J., Saerens, J., Van Putten, M. J., et al. (2014). Subcortical vascular cognitive impairment, no dementia: EEG global power independently predicts vascular impairment and brain symmetry index reflects severity of cognitive decline. *J. Clin. Neurophysiol.* 31, 422–428. doi: 10.1097/WNP.0000000000000060

Shibata, T., Musha, T., Kubo, M., Horie,Y., Asahi, T., Kuwayama, N., et al. (2014). Neuronal activity topography parameters as a marker for differentiating vascular cognitive impairment in carotid stenosis. *J. Stroke Cerebrovasc. Dis.* 23, 2384–2390. doi: 10.1016/j.jstrokecerebrovasdis.2014.05.022

Sztriha, L. K., Nemeth, D., Sefcsik, T., and Vecsei, L. (2009). Carotid stenosis and the cognitive function. *J. Neurol. Sci.* 283, 36–40. doi: 10.1016/j.jns.2009.02.307

Takaiwa, A., Hayashi, N., Kuwayama, N., Akioka, N., Kubo, M., and Endo, S. (2009). Changes in cognitive function during the 1-year period following endarterectomy and stenting of patients with high-grade carotid artery stenosis. *Acta Neurochir. (Wien)* 151, 1593–1600. doi: 10.1007/s00701-009-0420-4

Takaiwa, A., Kuwayama, N., Hayashi, N., Kubo, M., Matsui, M., and Endo, S. (2006). Cognitive function in patients with severe carotid stenosis–evaluation of RBANS, WAIS-R and NART before treatment of carotid revascularization. *No To Shinkei* 58, 681–686.

Van, O. M., De, Jong, F. J., Witteman, J. C., Hofman, A., Koudstaal, P. J., and Breteler, M. M. (2007). Atherosclerosis and risk for dementia. *Ann. Neurol.* 61, 403–410. doi: 10.1002/ana.21073

Wendell, C. R., Waldstein, S. R., Ferrucci, L., O'Brien, R. J., Strait, J. B., and Zonderman, A. B. (2012). Carotid atherosclerosis and prospective risk of dementia. *Stroke* 43, 3319–3324. doi: 10.1161/STROKEAHA.112.672527

20

Cognitive Vulnerability in Aging may be Modulated by Education and Reserve in Healthy People

María D. Roldán-Tapia*, Rosa Cánovas, Irene León and Juan García-Garcia*

Department of Psychology, University of Almería, Almería, Spain

*Correspondence:
María D. Roldán-Tapia
mdroldan@ual.es
Juan García-Garcia
jgarciag@ual.es

Aging is related to a deterioration of cognitive performance and to multiple alterations in the brain. Even before the beginning of a noticeable cognitive decline, the framework which holds cognitive function experiences these alterations. From a system-vulnerability point of view of cognition, the deterioration associated with age would be the collection of repercussions during a life. Brain function and structure are modified in a multidimensional way, which could concern different aspects like structural integrity, functional activity, connectivity, or glucose metabolism. From this point of view, the effects of aging could affect the most brain systems and their functional activity. In this study, we analyze the functional development of three cognitive domains in relation to aging, educational level, and cognitive reserve (CR). A total of 172 healthy subjects were divided into two age groups (young and old), and completed a battery of classic neuropsychological tests. The tests were organized and analyzed according to three cognitive domains: working memory and flexibility, visuoconstructive functions, and declarative memory. Subjects also completed a questionnaire on CR. Results showed that the performance in all cognitive domains decreased with age. In particular, tests related to working memory, flexibility, and visuoconstructive abilities were influenced by age. Nevertheless, this effect was attenuated by effects of education, mainly in visuoconstructive domain. Surprisingly, visual as well as verbal memory tests were not affected either by aging, education, or CR. Brain plasticity plays a prominent role in the aging process, but, as other studies have shown, the plasticity mechanism is quite different in healthy vs. pathological brains. Moreover, this plasticity brain mechanism could be modulated by education and CR. Specially, cognitive domains as working memory, some executive functions and the visuoconstructive abilities seem to be modulated by education. Therefore, it seems to be crucial, to propose mechanisms of maintenance of a healthy and enriched brain, since it promotes auto-regulatory mechanisms of well-aging.

Keywords: well-aging, educational attainment, cognitive reserve, brain compensation, neuroplasticity, cognitive domains

INTRODUCTION

As human life expectancy increases, maintaining cognitive function has become a target to pursue. It seems that a combination of educational and occupational fulfillment, recreational activities [all aspects included in the concept of cognitive reserve (CR)], and the biological process of aging itself could be the predictor of how to develop cognitive performance as we age.

In recent decades there has been an increasing interest in finding out why some older adults are able to maintain adequate cognitive abilities despite age, while others show clear cognitive decline with advancing age (Wilson et al., 2002). The concept of CR accounts for individual differences in which people with higher CR are able to enlarge the performance on cognitive tasks by recruiting different brain systems and/or using alternative cognitive strategies compared to individuals with lower CR (Stern et al., 2003; Stern, 2009; Tucker and Stern, 2011; Meng and D'Arcy, 2012).

In recent decades it has been demonstrated that age do not affect cognitive functions in the same way nor do they evolve at the same rate throughout life. Processing speed is one of the cognitive abilities that most consistently decline with age (Holdnack et al., 2013; Hong et al., 2015; Tam et al., 2015), even when motor dexterity is statistically controlled (Ebaid et al., 2017). Detriment with age in the case of working memory and inhibition has been also largely demonstrated (Turner and Spreng, 2012; Calso et al., 2016). With advancing age inhibitory mechanisms become increasingly less efficient and no longer prevent irrelevant information from saturating working memory capacity (De Beni et al., 2007). Normal aging seems also to be characterized by a general reduction in cognitive flexibility, defined as attention switching and task shifting. In fact, it has been argued that correlations between cognitive flexibility and primary mental abilities were relatively stable across the adult lifespan, suggesting that individual differences in cognitive flexibility could be responsible for age-related changes in other cognitive abilities (Hülür et al., 2016).

Finally, the extant literature regarding declarative memory indicates that episodic and semantic memory measures are associated with differential aging patterns across lifespan (Nyberg et al., 2012). Thus, several cross-sectional studies have stablished an early onset for episodic memory decline following a linear pattern that begins around the age of 20 or 30 years and results in as much as 1 standard deviation (SD) unit below peak level performance by the age of 60 years and 2 SD units at age 80 years (Schaie, 1994; Nilsson et al., 1997; Verhaeghen and Salthouse, 1997; Park et al., 2002). Longitudinal studies, however, suggest that episode memory decline begins by the age of 60 years followed by an accelerated deterioration (Schaie, 1994; Zelinski and Burnight, 1997). Nevertherless, that discrepancy may be explained by the increase of the educational level in the last decades. On the other hand, semantic memory or knowledge is among the more stable memory systems across the adult lifespan (Park and Reuter-Lorenz, 2009). Young to young–old adults (from age 35 to age 65 years) maintain or even slightly improve their semantic performance, and deficits appear only at very late ages in this domain (Kaufmann, 2001).

Advancing knowledge of influence of CR and educational attainment on aging can be very hopeful since, although the brain will be modified by age, there are numerous opportunities to adapt, restrict, or improve cognitive changes, allowing older adults continue to function independently. Therefore, the purpose of this study is to examine the effect of education and CR in the process of healthy brain aging. We seek to discover whether aging follows similar patterns in different cognitive domains, and how these variables might influence the aging process.

MATERIALS AND METHODS

The study was approved by the Ethics Committee of the University of Almería, and conducted in accordance with Helsinki declaration and Spanish legislation on personal data protection. Participation was voluntary and all subjects gave written consent.

Subjects

A sample of 140 subjects was recruited from social clubs, entertainment centers, and the University of Almería's Center for Adult Education.

The sample was divided into two age groups according to the traditional Spanish retirement age (65 years): adults (aged 36–64 years) and elderly adults (≥65 years). None of them had a history of psychiatric or neurological disorders, drug consumption, or head injury that could potentially affect their cognitive performance. Besides, for all subjects older than 64 years a score of 27 or lower in the *Mini-Examen Cognoscitivo* [Mini-Mental State Examination (Lobo et al., 2002)] was a criterion of exclusion. Following these criteria, three men were excluded and four women (one of them with fibromyalgia diagnosis) under the suspicion of suffering Mild Cognitive Impairment. Additionally, the elderly adults completed the Barthel index (Mahoney and Barthel, 1965). **Table 1** shows the sociodemographic characteristics of the participants.

Methods

Subjects completed the cognitive reserve scale (CRS), developed by the authors, that measures the reserve throughout a person's lifetime by means of taking part in cognitively stimulating activities (reading, playing a musical instrument, collecting things, speak several languages or dialects, traveling, or play sports) (León-Estrada et al., 2017). Each item was completed several times about different age periods: the older the participant, the more times each item had to be completed. A Likert-type scale of 0–4 points was used and the total CRS score was the sum of the mean scores for each item (24 items). The

TABLE 1 | Participant demographics, cognitive reserve scale (CRS) scores (León et al., 2014), and descriptive scores for elderly adults.

		Age group (years)	
		Adults (*n* = 98)	Elderly adults (*n* = 42)
Gender	Male	34	13
	Female	64	29
Age (years)		49.15 (7.18)	71.88 (5.62)
Level of education (years)		13.79 (4.71)	10.12 (5.12)
Mini-Examen Cognoscitivo		–	33.7 (1.67)
Barthel index		–	100 (0.0)
CRS		52.98 (10.15)	52.22 (12.58)

CRS gave scores ranging from 0 to 96, with higher CRS scores indicating more frequent participation. The CRS is available upon request from the authors and additionally, it is available on the Internet: http://www2.ual.es/CognitiveReserveScale/the-cognitive-reserve-scale-crs/.

Neuropsychological Assessment

A trained psychologist carried out the neuropsychological assessments in several cognitive domains: Working memory and flexibility, Digit Span subtest (backward) (Peña-Casanova et al., 2009c), the Stroop test (Peña-Casanova et al., 2009b), TMT-B (Peña-Casanova et al., 2009c), Controlled Oral Word Association Test (COWAT) (Benton and Hamsher, 1989), and the Corsi Block task (backward) (Peña-Casanova et al., 2009c), visuoconstructive abilities: matrix reasoning and Block Design subtests (Wechsler, 1993), and Rey–Osterrieth Complex Figure Test (ROCF) (quality of copy) (Peña-Casanova et al., 2009a), and declarative memory: Verbal Learning Spanish–Complutense Test TAVEC (Benedet and Alejandre, 1968), sum of the learning slope, short-term recall and delayed-memory, and ROCF short-term recall and delayed-memory. **Table 2** shows the main scores of neuropsychological tests.

In addition, subjects' IQ score was estimated by Vocabulary subtest (Wechsler, 1993). All the tests are translated and validated in Spanish and the raw scores of all tests were converted to standard scores adjusted for age and educational level (scale scores, z-scores, or percentile scores) following Spanish normative studies, except for COWAT, which was standardized following a normative study in an English population (Benton and Hamsher, 1989).

Statistical Analysis

In the present study, data were analyzed with multivariate analyses of covariance (MANCOVA). A total of three MANCOVAs were conducted separately to investigate the effect of age on the cognitive domains. Three dependent variables were used: the neuropsychological performance in the cognitive domains previously mentioned. Years of formal education and CR were entered as covariates for all statistical analyses to control for individual differences. Age was used as independent variable and divided into two age groups: adults (36–64 years) and elderly adults ($\geq$65 years).

As statistical assumptions underlying the MANCOVAs were not fully met, the estimation of the parameters in the linear model was analyzed using the resampling method of simple bootstrapping with 1000 bootstrap samples. The bootstrap bias-corrected accelerated method was used as a corrective method. Analyses were carried out using statistical package IBM-SPSS 22.0 for Windows (IBM Corp., 2013).

Results with $p < 0.05$ were considered statistically significant. The effect size was obtained by using the partial eta squared (η_p^2) and r of regression coefficient (B).

RESULTS

In relation to working memory and cognitive flexibility [Digit Span subtest (backward), the Stroop test, TMT-B, COWAT, and the Corsi Block task (backward)], there were significant differences between adults and elderly adults ($\Lambda_{\text{Wilks}} = 0.874$,

TABLE 2 | Multivariate analyses of covariance (MANCOVA) classified according to the three functional areas (anterior, posterior and temporal).

Functional areas, Mean (SD)	Age group (years)		p	η_p^2	Covariates			
	Adults (n = 98)	Elderly adults (n = 42)			Education		CR	
					p	r	p	r
Working memory and flexibility			0.003	0.126	NS	NS	NS	NS
Digit Span subtest (backward)	10.50 (2.62)	11.50 (1.92)	NS	NS	NS	NS	NS	NS
The Stroop test	9.24 (2.67)	11.00 (2.38)	0.001	0.28	0.049	0.16	0.007	0.23
TMT-B	8.96 (2.55)	10.02 (2.58)	NS	NS	NS	NS	NS	NS
COWAT	42.25 (28.20)	54.22 (27.24)	0.019	0.20	NS	NS	NS	NS
Corsi Block task (backward)	9.32 (2.25)	8.60 (1.34)	0.07	0.15	NS	NS	NS	NS
Visuoconstructive abilities			<0.01	0.15	<0.01	0.278	NS	NS
Matrix reasoning subtest	11.45 (2.79)	12.76 (2.99)	0.001	0.28	0.007	0.23	NS	NS
Block Design subtest	10.76 (2.65)	12.44 (2.68)	0.001	0.28	0.001	0.28	NS	NS
ROCF (quality of copy)	6.77 (2.67)	7.85 (2.43)	NS	NS	0.001	0.28	NS	NS
Declarative memory			NS	NS	NS	NS	NS	NS
TAVEC sum	0.39 (0.82)	0.44 (1.14)	NS	NS	NS	NS	0.045	0.17
TAVEC short-term recall memory	0.46 (0.95)	0.28 (1.07)	NS	NS	NS	NS	0.014	0.21
TAVEC delayed memory	0.40 (1.03)	0.28 (1.23)	NS	NS	NS	NS	0.036	0.18
ROCF short-term recall	8.90 (5.21)	9.54 (2.65)	NS	NS	NS	NS	NS	NS
ROCF delayed memory	8.31 (2.69)	9.49 (2.86)	NS	NS	0.005	0.24	NS	NS

Years of formal education and cognitive reserve were entered as covariates for all statistical analyses to control for individual differences. Age was used as independent variable and divided into two age groups: adults (36–64 years) and elderly adults (≥65 years). TMT-B, trail making test part B; COWAT, controlled oral word association test; ROCF, Rey–Osterrieth complex figure test; TAVEC, Verbal Learning Spanish-Complutense Test; CR, cognitive reserve; NS, non-significant.

$F_{5,130} = 3.735$; $p = 0.003$; $\eta_p^2 = 0.126$). The global effect of the covariates (education and CR) was not statistically significant.

Additionally, estimation of the effect of the independent variables and covariates on the dependent variables showed significant relationships between the Stroop test and age group ($B = -1.427$; $p = 0.001$; $r = 0.28$), education ($B = -0.098$; $p = 0.049$; $r = 0.16$), and CR ($B = 0.49$; $p = 0.007$; $r = 0.23$), as well as between COWAT and age group ($B = -13.70$; $p = 0.019$; $r = 0.20$), and the Corsi Block task (backward) and age group ($B = 0.98$; $p = 0.07$; $r = 0.15$) (**Table 2**).

In the case of the visuoconstructive abilities [the Matrix Reasoning, Block Design, and ROCF (quality of copy)], there were statistically significant differences between adults and elderly adults ($\Lambda_{Wilks} = 0.847$, $F_{3,130} = 7,817$; $p < 0.01$; $\eta_p^2 = 0.15$). The effect of education was significant ($\Lambda_{Wilks} = 0.722$, $F_{3,130} = 16.645$; $p < 0.01$; $\eta_p^2 = 0.278$), but no significant effect from CR.

The estimation of the effect of the independent variables and covariates on the dependent variables using simple bootstrapping disclosed significant relationships between the Matrix Reasoning subtest and age group ($B = -1.75$; $p = 0.001$; $r = 0.28$) and education ($B = 0.14$; $p = 0.007$; $r = 0.23$); the Block Design subtest and age group ($B = -2.45$; $p = 0.001$; $r = 0.28$) and education ($B = -0.187$; $p = 0.001$; $r = 0.28$), and the ROCF (copy) and education ($B = -0.231$; $p = 0.001$; $r = 0.28$) (**Table 2**).

Regarding the memory tests (TAVEC sum, TAVEC short-term recall, TAVEC delayed recall, and ROCF short-term recall and long-term recall), there were no significant differences between adults and elderly adults. Besides, the effect of the two covariates (education and CR) was not statistically significant.

Finally, estimation of the effect of the independent variables and covariates on the dependent variables using simple bootstrapping revealed significant relationships between TAVEC-sum and CR ($B = 0.017$; $p = 0.045$; $r = 0.17$), TAVEC short-term recall and CR ($B = 0.021$; $p = 0.014$; $r = 0.21$), TAVEC delayed recall and CR ($B = 0.019$; $p = 0.036$; $r = 0.18$), and ROCF delayed recall and education ($B = -0.149$; $p = 0.005$; $r = 0.24$) (**Table 2**).

DISCUSSION

In the present study, a functional analysis of brain has been performed using neuropsychological tests in two age-differentiated populations. The aim was to assess the evolution of cognitive changes across the life cycle and their relation to educational level and CR.

Our results, generally speaking, show a large influence of aging on inhibition, flexibility, working memory, and visuoperceptive functions, although there is also an important contribution of education in these domains. However, surprisingly, the same pattern was not found in declarative memory tasks where the effect of education and CR but not of aging could be verified. It seems clear that at least in a healthy population, an enriched environment allows us to face the tasks of flexibility, updating, monitoring, or memory as we get old.

Given our results in cognitive domains related to the frontal region, the data in the flexibility, inhibition, and spatial working memory tests have shown an influence of aging, while in inhibition tasks there is also a significant influence of education and reservation.

In the case of frontal areas, it is now well-established that normal aging is associated with cognitive decline (Craik and Salthouse, 2000; Rypma and D'Esposito, 2000; Kennedy et al., 2009), particularly in tasks involving executive functions (Salthouse et al., 2003; Podell et al., 2012). However, all executive functions do not decline in the same way with advanced age (Collette and Salmon, 2014). A previous study from our group (Roldán-Tapia et al., 2012) reported that the "performance of functions related to the dorsolateral prefrontal cortex (PFC) (verbal fluency, behavioral spontaneity, reasoning, divided and complex attention, and working memory) was associated with aging." Or, for example, regarding to shifting abilities, older people would show difficulties to maintain and to manipulate two mental plans but not to alternate between both of them (Kray et al., 2004). However, these results are not consistent with Schaie (1958, 1994) and Stawski et al. (2013) works, that show a stable performed in flexibility during lifespan (although it is true that they did an intra-subjects analyses).

In addition, numerous researches have shown how CR and education exert a protective effect on the decline associated with age in executive functions (Ardila et al., 2000; Opdebeeck et al., 2016).

On the other hand, the effect of aging on the visuoconstructive domains has also been demonstrated earlier, mainly in face recognition, mental rotation, and visuospatial abilities (Adduri and Marotta, 2009; Iachini et al., 2009; Daniel and Bentin, 2012). It seems that the occipital decrement and sensory deficits are consistent with perceptual processing declines as a function of aging (Zhuravleva et al., 2014).

The relationship between cognitive decline that occurs in the elderly, and age-related changes that take place in brain morphology and functioning, is still being documented.

Virtually no area of the brain is fully spared from the effects of aging, although certain brain systems seem to be particularly vulnerable to aging effects, which takes place earlier and in greater degree (Raz, 2000). From a system-vulnerability approach, the deterioration associated to age would be the collection of repercussions during a life. Brain structure and function are modified in a multidimensional way, which could affect different aspects such as structural integrity, functional activity, and connectivity, as a result of continuous interactions between endogenous and exogenous factors (Khachaturian, 2011; Jagust, 2013). The areas found to be most vulnerable to normal age changes are the PFC and the medial temporal cortex (Raz, 2000, 2004; Buckner, 2004; Hedden and Gabrieli, 2004).

But perhaps the most relevant fact is the influence of education on complex visuoconstructive tasks such as spatial reasoning, visuoconstruction, and the grafomotor integration of a complex design. Our data are in line with previous studies such as that of Ardila et al. (2000) which points out the importance of education for the execution of cognitive processes, especially in older people and even seems to play a relevant role in elderly "illiterates."

The results of the present study are also supported by data from other studies. For example, Kim et al. (2015) demonstrated a protective effect of education on the cortical thinning in cognitive normal older individuals. According to the authors, this protective effect could be achieved by increasing resistance to structural loss from aging.

In memory domains, our results point to the idea of certain stability across different age periods. This result is not new; other studies have supported the idea of maintenance of different types of memory (semantic memory) in healthy subjects (Park and Reuter-Lorenz, 2009). For example, the perirhinal cortex appears to undergo little age-related atrophy (Insausti et al., 1998). Also, performance in older adults seem be associated with the recruitment of additional brain regions in the medial temporal lobe and in frontal regions (Cabeza, 2001; Maguire and Frith, 2003; Giovanello and Schacter, 2012). It is no less true, however, that a group of studies have shown hippocampal degeneration (Raz, 2004; Raz and Rodrigue, 2006) or a reduction in BOLD signal in the medial temporal lobe (Maguire and Frith, 2003).

While in the case of the working memory, flexibility, and visuoconstructive domains, we do not find any relevant influence from CR in the aging process, the same cannot be said for mnesic processes. Structural MRI studies in healthy aging consistently reported positive associations between CR and increased gray and white matter volumes in associative frontal and temporoparietal cortices, as well as reduced mean diffusivity in the bilateral hippocampus (Akbaraly et al., 2009; Marioni et al., 2012). Declarative memory is greatly influenced by education, primarily, and also by CR, as well in short-term memory and delayed recall, as using visual and verbal stimuli. Valenzuela et al. (2008) found that hippocampal decline occurs more slowly in normal aging when performing cognitive challenging life.

It has also been shown that greater CR contributes to delay or attenuate pathological changes such as those that occur in Alzheimer's disease (Carnero-Pardo and Del Ser, 2007), vascular injury (Dufouil et al., 2003; Elkins et al., 2006), Parkinson's disease (Glatt et al., 1996), traumatic brain injury (Kesler et al., 2003), neuropsychiatric disorders (Barnett et al., 2006), and multiple sclerosis (Sumowski et al., 2009); greater CR may even prevent accumulation of amyloid plaque (Landau et al., 2012). Observations using cerebral blood flow (CBF) have found that Alzheimer's disease patients with higher education have a lower resting rCBF (Stern et al., 1992).

In individuals with AD and mild cognitive impairment, higher education and occupation (as proxies of CR) are correlated to more severe hypometabolism in temporoparietal areas (memory and visual abilities) and in the precuneus (Garibotto et al., 2008). Moreover, they are associated with an increased metabolism in the dorsolateral PFC (working memory and flexibility), suggesting a compensatory mechanism against AD-related cerebral neurodegeneration (Grady et al., 1994). A review paper calculated that a higher CR reduced the chances of suffer dementia by 46% (Valenzuela and Sachdev, 2005). However, even higher CR cannot maintain functions when pathology turns very severe.

Could it be that education affects cognitive abilities (processing speed, working memory, verbal fluency, or verbal episodic memory) differently?

Maybe, in demanding memory or complex visuoperceptive tasks, the influence of variables such as reserve and education is more marked in the case of healthy aging or even more visible in the case of pathological aging than in other cognitive domains. The domain of memory could be more sensitive to the effect of training, education, and lifestyle.

Our results show that, in healthy people, if we keep level of education and CR constant, the only variable that can influence the neuropsychological outcome in flexibility, working memory, and visuoconstructive domain, seems to be aging. Nevertheless, our data are collected from subjects who were healthy and not very advanced in age. It may be that the possible effect of CR depends on the baseline of normal versus pathological brain conditions. From this point of view Hayden et al. (2011) defined "reserve" as "the difference between cognitive performance as predicted by an individual's brain pathology and that individual's observed cognitive performance." Thus, people whose measured cognitive performance is better than predicted by their pathology have high reserve, whereas those who perform worse than predicted have low reserve.

Regarding the age of our study participants, a 15-year longitudinal study among elderly Catholic clergy members who were participating in the religious Orders (healthy aging) showed a typical profile of extraordinarily slow deterioration of cognitive functions, which last for decades. These findings suggest that cognitive changes associated with aging may be minimal when the process is not associated with a neurodegenerative disease (Christensen et al., 1994; Hayden et al., 2011; Reed et al., 2011).

Both our results and those from morphological and cognitive studies lead us to the idea that "brain aging" is an interactive and synergistic process in which several variables play an important role.

For example, the health condition versus pathology, the genetic load, and the influence of an enriched environment (CR and education). A good method to further investigate this interactive process is the use of brain mapping approaches to complete information obtained through the neuropsychological assessment of cognitive domains (Agis and Hillis, 2016) such as the ones described in the present study (working memory, flexibility, visuoconstructive functions, and declarative memory).

Additionally, the new developments of neuropsychological brain mapping batteries seem to contribute to enhance clinical diagnosis, pre-surgical mapping, and follow-up (Karakas et al., 2013). Hence, advances in the knowledge of neural substrates involved in cognitive tests and revealed by the interpretation of human brain mapping studies represent a strong resource to increase the comprehension of brain and how age and different levels of education or CR might affect cognitive vulnerability.

Limitations

Limitations of the current study are the size of the sample and the lack of inclusion of people with presumably low reserve (without access to education or social club). The present sample seem likely to have a higher than average CR, but the CRS includes a high variety of different activities that are not limited exclusively to the centers where the participants were recruited. Besides, in the elderly adults, the SD related to the years of formal education reflects variability among them (from just 5–15 years of formal education). However, future studies should include an older sample, as well as specific experimental tasks, to help discern the real influence of CR in healthy aging populations.

As a final conclusion, regarding the importance of CR in the domain of memory, its limited effect on fluency, divided attention, interference, spatial reasoning, and visuospatial tasks may be due to the brain's own compensation mechanism, which under healthy conditions, makes it independent of education or CR. It is the effect of CR could be quite different depending of the brain status: pathological or healthy.

REFERENCES

Adduri, C. A., and Marotta, J. J. (2009). Mental rotation of faces in healthy aging and Alzheimer's disease. *PLOS ONE* 4:e6120. doi: 10.1371/journal.pone.0006120

Agis, D., and Hillis, A. E. (2016). The cart before the horse: when cognitive neuroscience precedes cognitive neuropsychology. *Cogn. Neuropsychol.* doi: 10.1080/02643294.2017.1314264 [Epub ahead of print].

Akbaraly, T. N., Portet, F., Fustinoni, S., Dartigues, J. F., Artero, S., Rouaud, O., et al. (2009). Leisure activities and the risk of dementia in the elderly: results from the three-city study. *Neurology* 73, 854–861. doi: 10.1212/WNL.0b013e3181b7849b

Ardila, A., Ostrosky-Solis, F., Roselli, M., and Gómez, C. (2000). Age-related cognitive decline during normal aging: the complex effect of education. *Arch. Clin. Neuropsychol.* 15, 495–513. doi: 10.1016/S0887-6177(99)00040-2

Barnett, J. H., Salmond, C. H., Jones, P. B., and Sahakian, B. J. (2006). Cognitive reserve in neuropsychiatry. *Psychol. Med.* 36, 1053–1064. doi: 10.1017/S0033291706007501

Benedet, M. J., and Alejandre, M. A. (1968). *Test de Aprendizaje Verbal España Complutense (TAVEC)*. Madrid: Publicaciones de Psicología Aplicada.

Benton, A. L., and Hamsher, K. (1989). *Multilingual Aphasia Examination*, 2nd Edn. Iowa City, IA: The University of Iowa.

Buckner, R. L. (2004). Memory and executive function in aging and AD: multiple factors that cause decline and reserve factors that compensate. *Neuron* 44, 195–208. doi: 10.1016/j.neuron.2004.09.006

Cabeza, R. (2001). Cognitive neuroscience of aging: contributions of functional neuroimaging. *Scand. J. Psychol.* 42, 277–286. doi: 10.1111/1467-9450.00237

Calso, C., Besnard, J., and Allain, P. (2016). Normal aging of frontal lobe functions. *Geriatr. Psychol. Neuropsychiatr. Vieil.* 14, 77–85. doi: 10.1684/pnv.2016.0586

Carnero-Pardo, C., and Del Ser, T. (2007). Education provides cognitive reserve in cognitive deterioration and dementia. *Neurologia* 22, 78–85.

Christensen, H., Jorm, A. F., Henderson, A. S., Mackinnon, A. J., Korten, A. E., and Scott, L. R. (1994). The relationship between health and cognitive functioning in a sample of elderly people in the community. *Ageing* 23, 204–212. doi: 10.1093/ageing/23.3.204

Collette, F., and Salmon, E. (2014). The effect of normal and pathological aging on cognition. *Rev. Med. Liege* 69, 265–269.

Craik, F. I. M., and Salthouse, T. A. (2000). *The Handbook of Aging and Cognition*, 2nd Edn. Mahwah, NJ: Lawrence Erlbaum Associates.

Daniel, S., and Bentin, S. (2012). Age-related changes in processing faces from detection to identification: ERP evidence. *Neurobiol. Aging* 33, 206.e1–228.e1. doi: 10.1016/j.neurobiolaging.2010.09.001

De Beni, R., Borella, E., and Carretti, B. (2007). Reading comprehension in aging: the role of working memory and metacomprehension. *Neuropsychol. Dev. Cogn. B Aging Neuropsychol. Cogn.* 14, 189–212. doi: 10.1080/13825580500229213

Dufouil, C., Alperovitch, A., and Tzourio, C. (2003). Influence of education on the relationship between white matter lesions and cognition. *Neurology* 60, 831–836. doi: 10.1212/01.WNL.0000049456.33231.96

Ebaid, D., Crewther, S. G., MacCalman, K., Brown, A., and Crewther, D. P. (2017). Cognitive processing speed across the lifespan: beyond the influence of motor speed. *Front. Aging Neurosci.* 9:62. doi: 10.3389/fnagi.2017.00062

Elkins, J. S., Longstreth, W. T., Manolio, T. A., Newman, A. B., Bhadelia, R. A., and Johnston, S. C. (2006). Education and cognitive decline associated with MRI-defined brain infarct. *Neurology* 67, 435–440. doi: 10.1212/01.wnl.0000228246.89109.98

Garibotto, V., Borroni, B., Kalbe, E., Herholz, K., Salmon, E., Holtoff, V., et al. (2008). Education and occupation as proxies for reserve in aMCI converters and AD: FDG-PET evidence. *Neurology* 71, 1342–1349. doi: 10.1212/01.wnl.0000327670.62378.c0

Giovanello, K. S., and Schacter, D. L. (2012). Reduced specificity of hippocampal and posterior ventrolateral prefrontal activity during relational retrieval in normal aging. *J. Cogn. Neurosci.* 24, 159–170. doi: 10.1162/jocn_a_00113

Glatt, S. L., Hubble, J. P., Lyons, K., Paolo, A., Troster, A., Hassanein, R. E., et al. (1996). Risk factors for dementia in Parkinson's disease: effect of education. *Neuroepidemiology* 15, 20–25. doi: 10.1159/000109885

Grady, C. L., Maisog, J. M., Horwitz, B., Ungerleider, L. G., Mentis, M. J., Salerno, J. A., et al. (1994). Age-related changes in cortical blood flow activation during visual processing of faces and location. *J. Neurosci.* 14, 1450–1462.

Hayden, K. M., Reed, B. R., Manly, J. J., Tommet, D., Pietrzak, R. H., Chelune, G. J., et al. (2011). Cognitive decline in the elderly: an analysis of population heterogeneity. *Ageing* 40, 684–689. doi: 10.1093/ageing/afr101

Hedden, T., and Gabrieli, J. D. (2004). Insights into the ageing mind: a view from cognitive neuroscience. *Nat. Rev. Neurosci.* 5, 87–96. doi: 10.1038/nrn1323

Holdnack, J. A., Drozdick, L., Weiss, L. G., and Iverson, G. L. (2013). *WAIS-IV, WMS-IV, and ACS: Advanced Clinical Interpretation*. Sandiago, CA: Academic Press.

Hong, Z., Ng, K. K., Sim, S. K., Ngeow, M. Y., Zheng, H., Lo, J. C., et al. (2015). Differential age-dependent associations of gray matter volume and white matter integrity with processing speed in healthy older adults. *Neuroimage* 123, 42–50. doi: 10.1016/j.neuroimage.2015.08.034

Hülür, G., Nilam, R., Willis, S. L., Schaie, W. K., and Gerstorf, D. (2016). Cognitive aging in the Seattle Longitudinal Study: within-person associations of primary mental abilities with psychomotor speed and cognitive flexibility. *J. Intell.* 4:12. doi: 10.3390/jintelligence4030012

Iachini, I., Iavarone, A., Senese, V. P., Ruotolo, F., and Ruggiero, G. (2009). Visuospatial memory in healthy elderly, AD and MCI: a review. *Curr. Aging Sci.* 2, 43–59. doi: 10.2174/1874609810902010043

IBM Corp. (2013). *IBM SPSS Statistics for Windows, Version 22.0*. Armonk, NY: IBM Corp.

Insausti, R., Juottonen, K., Soininen, H., Insausti, A. M., Partanen, K., Vainio, P., et al. (1998). MR volumetric analysis of the human entorhinal, perirhinal, and temporopolar cortices. *Am. J. Neuroradiol.* 19, 659–671.

Jagust, W. (2013). Vulnerable neural systems and the borderland of brain aging and neurodegeneration. *Neuron* 77, 219–234. doi: 10.1016/j.neuron.2013.01.002

Karakas, S., Baran, Z., Ceylan, A. O., Tileylioglu, E., Tali, T., and Karakas, H. M. (2013). A comprehensive neuropsychological mapping battery for functional magnetic resonance imaging. *Int. J. Psychophysiol.* 90, 215–234. doi: 10.1016/j.ijpsycho.2013.07.007

Kaufmann, A. S. (2001). WAIS-III IQs, Horn's theory, and generational changes from young adulthood to old age. *Intelligence* 29, 131–167. doi: 10.1016/S0160-2896(00)00046-5

Kennedy, K.-M., Rodrigue, K. M., Head, D., Gunning-Dixon, F., and Raz, N. (2009). Neuroanatomical and cognitive mediators of age-related differences in perceptual priming and learning. *Neuropsychology* 23, 475–491. doi: 10.1037/a0015377

Kesler, S. R., Adams, H. F., Blasey, C. M., and Bigler, E. D. (2003). Premorbid intellectual functioning, education, and brain size in traumatic brain injury: an investigation of the cognitive reserve hypothesis. *Appl. Neuropsychol.* 10, 153–162. doi: 10.1207/S15324826AN1003_04

Khachaturian, Z. S. (2011). Revised criteria for diagnosis of Alzheimer's disease: National Institute on Aging-Alzheimer's Association diagnostic guidelines for Alzheimer's disease. *Alzheimers Dement.* 7, 253–256. doi: 10.1016/j.jalz.2011.04.003

Kim, J. P., Seo, S. W., Shin, H. Y., Ye, B. S., Yang, J. J., Kim, C., et al. (2015). Effects of education on aging-related cortical thinning among cognitively normal individuals. *Neurology* 85, 806–812. doi: 10.1212/WNL.0000000000001884

Kray, J., Eber, J., and Lindenberger, U. (2004). Age differences in executive functioning across the lifespan: the role of verbalization in task preparation. *Acta Psychol.* 115, 143–165. doi: 10.1016/j.actpsy.2003.12.001

Landau, S. M., Marks, S. M., Mormino, E. C., Rabinovici, G. D., Oh, H., O'Neil, J. P., et al. (2012). Association of lifetime cognitive engagement and low beta-amyloid deposition. *Arch. Neurol.* 69, 623–629. doi: 10.1001/archneurol.2011.2748

León-Estrada, I., García-Garcia, J., and Roldán-Tapia, L. (2017). Escala de reserva cognitiva: ajuste del modelo teórico y baremación. *Rev. Neurol.* 64, 7–16.

León, I., García-García, J., and Roldán-Tapia, L. (2014). Estimating cognitive reserve in healthy adults using the cognitive reserve scale. *PLOS ONE* 9:e102632. doi: 10.1371/journal.pone.0102632

Lobo, A., Saz, P., Marcos, G., Grupo, and de Trabajo, Z. A. R. A. D. E. M. P. (2002). *MMSE: Examen Cognoscitivo Mini-Mental.* Madrid: TEA Ediciones.

Maguire, E. A., and Frith, C. D. (2003). Aging affects the engagement of the hippocampus during autobiographical memory retrieval. *Brain* 126, 1511–1523. doi: 10.1093/brain/awg157

Mahoney, F. I., and Barthel, D. (1965). Functional evaluation: the Barthel Index. *Md. State Med. J.* 14, 61–65.

Marioni, R. E., Van den Hout, A., Valenzuela, M. J., and Brayne, C. (2012). Active cognitive lifestyle associates with cognitive recovery and a reduced risk of cognitive decline. *J. Alzheimers. Dis.* 28, 223–230. doi: 10.3233/JAD-2011-110377

Meng, X., and D'Arcy, C. (2012). Education and dementia in the context of the cognitive reserve hypothesis: a systematic review with meta-analyses and qualitative analyses. *PLOS ONE* 7:e38268. doi: 10.1371/journal.pone.0038268

Nilsson, L. G., Bäckman, L., Erngrund, K., Nyberg, L., Adolfsson, R., Bucht, G., et al. (1997). The Betula prospective cohort study: memory, health, and aging. *Aging Neuropsychol. Cogn.* 4, 1–32. doi: 10.1080/13825589708256633

Nyberg, L., Lovden, M., Riklund, K., Lindenberger, U., and Backman, L. (2012). Memory aging and brain maintenance. *Trends Cogn. Sci.* 16, 292–305. doi: 10.1016/j.tics.2012.04.005

Opdebeeck, C., Martyr, A., and Clare, L. (2016). Cognitive reserve and cognitive function in healthy older people: a meta-analysis. *Neuropsychol. Dev. Cogn. B Aging Neuropsychol. Cogn.* 23, 40–60. doi: 10.1080/13825585.2015.1041450

Park, D., and Reuter-Lorenz, P. A. (2009). The adaptive brain: aging and neurocognitive scaffolding. *Annu. Rev. Psychol.* 60, 173–196. doi: 10.1146/annurev.psych.59.103006.093656

Park, D. C., Lautenschlager, G., Hedden, T., Davidson, N. S., Smith, A. D., and Smith, P. K. (2002). Models of visuospatial and verbal memory across the adult life span. *Psychol. Aging* 17, 299–320. doi: 10.1037/0882-7974.17.2.299

Peña-Casanova, J., Gramunt-Fombuena, N., Quiñones-Ubeda, S., Sánchez-Benavides, G., Aguilar, M., Badenes, D., et al. (2009a). Spanish multicenter normative studies (NEURONORMA Project): norms for the Rey-Osterrieth complex figure (copy and memory), and free and cued selective reminding test. *Arch. Clin. Neuropsychol.* 24, 371–393. doi: 10.1093/arclin/acp041

Peña-Casanova, J., Quiñones-Ubeda, S., Gramunt-Fombuena, N., Quintana, M., Aguilar, M., Molinuevo, J. L., et al. (2009b). Spanish multicenter normative studies (NEURONORMA Project): norms for the Stroop color-word interference test and the Tower of London-Drexel. *Arch. Clin. Neuropsychol.* 24, 413–429. doi: 10.1093/arclin/acp043

Peña-Casanova, J., Quiñones-Ubeda, S., Quintana-Aparicio, M., Aguilar, M., Badenes, D., Molinuevo, J. L., et al. (2009c). Spanish multicenter normative studies (NEURONOMRA Project): norms for verbal span, visuospatial span,

letter and number sequencing, trail making test, and symbol digit modalities test. *Arch. Clin. Neuropsychol.* 24, 321–341. doi: 10.1093/arclin/acp038

Podell, J. E., Sambataro, F., Murty, V. P., Emery, M. R., Tong, Y., Das, S., et al. (2012). Neurophysiological correlates of age-related changes in working memory updating. *Neuroimage* 62, 2151–2160. doi: 10.1016/j.neuroimage.2012.05.066

Raz, N. (2000). "Aging of the brain and its impact on cognitive performance: integration of structural and functional findings," in *Handbook of Aging and Cognition—II*, eds F. I. M. Craik and T. A. Salthouse (Mahwah, NJ: Erlbaum), 1–90.

Raz, N. (2004). "The aging brain observed in vivo: differential changes and their modifiers," in *Cognitive Neuroscience of Aging: Linking Cognitive and Cerebral Aging*, eds R. Cabeza, L. Nyberg, and D. C. Park (New York, NY: Oxford University Press).

Raz, N., and Rodrigue, K. M. (2006). Differential aging of the brain: patterns, cognitive correlates and modifiers. *Neurosci. Biobehav. Rev.* 30, 730–748. doi: 10.1016/j.neubiorev.2006.07.001

Reed, B. R., Dowling, M., Tomaszewski, Farias S, Sonnen, J., Strauss, M., Schneider, J. A., et al. (2011). Cognitive activities during adulthood are more important than education in building reserve. *J. Int. Neuropsychol. Soc.* 17, 615–624. doi: 10.1017/S1355617711000014

Roldán-Tapia, L., García, J., Cánovas, R., and León, I. (2012). Cognitive reserve, age, and their relation to attentional and executive functions. *Appl. Neuropsychol.* 19, 2–8. doi: 10.1080/09084282.2011.595458

Rypma, B., and D'Esposito, M. (2000). Isolating the neural mechanisms of age-related changes in human working memory. *Nat. Neurosci.* 3, 509–515. doi: 10.1038/74889

Salthouse, T. A., Atkinson, T. M., and Berish, D. E. (2003). Executive functioning as a potential mediator of age-related cognitive decline in normal adults. *J. Exp. Psychol. Gen.* 132, 566–594. doi: 10.1037/0096-3445.132.4.566

Schaie, K. W. (1958). Rigidity-flexibility and intelligence: a cross-sectional study of the adult lifespan from 20 to 70 years. *Psychol. Monogr.* 72, 1–26. doi: 10.1037/h0093788

Schaie, K. W. (1994). The course of adult intellectual development. *Am. Psychol.* 49, 304–313. doi: 10.1037/0003-066X.49.4.304

Stawski, R. S., Sliwinski, M. J., and Hofer, S. M. (2013). Between-person and within-person associations among processing speed, attention switching, and working memory in younger and older adults. *Exp. Aging Res.* 39, 194–214. doi: 10.1080/0361073X.2013.761556

Stern, Y. (2009). Cognitive reserve. *Neuropsychologia* 47, 2015–2028. doi: 10.1016/j.neuropsychologia.2009.03.004

Stern, Y., Alexander, G. E., Prohovnik, I., and Mayeux, R. (1992). Inverse relationship between education and parietotemporal perfusion deficit in Alzheimer's disease. *Ann. Neurol.* 32, 371–375. doi: 10.1002/ana.410320311

Stern, Y., Zarahn, E., Hilton, H. J., Flynn, J., DeLaPaz, R., and Rakitin, B. (2003). Exploring the neural basis of cognitive reserve. *J. Clin. Exp. Neuropsychol.* 25, 691–701. doi: 10.1076/jcen.25.5.691.14573

Sumowski, J. F., Chiaravalloti, N., and Deluca, J. (2009). Cognitive reserve protects against cognitive dysfunction in multiple sclerosis. *J. Clin. Exp. Neuropsychol.* 31, 913–926. doi: 10.1080/13803390902740643

Tam, H. M., Lam, C. L., Huang, H., Wang, B., and Lee, T. M. (2015). Age-related difference in relationships between cognitive processing speed and general cognitive status. *Appl. Neuropsychol. Adult* 22, 94–99. doi: 10.1080/23279095.2013.860602

Tucker, A. M., and Stern, Y. (2011). Cognitive reserve in aging. *Curr. Alzheimer Res.* 8, 354–360. doi: 10.2174/156720511795745320

Turner, G. R., and Spreng, R. N. (2012). Executive functions and neurocognitive aging: dissociable patterns of brain activity. *Neurobiol. Aging* 33, 1–13. doi: 10.1016/j.neurobiolaging.2011.06.005

Valenzuela, M. J., and Sachdev, P. (2005). Brain reserve and dementia: a systematic review. *Psychol. Med.* 25, 441–454. doi: 10.1017/S0033291705006264

Valenzuela, M. J., Sachdev, P., Wen, W., Chen, X., and Brodaty, H. (2008). Lifespan mental activity predicts diminished rate of hippocampal atrophy. *PLOS ONE* 3:e2598. doi: 10.1371/journal.pone.0002598

Verhaeghen, P., and Salthouse, T. A. (1997). Meta-analyses of age-cognition relations in adulthood: estimates of linear and nonlinear age effects and structural models. *Psychol. Bull.* 122, 231–249. doi: 10.1037//0033-2909.122.3.231

Wechsler, D. (1993). *Escala de Inteligencia de Wechsler Para Adultos*. Madrid: TEA.

Wilson, R. S., Mendes de Leon, C. F., Barnes, L., Schneider, J. A., Bienias, J. L., Evans, D. A., et al. (2002). Participation in cognitively stimulating activities and risk of incident Alzheimer's disease. *JAMA* 287, 742–748. doi: 10.1001/jama.287.6.742

Zelinski, E. M., and Burnight, K. P. (1997). Sixteen-year longitudinal and time lag changes in memory and cognition in older adults. *Psychol. Aging* 12, 503–513. doi: 10.1037/0882-7974.12.3.503

Zhuravleva, T. Y., Alperin, B. R., Haring, A. E., Rentz, D. D., Holcomb, P. J., and Daffner, K. R. (2014). Age-related decline in bottom-up processing and selective attention in the very old. *J. Clin. Neurophysiol.* 31, 261–271. doi: 10.1097/WNP.0000000000000056

Permissions

The contributors of this book come from diverse backgrounds, making this book a truly international effort. This book will bring forth new frontiers with its revolutionizing research information and detailed analysis of the nascent developments around the world.

We would like to thank all the contributing authors for lending their expertise to make the book truly unique. They have played a crucial role in the development of this book. Without their invaluable contributions this book wouldn't have been possible. They have made vital efforts to compile up to date information on the varied aspects of this subject to make this book a valuable addition to the collection of many professionals and students.

This book was conceptualized with the vision of imparting up-to-date information and advanced data in this field. To ensure the same, a matchless editorial board was set up. Every individual on the board went through rigorous rounds of assessment to prove their worth. After which they invested a large part of their time researching and compiling the most relevant data for our readers.

The editorial board has been involved in producing this book since its inception. They have spent rigorous hours researching and exploring the diverse topics which have resulted in the successful publishing of this book. They have passed on their knowledge of decades through this book. To expedite this challenging task, the publisher supported the team at every step. A small team of assistant editors was also appointed to further simplify the editing procedure and attain best results for the readers.

Apart from the editorial board, the designing team has also invested a significant amount of their time in understanding the subject and creating the most relevant covers. They scrutinized every image to scout for the most suitable representation of the subject and create an appropriate cover for the book.

The publishing team has been an ardent support to the editorial, designing and production team. Their endless efforts to recruit the best for this project, has resulted in the accomplishment of this book. They are a veteran in the field of academics and their pool of knowledge is as vast as their experience in printing. Their expertise and guidance has proved useful at every step. Their uncompromising quality standards have made this book an exceptional effort. Their encouragement from time to time has been an inspiration for everyone.

The publisher and the editorial board hope that this book will prove to be a valuable piece of knowledge for researchers, students, practitioners and scholars across the globe.

List of Contributors

Fanny Quandt, Marlene Bönstrup, Robert Schulz and Jan E. Timmermann
BrainImaging and NeuroStimulation Laboratory, Department of Neurology, University Medical Center Hamburg-Eppendorf, Hamburg, Germany

Maximo Zimerman
Institute of Neuroscience, Favaloro University, Buenos Aires, Argentina
Institute of Cognitive Neurology, Buenos Aires, Argentina

Guido Nolte
Department of Neurophysiology, University Medical Center Hamburg-Eppendorf, Hamburg, Germany

Friedhelm C. Hummel
BrainImaging and NeuroStimulation Laboratory, Department of Neurology, University Medical Center Hamburg-Eppendorf, Hamburg, Germany
Institute of Neuroscience, Favaloro University, Buenos Aires, Argentina
Clinical Neuroengineering, Brain Mind Institute and Centre of Neuroprosthetics (CNP), Swiss Federal Institute of Technology (EPFL), Geneva, Switzerland
Clinique Romande de Réadaptation, Swiss Federal Institute of Technology (EPFL Valais), Sion, Switzerland

Jose A. Santiago, Virginie Bottero and Judith A. Potashkin
Department of Cellular and Molecular Pharmacology, The Chicago Medical School, Rosalind Franklin University of Medicine and Science, North Chicago, IL, United States

Xia Wu and Li Yao
College of Information Science and Technology, Beijing Normal University, Beijing, China
State Key Laboratory of Cognitive Neuroscience and Learning, Beijing Normal University, Beijing, China

Qing Li, Xinyu Yu, Xiaojuan Guo and Jiacai Zhang
College of Information Science and Technology, Beijing Normal University, Beijing, China

Kewei Chen and Eric M. Reiman
Banner Alzheimer's Institute and Banner Good Samaritan PET Center, Phoenix, AZ, USA

Adam S. Fleisher
Banner Alzheimer's Institute and Banner Good Samaritan PET Center, Phoenix, AZ, USA
Eli Lilly and Company, Indianapolis, IN, USA

Rui Li
Center on Aging Psychology, Key Laboratory of Mental Health, Institute of Psychology, Chinese Academy of Sciences, Beijing, China

Meret Branscheidt
Department of Neurology, University Hospital Zurich, Zurich, Switzerland

Julia Hoppe
Department of Neurology, University Medical Center Hamburg-Eppendorf, Hamburg, Germany

Nils Freundlieb
Department of Neurology, University Medical Center Hamburg-Eppendorf, Hamburg, Germany
Brain Stimulation, Department of Psychiatry and Psychotherapy, University Medical Center Hamburg-Eppendorf, Hamburg, Germany

Pienie Zwitserlood
Department of Psychology, University of Münster, Münster, Germany

Gianpiero Liuzzi
Department of Neurology, University Hospital Zurich, Zurich, Switzerland
Department of Neurology, University Medical Center Hamburg-Eppendorf, Hamburg, Germany

Zoe Gallant and Roderick I. Nicolson
Department of Psychology, University of Sheffield, Sheffield, United Kingdom

Styliani Douka and Olympia Lilou
Laboratory of Sports, Tourism and Recreation Management, School of Physical Education and Sport Science, Aristotle University of Thessaloniki, Thessaloniki, Greece

Vasiliki I. Zilidou
Laboratory of Sports, Tourism and Recreation Management, School of Physical Education and Sport Science, Aristotle University of Thessaloniki, Thessaloniki, Greece
Laboratory of Medical Physics, Medical School, Aristotle University of Thessaloniki, Thessaloniki, Greece

Magda Tsolaki
Department of Neurology, Medical School, Aristotle University of Thessaloniki, Thessaloniki, Greece

Zhe Li
Department of Neurology, The First Affiliated Hospital, Guangzhou Medical University, Guangzhou, China
Department of Neurology, The Second Affiliated Hospital, Guangzhou University of Chinese Medicine, Guangzhou, China

Jun Chen, Bo Liu and Xian Liu
Department of Radiology, The Second Affiliated Hospital, Guangzhou University of Chinese Medicine, Guangzhou, China

Jianbo Cheng
Department of Radiology, The People's Hospital of Gaozhou, Gaozhou, China

Sicong Huang
Department of Laboratory, The Second Affiliated Hospital, Guangzhou Medical University, Guangzhou, China

Yingyu Hu
Department of Business Development, Zhujiang Hospital, Southern Medical University, Guangzhou, China

Yijuan Wu, Guihua Li, Wenyuan Guo, Shuxuan Huang, Miaomiao Zhou and Pingyi Xu
Department of Neurology, The First Affiliated Hospital, Guangzhou Medical University, Guangzhou, China

Xiang Chen and Yousheng Xiao
Department of Neurology, The First Affiliated Hospital, Sun Yat-sen University, Guangzhou, China

Chaojun Chen
Department of Neurology, Guangzhou Hospital of Integrated Traditional and West Medicine, Guangzhou, China

Junbin Chen
Department of Neurology, Yuebei People's Hospital, Shaoguan, China

Xiaodong Luo
Department of Neurology, The Second Affiliated Hospital, Guangzhou University of Chinese Medicine, Guangzhou, China

Sinan Zhao
AU MRI Research Center, Department of Electrical and Computer Engineering, Auburn University, Auburn, AL, United States

D Rangaprakash
AU MRI of Electrical and Computer Engineering, Auburn University, Auburn, AL, United States
Department of Psychiatry and Biobehavioral Sciences, University of California, Los Angeles, Los Angeles, CA, United States

Archana Venkataraman
Department of Electrical and Computer Engineering, Johns Hopkins University, Baltimore, MD, United States

Peipeng Liang
Department of Radiology, Xuanwu Hospital, Capital Medical University, Beijing, China
Beijing Key Laboratory of Magnetic Resonance Imaging and Brain Informatics, Beijing, China
Key Laboratory for Neurodegenerative Diseases, Ministry of Education, Beijing, China

Gopikrishna Deshpande
AU MRI of Electrical and Computer Engineering, Auburn University, Auburn, AL, United States
Department of Psychology, Auburn University, Auburn, AL, United States
Alabama Advanced Imaging Consortium, Auburn University and University of Alabama Birmingham, Auburn, AL, United States

Rui Li, Xinyi Zhu, Pengyun Wang, Zhiwei Zheng, Ya-Nan Niu and Xin Huang
CAS Key Laboratory of Mental Health, Institute of Psychology, Beijing, China
Department of Psychology, University of Chinese Academy of Sciences, Beijing, China

Shufei Yin
Department of Psychology, Faculty of Education, Hubei University, Wuhan, China

Weicong Ren
CAS Key Laboratory of Mental Health, Institute of Psychology, Beijing, China
Department of Education, Hebei Normal University, Shijiazhuang, China

Jing Yu
CAS Key Laboratory of Mental Health, Institute of Psychology, Beijing, China
Faculty of Psychology, Southwest University, Chongqing, China

Keith M. McGregor, Bruce Crosson and Joe R. Nocera
VA Rehabilitation R&D Center for Visual and Neurocognitive Rehabilitation, Atlanta VA Medical Center, Decatur, GA, United States
Department of Neurology, Emory University School of Medicine, Atlanta, GA, United States

Kevin Mammino and Javier Omar
VA Rehabilitation R&D Center for Visual and Neurocognitive Rehabilitation, Atlanta VA Medical Center, Decatur, GA, United States

Juan Li
CAS Key Laboratory of Mental Health, Institute of Psychology, Beijing, China
Department of Psychology, University of Chinese Academy of Sciences, Beijing, China
Magnetic Resonance Imaging Research Center, Institute of Psychology, Chinese Academy of Sciences, Beijing, China
State Key Laboratory of Brain and Cognitive Science, Institute of Biophysics, Chinese Academy of Sciences, Beijing, China

Paul S. García
VA Rehabilitation R&D Center for Visual and Neurocognitive Rehabilitation, Atlanta VA Medical Center, Decatur, GA, United States
Department of Anesthesiology, Emory University School of Medicine, Atlanta, GA, United States

Isabella K. Wiesmeier, Daniela Dalin, Joerg Dietterle, Cornelius Weiller and Christoph Maurer
Department of Neurology and Neurophysiology, University Hospital Freiburg, Freiburg, Germany

Anja Wehrle
Institute for Sports and Sport Science, University of Freiburg, Freiburg, Germany
Department of Internal Medicine, Institute for Exercise and Occupational Medicine, University Hospital Freiburg, Freiburg, Germany

Urs Granacher
Division of Training and Movement Science, University of Potsdam, Potsdam, Germany

Thomas Muehlbauer
Division of Movement and Training Sciences, Biomechanics of Sport, Institute of Sport and Movement Sciences, University Duisburg-Essen, Essen, Germany

Albert Gollhofer
Institute for Sports and Sport Science, University of Freiburg, Freiburg, Germany

Cheng-Ya Huang
School and Graduate Institute of Physical Therapy, College of Medicine, National Taiwan University, Taipei, Taiwan
Physical Therapy Center, National Taiwan University Hospital, Taipei, Taiwan

Elena Solesio-Jofre
Movement Control and Neuroplasticity Research Group, Department of Movement Sciences, KU Leuven, Leuven, Belgium
Department of Biological and Health Psychology, Autonomous University of Madrid, Madrid, Spain

Linda L. Lin
Institute of Physical Education, Health and Leisure Studies, National Cheng Kung University, Tainan, Taiwan

Ing-Shiou Hwang
Institute of Allied Health Sciences, College of Medicine, National Cheng Kung University, Tainan, Taiwan
Department of Physical Therapy, College of Medicine, National Cheng Kung University, Tainan, Taiwan

Iseult A. M. Beets, Daniel G. Woolley, Lisa Pauwels and Sima Chalavi
Movement Control and Neuroplasticity Research Group, Department of Movement Sciences, KU Leuven, Leuven, Belgium

Dante Mantini
Movement Control and Neuroplasticity Research Group, Department of Movement Sciences, KU Leuven, Leuven, Belgium
Department of Health Sciences and Technology, ETH Zurich, Zurich, Switzerland
Department of Experimental Psychology, University of Oxford, Oxford, United Kingdom

Stephan P. Swinnen
Movement Control and Neuroplasticity Research Group, Department of Movement Sciences, KU Leuven, Leuven, Belgium
Leuven Research Institute for Neuroscience and Disease, KU Leuven, Leuven, Belgium

Luyao Wang
Intelligent Robotics Institute, School of Mechatronical Engineering, Beijing Institute of Technology, Beijing, China

Wenhui Wang and Tianyi Yan
School of Life Science, Beijing Institute of Technology, Beijing, China

Jiayong Song
The Affiliated High School of Peking University, Beijing, China

Weiping Yang
Department of Psychology, Hubei University, Wuhan, China

Ritsu Go and Jinglong Wu
Intelligent Robotics Institute, School of Mechatronical Engineering, Beijing Institute of Technology, Beijing, China
International Joint Research Laboratory of Biomimetic Robots and Systems, Ministry of Education, Beijing, China

Bin Wang
College of Computer Science and Technology, Taiyuan University of Technology, Shanxi, China

Qiang Huang
Intelligent Robotics Institute, School of Mechatronical Engineering, Beijing Institute of Technology, Beijing, China
Key Laboratory of Biomimetic Robots and Systems, Ministry of Education, Beijing, China

Alexandru D. Iordan, Katherine A. Cooke, John Jonides, Thad A. Polk and Patricia A. Reuter-Lorenz
Department of Psychology, University of Michigan, Ann Arbor, MI, United States

Kyle D. Moored
Department of Mental Health, Bloomberg School of Public Health, Johns Hopkins University, Baltimore, MD, United States

Benjamin Katz
Department of Human Development and Family Science, Virginia Tech, Blacksburg, VA, United States

Martin Buschkuehl
MIND Research Institute, Irvine, CA, United States

Susanne M. Jaeggi
School of Education, University of California, Irvine, Irvine, CA, United States

Scott J. Peltier
Functional MRI Laboratory, Department of Biomedical Engineering, University of Michigan, Ann Arbor, MI, United States

Bo Shen, Liyu Lu, Jun Zhu, Yang Pan, Wenya Lan and Li Zhang
Department of Geriatrics, Affiliated Brain Hospital of Nanjing Medical University, Nanjing, China

Yang Gao
Department of Computer Science and Technology, Nanjing University, Nanjing, China

Wenbin Zhang
Department of Neurosurgery, Affiliated Brain Hospital of Nanjing Medical University, Nanjing, China

Qun Yao, Donglin Zhu, Feng Li, Xingjian Lin and Jingping Shi
Department of Neurology, Affiliated Brain Hospital of Nanjing Medical University, Nanjing, China

Chaoyong Xiao and Qingling Huang
Department of Radiology, Affiliated Brain Hospital of Nanjing Medical University, Nanjing, China

Jennifer L. O'Brien
Department of Psychology, University of South Florida St. Petersburg, St. Petersburg, FL, United States

Jennifer J. Lister and Gregory K. Clifton
Department of Communication Sciences and Disorders, University of South Florida, Tampa, FL, United States

Bernadette A. Fausto
School of Aging Studies, University of South Florida, Tampa, FL, United States

Jerri D. Edwards
Department of Psychiatry and Behavioral Neurosciences, College of Medicine, University of South Florida, Tampa, FL, United States

Takashi Shibata, Michiya Kubo and Yukio Horie
Department of Neurosurgery, Stroke Center, Saiseikai Toyama Hospital, Toyama, Japan

Toshimitu Musha, Yukio Kosugi, Yohei Kobayashi and Mieko Tanaka
Brain Functions Laboratory Inc., Yokohama, Japan

Naoya Kuwayama and Satoshi Kuroda
Department of Neurosurgery, Graduate School of Medicine and Pharmacological Science, University of Toyama, Toyama, Japan

Karin Hayashi
Department of Neuropsychiatry, Toho University Medical Center Sakura Hospital, Chiba, Japan

Haruyasu Matsuzaki
Brain Functions Laboratory Inc., Yokohama, Japan
Department of Medical Course, Teikyo Heisei University, Tokyo, Japan

Kiyotaka Nemoto
Department of Neuropsychiatry, Institute of Clinical Medicine, University of Tsukuba, Tsukuba, Japan

Takashi Asada
Department of Neuropsychiatry, University of Tokyo Medical and Dental University, Tokyo, Japan

María D. Roldán-Tapia, Rosa Cánovas, Irene León and Juan García-Garcia
Department of Psychology, University of Almería, Almería, Spain

Index